Lecture Notes in Computer Science 9745

Commenced Publication in 1973
Founding and Former Series Editors:
Gerhard Goos, Juris Hartmanis, and Jan van Leeuwen

More information about this series at http://www.springer.com/series/7409

Vincent G. Duffy (Ed.)

Digital Human Modeling

Applications in Health, Safety, Ergonomics and Risk Management

7th International Conference, DHM 2016
Held as Part of HCI International 2016
Toronto, ON, Canada, July 17–22, 2016
Proceedings

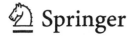 Springer

Editor
Vincent G. Duffy
Purdue University
West Lafayette, IN
USA

ISSN 0302-9743   ISSN 1611-3349   (electronic)
Lecture Notes in Computer Science
ISBN 978-3-319-40246-8   ISBN 978-3-319-40247-5   (eBook)
DOI 10.1007/978-3-319-40247-5

Library of Congress Control Number: 2016940816

LNCS Sublibrary: SL3 – Information Systems and Applications, incl. Internet/Web, and HCI

Printed on acid-free paper

This Springer imprint is published by Springer Nature
The registered company is Springer International Publishing AG Switzerland

Foreword

The 18th International Conference on Human-Computer Interaction, HCI International 2016, was held in Toronto, Canada, during July 17–22, 2016. The event incorporated the 15 conferences/thematic areas listed on the following page.

A total of 4,354 individuals from academia, research institutes, industry, and governmental agencies from 74 countries submitted contributions, and 1,287 papers and 186 posters have been included in the proceedings. These papers address the latest research and development efforts and highlight the human aspects of the design and use of computing systems. The papers thoroughly cover the entire field of human-computer interaction, addressing major advances in knowledge and effective use of computers in a variety of application areas. The volumes constituting the full 27-volume set of the conference proceedings are listed on pages IX and X.

I would like to thank the program board chairs and the members of the program boards of all thematic areas and affiliated conferences for their contribution to the highest scientific quality and the overall success of the HCI International 2016 conference.

This conference would not have been possible without the continuous and unwavering support and advice of the founder, Conference General Chair Emeritus and Conference Scientific Advisor Prof. Gavriel Salvendy. For his outstanding efforts, I would like to express my appreciation to the communications chair and editor of *HCI International News*, Dr. Abbas Moallem.

April 2016   Constantine Stephanidis

HCI International 2016 Thematic Areas and Affiliated Conferences

Thematic areas:

- Human-Computer Interaction (IICI 2016)
- Human Interface and the Management of Information (HIMI 2016)

Affiliated conferences:

- 13th International Conference on Engineering Psychology and Cognitive Ergonomics (EPCE 2016)
- 10th International Conference on Universal Access in Human-Computer Interaction (UAHCI 2016)
- 8th International Conference on Virtual, Augmented and Mixed Reality (VAMR 2016)
- 8th International Conference on Cross-Cultural Design (CCD 2016)
- 8th International Conference on Social Computing and Social Media (SCSM 2016)
- 10th International Conference on Augmented Cognition (AC 2016)
- 7th International Conference on Digital Human Modeling and Applications in Health, Safety, Ergonomics and Risk Management (DHM 2016)
- 5th International Conference on Design, User Experience and Usability (DUXU 2016)
- 4th International Conference on Distributed, Ambient and Pervasive Interactions (DAPI 2016)
- 4th International Conference on Human Aspects of Information Security, Privacy and Trust (HAS 2016)
- Third International Conference on HCI in Business, Government, and Organizations (HCIBGO 2016)
- Third International Conference on Learning and Collaboration Technologies (LCT 2016)
- Second International Conference on Human Aspects of IT for the Aged Population (ITAP 2016)

Conference Proceedings Volumes Full List

1. LNCS 9731, Human-Computer Interaction: Theory, Design, Development and Practice (Part I), edited by Masaaki Kurosu
2. LNCS 9732, Human-Computer Interaction: Interaction Platforms and Techniques (Part II), edited by Masaaki Kurosu
3. LNCS 9733, Human-Computer Interaction: Novel User Experiences (Part III), edited by Masaaki Kurosu
4. LNCS 9734, Human Interface and the Management of Information: Information, Design and Interaction (Part I), edited by Sakae Yamamoto
5. LNCS 9735, Human Interface and the Management of Information: Applications and Services (Part II), edited by Sakae Yamamoto
6. LNAI 9736, Engineering Psychology and Cognitive Ergonomics, edited by Don Harris
7. LNCS 9737, Universal Access in Human-Computer Interaction: Methods, Techniques, and Best Practices (Part I), edited by Margherita Antona and Constantine Stephanidis
8. LNCS 9738, Universal Access in Human-Computer Interaction: Interaction Techniques and Environments (Part II), edited by Margherita Antona and Constantine Stephanidis
9. LNCS 9739, Universal Access in Human-Computer Interaction: Users and Context Diversity (Part III), edited by Margherita Antona and Constantine Stephanidis
10. LNCS 9740, Virtual, Augmented and Mixed Reality, edited by Stephanie Lackey and Randall Shumaker
11. LNCS 9741, Cross-Cultural Design, edited by Pei-Luen Patrick Rau
12. LNCS 9742, Social Computing and Social Media, edited by Gabriele Meiselwitz
13. LNAI 9743, Foundations of Augmented Cognition: Neuroergonomics and Operational Neuroscience (Part I), edited by Dylan D. Schmorrow and Cali M. Fidopiastis
14. LNAI 9744, Foundations of Augmented Cognition: Neuroergonomics and Operational Neuroscience (Part II), edited by Dylan D. Schmorrow and Cali M. Fidopiastis
15. LNCS 9745, Digital Human Modeling and Applications in Health, Safety, Ergonomics and Risk Management, edited by Vincent G. Duffy
16. LNCS 9746, Design, User Experience, and Usability: Design Thinking and Methods (Part I), edited by Aaron Marcus
17. LNCS 9747, Design, User Experience, and Usability: Novel User Experiences (Part II), edited by Aaron Marcus
18. LNCS 9748, Design, User Experience, and Usability: Technological Contexts (Part III), edited by Aaron Marcus
19. LNCS 9749, Distributed, Ambient and Pervasive Interactions, edited by Norbert Streitz and Panos Markopoulos
20. LNCS 9750, Human Aspects of Information Security, Privacy and Trust, edited by Theo Tryfonas

Digital Human Modeling and Applications in Health, Safety, Ergonomics and Risk Management

Program Board Chair: **Vincent G. Duffy**, USA

- Norman I. Badler, USA
- Elsbeth de Korte, The Netherlands
- H. Onan Demirel, USA
- Afzal A. Godil, USA
- Ravindra Goonetilleke, Hong Kong, China
- Akihiko Goto, Japan
- Hiroyuki Hamada, Japan
- Dan Högberg, Sweden
- Satoshi Kanai, Japan
- Min Soon Kim, USA
- Noriaki Kuwahara, Japan
- Byung Cheol Lee, USA
- Kang Li, USA
- Tim Marler, USA
- Hamid Mcheick, Canada
- Ezutah Udoncy Olugu, Malaysia
- Caterina Rizzi, Italy
- Beatriz Sousa Santos, Portugal
- Leonor Teixeira, Portugal
- Renran Tian, USA
- Mihaela Vorvoreanu, USA
- Anita Woll, Norway
- Kuan Yew Wong, Malaysia
- James Yang, USA

The full list with the program board chairs and the members of the program boards of all thematic areas and affiliated conferences is available online at:

http://www.hci.international/2016/

HCI International 2017

The 19th International Conference on Human-Computer Interaction, HCI International 2017, will be held jointly with the affiliated conferences in Vancouver, Canada, at the Vancouver Convention Centre, July 9–14, 2017. It will cover a broad spectrum of themes related to human-computer interaction, including theoretical issues, methods, tools, processes, and case studies in HCI design, as well as novel interaction techniques, interfaces, and applications. The proceedings will be published by Springer. More information will be available on the conference website: http://2017. hci.international/.

General Chair
Prof. Constantine Stephanidis
University of Crete and ICS-FORTH
Heraklion, Crete, Greece
E-mail: general_chair@hcii2017.org

http://2017.hci.international/

Contents

Motion Prediction and Recognition

Quality and Safety in Healthcare

Design for Health

Work Design and Support

Modelling Human Behaviour and Cognition

Anthropometry, Ergonomics, Design and Comfort

Experimental Research of Range
of Motion About Wrist Joint

Wen-Yu Fu, Guang Cheng, Yu-Feng Ma, and Ai-Ping Yang[(⊠)]

College of Mechanical and Electrical Engineering,
Beijing Union University, Beijing 100020, China
jdtaiping@buu.edu.cn

Abstract. Objective: To investigate the range of motion (ROM) of wrist joint in human body, and the difference about ROMs between man and woman in subgroups and how it relates to age itself;

Methods: One hundred healthy and no movement disorders volunteers from 18–60 years old were recruited to complete the study. They were divided into 2 groups, and half of them are male. The VICON motion capture system was used to measure ROMs of wrist joint. The average value of wrist joint ROMs for each age groups were calculated; The change in the ROM for each age group was compared; The difference in the ROM between male and female was compared, and the difference in the ROMs of wrist joint on the left and right was compared too.

Results: ROMs of wrist palmar flexion and dorsiflexion decreased with the increasing of the age. The difference about ROMs in groups was not significant. Conclusion: The ROMs of wrist palmar flexion and dorsiflexion for normal human decreased with the increasing of the age, but the difference in groups was small.

Keywords: Range of motion · Wrist joint · Motion capture system

1 Introduction

Function sizes of human body should be considered in design of structure and location in various products, so that the operation of products is simple and easy. The function size of human body is produced by the coordinating between the joint rotation angle and the length of limbs. The function size of the human body is determined by the ROM of the human joints on the condition that the length of the limbs is fixed. So far, some Chinese scholars studied the ROMs of the human body, and obtaining some data about ROMs. But these data were measured 10 years ago [1–5]. With the improvement of the Chinese people's living standard, physique and function size may also change; especially for the labor from 18 to 60 these changes may be bigger. Therefore, it is necessary to measure and analyze ROMs of human limb joints again and provide new reliable value about ROMs for the product design with related industries.

ROMs are the measurement of movement around a specific joint of human body [6]. The change in value of published data about ROM is bigger, because it is affected by

© Springer International Publishing Switzerland 2016
V.G. Duffy (Ed.): DHM 2016, LNCS 9745, pp. 3–12, 2016.
DOI: 10.1007/978-3-319-40247-5_1

many factors, such as age, gender, physical condition, obesity, nationality, race, occupation and exercise habits. It is also restricted by age, disease and trauma [7]. Activities of joints can be divided into two categories: active and passive. Therefore ROM has two types. One is active ROM, and the other is passive ROM. Active ROM refers to movement of a joint provided entirely by the individual performing the exercise. The human body is in active state when they operate various machines. Therefore active ROM is studied in this paper. Because of the limitation of length, measurement and data analysis about ROM of adult human wrist joint were introduced mainly in this paper.

2 Method

2.1 Subjects

One hundred healthy people agreed to participate in this study. Half of the subjects were male. All subjects were healthy, without limb dysfunction and sports injury. They were divided into two groups: young, middle-aged and elderly. Information of the number of subjects, gender and age was shown in Table 1.

Table 1. Information about subjects

Number of subjects Ages	18 -40	41 -60
male	40	10
female	40	10

2.2 Measurement Items

In this study ROMs of human wrists was measured. These include wrist palmar flexion, wrist dorsiflexion, wrist radial deviation, wrist ulnar deviation.

ROM of human body joints was measured by using VICON motion capture system of British Oxford Metrics Limited Company [8–10]. Kinestate of moving objects can be captured by the multiple cameras distributed in space of this system and stored in the form of image. Then these image data will be processed. At last coordinates of moving objects in space at different moments will be gotten. To obtain the location of mark point when measuring ROM of wrist joint, preliminary experiments were performed based on the characteristics of human wrist joint activities. To different ROM of joint, witch ball will be stuck to the location of subject's joint when measuring ROM. To each ROM of joint a corresponding motion template will be established in VICON system. In the VICON system operation for each template of motion establishes a corresponding movement. An example of wrist palmar flexion was shown in Fig. 1 to illustrate the location of witch ball, the location of marker points in VICON system and the template of the motion model.

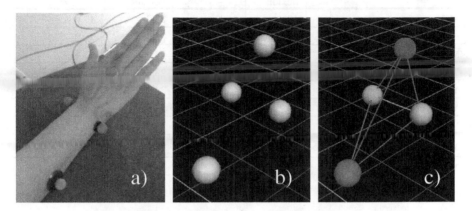

Fig. 1. A sketch about positions of marker points on the human body, the location of witch ball, and movement template when measuring wrist palmar flexion

To each joint ROM, it has definite starting position and its end position based on the characteristics of human activities. To ensure the reliable and unified of experimental data, measurement was repeated three times. For example, when measuring flexion of the wrist, according to the staring position and end position of witch ball (corresponding to the staring position and end position of joint), mathematical model will be established (namely: the angle between two planes. One plane is composed of red, yellow and green ball, and the other is composed of yellow, green and blue ball). Then joint ROM is obtained by solving this mathematical model.

3   Measurement Results

Tables 2 and 3 showed the test results:

(1) For different ROM of wrist joints, the left and right of ROM are different. But the difference between the left and the right is small;
(2) For ROM of radial deviation and ulnar deviation, ROM of the elderly is slightly greater than the young;
(3) Individual difference of ROM is bigger (the range of ROM for dorsiflexion on the left side is from 19.3° to 88.5°, and the difference between the maximum value and the minimum value is 69.2°);
(4) For the men and women of the same age, ROM for wrist joint is different. But the difference is small;

Table 2. ROM of left wrist joint

Joint / Average value	Wrist(left)			
	Palmar flexion	Dorsiflexion	Radial deviation	Ulnar deviation
Male and female	40.8	56.1	23.3	17.6
Female	41.0	54.0	23.3	17.0
Male	40.6	58.3	23.3	17.9
Young	42.1	57.8	23.6	17.0
Young female	43.4	54.0	24.1	16.9
Young male	40.9	61.8	23.0	17.1
Middle-aged and elderly	38.1	53.2	22.7	18.4
Middle-aged and elderly female	36.3	53.8	21.6	17.2
Middle-aged and elderly male	40.0	52.7	24.0	19.8

Table 3. ROM of right wrist joint (degree)

Joint / Average value	Wrist(right)			
	Palmar flexion	Dorsiflexion	Radial deviation	Ulnar deviation
Male and female	40.1	59.1	26.2	16.6
Female	39.7	58.5	25.3	16.2
Male	40.4	59.7	27.1	17.0
Young	41.3	60.2	25.9	15.5
Young female	40.4	58.9	24.8	15.3
Young male	42.3	61.6	27.0	15.7
Middle-aged and elderly	37.8	57.2	26.8	18.7
Middle-aged and elderly female	38.3	58.9	26.3	17.8
Middle-aged and elderly male	37.4	56.7	27.4	19.6

As shown in Fig. 2, the median of ROM of left ulnar deviation is 17.4°, and most data concentrate around it. The deviation in the results is 4.7°; the upper bound and the lower bound of the results are given based on it. About 97 percent of the subjects are in this range. As shown in Fig. 3, the median of ROM of left dorsiflexion deviation is 57.3°, and most data concentrate around it. The deviation in the results is 12.7°; the upper bound and the lower bound of the results are given based on it. About 95 percent of the subjects are in this range. As shown in Fig. 4, the median of ROM of left radial deviation is 22.7°, and

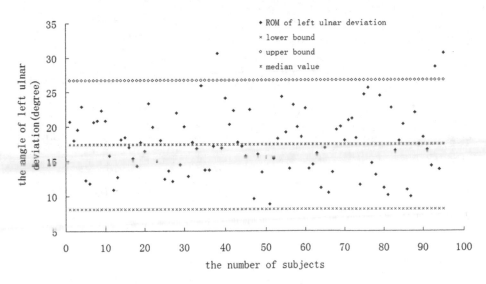

Fig. 2. The angle of left ulnar deviation

most data concentrate around it. The deviation in the results is 6.4°; the upper bound and the lower bound of the results are given based on it. About 97 percent of the subjects are in this range. As shown in Fig. 5, the median of ROM of left palmar flexion is 40.2°, and most data concentrate around it. The deviation in the results is 9.4°; the upper bound and the lower bound of the results are given based on it. About 97 percent of the subjects are in this range. Results that lie outside the upper bound and the lower bound in Figs. 2, 3, 4 and 5 could be abnormal data caused by the individual difference (the age or special professional background).

As shown in Fig. 6, the median of ROM of right ulnar deviation is 16.2°, and most data concentrate around it. The deviation in the results is 5.7°; the upper bound and the lower bound of the results are given based on it. About 98 percent of the subjects are in this range. As shown in Fig. 7, the median of ROM of right dorsiflexion is 60.5°, and most data concentrate around it. The deviation in the results is 12.2°; the upper bound and the lower bound of the results are given based on it. About 96 percent of the subjects are in this range. As shown in Fig. 8, the median of ROM of right radial deviation is 26.1°, and most data concentrate around it. The deviation in the results is 8.3°; the upper bound and the lower bound of the results are given based on it. About 95 percent of the subjects are in this range. As shown in Fig. 9, the median of ROM of right radial deviation is 39.7°, and most data concentrate around it. The deviation in the results is 10.6°; the upper bound and the lower bound of the results are given based on it. About 95 percent of the subjects are in this range. Results that lie outside the upper bound and the lower bound in Figs. 6 and 7 could be abnormal data caused by the individual difference (the age or special professional background).

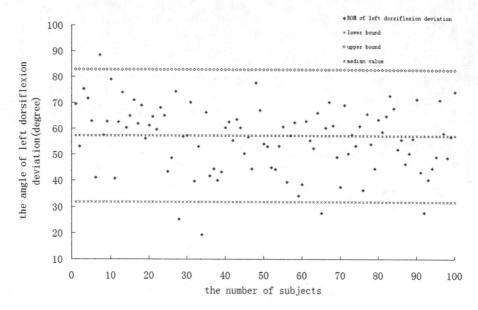

Fig. 3. The angle of left dorsiflexion

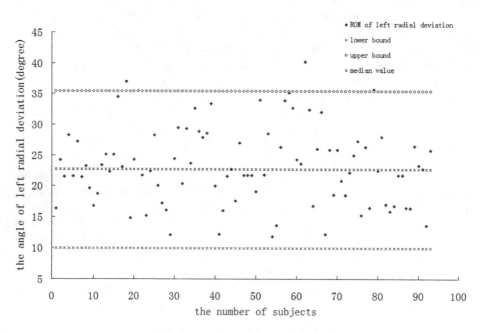

Fig. 4. The angle of left radial deviation

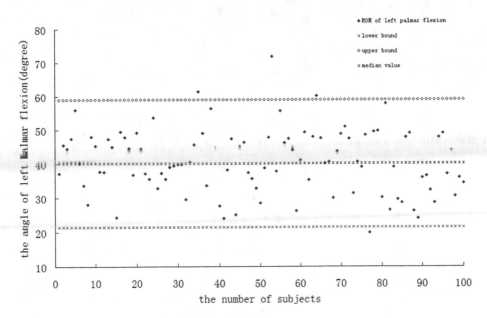

Fig. 5. The angle of left palmar flexion

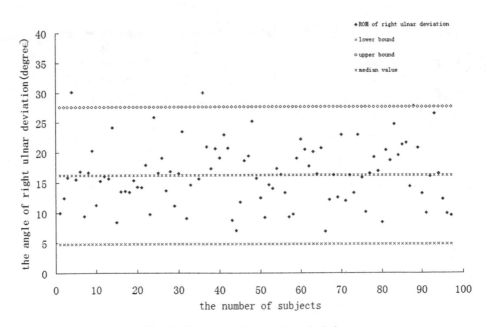

Fig. 6. The angle of right ulnar deviation

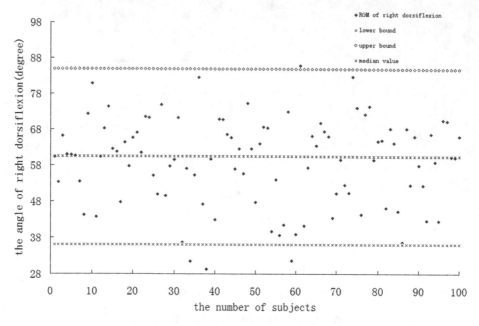

Fig. 7. The angle of right dorsiflexion

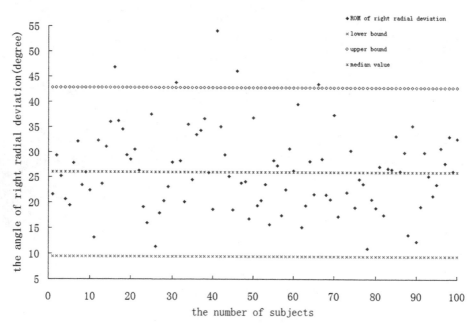

Fig. 8. The angle of right radial deviation

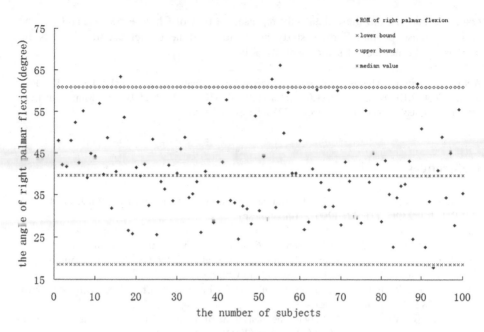

Fig. 9. The angle of right palmar flexion

4   Discussions

In this study the ROM of wrist joints in human body was investigated. The difference about ROM between man and woman in subgroups was analyzed and how it changes with age; One hundred volunteers were recruited. They were divided into 2 groups, and half of them are male. VICON motion capture system was used to measure ROM of wrist joint. The average value of wrist joint ROM for each age groups were obtained; The change in the ROM for each age group was compared; The difference in the ROM between male and female was compared, and the difference in the ROM of wrist joint on the left and right was compared too.

Previous study shows that wrist joint ROM was influenced by the age and sex of subjects [1]. With increasing age, aging occurs in the human body and the skeletons, muscles atrophy occurs and the extent of male is bigger than female. All these decrease wrist joint ROM and the decreased extent of male is bigger than female. In this study the change of ROM for palmar flexion and dorsiflexion with the age is the same as the previous study. But the change of ROM for radial deviation and ulnar deviation with the age had no obvious laws, and the change of magnitude is small. It may be related to the less number of subjects in this study, and it may also be related to the big individual's difference of ROM. But at least, in the general population, the ROM of radial deviation and ulnar deviation is not particularly close to the age (between 18 and 60 years old).

There are deficiencies in this experiment study. Due to the low number of subjects, subjects range in age from 18–60 years, and only 96 data are valid. Therefore, the results obtained from these data only represent a part of Chinese people, and not the entire Chinese people. Further study needs to be done to get accurate results by increasing the number of samples reasonably.

Acknowledgment. This research was supported by the National Key Technology R&D Program (2014BAK01B05, 2014BAK01B04 and 2014BAK01B02), 2015 Beijing Municipal Education Commission Research Project (12213991508101/008)

References

1. Kang, Y.H., Zhang, W.G., Qu, L.: Range of motion of healthy elders. Chin. J. Phys. Med. Rehabil. **23**(8), 221–223 (2001). (in Chinese)
2. Song, F., Wang, T., Li, J.A.: Influence of examiners and goniometers on measurement of range of motion. Chin. J. Clin. Rehabil. **6**(20), 3008–3009 (2002). (in Chinese)
3. Wang, J.W., Yu, X.J., Huang, P.H.: Unifying the scaling method of the loss of joint motion. J. Forensic Med. **24**(2), 138–142 (2008). (in Chinese)
4. Fan, Z.H.: Strength check and range of motion for joint check. Chin. J. Rehabil. Med. **2**(6), 277–282 (1987). (in Chinese)
5. Zhang, B., Wang, C.X.: A study on the measurement of movement range of the joints of the four limbs. Forensic Sci. Technol. **4**, 5–6 (2002). (in Chinese)
6. Department of Medical Administration, Ministry of Health of the People's Republic of China: Standard for Diagnosis and Treatment of Rehabilitation Medicine in China, pp. 27–32. Hua Xia Publishing House, Beijing (1998)
7. Joel, A.: Rehabilitation Medicine Principles and Practice, pp. 35–43, 354–355. JB Lippiincott, Philadelphia (1997)
8. Alexandra, K.M., Liam, E.A., Jace, R.D., Justin, G.K., Ross, A.C., Douglas, G.W.: Lower limb kinematics and physiological responses to prolonged load carriage in untrained individuals. Ergonomics **58**(5), 770–780 (2015)
9. Schall, M.C., Jr., Fethke, N.B., Chen, H., Oyama, S., Douphrate, D.I.: Accuracy and repeatability of an inertial measurement unit system for field-based occupational studies. Ergonomics (2015). doi:10.1080/00140139.2015.1079335
10. Amy, Y.C., Clark, R.D.: Determinants and magnitudes of manual force strengths and joint moments during two-handed standing maximal horizontal pushing and pulling. Ergonomics (2015). doi:10.1080/00140139.2015.1075605

The Study of Design of Children's Anti-lost Clothing Based upon Ergonomics

Xiaoping Hu[⊠] and Jiying Zhong

School of Design, Guangzhou Higher Education Mega Centre,
South China University of Technology, Panyu District,
Guangzhou 510006, People's Republic of China
huxp@scut.edu.cn

Abstract. Children belong to the distinctive group of population who has not yet obtained the complete perceptive ability, or full-fledged adaptability with the lack of self-protection. In recent years, due to the accelerated pace of life, parents' negligence in care for their children triggered a host of family tragedies, therefore provoking increasing emphasis upon the issue of children trafficking and missing children cases on the social media. This paper is to incorporate the latest intelligent tracking technology into the design of preventing lost clothing in accordance with different stages of developmental environment for children in order to reduce the likelihood of loss of a child. As the degree of integration between the technology and art design is on the rise, our attires as the necessities of our daily life are not simply a tool for keeping warm but also serve as a symbol of fashion and style. In the foreseeable future, it is inevitable to integrate ergonomics into the making of clothing with other elements of comfort and humanity.

Keywords: Children · Anti-lost · Design · Communication technology

1 Introduction

1.1 Purpose and Significance

This paper is to combine the human engineering and fashion design to apply in children's anti-lost clothing, in order to explore the needs of parents for children. Through the phased survey, I will statistics data and sum up the anti-lost clothing elements' which be suitable for children with different growth stage, in order to reduce or even eliminate the phenomenon of human-trafficking of children ensure the health of children's lives, and reduce the occurrence of family tragedies.

Children lost are the focus of social news in recent years. Distressed at the same time, we are supposed to focus on the source of the incident occurred to avoid the hidden dangers of children from the fundamental. Safety education for parents and the school is not enough to reduce the rate of lost, meanwhile busy living environment causes parents the negligence of care and feel powerless. Therefore, under such a passive environment, it has important significance to improve the healthy growth of children and the quality of social security by seeking a means of intelligent monitoring and master the children's position.

© Springer International Publishing Switzerland 2016
V.G. Duffy (Ed.): DHM 2016, LNCS 9745, pp. 13–21, 2016.
DOI: 10.1007/978-3-319-40247-5_2

1.2 Research Status

The purpose of this paper is to embed the positioning electronic components into clothing, and through the way of information feedback to remind, inform the parents of children's situation. At present, both domestic and foreign research on smart wear intensified, however, failure to conceal and lack of stealth characterize those corresponding devices, thereby enabling the traffickers to remove them easily when children encounter human trafficking. On the one hand, older adolescents may not favor the shape of the watch: the reluctance to wear it also poses a barrier. With regards to younger children, it is likely to lead to the accidental swallowing of the tiny objects. On the other hand, as to the majority of watches and bracelets with plastic straps and belts, allegedly there is seldom a pleasure for children to wear. But this can be solved via the solution that the device be embedded into clothing to enhance users' experience.

2 Survey Results of Children's Actual Situation

2.1 Children's Physical Characteristics Overview in Stages

Clothing, as a production of life necessities, its design must follow the "people-oriented" protocol, in the experimental study, we must consider both the objective existence of the data, and to understand the needs of their parents. In this study we randomly collect a questionnaire survey of one hundred cases of 23 to 40 years old children's parents. As the child's development dynamic speed change quickly, we made a segmented survey for parents to adapt to the children in different growth period to make the anti-lost clothes. According to different physiological and psychological characteristics, the fundamental research object can be divided into infancy, early childhood, preschool age, and school age.

First, Infancy (0 to 1 Year Old). Baby's early period basic static is sleep stage; this is the most significant children's physical growth and development period. During this period, the baby's functions are also gradually developed, from the 10th to 12th month they learn to walk, or walking upright.

Second, Early Childhood (1–3 Years Old). Child's weight and height are developing rapidly in this period. The shape characteristic is a big head, a short neck, a tall, straight body, and an abdominal convex. Children start learning to walk, speak, and have certain ability to imitate, doing simple things and get extreme attention to bold color and activity.

Third, Preschool Age (4 to 6 Years Old). The children's physique characteristic of this stage is quite narrow waist, protruding abdomen, shoulders, short limbs, bosom, waist; hip three surrounded degree of the size is not big. Their body grows faster, and surrounded degree increase slowly. The mental and physical development of children in this stage is very speedy. They can easily run and jump, and have certain ability of express languages.

Fourth, School Age (6 to 12 Years Old). This is a significant period of motor function and intellectual development. Children gradually moved away from childish feeling, have the certain imagination and judgment, but has not yet formed independent point of view. Life range from family, kindergarten to the school of and collective. Physical differences in boys and girls become increasingly obvious, there appear to be a circumference difference on the girls' busts and chests, their waists become slimmer than their buts.

2.2   Survey Results of Fabrics, Colors, and Styles of Anti-lost Clothing

In addition to distinguish the various stages of children's body characteristic, the investigation content also includes classifications of fabrics, color, and style for parents' aspects. Considering the elements may affect the children's stretching, we also should give full consideration to the placement of positioning components, method of use requirements, and give full solutions to the application.

Through the questionnaire survey, we concluded that the parents' requirements of fabric tend to be: elasticity, comfortable, soft, and without toxic characteristics; of the color tend to: bright, conspicuous, conducive to the development of children's intelligence and creativity; of style, consider more on loose, introduction, and leisure style.

Therefore we concluded that, under the comprehensive consideration for children's delicate skin, and because they are sensitive to external stimulation, prone to infections and skin rash. And thus anti-lost clothes should choose elastic fabric; use its soft and wet absorption, air exchanging, natural cellulose and good warmth retention property. So while using the fabrics, we should give priority to the knitting fabric. Using a soft, elastic and unique knitting fabric with good characteristic wrinkle resistance and resilience. On the one hand, to dress in the process of technology application design, combine the positioning device integrated with the fabric performance; On the other hand, to ensure the rationality of fabrics and clothing garment structure during the design process.

In addition, the bright color can be visible enough to help us quickly find the child in the crowd, but in order to prevent the fabric fade from causing damage to the skin, Plain and elegant color should be chosen in deciding the clothing color, such as light pink, light blue, yellow, etc.

As one of the three elements in design style, style is quite significant in designing clothes, especially in children's clothing design. Not only should we stick on the basic principle of design, but also must do the fundamental basis for the design of children's body and its activities. Thus, in the style design, we must master the clothes' restricting factors for children's activities. At the same time, we should pay close attention to the functional requirements of the clothes in the market and the popular trend of product design, ensure it is attractive both on the function and design development.

Considering the difference of peoples' understanding and requirements on the positioning of functional clothing, the questionnaire provides several different styles of clothing including basic style, casual style sports style and adult style to summarize the parents' preferences. The results show that the casual and sports style popularity rages highest in the survey while the adult style selected proportion is almost zero, basic design is under investigation for identity is much lower than the casual and sports. As shown in Fig. 2, 50 % of respondents chose the casual style, 37 % of respondents chose the sport style. Figure 1 shows that respondent parents under aged 35, while being active, have a higher level of education, and concern more about the fashion and leisure issues, are affected by the style of leisure and sports deeper. And as the age increasing, the respondents over the age of 35 has lower pursuit for fashion and sports, prefer mature, stable, comfortable and healthy style.

Therefore, we determine the anti-lost clothes to choose light knitted apparel leisure as the basic style.

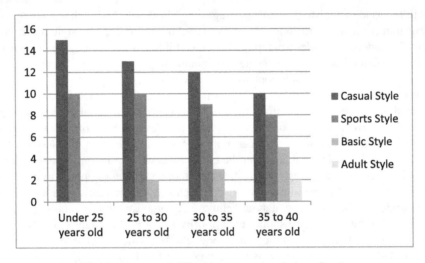

Fig. 1. Parents of different ages on the choice of style

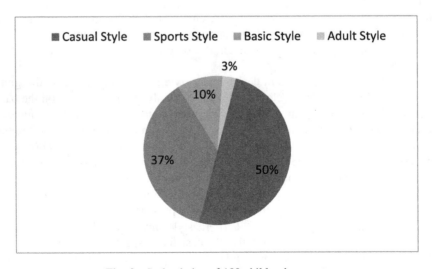

Fig. 2. Style choice of 100 children's parents

2.3   The Placement of Tracking Devices

The location design of components is the key point in the whole design of the garment. On the one hand, analysis from the perspective of the visual appearance, due to the limit of the element size and the requirements of physical performance factors in the position of design, size should not be too prominent to avoid combining effects and clothing aesthetics; On the other hand, from the angle of safety comfort analysis, the difference between properties of positioning component and textile fabrics is mainly manifested in the pliability, in design of position, I will fully consider the performance of comfort and safety on clothing, in order to avoid placing on the joint activities of the human body. In view of this, according to the requirements of the overall design, I determine the several different positions, namely Shoulder, Protothorax, Yoke, Hem, Medial suture, and investigate in the market, summarize their acceptance level.

The survey set double options. The research object is divided into two parts as a whole, a part of over the 30 years of age, a part of the under 30 year old. Parents who over 30 years of age have more abundant experience and understanding of children's activities which will give me a greater reference value.

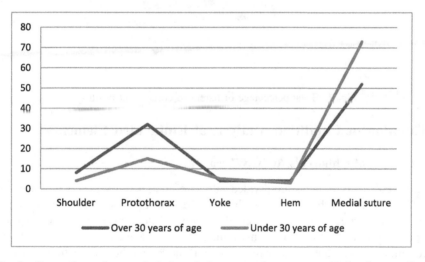

Fig. 3. Comparison of parents' choice of placement of components (Color figure online)

By the results of the survey analysis shows (As shown in Figs. 3 and 4), set the element in the protothorax and the medial suture are gain the more recognition. The degree of their preference is 24 % and 63 %. Figure 3 shows that the identity of shoulder position and yoke position is far lower than the protothorax position and the medial suture position, caused by the position of the joint active point, that is, the shoulder end and the back shoulder blade. Under normal circumstances, the greater human joints force, the higher the frequency of the positioning element and the more the human skin friction, to those will bring inconvenience to children's activities and make wearing uncomfortably. At the same time, due to the positioning element friction with the human body for a long time, the combination strength of the component and the fabric is reduced, and it's easy to cause the location of components defected from clothing, which will destroy use function. From the results of the survey analysis, the element in the position of hem of whole location design choice is insignificant, it means that parents mainly taking into account the appearance of the clothing and the influence factor of human activities. Overall, we should choose the medial suture position to meet the requirements of safety and comfortability.

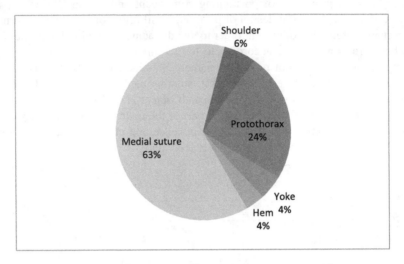

Fig. 4. Total percentage of parent to component position

3   Component Condition Analysis of Embedded Elements

3.1   Division of Children's Activity Area

The children's activity areas are divided into safe area, activity area, and detachment area. The safe area is the area in which the child is in the safe state of being accompanied; Activity area is the area for children to walk alone in a small range and play with peers; The detachment area is more than the area of the activity region. Through the communication status of the wireless network node and the information center is in the anti lost module, in order to judge the physical position and the movement tendency of the anti-lost element. When the element is fed back to the center that is about to enter the detachment zone, it will alarm timely, so as to realize the location of the wearer and monitoring, take the initiative to prevent the lost.

3.2   Sound Sensor

This type of sensor is mainly aimed at children in infancy, children in this period have not been developed fully with language ability and Mobility, and crying is one of the main signals of danger. Studies have shown that babies in different time ranges have different crying frequency, such as when the baby is sleepy crying frequency is approximately 6 kHz, and when the baby is hungry, crying frequency generally reach 15 kHz. After careful research and analysis, the frequency of a baby's cry almost $4 \sim 17$ kHz. So according to the different frequency sound, we can use the sound sensor to detect infant safety information which will be processed to send to the network to the guardian alarm. After these, positioning technology to track the location information of the baby can help Guardian find the baby successfully. So distinguish the baby's cry frequency range will appear in two cases: (1) The guardian can manually eliminate the wrong crying alarm information when the baby is around him; (2) The crying information collected by the guardian when the baby goes beyond his supervision range, is determined as the alarm information.

3.3 Types and Differences of Communication Technology

In terms of the communications technology, research has been underway to classify and categorize several widely employed technologies for tracking. According to its principle, I will analyze its pros and cons features in the respects of security, interference, involving distance range, relevant methodology and cost as well as the feasibility of embedment into clothing. While considering the problem of the clothing washing, equipment maintenance, and the condition of being fully enclosed or semi-enclosed, we will compare relevant data to select from these types of communications and electronic equipment applicable to each of the four stages of children (Fig. 5).

Bluetooth technology advantage: it is effective in the 2.4 GHz band which is a band that serves industry, technology, medical radio band without application license. Bluetooth technology has a wide range of applications, low power consumption, small size and low cost chip solutions that can be applied to very small devices.

Wireless Fidelity's outstanding advantages to be as follows: First, based on the Bluetooth technology of radio coverage is very small radius of about only about 50 feet, while the Wireless Fidelity coverage radius of up to 300 feet or so. Second, although its data security performance is worse than Bluetooth and transmission quality also needs to be improved, it's really speedy for data transfers.

The main purpose of Infrared communication technology is to replace the cables connecting the wireless data transmission. Its interface can save the cost of download or other information exchanges; Due to the need to transfer information docking, it has strong security. Relatively, its communication distance is short and in the process of communication cannot be moved. Moreover it will be interrupted in case of obstacles.

The advantages of ZigBee could be summarized as: By greatly protocol (less than 1/10 of the Bluetooth), the demand for communication controller can be reduced. ZigBee works in the low rate with 250 KBPS (2.4 GHz), 40 KBPS (915 MHz) and 20 KBPS (868 MHz) of raw data throughput, to meet the demand of low speed data transmission applications. ZigBee has a faster response speed. Only need 15 ms, it can be transferred from sleep to the working state, similarly, Just 30 ms, the node connection can enter the network. It can be argued that the above features are beneficial to further save the electricity.

Category / Condition	Bluetooth	Wireless Fidelity	Infrared	Zigbee
Transmission Speed	1.1Mb/s~2.1Mb/s(Even higher)	Can reach 54mbps.	4Mbps	10 ~ 250kb/ s
Transmission Distance	Generally within 10 meters.	Range of hundreds of feet.	Communication distance is short.	Transmission distance of 10 to 75 meters, after the expansion of up to a few hundred meters, or even thousands of meters
Standby Time	Several weeks	Hours	Longer than others	In a low power standby mode, two section No. 5 battery can support 1 node for 6 ~ 24 months or even longer.
Security	Can encrypt	Exist security risks	It has strong security.	Provides a three level security model.

Fig. 5. Comparison of the performance of Bluetooth, Wireless Fidelity, Infrared and ZigBee

ZigBee and Bluetooth are both used in the 2.4 GHz band, which relatively has weak ability through the wall. The difference is that ZigBee uses DSSS spread spectrum, while Bluetooth using FHSS spread spectrum. It depends on product positioning in the market to use DSSS or FHSS, because they can solve the transmission capacity and characteristics of the wireless local area network, which including the anti-interference ability, using distance range, broad frequency the size of the small and transmit data. DSSS technology is suitable for fixed environment or application of higher transmission quality requirements, therefore, wireless plant, wireless hospital and online communities, mostly using DSSS wireless technology products. While FHSS is mostly used in fast moving endpoint, such as mobile phone, the wireless transmission technology of using FHSS spread-spectrum technology.

4   Conclusion

Since to master and realize intelligent technology has a time limited, and my interdisciplinary knowledge structure system is not complete, especially the subject of positioning technology is not comprehensive, resulting in many problems and deficiencies in the research. Mainly embodied in the subject of the relevant professional knowledge structure, and the undetailed test, it is necessary to further improve and perfect the analysis. But I hope that through the investigation of parents and children's needs, as well as the communication technology of the data collection and comparison, we can find a suitable way for children to anti-lost. Also hope that I can do my own part of the strength to combine the clothing design and human engineering to solve the social problem of children lost.

References

1. Li, X., Zheng, C., et al.: Adult's response to baby cries and brain mechanisms. Prog. Psychol. Sci. **10**, 1770–1779 (2013)
2. Shou, H.: New intelligent positioning clothing. China. 202890499 u, 24 April 2013
3. Luo, W.: A new kind of Bluetooth technology, ultra-low power consumption Bluetooth technology. J. Mod. Telecommun. Technol. **10**, 31–38 (2010)
4. Hong, W.: Intelligent children near field oriented locating safety clothing (2014)
5. Guan, S.: 4 to 6 Years Old Preschool Children Size Research, pp. 63–80. Tianjin University of Technology Institute of Art and Clothing, Tianjin (2007)
6. Wei, X., Ren, T.: Dual mode based on single chip microcomputer control children lost prevention system design. Micro Comput. Appl. **6**, 86–89 (2012)
7. Pan, J.: Garment Ergonomics and Design, pp. 6–19, 76–88. China Light Industry Press, Beijing (2000)
8. Xiaoyi, Y., Wenjin, H., Shen, L., et al.: Based on the intelligent safety of children's wear evaluation system set up. J. Text. Rev. 66–68 (2014)

Study on Somatotype Characteristics and Differences of Female Youth from Liaoning Province and Guangdong Province in China

Xiaoping Hu[✉] and Jing Zhou

School of Design, Guangzhou Higher Education Mega Center,
South China University of Technology, Panyu District, Guangzhou 510006,
People's Republic of China
huxp@scut.edu.cn

Abstract. The purpose of this paper is to study the somatotype characteristics and differences of female youth from North and South China. We select the female youth aged 20 to 29 as the research objects, were measured by garment specialty students. The measure covered height, chest circumference, waist circumference, neck circumference, shoulder width, abdominal circumference and hip circumference. The somatotype data was collected from 102 different female youth. Half of them are from Liaoning province in north China and the other half are from Guangdong province in south China. Two area female youth's somatotype characteristic and difference were summarized based on descriptive statistics by SPSS software. The difference between chest circumference and abdominal circumference is the focus of this research. Not only can the study provide data for the costume design of north and south young females, but also provide reference data for subdivision garment size.

Keywords: Somatotype characteristic · Garment size · Female youth

1 Introduction

There are garment size for man, women and children, but there is no specific standard for female youth from different area, which leads to the clothing in the current market can't fit the different area female youth. So it is necessary to study the somatotype characteristic and difference between the north female youth and south female youth for garment design. Due to the acquired factors, such as genetic factors, physical growth, living habits, eating habits and routine work., the somatotype difference is obvious between north and south. Costumes need adapted to the human body, and researching for different periods, different regions and different age of human body is the basic subjects of clothing structure design. Based on this issue, the research of the body of the different area female and garment size is imperative.

© Springer International Publishing Switzerland 2016
V.G. Duffy (Ed.): DHM 2016, LNCS 9745, pp. 22–31, 2016.
DOI: 10.1007/978-3-319-40247-5_3

2 The Garment Classification About Somatotype in the Domestic and Overseas

2.1 The Garment Size in China

The Garment Size Classification is Simple. In China, the garment size standard about female only have 4 kinds of somatotype. The garment size standard is not in accordance with the age and geographical division. So it leads many consumers can't find suitable clothing in the market. At the same time, the classification of the garment size standard is detailed in many developed countries. For example, in Japan, the garment size standard divide the somatotype of adult into 7 kinds which included Y, YA, A, AB, B, BE, E. They also divided different age stage, for example, they divided female somatotype into 3 kinds which included the young girl somatotype, young women somatotype and women somatotype. The classification of garment size in Japan is very detail.

The Data is Old. In the late 1980s, China has carried out anthropological on a large scale and get the basic data of the garment size standard. The garment size standard GB/T1335-1991 were set out based on the data. Later on, there were appeared the 1997 edition and the 2008 edition. The 2008 edition is used by now. But these two edition were just slightly adjusted based on the 1991 edition, and they did not update the basic somatotype data. With the improvement of living conditions, the Chinese somatotype has changed in 20 years. So the data of the current garment size standard is old, which is lack of reference value to guide the clothing companies produced clothing for the consumer demands.

2.2 The Methods of the Classification About Somatotype in Domestic and Overseas

The partition of people's somatotype is the key to set out the standard of garment size. Many countries have different methods and index to divide the somatotype of the garment size standard. Overall, there are several kinds. Firstly, the partition based on the discrepancy of girth, mainly based on the discrepancy of chest circumference and waistline, the discrepancy of chest circumference and hip circumference and the discrepancy of waist circumference and hip circumference as the partitioning index. Secondly, the partition based on height, weight, age and chest circumference. Thirdly, the partition based on the index of the body, such as the index of stoop, the ratio of body and chest circumference and the ratio of chest circumference and waist circumference. Fourthly, the partition based on the index of the type of chest, waist and hip. The last, the partition based on clustering method, which is divided by selecting the classification of somatotype.

In China, the classification of somatotype is based on the partition of discrepancy of girth, mainly based on the discrepancy of chest circumference and waist circumference. However, with the change of the somatotype characteristics of the female youth, the discrepancy of chest circumference and waist circumference which as the basis to divide somatotype can't represent all kinds of somatotype characteristics. So, in this study, we measured data of the body of female youth who aged from 20 to 29 from north and south.

3 Experiment

3.1 Experiment Subject

All data collection used the random sampling method. The sample contains 108 female youth aged 20 to 29 years old from Liaoning province and Guangdong province. The experiment time is from January 10th 2016 to January 30th 2016.

3.2 The Measurement Parts

In order to combine purposes of research and requirements, we choose 10 kinds of representative measuring project based on the database require of somatotype in garment production, which include height, chest circumference, waist circumference, abdomen circumference, hip circumference, shoulder width, arm circumference, arm length, the length from neck to waist and neck circumference. These project covers the main control parts of the body and can satisfy all kinds of related analysis of the body type.

3.3 The Measurement Methods and Tools

The measurement method is traditional manual measurement. In order to ensure the data is accurate, we assign one professional person to operate in the whole process. The measured women wearing thin lingerie. They keep stand straight, visual front and arm natural prolapse. Finally, the surveyor use a tape to measure.

4 Data Analysis

4.1 The Data Prepossessing

The experiment measured 108 young women. In order to ensue the data accurately and reliably, we prepossessing the measured data. We removed some invited data after check the measure data. Then we get 102 valid data, the effective rate is 94 %.

4.2 The Analysis Methods

Use the SPSS software to analysis the mean and the standard deviation of the data. Then T test the sample, summary the somatotype characteristics in north and south. Compare the differences between north female youth and south female youth.

4.3   The Analysis of Data

After statistics and classified the data, we can know that the distribution of chest circumference, waist circumference and hip circumference. N stands for north and S stands for south. The figures as follow and the abscissa axis stands for number, the depth axis stands for girth. From the Figs. 1, 2 and 3, we can know that the chest circumference of north female youth mainly distribute in the range of 80–83 cm. The waist circumference of north female youth mainly distribute in the range of 68–71 cm. And the hip circumference of north female youth mainly distribute in the range of 82 101 cm, and the percentage is 88.2 %. From the Figs. 4, 5 and 6, we can know that the chest circumference of south female youth mainly distribute in the range of 82–89 cm, and the percentage is 74.5 %. The waist circumference of south female youth mainly distribute in the range of 63–70 cm, and the percentage is 76.5 %. And the hip circumference of south female youth mainly distribute in the range of 86–95 cm, and the percentage is 80 %. Compared with the chest circumference, waist circumference and hip circumference of south female youth, the waist circumference and hip circumference of north female youth is clearly larger, but the chest circumference is smaller. This prove that north female youth is fatter, their fat accumulated at waist and hip, which is led the waist circumference and hip circumference larger.

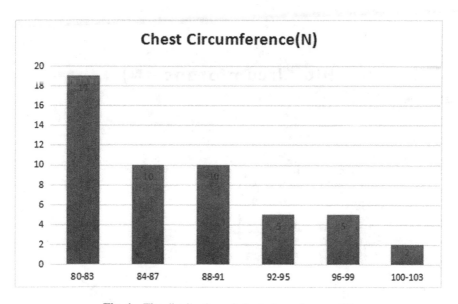

Fig. 1. The distribution of chest circumference (N)

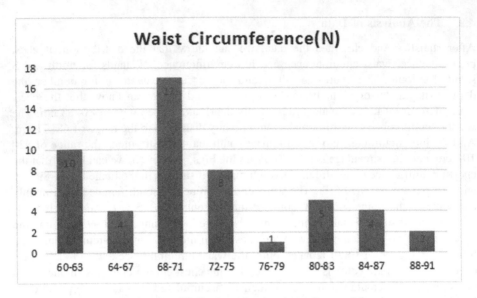

Fig. 2. The distribution of waist circumference (N)

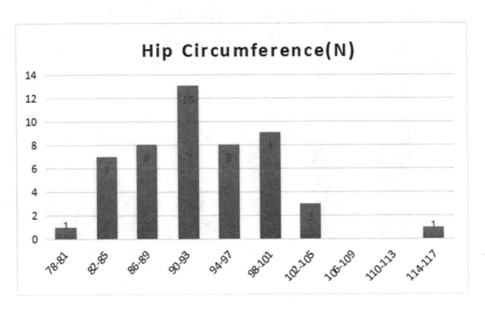

Fig. 3. The distribution of hip circumference (N)

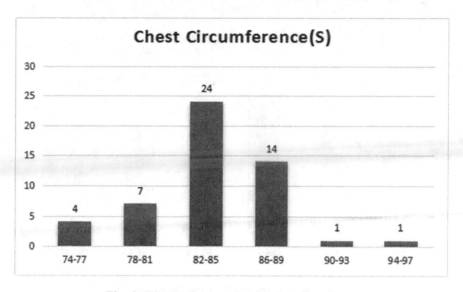

Fig. 4. The distribution of chest circumference (S)

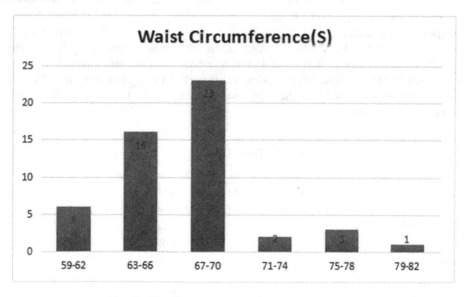

Fig. 5. The distribution of waist circumference (S)

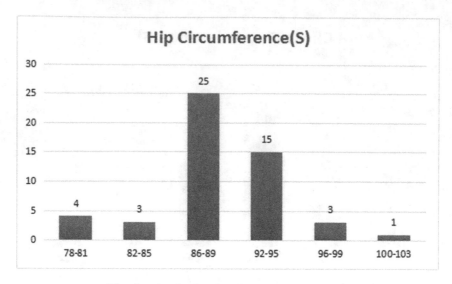

Fig. 6. The distribution of hip circumference (S)

4.4 The Analysis of Data Dispersion

The standard deviation reflects the trend of dispersion. The larger standard deviation, the larger degree of dispersion. On the contrary, the stand deviation is small, the degree of dispersion is concentrated. From the Table 1, the biggest standard deviation have 3 items as follows: the waist circumference of north female youth is 7.522 cm, the abdomen circumference of north female youth is 8.069 and the arm circumference of south female youth is 9.814. These evidence that north female youth have big changes in waist circumference and abdomen circumference, the south female youth have big changes in arm circumference.

Table 1.

	Native place	N	Mean	Std. deviation	Std. error mean
Height (cm)	N	51	165.38	4.560	.632
	S	51	159.92	4.685	.656
Chest circumference (cm)	N	51	87.37	5.726	.794
	S	51	83.88	3.897	.546
Waist circumference (cm)	N	51	71.51	7.522	1.043
	S	51	67.17	4.256	.596
Abdomen circumference (cm)	N	51	77.06	8.069	1.119
	S	51	72.24	5.237	.733
Hip circumference (cm)	N	51	92.83	6.744	.935
	S	51	90.23	3.867	.541
Neck circumference (cm)	N	51	33.09	6.840	.948

(*Continued*)

Table 1. (*Continued*)

	Native place	N	Mean	Std. deviation	Std. error mean
	S		32.31	1.005	.141
Arm circumference (cm)	N	51	26.56	4.815	.668
	S	51	25.83	9.814	1.374
Neck to Waist (cm)	N	51	38.19	.595	.083
	S	51	37.65	.744	.104
Arm length (cm)	N	51	52.66	3.255	.451
	S	51	52.47	4.456	.624
Shoulder width (cm)	N	51	38.21	.776	.108
	S	51	37.78	.923	.129

4.5 Independent-Samples T Test

In order to make the classification of somatotype can clearly reflect the study about the overall somatotype characteristics, there need to combine several investigate of index. In this paper, we use the independent-samples T test which is belong the part of SPSS to realize.

Table 2.

		Levene's test for equality of variances		T-test for equality of means						
		F	Sig.	T	df	Sig. (2-tailed)	Mean difference	Std. error difference	95 % confidence interval of the difference	
									Lower	Upper
Height (cm)	Equal variances assumed	.054	.818	5.997	101	.000	5.463	.911	3.656	7.270
	Equal variances not assumed			5.995	100.779	.000	5.463	.911	3.655	7.271
Chest circumference (cm)	Equal variances assumed	10.193	.002	3.602	101	.000	3.483	.967	1.565	5.401
	Equal variances not assumed			3.615	90.058	.000	3.483	.963	1.569	5.397
Waist circumference (cm)	Equal variances assumed	12.827	.001	3.597	101	.001	4.343	1.207	1.948	6.738
	Equal variances not assumed			3.615	80.936	.001	4.343	1.201	1.953	6.733
Abdomen circumference (cm)	Equal variances assumed	13.726	.000	3.590	101	.001	4.822	1.343	2.158	7.487
	Equal variances not assumed			3.605	87.708	.001	4.822	1.338	2.164	7.481
Hip circumference (cm)	Equal variances assumed	10.892	.001	2.395	101	.018	2.601	1.086	.447	4.756
	Equal variances not assumed			2.407	81.575	.018	2.601	1.081	.452	4.751

(*Continued*)

Table 2. (*Continued*)

		Levene's test for equality of variances		T-test for equality of means					95 % confidence interval of the difference	
		F	Sig.	T	df	Sig. (2-tailed)	Mean difference	Std. error difference	Lower	Upper
Neck circumference (cm)	Equal variances assumed	1.895	.172	.798	101	.426	.773	.968	−1.147	2.693
	Equal variances not assumed			.806	53.243	.424	.773	.959	−1.150	2.696
Arm circumference (cm)	Equal variances assumed	.007	.932	.477	101	.634	.724	1.519	−2.288	3.737
	Equal variances not assumed			.474	72.438	.637	.724	1.528	−2.321	3.770
Neck to waist (cm)	Equal variances assumed	4.543	.035	4.112	101	.000	.545	.133	.282	.808
	Equal variances not assumed			4.103	95.591	.000	.545	.133	.281	.809
Arm length (cm)	Equal variances assumed	.094	.760	.251	101	.802	.193	.768	−1.330	1.716
	Equal variances not assumed			.250	91.470	.803	.193	.770	−1.337	1.722
Shoulder width (cm)	Equal variances assumed	.806	.372	2.545	101	.012	.427	.168	.094	.760
	Equal variances not assumed			2.540	97.408	.013	.427	.168	.093	.761

If the significant level of Sig value of F test is greater than 0.05, it is homogeneous variance. Then chose the first line in equal variances assumed to observe the significant level of T test. If the Sig (2-tailed) is greater than 0.05, then there is no differences. Instead, there is differences. IF Sig value is less than 0.05. Then chose the second line in equal variances not assumed to observe the significant level of T test. If the Sig (2-tailed) is greater than 0.05, then there is no differences. Instead, there is differences.

Based on the independent-samples T test and the Table 2, we can know that:

1. There is significant differences between chest circumference of north female youth and chest circumference of south female youth.
2. There is significant differences between waist circumference of north female youth and waist circumference of south female youth.
3. There is significant differences between abdomen circumference of north female youth and abdomen circumference of south female youth.
4. There is significant differences between hip circumference of north female youth and hip circumference of south female youth.
5. There is no significant differences between neck circumference of north female youth and neck circumference of south female youth.
6. There is no significant differences between arm circumference of north female youth and arm circumference of south female youth.

7. There is significant differences between the length neck to waist of north female youth and the length neck to waist of south female youth.
8. There is no significant differences between arm length of north female youth and arm length of south female youth.
9. There is significant differences between shoulder width of north female youth and shoulder width of south female youth.
10. There is significant differences between height of north female youth and height of south female youth.

5 Conclusion

Based on the analysis of somatotype type about the female youth in north China and south China, we found that there is significant differences between the somatotype of the north female youth and the somatotype of the south female youth. Most of the somatotype data of the north female youth is greater than the south female youth. This study is offer some reference for the fashion designer and clothing enterprise of north female youth and south female youth. This research has a certain practical value, which is benefit for related products development. Some data also need pay much more attention and some related research need to deepen and expand.

References

Zhang, W.B., Chen, H.Y.: The Statistical Analysis of Practical Data and the Application of SPSS12.0. Beijing University of Posts and Telecommunications Press, Beijing (2006)
Zhang, J.X.: Human Ergonomics of Costume Design. China Light Industry Press, Beijing (2010)
Liu, R.P., Liu, W.H.: The Principle and Technique of Clothing Structure Design. The Textile Industry Press, Beijing (1993)
Zhang, Y.: The Statistical Software Applications. Intellectual Property Press, Beijing (2013)
Hu, X., Zhao, Y.: Study on the body shape of middle-aged and old women for garment design. In: Duffy, V.G. (ed.) DHM 2015. LNCS, vol. 9185, pp. 53–61. Springer, Heidelberg (2015)

Research on the Comfortable and Maximum Pedaling Forces of Chinese Population

Huiyu Luo[1], Chang Liu[2], Jing Zhang[1], Qing Ye[1], and Li Ding[1(✉)]

[1] School of Biological Science and Medical Engineering,
Beihang University, Beijing, China
ding1971316@buaa.edu.cn
[2] Pan-Asia Technical Automotive Center Co., Ltd., Shanghai, China

Abstract. With the fast development of the automotive designs, auto manufacturers have paid more and more attention to the comfort driving in recent years. Driving pedaling forces, referring to the forces exerted by the drivers on the brake, clutch, and accelerator pedals when they are driving cars, are ergonomic evaluation indices of human-vehicle interaction. Nowadays, there are few researches on the pedal comfort of the Chinese population. Therefore, this paper aims to study the Chinese drivers' pedaling force data and the factors influencing on it. The experiment facilities were designed to measure the pedaling forces. The research showed that: (1) The dissatisfaction of drivers with the brake pedal is much more than that with clutch, and accelerator pedal, from the view of pedaling forces. (2) The pedaling forces of the subjects show the basic normal distribution. (3) The gender difference has little impact on the comfortable pedaling forces, but there is remarkable difference on the maximum pedaling force acceptable between male and female. (4) The angle of elbow flexion joint has no significant influence on the comfortable pedaling forces, but with the increase of the elbow joint, the maximum pedaling forces acceptable declines.

Keywords: Ergonomics · Comfort driving · Pedaling force

1 Introduction

Automobile comfort research is a part of the fine design of automobile, and the research is significant for both automobile manufacturers and drivers. On the one hand, the automobile manufacturers can improve their market competitiveness by virtue of comfort research. On the other hand, comfortable driving research not only can make the drivers enjoy the driving pleasure of, but also has important significance for alleviating the car drivers' occupational disease.

Automobile comfort driving research mainly includes two aspects, (a) Adjust the drivers' posture to achieve comfortable driving based on the analysis of the human body and the subjective feelings of the comfortable driving position. In 1975, Rebiffe analysed the drivers' operation process, and calculated the driver comfortable driving angle by establishing the biomechanical model and theoretical analysis [1]. In 1980, Grandjean and Rebiffe did biomechanical analysis by limiting the position of the drivers' head,

© Springer International Publishing Switzerland 2016
V.G. Duffy (Ed.): DHM 2016, LNCS 9745, pp. 32–41, 2016.
DOI: 10.1007/978-3-319-40247-5_4

feet and hands, and worked out the joint angles of the drivers under comfortable driving posture [2]. In 1998, Porter and Gyi obtained the comfortable joint angle by testing 55 subjects, and compared with the data of Porter and Gyi [3]. In 2008, Ma et al. tested the driving comfortable angles (including the back angle, trunk thigh angle, knee angle) with PASSAT and POLO two models [4]. The studies above were carried out under the background that people adapt to the existing vehicles, and the results mainly depended on the subjects' subjective feeling. (b) The seat, steering wheel and pedals are most frequently-used when the drivers driving. Therefore, these three devices play an important role on the comfort driving, and there are many researches concerning the optimization of these three devices, especially the seat. Zhifei Zhang et al. researched on vehicle seat comfort based on the static and dynamic test of body pressure distribution, and compared the differences between dynamic and static pressure indicators. The features of the body pressure are got more clearly based on the research [5]. Matsuoka, who thought that passengers' seats and the drivers' seat should be paid equal attention to meet the comfortable driving and riding requirements, so they did the body pressure distribution researches, and determined the several factors of the comfort of seat design: minimum cushion angle, hip joint to allow the scope of activities, knee joint angle and ankle joint angle [6]. Liu Haoxue et al. provided a reference for the optimization design between brake and accelerator pedal by analyzing the relationship between the height difference of brake and accelerator pedal and the drivers' reaction time [7].

But there are rarely researches about automotive pedals comfort of Chinese population. According to our comfort driving survey in China, nearly half of the participants deemed that the pedaling force needed are too large or too small, which can't meet the requirement of the drivers. Accordingly, this paper aims to find out the comfortable pedaling force of Chinese and the reasons for recent dissatisfaction with the pedal design.

2 Methods

2.1 Research Equipments

The Violet ZG-601MDB driving simulator the Santana seat was used for simulating the driving environment. The pedaling forces are measured and recorded by the pressure measurement system, which consists of two sub-modules, the DAQ module and the software platform. The DAQ module included BD-4K pressure sensor, and in relation to software platform, the Kingview6.55 was adopted.

2.2 Subjects

According to the standard of human body size in China, 510 healthy Chinese drivers were selected to participate in this test, including 260 males and 250 females. Male subjects with an average height of 169.3 cm, maximum height for 195.0 cm, minimum height for 151.0 cm. Their average weight for 66.1 kg, and average driving experience is 6.1 years, longest driving experience for 37 years and shortest driving for 1 month;

right handedness for 239 people, left handedness is 9 and ambidextrous for 2 people. For the female subjects, the average height for 158.2 cm, maximum height for 174.6 cm, minimum height for 144.0 cm; average weight is 55.6 kg, average driving to 4.7 years, longest driving experience 24 years and shortest driving experience for half a month; right handedness for 249 people, left handedness for 10 people and ambidextrous for 1. And the height and weight reference for the subjects selection is shown in Table 1.

Table 1. The height and weight of the subjects

M	Height (m)	<1.540	1.540–1.591	1.591–1.610	1.610–1.693	1.693–1.773	1.773–1.797	1.797–1.854	>1.854
	Number	3	10	13	104	104	13	10	3
	Weight (kg)	<46	46–50.9	50.9–53.5	53.5–64.5	64.5–80.4	80.4–85.9	85.9–95.9	>95.9
	Number	3	10	13	104	104	13	10	3
F	Height (m)	<1.451	1.451–1.482	1.482–1.501	1.501–1.574	1.574–1.650	1.650–1.673	1.673–1.719	>1.719
	Number	2	9	12	102	102	12	9	2
	Weight (kg)	<40.4	40.4–43.6	43.6– 45.5	45.5–55.7	55.7– 69.5	69.5–73.8	73.8–82.0	>82
	Number	2	9	12	102	102	12	9	2

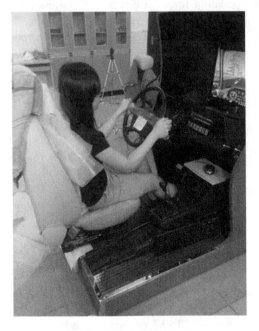

Fig. 1. Experimental scene

2.3 Testing Process

(a) The subjects were asked to adjust the seat to a comfortable position, and the testers recorded the driver's elbow joint, hip angle. (b) Guided the subjects to adapt to the driving environment, and reminded them to keep straight driving. (c) Started driving simulator with slow modules, medium vehicle. And the subjects would operate the clutch, accelerator pedal and the brake plate respectively. (d) When the subjects exerted the defined force, including maximum and comfortable force, they should keep the posture 10 s so that the testers could record data better (Fig. 1). (e) Measured the maximum acceptable stepping force with the same method, and lead subjects to adjust the angle of the elbow joint, including 90 DEG, 120 DEG and 150 DEG and 180 DEG.

3 Analysis and Results

This test was based on Chinese drivers' driving habits and experience, and the data could be applied to the Chinese drivers. Normally the drivers would be cautious in the acceleration process, so the stepping force exerted on the accelerator pedal was minimal, but for the clutch, the drivers need to step on the clutch to the low to complete the shift operation, so the stepping force exerted on the accelerator pedal was maximal. This paper mainly analyzed the subjective evaluation of the three pedals, the distribution characteristics of driving pedaling forces. In addition, the impacts of the different gender and angle of elbow joint on the pedaling force are analyzed respectively.

3.1 Dissatisfaction with the Three Pedals

In this test, the drivers were asked to point out the most uncomfortable pedal among clutch, accelerator pedal and brake pedal, and the evaluation results are shown in Fig. 2. The drivers thought that the most comfortable pedal was accelerator pedal. Only 4 % of the drivers thought that the accelerator pedal was uncomfortable, and the brake pedal and the clutch account for 64 % and 32 % respectively. By the analysis of the figure, the gender differences had no obvious effect on the satisfaction of the pedal.

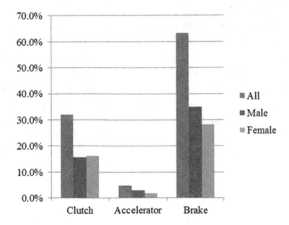

Fig. 2. The percentage of the pedals' dissatisfaction (Color figure online)

3.2 The Force Analysis Based on Gender Differences

Under comfortable sitting posture, the comfortable pedaling force for male is pretty much the same as that for female, but there is a significant different between the maximum pedaling forces acceptable of male and female. As shown in the Fig. 3, for male, the maximum pedaling forces acceptable exerted on the clutch, accelerator and the brake pedal are 148 N, 125 N, and 100 N higher than that of the female separately.

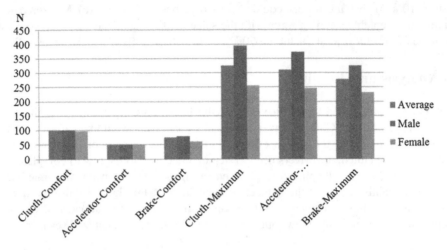

Fig. 3. The pedaling force analysis based on gender differences (Color figure online)

3.3 Data Distribution

In order to verify the data distribution characteristics of the pedaling force, SPSS statistical software is selected to analyze numerical data.

First of all, the normal distribution test was used for the data of the comfortable pedaling force of the clutch, and the figure P-P was shown in Fig. 4, which could prove the data basically fit the normal distribution. And the other pedals and conditions were basically coincident with Fig. 4.

Secondly, the normal distribution maps of the pedaling forces data from different pedals and conditions were shown in Figs. 5, 6, 7, 8, 9 and 10, the characteristic of the forces data distribution were shown clear. For the comfortable pedaling force, the data distribution of the clutch was relatively dispersed, and its average value was 100 N, the standard deviation was 38.6 N. For the accelerator pedal, the data distribution was intensive, and its average value was 52 N, the standard deviation was 19.0 N. The average value of the brake pedal was 78 N, and its standard deviation was 27.6 N. About the maximum acceptable pedaling force, the data distribution was more dispersed, and the numerical values were significantly greater than the comfortable pedaling force.

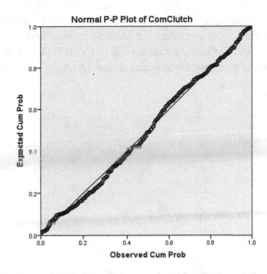

Fig. 4. Normal P-P plot of the comfortable clutch pedaling force

3.4   Pedaling Force Under Different Elbow Flexion Angles

In general, the drivers would exert the comfortable pedaling force on the pedals when they operated the devices, especially, when the drivers operated the accelerator pedal, they would be cautious to avoid accident, so that the stepping force exerted on the

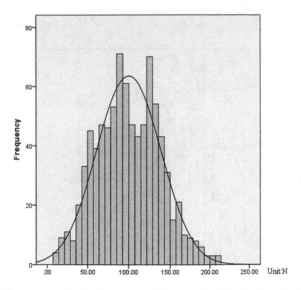

Fig. 5. The normal distribution map of the comfortable clutch pedaling force

accelerator pedal was minimal (see Table 2), for 51 N to 54 N. As the drivers need to step on the clutch to the low to complete the shift operation, and the value of which is about 96 N to 104 N, and the brake pedal for 76 N to 80 N. In addition, by analyzing the relationship between pedaling force under different angle of elbow joint, we found

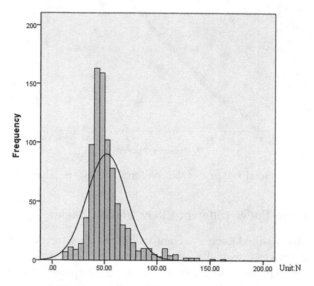

Fig. 6. The normal distribution map of the comfortable accelerator pedaling force

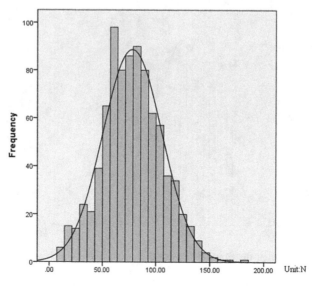

Fig. 7. The normal distribution map of the comfortable brake pedaling force

that the angle of elbow joint has no significant influence on the comfortable pedaling force. But with the angle of elbow joint changing from 90° to 180°, the maximum pedaling force acceptable declined.

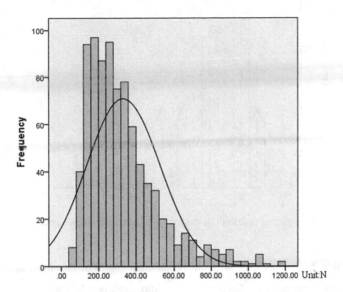

Fig. 8. The normal distribution map of the maximum clutch pedaling force

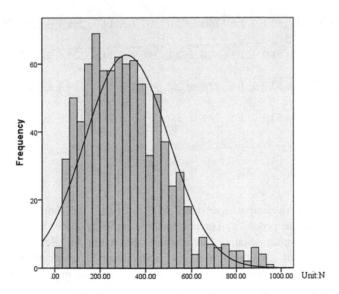

Fig. 9. The normal distribution map of the maximum accelerator pedaling force

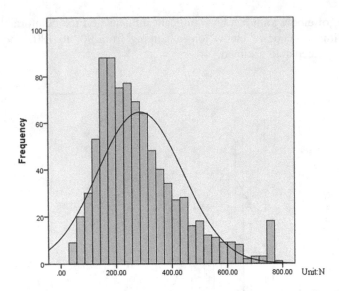

Fig. 10. The normal distribution map of the maximum brake pedaling force

Table 2. The pedaling force among different angles of the elbow joint

Degree	Comfortable pedaling force			Maximum pedaling force		
	Clutch	Accelerator	Brake	Clutch	Accelerator	Brake
Comfort DEG	99.9 ± 3.1	52.0 ± 1.3	77.9 ± 2.2	330.9 ± 13.2	317.9 ± 13.4	286.8 ± 11.1
180 DEG	96.3 ± 3.0	52.1 ± 1.5	76.1 ± 2.0	301.7 ± 14.0	298.4 ± 12.8	289.8 ± 11.7
150 DEG	99.8 ± 2.8	51.9 ± 1.3	80.4 ± 2.1	340.9 ± 14.8	324.4 ± 13.3	278.3 ± 10.2
120 DEG	103.3 ± 2.9	52.9 ± 1.6	77.8 ± 2.2	346.5 ± 15.3	329.3 ± 14.7	296.9 ± 12.4
90 DEG	97.21 ± 2.8	53.3 ± 1.5	79.8 ± 2.0	351.5 ± 15.9	338.9 ± 15.0	299.6 ± 12.2

Unit: N

4 Conclusion

(a) According to the subjective assessment of the drivers, they showed the least satisfaction with the brake pedal. (b) The comfortable pedaling forces on the three pedals are various; the maximum pedaling forces acceptable would be affected by the gender factor. (c) The angle of elbow joint had less connection with the comfortable pedaling force, yet the angle of elbow joint would affect the maximum acceptable pedaling forces.

Acknowledgements. The study was supported by the National Key Technology R&D Program (2014BAK01B05) and National Natural Science Foundation of China (51175021).

References

1. Rebiffe, M.P.: The driving seat: its adaptation to functional and anthropometric requirements. In: Proceedings of a Symposium on Sitting Posture, 132–147 (1969)
2. Grandjean, E.: Sitting posture of car drivers form the point of view of ergonomics. Hum. Factors Transp. Res. **2**, 205–213 (1980)
3. Porter, J.M., Gyi, D.E.: Exploring the optimum posture for driver comfort. Int. J. Veh. Des. **19** (1), 255–266 (1998)
4. Ma, M., Fan, R., Ruan, Y.: The test of comfortable driving posture and the fuzzy evaluation of the comfort. Eng. Manag. **2008**(13), 121–125 (2008). doi:10.3969/j.issn.1007-5429.2008.04. 025
5. Zhang, Z.F.: A Study on the Ride Comfort of Vehicle Seats Based on Body Pressure Distribution
6. Matsuoka, Y., Hanai, T.: Study of comfortable sitting posture. SAE paper no. 880054 (1988)
7. Liu, H.X.: A Study of the Effects on Working Efficiency of the Height Difference Between Acceleration Pedal and Brake Pedal

The Ten Characteristics of the Critical Task

Ergonomic Analysis of Vitality Requirements in Aortic Valve Surgery

René Patesson[1] and Eric Brangier[1,2(✉)]

[1] Université Libre de Bruxelles – CREATIC,
Campus du Solbosch. 44, Avenue Jeanne, 1050 Brussels, Belgium
[2] Université de Lorraine - PErSEUs, EA 7312. Sciences Humaines et Sociales.
Ile du Saulcy - CS 60228, 57045 Metz cedex 01, France
Eric.Brangier@univ-lorraine.fr

Abstract. This research forms a part of the design of a system for the resection and implantation of an aortic valve. Four transapical endovalve implantations are analyzed with a view to characterizing the exceptional criticality of this surgical procedure. We demonstrate that the surgeon's activity is largely cognitive, operational and social and requires mastery of a critical task, i.e. the performance and supervision of a risky, deliberately initiated procedure with an uncertain outcome. The concept of "critical task" is used to describe tasks combining potentially extreme seriousness and potential success, risk-taking with cure. The task is critical as its criticality is intentionally generated by the surgical team. In short, this paper defines the concept of critical task according to ten characteristics: Deliberate, Uniqueness, Learning restriction, Planning, Expertise, Preparation, Collective, Hazardous, Rigidity and Uncertain outcome; and supplies a number of ergonomic recommendations with a view to improvement.

Keywords: Critical task · Surgery · Design ergonomics · Medical device · Usability

1 Introduction

In ergonomics, it is seldom that interest is taken in one-minute tasks, the intensity and seriousness of which may change a life completely. The transapical implantation of an aortic valve is a task during which a heart surgeon may jeopardize the survival of a person whose heart is artificially sent into fibrillation for one minute, which is the time it takes to implant the new valve. This is a critical task, i.e. a task that can only be performed once and for which trial and error are therefore impossible. No repetition or adjustment is possible: this is what makes it a critical task.

The method habitually used for transapical valve implantation requires rapid ventricular pacing at 180–220 beats per minute, which lowers the systolic blood pressure to ≤60 mmHg. The heart then beats so fast that it "freezes" and the blood no longer circulates, which also blocks blood circulation in the brain. As a result, such

© Springer International Publishing Switzerland 2016
V.G. Duffy (Ed.): DHM 2016, LNCS 9745, pp. 42–53, 2016.
DOI: 10.1007/978-3-319-40247-5_5

blockage can only be very limited in time – to one minute – and that the surgeon is working within a highly restricted time frame.

Within the scope of a research project, the purpose of which was to define the ergonomics of a new system for the replacement of a stenosed and calcified aortic valve without opening the heart and without resorting to external blood circulation, i.e. on the beating heart and using a transcatheter transapical procedure, we analyzed the exact minute of fibrillation during which many technical, human and organizational factors combine to ensure high efficiency (or otherwise). This paper therefore has three complementary aims:

- To understand very short and vitally important tasks, to which we shall be referring as critical;
- To propose a definition of "critical tasks" by describing ten properties;
- To determine the ergonomic information supplied by such tasks concerning the operation.

To achieve these aims, we shall first present the characteristics of aortic valve implantation, and then perform a brief inventory of the state of the art of ergonomic approaches in surgery in order to raise the issue of the critical task. In this connection, we shall demonstrate that the concept of "critical task" remains as yet undeveloped. We shall then review four transapical endovalve implantation operations to extract relative qualitative and quantitative data. Finally, we shall propose and discuss a definition of "critical task" and supply a number of ergonomic recommendations to improve such work situations.

2 Transapical Aortic Valve Implantation

Aortic stenosis is the most frequent acquired heart disease, with a prevalence of 4.8 % in patients over 75, who account for over 60 % of indications for heart surgery in elderly patients. Despite the good results achieved with conventional aortic-replacement surgery in elderly patients, many patients are still denied this operation as the surgical risk can be high. In this vulnerable group, TAVI (Transcatheter Aortic Valve Implantation) may enable good results to be achieved while minimizing mortality and morbidity. Ideally, the combined use of surgery and radiological monitoring requires an operating room with fluoroscopic and echocardiogram equipment as well as a scanner. To implant an aortic valve, several approaches are possible; however, for the purpose of this study, the transapical approach has been selected.

In this case, using a left anterior small thoracotomy, the surgeon introduces a device into the heart which enables him/her to position, expand and implant an endovalve to replace the calcified valve; the latter is usually crushed by the expansion of the new valve. In surgical terms, the transapical method (Fig. 1) is more invasive than the femoral method and requires a general anaesthetic, but is more suitable in cases of peripheral vascular disease and aortic atherosclerosis. Moreover, the risk of stroke is lower. The short distance between the apex and the valve ensures more accurate manipulation than the transfemoral method.

The TAVI technique enables a balloon-expandable bioprosthesis to be used, without resection of the native aortic valve (Fig. 1). The chief difficulty of replacing the valve is that it requires that the heart be stopped by fibrillation for a maximum of one minute during the positioning and expansion of the endovalve, as this task must be performed without blood circulation to prevent the endovalve from coming loose, as well as embolisation during the crushing of the calcified valve.

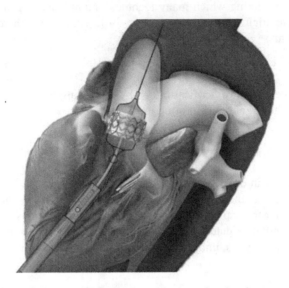

Fig. 1. Balloon inflation, expansion and positioning of endovalve at aortic root level

However, a number of complications are linked to the continued coexistence of the calcified and the new endovalve. With this in mind, the endovascular resection of the aortic valve prior to TAVI was developed and improved [3]. The purpose of this research is to perform remote resection of the diseased valve by catheter and remove it while implanting the new valve. All this had to be done in a single, critical minute, while the heart was fibrillating. From an ergonomic point of view, this is a particularly complex and delicate operation. It is a vital task and must be performed in a very short time (60 s). Hence, to procure as much relevant information as possible to design an ergonomic system, it was necessary to collect ergonomic information during surgical operations by describing the state of the art and performing an ergonomic analysis of transapical operations.

3   Theoretical Orientations

Ergonomics research in the area of surgery is often based on the quality of care model [8] used to draw up and update a model for the analysis of work situations in the area of healthcare [6], "Systems Engineering Initiative for Patient Safety (SEIPS)". This model focuses on the design of the work system and its impact on the induced processes and performances. It requires that the system characteristics, its components, the interactions between components, the safety of patients and persons and organizational results, including overall performance, be taken into account [5]. This model also emphasizes the importance of technology (IT, instruments, tools, processes and procedures), despite the fact that ergonomic characteristics relate more to the usability of medical systems [16, 18] and standards (e.g. ISO 62366). Generally speaking, there are two types of ergonomic knowledge. The first comprises precise and stabilized information, e.g. the results of the metrological measurement of noise in hospitals and recommendations concerning the usability testing of medical systems (Magnetic Resonance Imaging, ultrasound units, etc.). Nevertheless, despite the wealth of information it generates, such research does not really apply to operations, let alone heart operations and even less the critical tasks specific to such operations.

Mini-invasive surgery, much supported by laparoscopic systems, has introduced a new deal as far as operating methods and modes of work in operating rooms are concerned [12]. This change of scale in the actions of surgical teams has led to change in various areas:

- First of all, at the motor and physical level: the functions of the human locomotor apparatus required for mini-surgery are not the same as those required in open surgery [1]. Postures have changed, as have locations and the forces exerted and involved. Often, even the clothing has changed (lead aprons).
- The same applies to the perceptual and sensory level. The new systems have led to changes in the use of the senses and in perception: visual displays, touch screens and new sound formats [15, 17].
- At the cognitive and overall levels, the focus is on memory, information processing, learning, decision making and the ability to assess a situation. The new surgical systems have changed the knowledge used and therefore the treatment of information and knowledge in complex situations [10].
- At the socio-organizational level, the psychosocial factors which enhance – or diminish– skill in execution in the area of surgery are altered. New, non-technical skills [19], which are an essential factor in the performance of tasks and the safety of the system, are required of all staff working in the operating theatre. Such practices also appear to modify communication [14].
- At the time-related level, an overall concordance process is set up during an operation. However, this does not always resolve the issue of time regulation. A survey of anesthesia errors [7] showed that these were linked to noncompliance with the predetermined plan, i.e. that a person made a mistake when implementing a plan, prescription or procedure, causing desynchronization and serious errors.

When implanting a valve, fibrillation requires perfect organization of time to the very last second. The idea is to make a heart which is known to be very weak beat at 180/200 BPM. The surgeon is therefore generating a critical task and everyone must be synchronized. The synchronization of time, modes of operation, displays, communication and technologies is therefore critical.

The concept of "critical task" has not been developed in ergonomics. However, a number of studies have emphasized the analysis of criticality. The well-known critical-incident method [9, 13] incites individuals to tell their story and explore the elements of their work which have been memorized and can be verbally reactivated. Its premise is that an incident reveals the performance of the work and emphasizes the inadequacies and malfunctioning linked to specific tasks. However, this method is based on the premise that critical incidents can only be identified *after the event* and never *before the event*. Critical incidents are never deliberately generated, which is the exact opposite of the task we have set out to analyze.

4   The Analysis of Critical Task

In mini-invasive surgery, compared with traditional open-heart surgery, during which each person in the operating area saw everything, the surgeon perceives and absorbs all the useful information, e.g. the sensorimotor positioning feedback sent by the catheter. However, the positioning of the valve is a critical task, which needs to be accurate to the last millimeter and must be performed in a few seconds. As the system does not include an endoscope, the surgeon cannot directly view the area on which he/she is operating.

The main issue is therefore to identify and understand this critical task, which is linked to a complex, swift, collective, instrumented and risky process performed in a dynamic environment and is determined by both the surgeon's actions and goals and the behaviors of the staff, as well as by the interactions between the system elements which contribute to the modification of the situation.

4.1   Analysis Methods

Analysis of the activity requires the implementation of a number of methods for the observation, analysis, formalization and modeling of what actually occurs during work. Our observation techniques are traditionally used in ergonomics and involve the collection of data by various means:

- Direct observation in the operating room (during the 4 transapical TAVI operations, using several video cameras, photography and audio recordings (Fig. 2)).
- Study of traces, including recordings of previous operations and the related X-ray image videos.
- Utterances by the surgeon (outside the operating room and sometimes during the operation).
- Five focus groups and interviews with surgeons, cardiologists and anesthetists.

The four TAVI operations were filmed and analyzed using Actigram-Kronos software [11] so as to visualize the activity graphs for these operations. Statistical data were extracted to achieve as close as possible a characterization of the critical minute during which the patient was sent into fibrillation. A hierarchical model of the task was then created using K-Mad-e software [4].

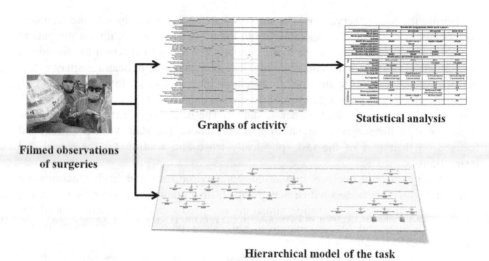

Filmed observations of surgeries

Graphs of activity

Statistical analysis

Hierarchical model of the task

Fig. 2. Synopsis of the analysis method (video, activity graphs, hierarchical analysis)

4.2   Some General Information Concerning Valve Implantation

Out of the 80 min of a transapical operation, three stages can be distinguished. The first is the preparation of the apical route and penetration into the heart. The second includes the actual implantation of the valve, which begins with the arrival of the system in the heart and ends with its withdrawal. During the third and final stage, the incisions are closed and the operation completed.

In this case, we shall be taking an interest only in the second, critical stage or task (Table 1), which is itself divided into three sub-stages with a total average duration of 5 min, 24 s and 8 tenths.

1. The arrival of the delivery system and its penetration into the heart (around 38 s);
2. The presence of the delivery system inside the heart (on average 3 min, 52 s and 8 tenths);
3. The withdrawal of the system (on average 53.2 s).

Table 1. Structure and duration of critical task during four operations

Task	Observation	Duration in %	Duration in minutes (average)
Implantation and withdrawal	Entry of delivery system into patient	12.0 %	38 s, 8 ds
	Delivery system in position in patient's heart	71.7 %	3 min, 52 s, 8 ds
	Withdrawal of delivery system from patient	16.4 %	53 s, 2 ds
Total		100 %	5 min, 24 s, 8 ds

During the four observations, the second phase includes changes to the technical and social environment. The operating-room lights focus more brightly on the patient and are dimmed in the rest of the room. Sound presence is focused on the sounds of physiological measurements and scanning. The physiological-indicator display monitors are placed next to the surgeon. In psychosocial terms, in all four cases, this task systematically began with a description by the surgeon of the procedure and of each person's role as soon as fibrillation was started. The behavior of each participant was orchestrated by the surgeon's signal to start fibrillation. The staff was very silent and focused on their part of the task, physically tense and waiting for the signal and instructions.

The surgeon only controls part of his/her environment and his/her actions are combined with other factors which may escape his/her control. The operation situation showed several times that change situations occurred outside the perimeter of the surgeon's actions and the physiological and electro-physiological reactions of the patient and occasionally of the team.

To implant the valve, the surgeon has only a very partial view of the heart (in 2D, in black and white, and for only five seconds). In order to act on the basis of this information, it would appear that the surgeon constructs a coherent representation of the overall situation and updates it continually according to the actions, the results and their repeated assessments. He/she combines new information with the existing knowledge in his/her working memory and constructs a gradual, composite and elaborate image of the valve's position as well as potential projections of the future fixation and operation of the valve. For this purpose, he/she continuously extracts medical, technical and psychosocial information which he/she endeavors to integrate in order to form a coherent and effective mental image for the purpose of implanting the valve. He/she may also use his/her past experiences and learning to enable earlier valve-positioning images to coincide with the images relating to the current operation.

However, the surgeon is not alone. This is a collective intervention. Within this overall representation, the surgeon needs to understand the way in which each team member is actually functioning compared with his/her expectations, determine their strengths and weaknesses, and, depending on the resulting image, delegate tasks with a varying degree of confidence or monitor their performance more closely [19]. In short, he/she endeavors to control the actions and, to the greatest possible extent, utilizes a fund of information which will prevent him/her from being taken by surprise and discomfited by uncontrollable and unforeseen events. Indeed, the purpose of the surgeon's activity is, as much as possible, to remain connected to his/her medical, human, technical and social environment in order to remove all uncertainty. In consequence, he/she endeavors to maintain a constant and clear mental image of the relevant information and the critical situation in order to avoid all threats.

4.3   Some Data Concerning the Sending of the Patient into Fibrillation

What does the surgical team do when the patient's heart is sent into fibrillation? Of course, the purpose of its actions is to implant the valve as well as possible. At the same time, everyone is aware of the criticality of the task.

Table 2 shows that Operation 2 posed a fibrillation problem as it had to be stopped twice before the valve was inserted. In the other cases, the implantation was performed within a period of 35 to 63 s – a truly critical duration.

Table 2. Extracts of actigram statistics relating to the sending of the patient into fibrillation during four operations.

Characteristics of pacing	Operations			
	1	2	3	4
Number of pacing by operations	1	3	1	1
Number of pacing operations ineffective for implantation	0	2	0	0
Total duration of each pacing	49.61 s	10.6 s + 4.12 s + 36.48 s	10.84 s + 52.84 s	35.39 s
Number of interruptions between pacing operations	0	2	0	0
Requests by the surgeon for acceleration of fibrillation	0	2	1	0
Duration of acceleration	0	11.44 s + 21.76 s	52.84 s	0
Duration of pacing used for implantation	49.61 s	36.48 s	63.68 s	35.39 s

This is a complex task which needs to be performed within a very short time (60 s). Some of its characteristics are those of high-risk situations, e.g. in particular those reviewed in work on human error in dynamic situations [2]. A dynamic situation is characterized by spontaneous development related to actions which momentarily escape the operator's (in this case, the surgeon's) control. It can therefore be said that it under the operator's partial control. Such situations therefore involve uncertainties which need to be reduced during the action.

In particular, the task involves unstructured and non-obvious problems; its aims may change instantaneously and in temporal competition; significant and potentially serious consequences; several actors cooperating with shared representation problems and experience which is both shared and variable as well as swift and imperative mutual adjustments. All these aspects are parameters which contribute (or otherwise) to the fulfillment of the vital requirement. The vital requirement depends on the regulation of the lethal risk by the surgeon. The latter uses a great many variables monitored in many different ways, including the simultaneous evolution of physiological data, palpation, the acquisition of visual information and action according to the circumstances. The valve must be implanted while managing a dynamic environment that comprises technologies, people and a patient. Each time, this environment is unique, and although formed specifically for an operation also changes during the operation, depending on a more or less shared awareness of the situation as well as changes to the situation.

From this point of view, the implantation of a valve is performed within a decision-making framework in which the primary endeavor is the assessment of time constraints and vital constraints, the latter being the determining structures for the modes of operation. Our general hypothesis is therefore that the vital constraints form the basis of a critical task which shapes the surgeon's modes of operation (Table 3).

Table 3. Characteristics of a critical task and related recommendations for the design and organization of critical situations.

Characteristics	Suggested ergonomic recommendations
Deliberate	Announce beginning of critical phase Have an information system concerning the launch of the critical phase
Uniqueness	Practice Supply clear procedures Assign and validate the roles of each participant Ensure redundancy and cross-monitoring Design a guidance system which enables proactive learning
Learning restriction	Supply the surgeon with a tool that increases his/her control and actions Favour systems which are easy to learn
Planning	Enable the team members to improve their ability to forecast and anticipate Concentrate on the various critical components (or critical stages) of the situation Set priorities among the possible actions, help people to understand the order of priority by supplying explanations
Expertise	Guarantee a high level of performance by the surgical team Ensure feedback and enable the team to share the expertise relating to valve implantation Validate the ability of the team members to monitor the performance of other people's tasks
Preparation	Use communication to share and therefore increase the team members' perception and understanding Ensure the accuracy and acceptance of the phases which precede the critical task
Collective	Be aware of the status of a specific event and share it with the others Maintain collective vigilance Increase awareness of the situation to ensure that the teams/assistants know what to expect and if necessary can coordinate and synchronize with each other

(Continued)

Table 3. (*Continued*)

Characteristics	Suggested ergonomic recommendations
	Ensure each team member has an idea of what valve implantation should look like
	Share information monitoring with the others
Hazardous	Do not use inappropriate resources
	Provide "safety nets" to prevent the team members from becoming mired in errors
Rigidity	Understand the operational issues which affect the team, in particular perception during TAVI
	Define stages step by step to validate the understanding of each stage by the entire team
Uncertain outcome	Design a tool which reduces dependence on the uncertainties of the situation
	Be aware of other people

5   Characteristics of the Critical Task

The concept of "critical task" identifies tasks which begin and end within a specific time frame, the performance of which is unique and the potential seriousness extreme. The task is critical as the criticality is deliberately generated by the surgical team. More broadly, a critical task can be described using the following 10 characteristics:

1. Deliberate: The critical task is decided upon deliberately. The risk it generates is not created by an error. The risk is accepted and presented as a prerequisite for success and therefore the patient's life.
2. Uniqueness: The critical task can only be performed once. There can be no second attempt. The critical task is defined by the fact that its performance must be achieved at the first attempt. There can be no false starts. Error generates catastrophe and both the operator and team are aware of the fact. Collective awareness of criticality is a fundamental component of the hazardousness of the work situation.
3. Learning restriction: As there is no opportunity for trial and error, the critical task is characterized by a serious learning constraint.
4. Planning: Critical tasks are subject to serious planning constraints. The goals are organized within a specific time frame and in a specific order. The list of actions to be performed is defined in advance and repeated prior to performance.
5. Expertise: Critical tasks are predicated on general skill and ability requirements. They involve expert skills and are performed by experts. Expertise is obviously a criterion for the quality of the knowledge and excellence of practices; it is also a factor in the social acceptance of risk. The creation of a high-risk situation is better tolerated and accepted when the associated risks are matched with acknowledged expertise.

6. Preparation: A critical task is always preceded by a preparatory task which organizes it so that all that is required for the operation is available in advance. The preparatory task is much longer than the actual critical task.
7. Collective: A critical task is collective, as it can only be successfully completed by an organized group with multiple skills.
8. Hazardous: Critical tasks always involve a high risk level. They are stopped when the perceived risk is high. This applies in particular to Operation 2, during which fibrillation was stopped twice as the physiological indicators were other than expected.
9. Rigidity: Once begun, a critical task allows little room for manoeuvre. The operator's discretionary margin is very small.
10. Uncertain outcome: Critical tasks are preceded by tasks involving the identification of potential weak points, the purpose of which is to reduce uncertainties:
    (a) Uncertainty relating to the dynamics of the patient's condition.
    (b) Uncertainty relating to the actions which can or must be performed.
    (c) Uncertainty concerning the manner in which the actions will be performed by the team (fear of delegating – and the surgeon is obliged to delegate tasks and coordinate them).
    (d) Uncertainty concerning the consequences of each action, its efficiency, accuracy and reliability (viz. search for reliable information and relevant visual information concerning valve positioning). In this case, the uncertainty is related to the low level or lack of predictability of certain data or actions.

The characteristics of a critical task emphasize that the organization and understanding of the development of these various dynamic processes are primordial, as this is required if the patient is to remain alive and healthy. The planning of the actions must be compatible with the successful implantation of the valve and therefore the desired future condition of the patient.

6 Suggestions and Recommendations for the Design of a System Dedicated to the Management of Critical Tasks

To a certain extent, a military operation, an anti-terrorist action or the management of a serious fire are fairly similar to heart-valve operations, in that they are based on critical tasks which deliberately place persons at risk despite the fact that ultimately they are designed to save these persons' lives.

The purpose of this paper was to characterize these tasks according to ten criteria concerning which ergonomic recommendations can also be deduced (Table 3).

The design of this system will enable the relevance of these recommendations to be assessed.

References

1. Albayrak, A., Snijders, C.J.: Basics of Surgery: Tools, Techniques, Attitude and Expertise, pp. 151–169. Maarssen, Elsevier, Gezondheidszorg (2007)
2. Amalberti, R.: La conduite de systèmes à risques, 2nd edn. PUF, Paris (2001)
3. Astarci, P., Glineur, D., Elkhoury, G., Raucent, B.: A novel device for endovascular native aortic valve resection for transapical transcatheter aortic valve implantation. Interact. CardioVasc. Thorac. Surg. **14**, 378–380 (2012)
4. Baron, M., Lucquiaud, V., Autard, D., Scapin, D.L.: K-MADe: un environnement pour le noyau du modèle de description de l'activité. In: Proceedings of the 2006 Conference of the Association Francophone d'Interaction Homme-Machine 2006, pp. 287–288 (2006). http://doi.acm.org/10.1145/1132736.1132786
5. Carayon, P.: Handbook of Human Factors and Ergonomics in Health Care and Patient Safety, 2nd edn, p. 876p. CRC Press, Boca Raton (2011)
6. Carayon, P., Schoofs Hundt, A., Karsh, B.-T., Gurses, A.P., Alvarado, C.J., Smith, M., Flatley Brennan, P.: Work system design for patient safety: the SEIPS model. Q. Saf. Health Care **15**(Suppl 1), 50–58 (2006)
7. De Keyser, V., Nyssen, A.S.: Les erreurs humaines en anesthésie. Le travail humain **56**(2–3), 233–241 (1993)
8. Donabedian, A.: The quality of care. JAMA **260**(12), 17–43 (1988)
9. Flanagan, J.: The critical incident. Psychol. Bull. **51**, 327–358 (1954)
10. Hanna, G.B., Cuschieri, A.: Image display technology and image processing. World J. Surg. **25**, 1419–1427 (2001)
11. Kerguelen, A.: «Actogram Kronos»: Un outil d'aide à l'analyse de l'activité. In: Norimatsu, H., Pigem, N. Les techniques d'observation en sciences humaines, pp. 142–158. Armand Colin (2008)
12. Liang, B., Qi, L., Yang, J., Cao, Z., Zu, X., Liu, L., Wang, L.: Ergonomic status of laparoscopic urologic surgery: survey results from 241 urologic surgeons in China. PLoS ONE **8**(7), e70423 (2013). doi:10.1371/journal.pone.0070423
13. Leplat, J.: De l'étude de cas à l'analyse de l'activité. Pistes **4**(2) (2002)
14. Mitchell, L., Flin, R.: Non-technical skills of the operating theatre nurse: literature review. J. Adv. Nurs. **63**, 15–24 (2008)
15. Van Det, M.J., Meijerink, W.J.H.J., Hoff, C., Totte, E.R., Pierie, J.P.E.N.: Optimal ergonomics for laparoscopic surgery in minimally invasive surgery suites: a review and guidelines. Surg. Endosc. **23**, 1279–1285 (2009). 10.1007/s00464-008-0148-x
16. Weinger, B.W., Wiklund, M.E., Gardner-Bonnerau, D.J.: Handbook of Human Factors in Medical Device Design, p. 844. CRC Press, Boca Raton (2011)
17. Wauben, L.S.G.L., van Veelen, M.A., Gossot, D., Goossens, R.H.M.: Application of ergonomic guidelines during minimally invasive surgery: a questionnaire survey of 284 surgeons. Surg. Endosc. **20**(8), 1268–1274 (2006). doi:10.1007/s00464-005-0647-y
18. Wiklund, M.E., Wilcox, J.: Designing Usability into Medical Device, p. 339. CRC Press, Boca Raton (2005)
19. Yule, S., Flin, R., Paterson-Brown, S., Maran, N.: Non-technical skills for surgeons in the operating room: a review of the literature. Surgery **139**(2), 140–149 (2006). doi:10.1016/j.surg.2005.06.017

Experimental Validation of a New Dynamic Muscle Fatigue Model

Deep Seth, Damien Chablat$^{(\boxtimes)}$, Sophie Sakka, and Fouad Bennis

IRCCyN, Ecole Centrale de Nantes, 1 Rue de la Noë, 44300 Nantes, France
{Deep.Seth,Damien.Chablat,Sophie.Sakka}@irccyn.ec-nantes.fr,
Fouad.Bennis@ec-nantes.fr

Abstract. Muscle fatigue is considered as one of the major risk factor causing Musculo-Skeletal Disorder (MSD). To avoid MSD the study of muscle fatigue is very important. For the study of muscle fatigue a new model is developed by modifying the Ruina Ma's dynamic muscle fatigue model and introducing the muscle co-contraction factor 'n' in this model. The aim of this paper is to experimentally validate a dynamic muscle fatigue model using Electromyography (EMG) and Maximum Voluntary Contraction (MVC) data. The data of ten subjects are used to analyze the muscle activities and muscle fatigue during the extension-flexion (push-pull) motion of the arm on a constant absolute value of the external load. The findings for co-contraction factor shows that the fatigue increases when co-contraction area decreases. The dynamic muscle fatigue model is validated using the MVC data, fatigue rate and co-contraction factor of the subjects.

Keywords: Muscle fatigue · Maximum Voluntary Contraction (MVC) · Muscle fatigue model · Co-contraction · Fatigue rate · Electromyography (EMG)

1 Introduction

In the field of industrial bio-mechanics, muscle fatigue is defined as "any reduction in the maximal capacity to generate the force and power output". In industries, mostly repetitive manual tasks leads to work related Musculo-Skeletal Disorder (MSD) problems [1,2]. Some times people have to work more on the same repetitive task which can be painful and leads to MSD due to muscle fatigue. MSD can cause pain [1,3,4] or temporary dysfunction of the affected muscles [5,6]. Muscle fatigue and uncomfortable working postures can cause drop in the productivity of human. To improve the performance and production, improvement in the work environment and ergonomics with the study of muscle fatigue are necessary that can reduce the chances of MSD [4].

Various static and dynamic muscle fatigue models are proposed earlier to study muscle fatigue [7–12]. Liang's fatigue model [9] have experiment validation for fatigue and effect of recovery in arm with static drilling posture.

© Springer International Publishing Switzerland 2016
V.G. Duffy (Ed.): DHM 2016, LNCS 9745, pp. 54–65, 2016.
DOI: 10.1007/978-3-319-40247-5_6

Silva [13] simulate the hill model and validate it using opensim. Some Dynamic fatigue models are also introduced [14–16]. A Dynamic Muscle Fatigue Model [17] has been proposed to describe the fatigue process of muscle groups. However, no consideration about the co-contraction of paired muscles is taken. Missenard [18] explains the effect of fatigue and co-contraction on the accuracy of arms motion.

The main objective of this study is to revise this dynamic muscle fatigue model by including the factor of co-contraction of paired muscles, as well as to validate it through mathematics and experiments. In this article, we are focusing on the study of muscle activity with co-contraction, using elbow joint's muscle groups as target. With the assistance of EMG, the function of co-contraction is confirmed and calculated. Using the MVC data calculated during the fatigue test experiments, we have validated the muscle fatigue model.

2   Dynamic Muscle Fatigue Model

The dynamic muscle fatigue model is applicable on the dynamic motion of the human body parts. The motions like push/pull operations of the arm, walking, pronation, supination etc. are examples of dynamic motion. A dynamic muscle fatigue model is proposed by Liang Ma [9,19] firstly applied on static drilling task. Ruina Ma [16,17] developed this model for the dynamic motions like push/pull operation of the arm. The Ruina Ma's model can be described by the Eqs. 1 and 2. However, the co-contraction of the muscles are not included in both the models.

$$\frac{d\Gamma_{cem}(t)}{dt} = -k\frac{\Gamma_{cem}}{\Gamma_{MVC}}\Gamma_{joint}(t) \tag{1}$$

and, if Γ_{Joint} and Γ_{MVC} held constant, the model can then simplify as follows:

$$\Gamma_{cem}(t) = \Gamma_{MVC}.e^{-k_{torque}Ct}, \quad \text{where} \ \ C = \frac{\Gamma_{Joint}}{\Gamma_{MVC}} \tag{2}$$

The parameters for this model is expressed in the Table 1

Table 1. Parameters of Ruina Ma's dynamic muscle fatigue model

Elements	Unit	Description
k	min^{-1}	Fatigue factor, constant
Γ_{MVC}	N.m	Maximum torque on joint
Γ_{Joint}	N.m	Torque from external load
Γ_{cem}	N.m	Current capacity of the muscle

2.1   Hypothesis for New Dynamic Muscle Fatigue Model

Muscle fatigue is directly proportional to the torque applied at the human joint. It is also inversely proportional to the maximum capacity (without fatigue) of muscle to generate a torque Γ_{MVC} (Maximum MVC). According to this model, the evolution of Γ_{cem} (Current capacity of the muscle) can be represented by a linear differential equation of the first order.

As we know, there are two major muscle groups for each joint motion, agonist and antagonist. For push motion, a muscle motivates the motion while antagonist muscle makes the motion accurate and stable. If the motion is reversed, i.e., pull cycles, agonist and antagonist muscles switch their roles. Co-operation of the two muscles is called co-contraction.

2.2 Proposed Dynamic Model of Muscular Fatigue

In dynamic muscle fatigue model [20], we select two parameters Γ_{joint} and Γ_{MVC} to build our muscle fatigue model. The hypotheses can then be incorporated into a mathematical model of muscle fatigue which is expressed as follows:

$$\frac{d\Gamma_{cem}(t)}{dt} = -k.n.\frac{\Gamma_{cem}}{\Gamma_{MVC}}\Gamma_{joint}(t) \tag{3}$$

where, k is the fatigue factor and n is the co-contraction factor.

And, if Γ_{Joint} and Γ_{MVC} held constant, the model can then simplify as follows:

$$\Gamma_{cem}(t) = \Gamma_{MVC}.e^{-k.n.Ct}, \quad \text{where} \quad C = \frac{\Gamma_{Joint}}{\Gamma_{MVC}} \tag{4}$$

$$k = \frac{-1}{n.Ct}.\ln\left(\frac{\Gamma_{cem}(t)}{\Gamma_{MVC}}\right) \tag{5}$$

The other parameters for this model are the same as in Table 1. We define n as the co-contraction factor.

2.3 Co-contraction Factor 'n'

The co-contraction is the simultaneous contraction of both the agonist and antagonist muscle around a joint to hold a stable position at a time. Assumptions made for finding co-contraction factor are as follows:

1. The co-contraction is the common intersecting area between the two groups of acting muscles.
2. The co-contraction factor will be the same for each agonist and antagonist activities.

The co-contraction area can be understand by the Fig. 1. This figure is just an example representation of a motion cycle. In this figure, we can introduce the common EMG activity between bicep and tricep muscle groups shown by the orange color, which is co-contraction area C_A. The formula for calculating the co-contraction area from EMG activities is given in Eq. 6. The trapezius activity shown along with the two muscles is co-activation.

$$C_A = \frac{\int_{t_0}^{t_{100}} EMG_{min} \times dt}{\int_{t_0}^{t_{100}} [EMG_{agonist} + EMG_{antagonist}] \times dt} \tag{6}$$

where, EMG_{min} is the common area share by the EMG activity of bicep and tricep, $EMG_{agonist}$ and $EMG_{antagonist}$ are the full activities of the bicep and triceps muscle's. The activities of the both the muscles are normalized with respect to the normalization value of the activities for the same muscle which can be calculated using the Eq. 10, it is because the absolute value of the external torque is same for push/pull operation.

The co-contraction area C_A can also be represented as follows:

C_A = common activities between the two muscle groups.

$$C_A = a.\exp b.x \qquad (7)$$

where, a and b are constant parameters and x is the time of the test.

In our model, the co-contraction factor represents the main activities of muscle in each dynamic cycle excludes the co-contraction area of the same cycle. So we can represent co-contraction factor n as follows.

$$n = 1 + C_A \qquad (8)$$

$$n = 1 + a.\exp b.x \qquad (9)$$

2.4   Push-Pull Operation and Muscles Activities

The push/pull motion of the arm is the flexion and extension of the arm about the elbow. The plane of the motion is vertical plane. The Push/pull activities with the muscle activation is shown in Fig. 3. In Ma's model there were no part of co-contraction and delay in the model which we have added in this new model.

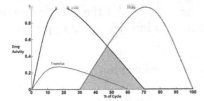 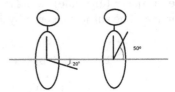

Fig. 1. A representative plot of EMG activity of bicep, triceps and trapezius normalized with the maximum value of each muscle's activity for one cycle (Color figure online)

Fig. 2. Arm movement range while flexion and extension in vertical plane

3   Methodology: Experiment and Data Processing

3.1   Experiment Protocol

1. The repetitive arm's flexion-extension in a vertical plane as shown in Fig. 2.
2. The motion range is seventy degrees. The test protocol repetition continues till exhaustion.
3. Each cycle (flexion + extension) should be completed within 3 seconds.
4. External load was 20 % of MVC. MVC was calculated every one min.

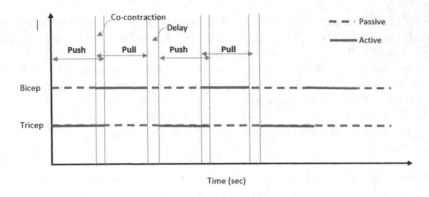

Fig. 3. Push/pull motion and muscles activities

3.2 Data Acquisition

A Biodex system 3 research (Biodex medical,shirley, NY) isokinetic dynamometer was used to measure the value of elbow angle, velocity and torque. The Electromyographic sensor electrodes were put on Biceps, Tricep and Trapezius muscles to record their electrical activities. The frequency of data acquisition was set at 2000 Hz so that most of the activities get recorded.

3.3 Subjects Description

The subjects (all male) details are given in the Table 2. All the subjects were sportive. The subjects were physically fit and had no injuries in the upper limb.

Table 2. Subjects anthropometric data and description

Subject	Age	Weight	Height	Upper arm	Forearm	Sports
1	28	89 kg	185 cm	29 cm	26.5 cm	Running
2	24	80.2 kg	183.5 cm	31.5 cm	28 cm	Musculation
3	20	69.8 kg	180.1 cm	30 cm	29.5 cm	Handball
4	20	80.9 kg	177 cm	29.8 cm	29 cm	Handball
5	21	62.2 kg	172.8 cm	29.2 cm	26.5 cm	Tennis
6	25	61.1 kg	164.8 cm	26 cm	24.5 cm	Rugby
7	26	74 kg	176 cm	28.5 cm	27 cm	Tennis
8	27	66 kg	181 cm	29.5 cm	26.5 cm	wall climb
9	23	66.3 kg	164 cm	27 cm	25.5 cm	Swimming
10	26	85 kg	184 cm	29 cm	26.5 cm	Football

3.4   Data Processing and Analysis

All the raw data were processed using standardized MATLAB program. Data
processing includes noise filtering from raw EMG data with the filter frequency
10 Hz for low pass filter and 400 Hz for high pass filter and normalization of the
data. The total number of cycles compared for all the ten subjects are 1998 cycles.
All the cycles are normalized on time scale and compared. The cycle selection
for flexion and extension phases is done according to the velocity change in each
cycle. The collective EMG plots for Biceps, Triceps and Trapezius muscle are
show in Fig. 4a and b for all the ten subjects and the collective comparison for
the mechanical data position, velocity and torque is shown in Fig. 5b and a for
all the ten subjects.

For Figs. 4a, b and 5a and b representations are as follows:
___ Blue color curve show mean EMG activity.
I Red bar plot on blue curve shows the standard deviation of all the EMG
activities along the mean.
− Black dotted curves shows the maximum and minimum reach from the EMG
activities. All the cycles are normalized according to the equation:

$$value_{Normalization} = value_{std}{}^{max} + 2\sigma \qquad (10)$$

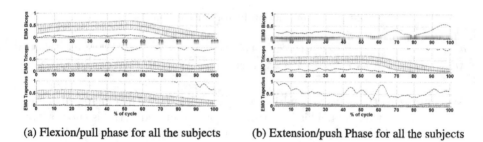

(a) Flexion/pull phase for all the subjects   (b) Extension/push Phase for all the subjects

Fig. 4. Mean and standard deviation plots for EMG data of bicep, triceps and
Trapezius

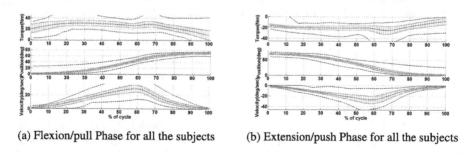

(a) Flexion/pull Phase for all the subjects   (b) Extension/push Phase for all the subjects

Fig. 5. Mean and standard deviation plots for velocity, position and torque

- $value_{Normalization}$: Normalization value for the EMG data.
- $value_{std}^{max}$: Maximum value of standard deviation along the mean.
- 2σ : σ values addition upto 2σ

4   Results and Discussion

The raw data obtained after the fatigue test is processed and the results and observations are discussed in this section. After processing the EMG data of all the muscle groups from Figs. 4 and 5 we can observe that when the biceps are active during flexion phase there are always some activities from the triceps and on the other hand when triceps are active during pull phase the biceps are almost passive or activities are very near to zero. We can also observe the co-activation of trapezius muscle with the activation of biceps. The activation of triceps with the biceps is co-contraction between two muscles during flexion phase.

The co-contraction area calculated by using Eq. 6 is fitted with the exponential Eq. 7 in Sect. 2.3. The Fig. 6 shows the fitted graphs for the co-contraction percentage for test cycles of all ten subjects. In Fig. 6 blue dots show the percentage area of contraction during each extension-flexion cycle and red curve shows the exponential fit for the percentage co-contraction. This shows that the co-contraction percentage for activity between the muscles reduces as the fatigue test proceed or the muscles gets fatigued. By the Eqs. 6 and 3 we can find n_i as shown in Table 3, where i is the subject number:

Table 3. Co-contraction factor for each subject

n_i	n_1	n_2	n_3	n_4	n_5	n_6	n_7	n_8	n_9	n_{10}
Mean co-contraction factor	1.4	1.45	1.33	1.4	1.41	1.35	1.36	1.26	1.5	1.3

We can notice that only the subject number 8 in Fig. 6h has increasing slope for the co-contraction area. This behavior can be associated with his sport activity which is wall climbing and very different from other subjects as shown in Table 2.

The co-activation of the trapezius muscle is observed mostly in the flexion phase. The MVC values are measured between each protocol of one minute. In Fig. 7 blue line shows the MVC measured for flexion and extension after each test protocol of 1 min. We can see in most of the cases MVC decreases as fatigue increases. The MVC is same as Γ_{cem} used in our model. The theoretical and experimental evolution of Γ_{cem} is on the basis of k (fatigue rate) using Eq. 4 and calculated n_i and $C = 0.2$. The evaluation of fatigue parameter 'k' for Γ_{cem} extension is shown in Fig. 7a, c, e, g, i, k, m, o, q and s. Similarly fatigue parameter 'k' evaluation for Γ_{cem} flexion is shown in Fig. 7b, d, f, h, j, l, n, p, r and t. The theoretical and experimental evolution of Γ_{cem} shows that the experimental values are well fit with in the theoretical model. The co-contraction factor have significant effect on the model. The fatigue rate increases with the input of co-contraction factor. The minimum, maximum and average value of 'k' for each subject are shown in Table 4.

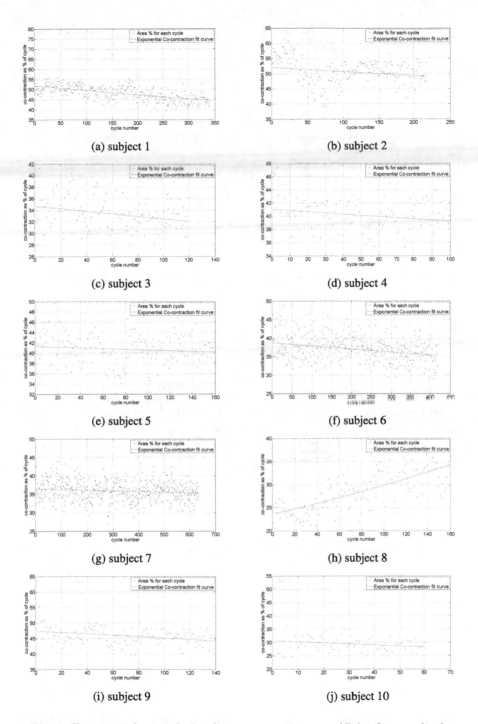

Fig. 6. Exponential curve fit for the co-contraction area (Color figure online)

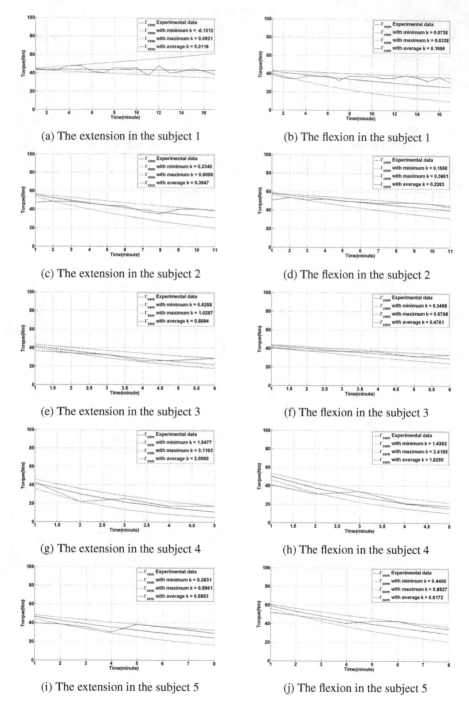

(a) The extension in the subject 1

(b) The flexion in the subject 1

(c) The extension in the subject 2

(d) The flexion in the subject 2

(e) The extension in the subject 3

(f) The flexion in the subject 3

(g) The extension in the subject 4

(h) The flexion in the subject 4

(i) The extension in the subject 5

(j) The flexion in the subject 5

Fig. 7. Theoretical evolution of Γ_{cem} and experimental data using different values of k (Color figure online)

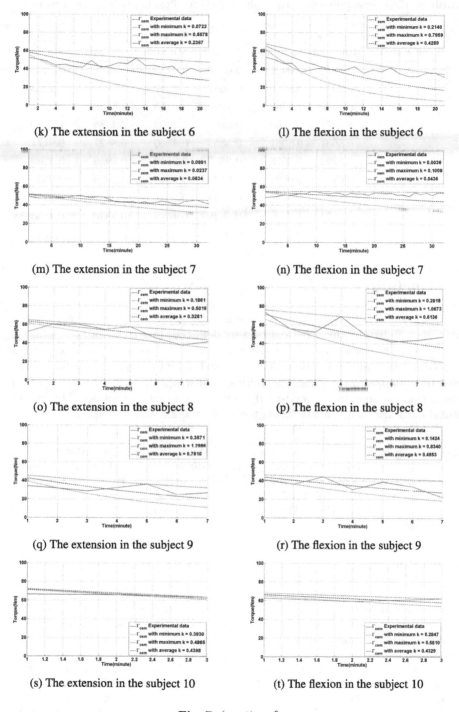

(k) The extension in the subject 6

(l) The flexion in the subject 6

(m) The extension in the subject 7

(n) The flexion in the subject 7

(o) The extension in the subject 8

(p) The flexion in the subject 8

(q) The extension in the subject 9

(r) The flexion in the subject 9

(s) The extension in the subject 10

(t) The flexion in the subject 10

Fig. 7. (*continued*)

Table 4. Experimentally calculated values of 'k' for flexion and extension motion

Subject number	$k_{extension}$			$k_{flexion}$		
	Minimum	Maximum	Average	Minimum	Maximum	Average
1	−0.1212	0.0921	0.0116	0.0738	0.5338	0.1995
2	0.2345	0.6085	0.3647	0.1558	0.3661	0.2263
3	0.5258	1.0287	0.8084	0.3498	0.6798	0.4761
4	1.5477	3.1993	2.0990	1.4302	2.4185	1.8250
5	0.3631	0.8961	0.5853	0.4400	0.8827	0.6172
6	0.0722	0.5578	0.2367	0.2140	0.7959	0.4289
7	0.0237	0.0991	0.0634	0.0036	0.1009	0.0436
8	0.1861	0.5061	0.3281	0.2018	1.0673	0.6136
9	0.3571	1.2996	0.7610	0.1424	0.8340	0.4853
10	0.3930	0.4865	0.4398	0.2847	0.5810	0.4329

5   Conclusions

The proposed model for dynamic muscle fatigue includes the co-contraction parameter, unlike in any other existing model according to the author's knowledge. The results and analysis of the experimental data validates the most of the assumptions made for the proposed model. EMG analysis along with MVC helps to understand the muscle activities, it justifies the significance of the co-contraction parameter in proposed dynamic muscle fatigue model. The experimental data also helps in validating the new dynamic muscle fatigue model.

Acknowledgments. The project is funded by the European Commission under the 'Erasmus Mundus Heritage Program', jointly coordinated by Ecole Centrale de Nantes, France and Indian institute of Technology Madras, India. The Experiments was performed in STAPS, University of Nantes, France. We are also thankful to Antoine Nordez and Marc Jubeau from UFR STAPS, France for assistance in preparing and conducting the experiments.

References

1. Nur, N.M., Md Dawal, S.Z., Dahari, M.: The prevelence of work related muscu-loscleletal disorders among workers performing industrial repetitive tasks in the automotive manufacturing companies. In: Proceedings of the 2014 International Conference on Inductrial Engineering and Operations Management, Bali, Indonesia (2014)
2. Punnett, L., Wegman, D.H.: Work related musculoskeletal disorders: the epidemiologic evidence and the debate. J. Electromyogr. Kinesiol. **14**, 13–23 (2004)
3. Huppe, A., Muller, K., Raspe, H.: Is the occurrence of back pain in germany decreasing? two regional postal surveys a decade apart. Eur. J. Public Health **17**, 318–322 (2006)

4. Lawrence, R.C., Helmick, C.G., Arnett, F.C., Deyo, R.A., Felson, D.T., Giannini, E.H., Heyse, S.P., Hirsch, R., Hochberg, M.C., Hunder, G.C., Liang, M.H., Pillemer, S.R., Steen, V.D., Wolfe, F.: Estimates of the prevalence of arthritis and selected musculoskeletal disorders in the united states. Arthritis Rheum. **41**(5), 778–799 (1998)
5. World Health Organization: Preventing musculoskeletal disorders in the workplace. Protecting workers 'Health series; no. 5', Geneva 27, Switzeland, 2003. ISBN 92 4 159053 X
6. Chaffin, D.B., Andersson, G.B.J., Martin, B.J.: Occupational Biomechanics, 3rd edn. Wiley-Interscience, New York (1999)
7. Ding, J., Wexler, A.S., Binder-Macleod, S.A.: Mathematical models for fatigue minimization during functional electrical simulation. J. Electromyogr. Kinesiol. **13**, 575–588 (2003)
8. Hill, A.V.: The heat of shortening and dynamic constant of muscle. Proc. R. Soc. Lond. B **126**, 136 195 (1930)
9. Ma, L., Chablat, D., Bennis, F., Zhang, W.: A new muscle fatigue and recovery model and its ergonomics application in human simulation. Virtual Phys. Prototyp. **5**, 123–137 (2008)
10. Galiamova, E.V., Syuzev, V.V., Gouskov, A.M.: Human skeletal muscle - mechanical and mathematical models. In: ICABB-2010, Venice, Italy (2010)
11. Vollestad, N.K.: Measurement of human muscle fatigue. J. Neurosci. Meth. **74**, 219–227 (1997)
12. Xia, T., Law, L.A.F.: A theoretical approach for modeling peripheral muscle fatigue and recovery. J. Biomech. **41**(14), 3046–3052 (2008)
13. Martins, J.M., Silva, M.T., Pereira, A.F.: An efficient muscle fatigue model for forward and inverse dynamic analysis of human movements. Procedia IUTAM **2**, 262–274 (2011)
14. Freund, J., Takala, E.-P.: A dynamic model of the forearm including fatigue. J. Biomech. **34**, 597–605 (2001)
15. Liu, J.Z., Brown, R.W., Yue, G.H.: A dynamical model of muscle activation, fatigue and recovery. Biophys. J. **82**, 2344–2359 (2002)
16. Ma, R., Chablat, D., Bennis, F.: Human muscle fatigue model in dynamic motions. In: Lenarcic, J., Husty, M. (eds.) Latest Advances in Robot Kinematics, pp. 349–356. Springer, Netherlands (2012)
17. Ma, R., Chablat, D., Bennis, F., Ma, L.: A framework of motion capture system based human behaviours simulation for ergonomic analysis. In: Stephanidis, C. (ed.) Posters, Part II, HCII 2011. CCIS, vol. 174, pp. 360–364. Springer, Heidelberg (2011)
18. Missenard, O., Mottet, D., Perrey, S.: Muscular fatigue increases signal-dependent noise during isometric force production. Neurosci. Lett. **437**, 154–157 (2008)
19. Ma, L., Chablat, D., Bennis, F., Zhang, W.: A new simple dynamic muscle fatigue model and its validation. Int. J. Ind. Ergonomics **39**(1), 211–220 (2009)
20. Ma, R., Chablat, D., Bennis, F.: A new approach to muscle fatigue evaluation for push/pull task. In: 19th CISM-IFToMM Symposium on Robot Design, Dynamics, and Control, Paris, France, pp. 1–8 (2012)

Experimental Study on Discrimination Thresholds for Haptic Perception of Size in Manual Operation

Ai-ping Yang[1], Guang Cheng[1], Wen-yu Fu[1], Hui-min Hu[2(✉)],
Xin Zhang[2], and Chau-Kuang Chen[3]

[1] Department of Industrial Engineering,
Beijing Union University, Beijing, China
[2] Ergonomics Laboratory, China National Institute of Standardization,
Beijing, China
huhm@cnis.gov.cn
[3] School of Graduate Studies and Research, Meharry Medical College,
Nashville, TN, USA

Abstract. Objective: This experimental study was designed to measure discrimination thresholds for haptic perception of size in manual operation. Methods: Common manual operation modes with finger pressing or pulling, three finger pinch or grip, and hand grip were used in this study. Taking the index finger pressing operation as an example, the distal phalanx finger length and the width of the index finger were measured in order to determine the size range of sample buttons. The assessment procedure along with the measurement data sheet of index finger regarding pressing operation was designed. Study subjects were recruited and discrimination thresholds for the size haptic perception of the index finger were measured and analyzed.

Results: The press operation assessment of index finger was performed on one-hundred subjects. By statistical analysis of valid data, the index finger size discrimination threshold of 1–2.5 mm was obtained. The discrimination threshold (2–2.5 mm) of male subjects was somewhat greater than that (1.5–2 mm) of female subjects. The size discrimination threshold in the elderly population was slightly larger than the young group.

Conclusion: The study results can provide basic data for the selection of sample size step of manual devices, thereby serving as the cornerstone of the effectiveness and accuracy in ergonomic design and assessment.

Keywords: Discrimination threshold · Size · Index finger pressing · Ergonomic design and assessment

1 Introduction

A lot of scholars have carried out the research on the haptic discrimination, which mainly includes the following: bimanual curvature discrimination of hand-sized surfaces [1], curvature affecting haptic length perception [2], haptic discrimination of

© Springer International Publishing Switzerland 2016
V.G. Duffy (Ed.): DHM 2016, LNCS 9745, pp. 66–72, 2016.
DOI: 10.1007/978-3-319-40247-5_7

bilateral symmetry in 2-dimensional and 3-dimensional unfamiliar displays [3], haptic curvature discrimination [4], haptic distal spatial perception mediated by strings [5], haptic perception of parallelity in the midsagittal plane [6], geographical slant perception [7], perception size and touch input behavior [8], peripheral neuropathy and object length perception by effortful (dynamic) touch [9], haptic two-dimensional angle categorization and discrimination [10], This study was designed to measure discrimination thresholds for haptic perception of size in manual operation.

During the study of human-machine adaptation for manual appliance, sample test or experimental method for simulating task scenario can be often used. The design of sample size step is usually given on the basis of experience while the number of samples is reduced by the limitation of the project cycle and research funding. Thus, the selection of sample step size will be adjusted and the validity and accuracy of the results can be eventually affected. The reasonable selection of sample size is the basis of ergonomics assessment research. Determining the step value of sample size based on discrimination thresholds is a necessary step in the assessment of ergonomics. Therefore, using the index finger pressing operation as an example, discrimination thresholds for haptic perception of size in the manual operation was performed to provide basic data for the evaluation of human-machine adaptation of manual appliance.

The main contents of this study were as follows:

1. The length and width of distal phalanx finger of the right index finger were measured;
2. Combined with the button size range and pressing force of manual ergonomics standards, the size range of the test buttons were determined; the button assembly was also developed and adjusted to the same displacement and the same pressing force; and
3. One-hundred healthy and non-dyskinesia subjects were recruited, and discrimination thresholds for size haptic perception concerning the right index finger was assessed, which resulted in a threshold value of 1–2.5 mm. The size discrimination threshold of the index finger was affected by gender and age. The size discrimination threshold of male subjects was mostly 2–2.5 mm, compared to the female size discrimination threshold of 1.5–2 mm. The size discrimination threshold in the elderly population was slightly larger than the younger group.

2 Experiment of Forefinger Discrimination Threshold for Size

The size range of button samples was determined based on the hand size and related standards of manual operation ergonomics. The button assembly was designed and manufactured; the test bench was built; the testing process and data record sheets were designed; study subjects were recruited; and assessment procedure was performed. By statistical analysis of valid data, the discrimination threshold of the right index finger for size was obtained. Specific contents were as follows:

2.1 Size Range of Button Samples

The main factors affecting the operation of the index finger pressing operation included: the abdominal width and length of the distal end of the index finger, shape and size of button, installation position, material for button, etc. In this study, samples were made of nylon material. A more common round button shape was selected although the shapes generally were either round, square, or rectangular. Pressing operation was usually divided into certain categories regarding the index finger, thumb, and palm. In this study, the index finger pressing action was used. Throughout the experiment, the width and length of the distal end of the index finger of 30 adult men and women were measured and analyzed. Referring to the dimension range of the circular button in the related ergonomics standards, the circular button sample size range was determined as 6–12 mm, and the step sizes were 0.5 and 1 mm.

2.2 Experiment Scheme

(1) Assembly and Development of Button Sample.

The circular pressing head of button samples were produced, and the ranges of the diameter were 6–12 mm. Specific diameters included: 6 mm, 7 mm, 7.5 mm, 8 mm, 9.5 mm, 10 mm, 9 mm, 9.5 mm, 10 mm, 11 mm, and 12 mm. The finished products are shown in Fig. 1.

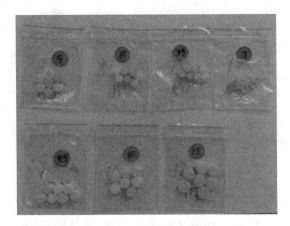

Fig. 1. Button head samples

The press body assembly consisted of press head, supporting rod, fixing sleeve, spring, pre tightening sleeve, shell, nut and adjusting rod as shown in Fig. 2. The three regulation functions of this mechanism were the pressing force adjustment, the pressing displacement adjustment, and the replacement function of pressing head.

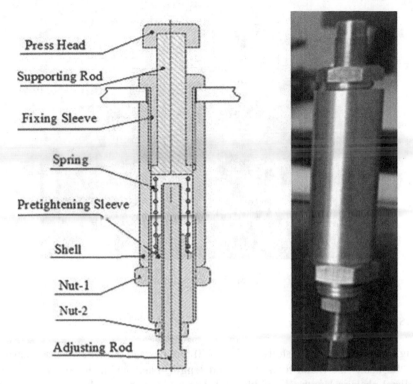

Fig. 2. The button body assembly (the left shows the design chart, the right shows the button sample)

(2) Test procedure and specification.

In a comfortable standing position, the subjects pushed the button at a normal rate with the right hand index finger. (Note: The distance between the subjects and the test bench was adjusted by the subjects themselves with the experiment table height taken below 5 cm of the standing elbow height of the people in the 50th percentile). The subjects made judgments about the diameter of the circular button head, which were either the same or different.

Thus, all data were recorded in the corresponding table featuring the three symbols as follows:

1. The tick symbol √, which showed the subject accurately distinguishing the size;
2. X symbol, which displayed subjects incapable of distinguishing the size or error; and
3. ? Symbol, which indicated subject being in the middle of the other two symbols, which was equivalent to the fuzzy perception. Test scenarios were shown in Fig. 3.

The experimental specification consisted of three points:

4. The subject's eyes needed to be occluded when the test was performed;
5. The step size was determined randomly when the test was performed;
6. Each test should be repeated two times to eliminate the process error.

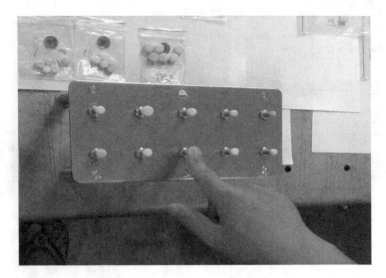

Fig. 3. Testscenarios

3 Results

The height and weight of the study subjects (50 females and 50 males) were measured, so was the hand size (hand thickness, hand length, hand width, index finger length, finger distal phalanx length and width). All data were used to analyze the relationship between hand discrimination threshold for size and related anthropometric dimensions.

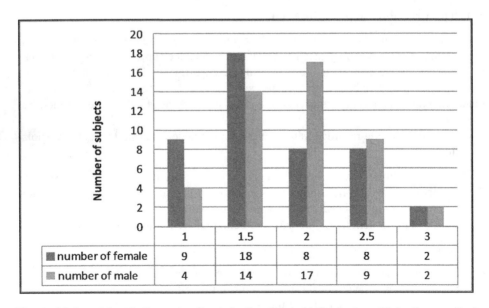

Fig. 4. Male and female finger size discrimination threshold distributions (Color figure online)

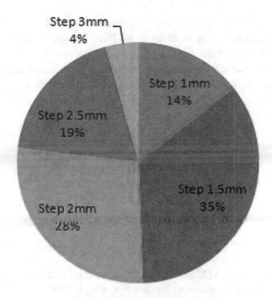

Fig. 5. The proportional distribution of various sensing steps of the index finger

Of the one-hundred subjects used in this study, 91 (46 males and 45 females) provided the most valid data (as shown in Figs. 4 and 5). The size discrimination threshold of the right hand index finger was about 1–2.5 mm, about 96 % of the total subjects chose this range, and the number of people who selected 1.5–2 mm was about 63 %.

For male subjects, 17 selected the maximum of 2 mm as step size, and 14 picked 1.5 mm (67.4 %). For female subjects, 18 adopted the maximum steps size of 1.5 mm while 9 chose 1 mm and 8 selected 2 mm. Overall, 78 % of the female subjects selected 1–2 mm as a step size.

4 Conclusions

(1) The experimental study was conducted to measure discrimination thresholds for haptic perception of size in manual operation. The press operation assessment of index finger was performed on one-hundred subjects. Forty percent (40 %) of the female subjects chose a maximum of 1.5 mm as a step size while 37 % of the male subjects selected a maximum of 2 mm as a step size. The size discrimination threshold values of female group regarding the right hand index finger were slightly lower than those of male group, indicating that females were more sensitive to touch than males.

(2) As indicated in the assessment results, the number of people who chose 3 mm as a step size was only 4 % of the total number of study subjects, indicating that the size discrimination threshold value of index finger size category was less than 3 mm for ordinary people.

(3) The weakness of this study included a low sample size in which only 27 % were an older age. Because of the sensitivity of the young man and the small size of their hands, the study results regarding the size discrimination threshold might be smaller. However, the size discrimination threshold value might be slightly larger when used in practice. Therefore, the increment of the number of study subjects was highly recommended in order to obtain more accurate results of the index finger discrimination threshold for size.

Acknowledgment. This research was supported by the National Key Technology R&D Program (2014BAK01B02, 2014BAK01B04, and 2014BAK01B05), 2015 Beijing Municipal Education Commission Research Project (12213991508101/008).

References

1. Sanders, A.F.J., Kappers, A.M.L.: Bimanual curvature discrimination of hand-sized surfaces placed at different positions. Percept. Psychophys. **68**(7), 1094–1106 (2006)
2. Sanders, A.F.J., Kappers, A.M.L.: Curvature affects haptic length perception. Acta Psychol. **129**, 340–351 (2008)
3. Ballesteros, S., Manga, D., Reales, J.M.: Haptic discrimination of bilateral symmetry in 2-dimensional and 3-dimensional unfamiliar displays. Percept. Psychophys. **59**(l), 37–50 (1997)
4. Pont, S., Kappers, A.M.L., Koenderink, J.J.: Haptic curvature discrimination at several regions of the hand. Percept. Psychophys. **59**(8), 1225–1240 (1997)
5. Cabe, P.A.: Haptic distal spatial perception mediated by strings: size at a distance and egocentric localization based on ellipse geometry. Atten. Percept. Psychophys. **75**, 358–374 (2013)
6. Kappers, A.M.L.: Haptic perception of parallelity in the midsagittal plane. Acta Psychol. **109**, 25–40 (2002)
7. Durgin, F.H., Hajnal, A., Li, Z., Tonge, N., Stigliani, A.: Palm boards are not action measures: an alternative to the two-systems theory of geographical slant perception. Acta Psychol. **134**, 182–197 (2010)
8. Jung, E.S., Im, Y.: Touchable area: an empirical study on design approach considering perception size and touch input behavior. Int. J. Ind. Ergon. **49**, 21–30 (2015)
9. Carello, C., Kinsella-Shaw, J., Amazeen, E.L., Turvey, M.T.: Peripheral neuropathy and object length perception by effortful (dynamic) touch: a case study. Neurosci. Lett. **405**, 159–163 (2006)
10. Toderita, I., Bourgeon, S., Voisin, J.I.A., Chapman, C.E.: Haptic two-dimensional angle categorization and discrimination. Exp. Brain Res. **232**, 369–383 (2014)

Physiology and Anatomy Models

Automatic Below-Knee Prosthesis Socket Design:
A Preliminary Approach

Giorgio Colombo[1], Giancarlo Facoetti[2(✉)], and Caterina Rizzi[3]

[1] Department of Mechanical Engineering, Polytechnic of Milan, Milan, Italy
giorgio.colombo@polimi.it
[2] BigFlo s.r.l. (BG), Dalmine, Italy
giancarlo.facoetti@bigflo.it
[3] Department of Management, Information and Production Engineering,
University of Bergamo (BG), Dalmine, Italy
caterina.rizzi@unibg.it

Abstract. In this work we present a preliminary study on a system able to design automatically sockets for lower-limb prosthesis. The socket is the most important part of the whole prosthesis and requires a custom design specific for the patient's characteristics and her/his residuum morphology. The system takes in input the weight and the lifestyle of the patient, the tonicity level and the geometry file of the residuum, and creates a new model applying the correct geometric deformations needed to create a functional socket. In fact, in order to provide the right fit and prevent pain, we need to create on the socket load and off-load zones in correspondence of the critical anatomical areas. To identify the position of such critical areas, several neural networks have been trained using a dataset generated from real residuum models.

Keywords: Lower limb prosthesis · Neural network · Prosthetic socket · CAD

1 Introduction

The most important part of a lower-limb prostheses is the socket. The socket is the component that links the patient's residual limb to the whole prosthesis. A correct socket geometry is fundamental to provide the right comfort and mobility level to the patient. Thus, particular care is necessary during the design of this component since it, requires a custom design; in fact, the socket has to be realized starting from the specific patient's anatomy.

The socket should fit the patient's residuum and create load and off-load zones. Load zones are required to provide the right pressure and stability during daily activities, while off-load zones are needed on specific anatomical areas, in order to prevent pain [1]. Figure 1 shows the correct load and off-load zones on a below-knee residuum. As we can see in the Fig. 1, we need to lower the pressure on the crest and the terminal of the tibia, on the head of the fibula and on the lateral femoral condyle, while we need to apply a certain pressure on the areas marked in green that usually depends on the residuum tonicity [3].

Furthermore, in order to create the right fit between the residuum and the socket, the socket has to be smaller than the residuum. This size difference depends on the patient's weight and lifestyle.

© Springer International Publishing Switzerland 2016
V.G. Duffy (Ed.): DHM 2016, LNCS 9745, pp. 75–81, 2016.
DOI: 10.1007/978-3-319-40247-5_8

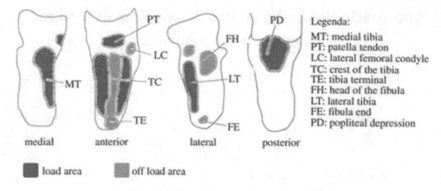

Fig. 1. Anatomical zones of below knee residuum

The traditional prosthesis design process is mostly hand-made, through a set of positive and negative plaster casts, and strongly depends on the technician's skills and experience, following a trial and error approach.

To improve the whole process, in previous works we proposed a new design framework [1] where is possible to design and validate lower limb prosthesis, below and above-knee both, in a virtual environment, with a set of CAD-CAE tools that permit to replicate all the traditional design steps. The new framework focuses on the patient characteristics and guides the orthopedic technician through a semi-automatic workflow that embeds domain knowledge and design rules. Furthermore, the system uses FEM analysis and virtual humans simulation to validate the generated models.

2   Automatic Socket Creation

In this work, we focused the attention on the automation of the socket geometry design to make this important phase a predictable and repeatable process. We are developing a system that takes in input some patient's characteristics and his/her residuum geometry, and automatically generates a socket applying the correct geometric operations. The workflow of the procedure is based on the following steps (Fig. 2):

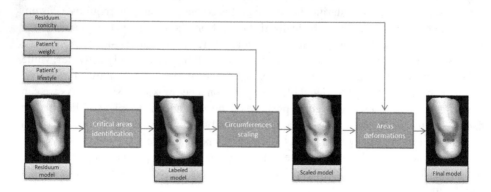

Fig. 2. Workflow of the system

- Identification of the critical anatomic areas;
- Circumference scaling;
- Application of the correct deformation on the critical anatomic areas.

The size of the circumference scaling and the depth of the deformations are determined by the residuum tonicity and by patient's weight and life style. In particular:

1. **Patient's residuum tonicity** that is divided in 4 qualitative levels. In the traditional socket manufacturing process, this value is used to size the depth of the deformations on the load and off-load zones. The more the deformation is depth, the more the pressure will be high. Deformations are also created on the off-load zones, in order to lower the pressure in such areas. Table 1 shows the relation between tonicity level and the deformations depth required.

Table 1. Tonicity - deformation depth relations

Tonicity	Deformation depth [mm]
Low	1–2
Normal	3–4
Good	5–6
Very good	7–8

2. **Patient's weight and life-style.** These two parameters determine the size of circumference scaling, which usually spans from 1 % to 6 %. The scaling is not uniform, but starts with 1 % at 4 cm over the residuum top, and it increases gradually going up to the residuum upper part. Patient life-style is represented with the K-levels ranking system published by the US Health Care Financing Administration's (HCFA). Table 2 shows the relation among patient's weight-lifestyle and the circumference scaling required.

Table 2. Patient's weight-lifestyle and circumference scaling required

		Circumference scaling %			
		1%-2%	2%-3%	3%-5%	4%-6%
Weight	< 75 Kg				
	75 - 100 Kg				
	100 - 125 Kg				
	> 125 Kg				
Lifestyle	K1				
	K2				
	K3				
	K4				

Finally, the **patient's residuum geometry** is acquired from MRI or laser scanning, reconstructed and converted in STL file format.

3 Anatomical Zones Recognition

First, the system exploits a neural network trained to identify on the patient's residuum geometry the location of the anatomical areas on which to apply the load and off-load zones [4, 5]. To this end, we expanded a prototype system presented in a previous work, in which we showed how to convert a 3D shape in an input suitable for a neural network, through a ray-casting process [2].

We created the dataset needed to train the neural network as follows: we used 5 STL files acquired from 5 different below-knee amputees, and labeled by human experts. In the labeling phase the experts was asked to put on the residuum model 4 different markers representing the perimeters of a given area. In particular, in this preliminary study we focused on the crest of the tibia, the patella and the patella tendon (Fig. 3).

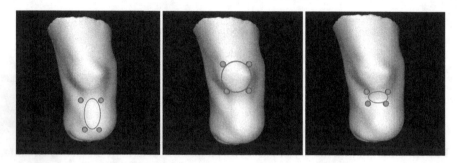

Fig. 3. Crest of tibia, patella and patella tendon critical areas

The 3d geometry has been converted in a grid of points on its surface, and the input feature vector of the network has been composed of the normalized distances of these points from a reference plane (Fig. 4).

As the size of the dataset was quite small, we generated a new synthetic training dataset using the 5 labeled original models as starting seed for the creation of new labeled

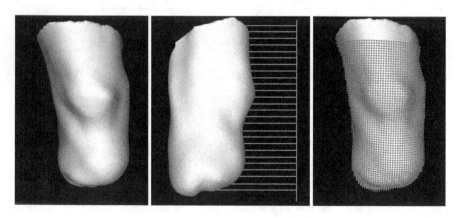

Fig. 4. 3d geometry - grid points conversion

geometries, through geometrical transformation operations such as scaling, skewing and rotation. This technique is often used in classification system for optical character recognition [6]. Finally, the artificial neural network has been trained with the back-propagation algorithm.

The neural network architecture consists of 1 input layer, 1 hidden layer, and 1 output layer. The input layer has 600 nodes corresponding to the 600 (30 * 20) points of the grid. In particular, the input value of each node consists of the distance of the residuum surface in that point from the reference place that lies in front of the residuum (Fig. 3). The distances have been normalized in range $(-1, +1)$.

The output layer has 8 nodes, corresponding to the x and y coordinates of each of the four marker used by the experts to label the model. (x1, y1, x2, y2, y3, x,3, y4, x4).

Regarding the number of nodes of the hidden layer, generally, there are no strict rules for deciding how many nodes it's necessary to assign to the hidden layer. Too few nodes could lead to a high error during the prediction phase, while too much nodes could create a model that can't generalize well (overfitting).

One design best practice suggests to use, for the hidden layer, a number of nodes that is equal to the geometric mean between the number of the input layer and the number of the output layer. In this specific case, we found out that the number of hidden layer that leads to the minimum test error and then provides better results is 70 (Fig. 5).

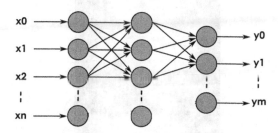

Fig. 5. Neural network architecture: Input layer (600 nodes), 1 hidden layer (70 nodes) and 1 output layer (8 nodes).

The final training dataset was composed of 400 labeled models of below knee residuum. In this study we trained a single neural network for a single critical area to be identified. Thus we have a neural network trained to recognize the area of the patella, one for the patella tendon, and another for the crest of the tibia.

Table 3. Final test errors

Anatomical area	Mean test squared error
Patella	62.15
Patella tendon	64.022
Tibia crest	60.25

The dataset has been split randomly into two parts: 80 % for the training set and 20 % for the validation set. The algorithm for the training has been the back-propagation with early stopping. Finally, the performance of the network has been tested on another residuum model, never used during the training phase. Final test errors are represented in Table 3.

4   Load and Off-Load Zones Creation

Once the geometry residuum areas have been identified, the system performs geometric deformations to create the required load and off-load zones. As previously said, the depth of the deformation is driven by the residuum tonicity that is divided in four levels: low, normal, good and very good.

Depending on the tonicity value, the deformations depth spans from 1 to 8 mm. A residuum with a good tonicity requires a less tight socket than a residuum with low tonicity. The deformations are smooth without hard steps and are generated by a Gaussian function with high variance. Figure 6 shows the example where the red zone is the created load zone for the patella tendon critical area.

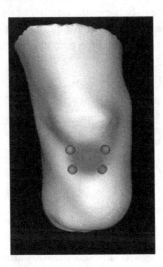

Fig. 6. Load zone creation on the patella tendon area

The final outcome is a new geometric model that replicates the shape of the residuum, except the areas in which deformations have been applied and load and off-load zones have been created. This new geometry represents the internal surface of the prosthesis socket. By adding a uniform thickness we can generate the final socket model.

5   Results, Conclusions and Future Steps

This work is a preliminary test to verify the feasibility of the approach. To validate the automatic deformation, we compared the output of the system with a validation dataset.

It consists of 5 sockets designed manually by professional technicians through a commercial prosthetic CAD system.

Results are promising, but there are several issues to be addressed in the future. First, we need to improve the precision of the identification algorithm. The total cumulative squared mean error is about 60 squared mm; this error is the sum of the errors of the 4 markers positions, this means that each marker is placed with a mean error of about 3.8 mm, this could be acceptable but expanding the dataset with new case studies could lead to a better predictive model. Secondly, we need to deal with the shaping of the upper border of the socket. Some commercial prosthetic CAD systems use reference templates as starting shape, but we have planned to investigate the possibility to apply automatic procedures also to this design phase.

References

1. Buzzi, M., Colombo, G., Facoetti, G., Gabbiadini, S., Rizzi, C.: 3D modelling and knowledge: tools to automate prosthesis development process. Int. J. Interact. Des. Manuf. **6**(1), 41–53 (2012)
2. Colombo, G., Facoetti, G., Rizzi, C., Vitali, A.: Automatic identification of below-knee residuum anatomical zones. In: Duffy, V.G. (ed.) DHM 2015. LNCS, vol. 9185, pp. 327–335. Springer, Heidelberg (2015)
3. Lee, W.C., Zhang, M., Mak, A.F.: Regional differences in pain threshold and tolerance of the transtibial residual limb: including the effects of age and interface material. Arch. Phys. Med. Rehabil. **86**, 641–649 (2005)
4. Haykin, S.: Neural Networks and Learning Machines – Pearson. Prentice Hall, USA (2008)
5. Bishop, C.M.: Pattern Recognition and Machine Learning Information Science and Statistics. Springer, Heidelberg (2006)
6. Jadeberg, M., Simonyan, K., Vedaldi, A., Zisserman, A.: Synthetic data and artificial neural networks for natural scene text recognition. In: Workshop on Deep Learning and Representation Learning (2014)

Development of Musculoskeletal Model to Estimate Muscle Activities During Swallowing

Takuya Hashimoto[1(✉)], Atsuko Murakoshi[1], Takahiro Kikuchi[2],
Yukihiro Michiwaki[2], and Takuji Koike[1]

[1] The University of Electro-Communications, Tokyo, Japan
hashi.tak@uec.ac.jp
[2] Japanese Red Cross Musashino Hospital, Tokyo, Japan

Abstract. Swallowing, or deglutition, is well known as a process to transport bolus of food from mouth to stomach, whereas it is difficult to understand its physiological mechanism because it involves in complex neuromuscular coordination. In order to understand swallowing mechanism in terms of muscle activity, we develop a musculoskeletal model in which muscles around the hyoid bone and the thyroid cartilage are represented as wire actuators. The changes of muscle lengths are calculated to estimate muscle activities during normal swallowing as a static analysis using the musculoskeletal model. The results of this study would contribute to provide greater insight into swallowing and to improve treatments for dysphagia.

Keywords: Swallowing · Musculoskeletal analysis

1 Introduction

Swallowing, or deglutition, is well known as a process to transport bolus of food from mouth to stomach. The process requires complex neuromuscular coordination because it involves voluntary control and reflexive motion of more than 30 nerves and muscles [1]. Therefore, neuromuscular disorders affect swallowing function and are highly associated with difficulty of swallowing, called dysphagia. Dysphagia also can lead to aspiration pneumonia, malnutrition, dehydration, weight loss, and airway obstruction. Aspiration pneumonia is particularly a big health concern in aging societies in terms of high mortality and long hospitalization period. In fact, the number of pneumonia patients has been actually increased with increasing of aging population [2], and now pneumonia has been the third leading cause of death in Japan. Because most of pneumonia of elderly people are said to be aspiration pneumonia caused by dysphagia, prevention and treatment of dysphagia would contribute to extending healthy-life span and increasing quality of social welfare. Therefore, it is very important to assess swallowing disorders accurately at an early stage.

Videofluoroscopic examination (VF) [3] which uses a real-time x-ray called fluoroscopy has been generally considered as the gold standard method to evaluate patient's ability to swallow because of its comprehensive information, but it requires

© Springer International Publishing Switzerland 2016
V.G. Duffy (Ed.): DHM 2016, LNCS 9745, pp. 82–91, 2016.
DOI: 10.1007/978-3-319-40247-5_9

special facilities and the use of a radiology equipment. Videoendoscopic examination (VE) [4] is also conducted as a reliable and portable method that can be done at bedside. However, these examinations mainly provide qualitative information on the movement of anatomical structure during swallowing. In order to evaluate swallowing function quantitatively, the use of a surface electromyography (sEMG) [5, 6] and swallowing sound [7] have been proposed. Because most of muscles related to swallowing construct a layered structure, sEMG measurement cannot avoid cross-talk effect even though sEMG measurement is considered as a reliable method to estimate muscle activities. In addition, the swallowing sound measurement cannot detect muscle activities. Therefore, it is difficult to understand muscle activities quantitatively during swallowing even though swallowing consists of complex neuromuscular coordination.

In this study, we develop a musculoskeletal model of swallowing to investigate swallowing function quantitatively in terms of muscle activity. The musculoskeletal model includes the hyoid bone and the thyroid cartilage as skeletal objects. Muscles around the hyoid bone and thyroid cartilage are also modeled as wire actuators based on anatomical knowledge. In order to investigate muscle activities during swallowing, we first analyzed the movements of the hyoid bone and thyroid cartilage during normal swallowing of a healthy subject. We then calculated the changes of muscle lengths as a static analysis based on analysis results.

2   Development of Musculoskeletal Model of Swallowing

In order to investigate muscle activities statically and dynamically, we develop a musculoskeletal model of swallowing. In the musculoskeletal model, the skeleton consists of three parts: hyoid bone, thyroid cartilage, a set of skull and cervical spine. A CT-data obtained from a healthy 20's male was used to create the skeleton data. The hyoid bone and the thyroid cartilage are treated as rigid bodies with mass and inertia. In addition, the cricoid cartilage is treated as a part of the thyroid cartilage. Muscle is simplified as a kind of a wire actuator which generates only contractive force by reference to the previous study [8]. The musculoskeletal model of swallowing includes 10 kinds of muscles acting on the hyoid bone and/or the thyroid cartilage: (1) middle constrictor muscle of pharynx, (2) inferior constrictor muscle of pharynx, (3) digastric muscle, (4) stylohyoid muscle, (5) geniohyoid muscle, (6) mylohyoid muscle, (7) sternohyoid muscle, (8) superior belly of the omohyoid muscle, (9) thyrohyoid muscle, (10) sternothyroid muscle. The detailed description of each muscle model is described below.

(1) *Middle constrictor muscle of pharynx from greater horn and lesser horn: PG, PL*

The middle constrictor muscle of pharynx is a kind of a fan-shaped muscle which partly forms the posterior wall of the pharynx as shown in Fig. 1(a). This muscle is divided into two parts according to attachment sites. One of them arises from the pharyngeal raphe and ends up with the greater horn (cornu) of the hyoid, and it is named PG in this paper. The other one also arises from the pharyngeal raphe and ends up with the lessor horn (cornu), and it is named PL. In our model, each muscle is represented with four wires (PG1 and PL1 for upper part, PG2 and PL2 for lower part), because they are wide-spanned muscle.

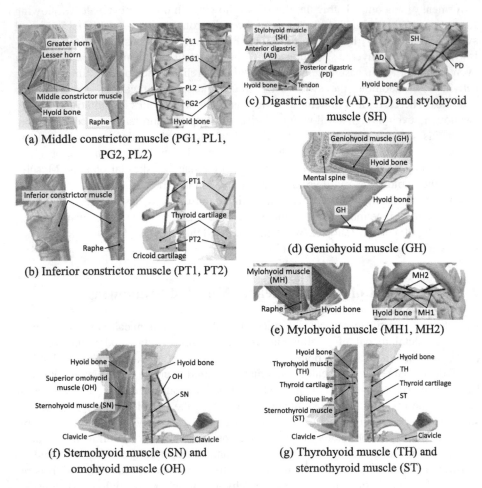

(a) Middle constrictor muscle (PG1, PL1, PG2, PL2)

(b) Inferior constrictor muscle (PT1, PT2)

(c) Digastric muscle (AD, PD) and stylohyoid muscle (SH)

(d) Geniohyoid muscle (GH)

(e) Mylohyoid muscle (MH1, MH2)

(f) Sternohyoid muscle (SN) and omohyoid muscle (OH)

(g) Thyrohyoid muscle (TH) and sternothyroid muscle (ST)

Fig. 1. Anatomical images [9] and wire models of muscles around the hyoid bone and the thyroid cartilage.

(2) *Inferior constrictor muscle of pharynx: PT1, PT2*

Similarly to the middle constrictor muscle, the inferior constrictor muscle of pharynx is the part of posterior wall of the pharynx as shown in Fig. 1(b). This muscle is composed of two parts and both of them arise from the pharyngeal raphe. One of them ends up with the thyroid cartilage and the other ends up with the cricoid cartilage. In this study, only the muscle whose insertion is the thyroid cartilage is included. This muscle is represented with two wires (PT1 for upper part and PT2 for lower part).

(3) *Digastric muscle: AD, PD*

The digastric muscle is a slender muscle located under the jaw as shown in Fig. 1(c). This muscle is divided into two muscles by an intermediate tendon. One of them is the posterior belly which arises from the mastoid process of the temporal bone and inserts into the intermediate tendon. The other one is the anterior belly which arises from the intermediate tendon and inserts into the inner surface of the lower border of the mandible. In our model, each muscle is represented as a simple wire (AD, PD) and the intermediate tendon is assumed as a via-point [8].

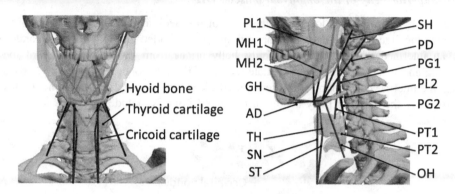

Fig. 2. Musculoskeletal model of swallowing

(4) *Stylohyoid muscle: SH*

As shown in Fig. 1(c), the stylohyoid muscle is a slender muscle which arises from the posterior surface of the styloid process of the temporal bone and inserts into the greater horn of the hyoid bone. A wire actuator, named SH, is assigned for this muscle.

(5) *Geniohyoid muscle: GH*

The geniohyoid muscle is a fusiform muscle passing parallel to the midline in an anterior-posterior direction as shown in Fig. 1(d). Its origin is the mental spine which located on the back of the madible, and the insertion is an anterior surface of the hyoid bone. This muscle is represented as a simple wire actuator, named GH.

(6) *Mylohyoid muscle: MH1, MH2*

The mylohyoid muscle is a flat and triangular muscle which runs from the mandible to the hyoid bone. As shown in Fig. 1(e), this muscle forms the floor of oral cavity. Its origin is the mylohyoid line and the sublingual fossa of mandible. The insertion is an anterior surface of the hyoid bone and a midline raphe which connects the mental spine and the hyoid bone. Our model represents only a muscle whose origin is the hyoid, but a muscle whose origin is the midline raphe is not included for simplicity. This muscle is modeled as two wires (MH1, MH2).

(7) *Sternohyoid muscle: SN*

The sternohyoid muscle is a paired muscle in the superficial layers of the neck and runs parallel to the midline as shown in Fig. 1(f). The origin is the posterior part of the manubrium of sternum, the sternoclavicular articulation, and the first costal cartilage. The insertion is the lower border of the hyoid bone. In our model, the origin is defined as the posterior part of the manubrium of sternum because the skeleton data contains only an upper part of the collarbone. This muscle is simplified as a wire actuator, named SN.

(8) *Superior belly of the omohyoid muscle: OH*

The omohyoid muscle is located at the front of the neck as shown in Fig. 1(f). Similarly to the digastric muscle, the omohyoid muscle is divided into two bellies separated by an intermediate tendon. The inferior belly arises from the upper border of the scapula and inserts into the intermediate tendon. The other one, superior belly, arises from the intermediate tendon and inserts into the lower border of the hyoid bone. In this study, only the superior belly acting on the hyoid bone is included as OH.

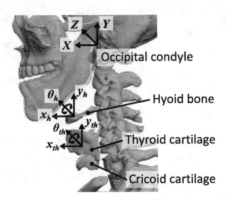

Fig. 3. Global and local coordinate systems

(9) *Thyrohyoid muscle: TH*

The thyrohyoid muscle is a thin muscle which connects the hyoid bone and the thyroid cartilage, and it runs parallel to the sternothyroid muscle as shown in Fig. 1(g). The origin is the oblique line on the thyroid cartilage, and the insertion is the lower border of the greater cornu of the hyoid bone. This muscle is represented as a simple wire, named TH.

(10) *Sternothyroid muscle: ST*

The sternothyroid muscle is a thin muscle located under the sternohyoid muscle (Fig. 1 (g)). The origin is the posterior part of the manubrium of sternum and the first costal cartilage, but the origin is defined as the manubrium of sternum as well as the sternohyoid muscle in this study. The insertion is defined as the oblique line on the thyroid cartilage. This muscle modeled as a simple wire, named ST.

In this way, muscles are represented as wire actuators as shown in Fig. 2 based on anatomical knowledge [9] and the CT data. Arrangement of muscles in left and right sides is symmetrical about the sagittal plane for simplicity. In total, the number of muscle is 32 (N = 32). To describe the positions of muscles, the global coordinate system is defined at the center of left-right occipital condyles. The local coordinate systems are defined at the center of gravity of the hyoid bone and the center of gravity of the thyroid cartilage as shown in Fig. 3, respectively.

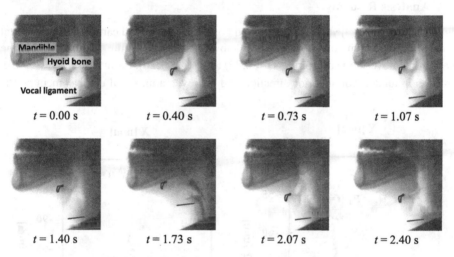

Fig. 4. Video fluoroscopic image of swallowing

3 Motion Analysis of the Hyoid Bone and the Thyroid Cartilage

The normal swallowing process is classified into three phase according to the location of bolus: oral phase, pharyngeal phase, and esophageal phase. The pharyngeal phase is particularly important, which transports bolus into the stomach from the pharynx. In this phase, the hyoid bone and the larynx move upward and forward. The thyroid cartilage is also elevated in association with hyoid motion. At that time, the posterior part of tongue moves in a posteroinferior direction. When the larynx and the posterior part of tongue move, the epiglottis falls down to prevent bolus from going into the trachea and instead propels it into the esophagus. If this process is not performed adequately, food and drink go into the trachea and it may cause dysphagia. Because this process is driven by muscles attaching to the hyoid bone and the thyroid cartilage, to analyze movements of the hyoid bone and the thyroid cartilage is important to evaluate swallowing function.

3.1 Analysis Method

We used a VF video to analyze two-dimensional movements of the hyoid bone and the thyroid cartilage. The video has been obtained from a video fluoroscopic examination of a healthy 20's male. In analysis, we manually extracted the region of hyoid bone and the vocal ligament of thyroid cartilage frame-by-frame as shown in Fig. 4. Displacements and posture of each object were measured based on each initial position and posture. Then, measured displacements and posture were transformed to the global coordinate system. In addition, the volumes of the hyoid bone and the thyroid cartilage were estimated from a skeletal data obtained from CT-data of the same male.

3.2 Analysis Results

Figure 5 shows the trajectories of the hyoid bone and the thyroid cartilage in the sagittal plane, which were smoothed by a simple moving average. Figure 5(a) shows that the hyoid bone moves upward from P_s^h ($t = 0.83$) to P_1^h ($t = 1.20$). From P_1^h to P_2^h ($t = 1.70$), it moves in an anterior-superior direction and achieves a maximal displacement at P_2^h.

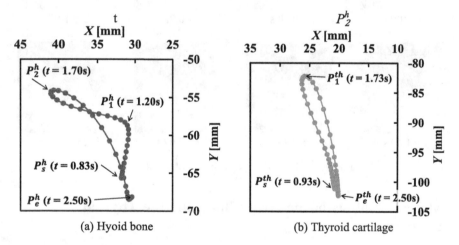

(a) Hyoid bone   (b) Thyroid cartilage

Fig. 5. Trajectories of the hyoid bone and the thyroid cartilage

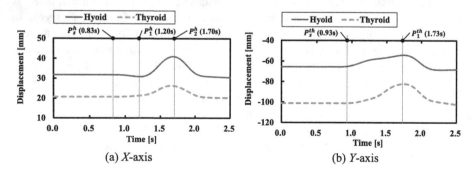

(a) X-axis   (b) Y-axis

Fig. 6. Displacements of the hyoid bone and the thyroid cartilage in X- or Y-axis.

Then, it returns to an initial position from P_2^h to P_e^h ($t = 2.50$). Figure 5(b) shows that the thyroid cartilage mainly moves in an superior direction from P_s^{th} ($t = 0.93$) to P_1^{th} ($t = 1.73$). The thyroid cartilage achieves a maximal displacement along with the hyoid bone at P_1^{th}. From P_1^{th} to P_e^{th} ($t = 2.50$), it returns to an initial position. Figure 6 shows the displacements of the hyoid bone and the thyroid cartilage in X- or Y-axis.

4   Estimation of Muscle Activities During Swallowing

4.1   Method

In this analysis, the change of muscle length was calculated to estimate muscle activity using the musculoskeletal model as a static analysis, because muscle length would reflect a part of muscle activity. Muscle length is defined as the distance between the origin and insertion of a muscle, which is given by

$$l_i = \sqrt{(O_i^x - I_i^x)^2 + (O_i^y - I_i^y)^2 + (O_i^z - I_i^z)^2} \quad i = 1, 2, 3, \ldots, N \qquad (1)$$

Here, l_i is muscle length of i-th muscle. O_i^x, O_i^y, O_i^z, I_i^x, I_i^y, and I_i^z represent the positions of origin and insertion of i-th muscle in the global coordinate system, respectively. The lengths of all muscles included in the musculoskeletal model were calculated three-dimensionally along with the movements of the hyoid bone and the thyroid cartilage. Finally, each muscle length was normalized by each initial length as below:

$$L_i = \frac{l_i}{l_i^0} \qquad (2)$$

Here, L_i and l_i^0 are the normalized and initial length of i-th muscle, respectively.

4.2   Results and Discussions

Figure 7 shows the calculation results. The mylohyoid muscle (MH1, MH2), the sty-lohyoid muscle (SH), the posterior belly of the digastric muscle (PD), and the upper part of the middle constrictor muscle (PG1, PL1) shortened along with the elevation of the hyoid bone. The thyrohyoid muscle (TH) stretched in the initial period of the elevation of the hyoid bone, but it shortened when the thyroid cartilage elevated followed by the hyoid bone. In addition, the upper part of the inferior constrictor muscle of pharynx (PT1) shortened simultaneously. The geniohyoid muscle (GH) and the anterior belly of the digastric muscle (AD) shortened when the hyoid bone moved forward. As the result, the following predictions are obtained:

- The mylohyoid muscle (MH1, MH2), the stylohyoid muscle (SH), the posterior belly of the digastric muscle (PD), and the upper part of the constrictor muscle (PG1, PL1) contribute to upward movement of the hyoid bone

- The geniohyoid muscle (GH) and the anterior belly of the digastric muscle (AD) contribute to forward movement of the hyoid bone
- The thyrohyoid muscle (TH) and the upper part of the inferior constrictor muscle (PT1) contribute to upward movement of the thyroid cartilage

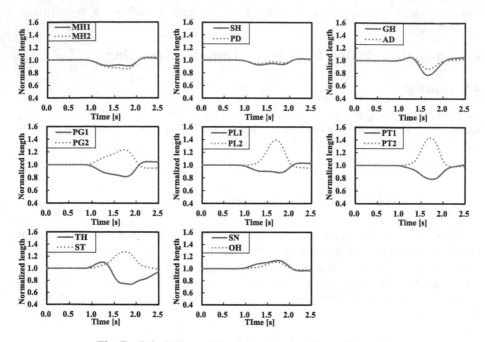

Fig. 7. Calculation results of the changes of muscle lengths

5 Conclusion

We developed the musculoskeletal model of swallowing based on anatomical knowledge to investigate swallowing function quantitatively in terms of muscle activity. In the musculoskeletal model, muscles around the hyoid bone and thyroid cartilage are modeled as wire actuators. In order to investigate muscle activities during swallowing, we calculated the changes in length of the muscle as a static analysis using the musculoskeletal model.

One of our future works is to realize dynamic analysis to estimate individual muscle force in swallowing by using inverse dynamics computation and optimization program [10]. In addition, it is important to verify the reliability of force estimation result by comparing with biological signal such as a surface electromyography (sEMG). To consider viscoelastic properties of physiological tissue including muscle is also important for dynamic analysis.

References

1. Jones, B. (ed.): Normal and Abnormal Swallowing: Imaging in Diagnosis and Therapy. Springer, New York (2003)
2. Fernandez-Sabe, N., Carratala, J., Roson, B., Dorca, J., Verdaguer, R., Manresa, F., Gudiol, F.: Community-acquired pneumonia in very elderly patients: causative organisms, clinical characteristics, and outcomes. Medicine 82(3), 159–169 (2003)
3. Palmer, J.B., Kuhlemeier, K.V., Tippett, D.C., Lynch, C.: A protocol for the videofluorographic swallowing study. Dysphagia 8(3), 209–214 (1993)
4. Leder, S.B., Sasaki, C.T., Burrell, M I · Fiberoptic endoscopic evaluation of dysphagia to identify silent aspiration. Dysphagia 13(1), 19–21 (1998)
5. Neis, L.R., Logemann, J., Larson, C.: Viscosity effects on EMG activity in normal swallow. Dysphagia 9(2), 101–106 (1994)
6. Crary, M.A., Baldwin, B.O.: Surface electromyographic characteristics of swallowing in dysphagia secondary to brainstem stroke. Dysphagia 12(4), 180–187 (1997)
7. Nagae, M Suzuki, K.: A neck mounted interface for sensing the swallowing activity based on swallowing sound. In: Proceedings of the 2011 Annual International Conference of the IEEE Engineering in Medicine and Biology Society, pp. 5224–5227 (2011)
8. Nakamura, Y., Yamane, K., Fujita, Y., Suzuki, I.: Somatosensory computation for man-machine interface from motion-capture data and musculoskeletal human model. IEEE Trans. Rob. 21(1), 58–66 (2005)
9. McFarland, D.H.: Netter's Atlas of Anatomy for Speech, Swallowing, and Hearing. Elsevier Health Sciences, New York (2008)
10. Ueda, J., Ding, M., Krishnamoorthy, V., Shinohara, M., Ogasawara, T.: Individual muscle control using an exoskeleton robot for muscle function testing. IEEE Trans. Neural Syst. Rehabil. Eng. 18(4), 339–350 (2010)

Combination of Non Invasive Medical Imaging Technologies and Virtual Reality Systems to Generate Immersive Fetal 3D Visualizations

Jorge Roberto Lopes dos Santos[1,2(✉)], Heron Werner[3], Gerson Ribeiro[1,2], and Simone Letícia Belmonte[1,2]

[1] Arts and Design Department - Núcleo de Experimentação Tridimensional, Pontifícia Universidade Católica do Rio de Janeiro, Rio de Janeiro, Brazil
jorge.lopes@puc-rio.br
[2] Laboratório de Modelos Tridimensionais, Ministério da Ciência Tecnologia e Inovação - Instituto Nacional de Tecnologia, Rio de Janeiro, Brazil
[3] Clínica de Diagnóstico Por Imagem – CDPI, Rio de Janeiro, Brazil

Abstract. Advances in imaging technology have led to vast improvements in fetal evaluation. Ultrasound examination is the primary method of fetal assessment because it is patient friendly, effective, and cost efficient and is considered to be safe. Magnetic resonance imaging is generally used when ultrasound cannot provide sufficiently high-quality images. It offers high-resolution fetal and placental imaging with excellent contrast. The objective here is to describe the combination of non-invasive medical imaging technologies and virtual reality systems in fetal medicine.

Keywords: Fetal medicine · Virtual reality · Magnetic resonance imaging · Ultrasound 3D · CT scanner

1 Introduction

The purpose of this work is to present a study related to the combination of non-invasive medical imaging technologies and Virtual Reality (VR) immersive technologies as a complementary tool to assist fetal medicine studies (Fig. 1).

Advances in image-scanning technology have led to vast improvements in medicine, especially in the diagnosis of fetal anomalies. In general, two main technologies can be used to visualize and, as a result, obtain inner images of the maternal body during pregnancy: Ultrasonography (USG) and Magnetic Resonance Imaging (MRI) (Fig. 2).

Apart from the technical differences, an interesting obvious difference between the technologies is related to the portability of USG equipment compared to MRI, which is carried out inside a tubular format, making it necessary for the patient to be positioned inside the equipment. The portability of some USG apparatus makes it possible for the equipment to travel to the patient, while for MRI scans the patient has to go to the equipment (Fig. 3).

© Springer International Publishing Switzerland 2016
V.G. Duffy (Ed.): DHM 2016, LNCS 9745, pp. 92–99, 2016.
DOI: 10.1007/978-3-319-40247-5_10

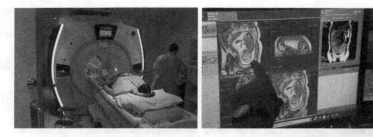

Fig. 1. Patient ready to start the magnetic resonance imaging scan and a radiologist analysing the MRI files during the scanning process.

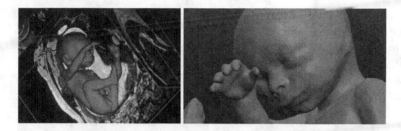

Fig. 2. 3D model of the fetus generated from MRI DICOM (Digital Communication in Medicine protocol) files.

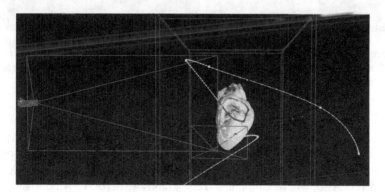

Fig. 3. Screen of the software "Unreal Engine" from Epic Games, the 3D model generated from the slices obtained on the non-invasive image technology to then apply the texture and lights and create the paths for the fly-through VR navigation.

Computed tomography (CT) is used only in specific cases of suspected fetal malformation, particularly those related to the skeleton, because of potential risks associated with exposure of the fetus to radiation. Its use during pregnancy must be adequately justified and its application is limited to specific pathologies such as bone dysplasia, which can, in some cases, be difficult to diagnose by USG, especially in the absence of

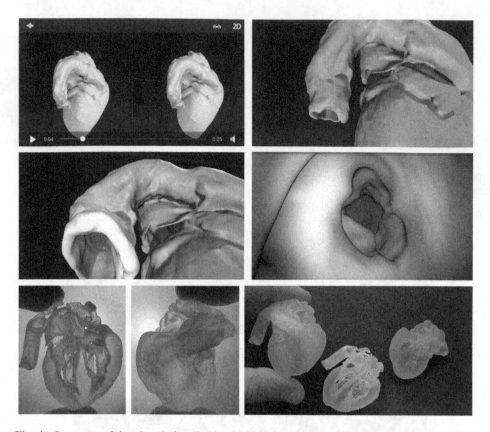

Fig. 4. Sequence of the virtual visualization inside a fetal heart at 38 weeks, after autopsy, from Micro-CT scanner (Zeiss Xradia Versa 510), and 3D printed full scale physical models (Projet 3510 HD Plus)

a family history of the disease. CT can also be used (after the birth, due to the X Ray radiation) and its physical principles are based on the amount of radiation absorbed by each body part, which means that tissues with different composition absorb X-rays in different ways. Also, Micro Computed Tomography (MicroCT) which has a higher image resolution can be used in cases of autopsy analysis (Fig. 4).

USG is the primary fetal monitoring method during pregnancy, and also the most commonly-used method, given its long record of safety, usefulness, and cost-effectiveness. The development of USG scanning during the 1960s opened a new window into the study of the fetus. Its applications are based on the detection and representation of acoustic waves reflected by interfaces within the body, providing the information needed to generate greyscale images of the uterine content (Fig. 5).

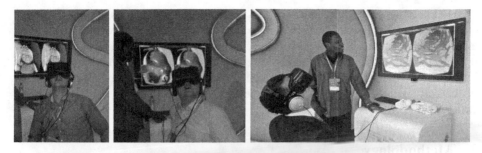

Fig. 5. Pictures taken in September 2015 during the "Hospital Innovation Show" in São Paulo, Brasil where the project was presented for many physicians.

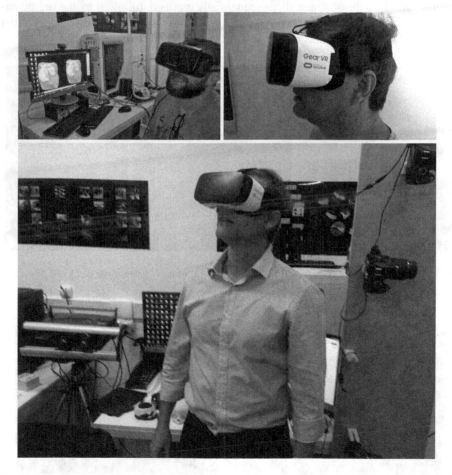

Fig. 6. Two fathers having the opportunity to participate on the experiment visualizing their unborn babies during the pregnancy and the fetal medicine specialist Dr. Heron Werner during the equipment tests.

MRI is a non-invasive method that has been used in obstetrics since the 1980s. It offers high-resolution fetal images with excellent contrast that allow visualization of internal tissues. When USG yields unexpected results, MRI is generally used, because it provides additional information about fetal abnormalities and conditions for which USG cannot provide high-quality images. MRI files can generate detailed characteristics of the soft tissues of the fetus body as the face, hands or feet as well internal body structures as aerial paths [2].

2 Methodology

The construction process of the 3D accurate virtual model starts with the 3D modeling volume built from the obtained slices sequentially grouped, followed by the segmentation process where the Physician selects the important body parts to be visualized that will be then accurately reconstructed in 3D (Fig. 6).

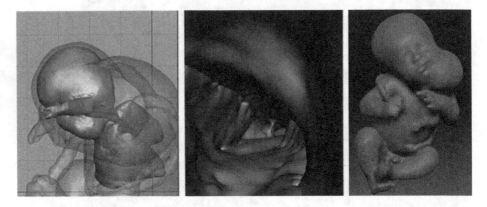

Fig. 7. 3D view obtained from MRI of fetal cervical tumor at 37 gestational weeks of gestation.

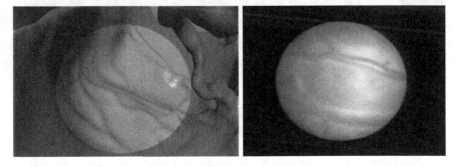

Fig. 8. Virtual fetoscopy highlights area of placenta.

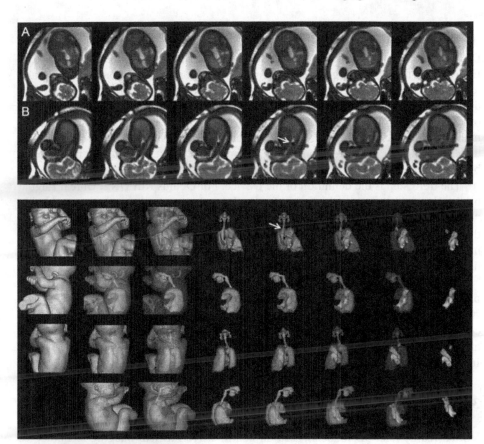

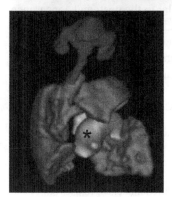

Fig. 9. Virtual fetoscopy after MRI highlights airway path in a fetus (28 weeks) with Diaphragmatic Hernia. In this case, MRI was performed after fetal surgery. The arrow shows the red structure corresponding to Balloon inflated inside the trachea. Note the presence of the stomach inside the thorax (*).

Having the accurate 3D model (womb, umbilical, cord, placenta and fetus) the final stage is the programming of the virtual reality (VR) for different devices as Oculus Rift DK2 and Samsung Gear VR. Through the use of the software "Unreal Engine" from Epic Games, the 3D model generated from the slices obtained on the non-invasive image technology as MRI, to then apply the texture and lights and create the paths for the fly-through VR navigation. According to Riva and Davide, VR can be used to explore the organs by "flying" around, behind, or even inside them. In this sense virtual environments can be used both as didactic and experiential educational tools, allowing a deeper understanding of the interrelationship of anatomical structures that cannot be achieved by any other means [3] (Fig. 7).

The third step is the definition of the Device. For Oculus Rift DK2, Unreal Engine have a plug-in that prepare the project for Oculus and we compile in one executable file "*.exe". For Samsung Gear VR, the third step is render the project in a panoramic video that will be convert in 360° video on the device (this conversion is necessary because mobiles phones have limited graphic hardware). In this engine, we can include also the heartbeat sounds of the fetus to improve the immersive sensation (Fig. 8).

Important to observe that the navigation through internal paths should be pre-defined by the physician responsible for the patient in order to highlight the main subjects to be studied by the fetal medicine team as well for parents understanding. So far seven complete different studies have been developed to attend physicians in Fetal Medicine and Cardiology and the project was presented on September 2015 during the "Hospital Innovation Show" in São Paulo, Brasil (Fig. 9).

3 Conclusion

Virtual reality fetal 3D models based on non-invasive medical imaging technologies were successfully generated. They were remarkably similar to the postnatal appearance of the newborn baby, especially in cases with pathology, increasing the possibilities of digital tools to help fetal medicine researches. The 3D fetal models applied on virtual reality immersive technologies may improve our understanding of fetal anatomical characteristics, and can be used for educational purposes and as a method for parents to visualize their unborn baby.

References

1. Pensieri, C., Pennacchini, M.: Overview: virtual reality in medicine. J. Virtual Worlds Res. 7(1), 1–36 (2014)
2. Santos, J.L., Werner, H., Fontes, R., et al.: Additive manufactured models of fetuses built from 3D ultrasound, magnetic resonance imaging and computed tomography scan data. In: Hoque, M.E. (ed.) Rapid Prototyping Technology Principles and Functional Requirements, pp. 179–192. InTech, Rijeka (2011)
3. Riva, G., Gamberini, L.: Virtual reality in telemedicine. In: Riva, G., Davide, F. (eds.) Communications Through Virtual Technology: Identity Community and Technology in the Internet Age, p. 109. IOS Press, Amsterdam (2003)

4. Fiorini, S.T., Frajhof, L., de Azevedo, B.A., dos Santos, J.R., Werner, H., Raposo, A., de Lucena, C.J.P.: Three-dimensional models and simulation tools enabling interaction and immersion in medical education. In: Marcus, A. (ed.) DUXU 2015. LNCS, vol. 9188, pp. 662–671. Springer, Heidelberg (2015)
5. Werner, H., Lopes, J., Tonni, G., Junior, E.A.: Physical model from 3D ultrasound and magnetic resonance imaging scan data reconstruction of lumbosacral myelomeningocele in a fetus with Chiari II malformation. Childs Nerv. Syst. **31**, 511 (2015)

Computational Modeling for Simulating Obstructive Lung Diseases Based on Geometry Processing Methods

Stavros Nousias[✉], Aris S. Lalos, and Konstantinos Moustakas

Department of Electrical and Computer Engineering,
University of Patras, Patras, Greece
{nousias,aris.lalos,moustakas}@ece.upatras.gr

Abstract. Obstructive lung diseases (e.g. asthma & COPD) are life-long inflammatory diseases that result in narrowing of the lung airways, reducing the airflow that reaches the oxygen exchanging areas. The knowledge and understanding of the pathophysiology behind these diseases could lead to improved diagnosis and assessment, through the development of computational models that take into account details related to lung geometry, lung mechanical features and the dynamics of the fluid motion inside the lungs. Although there are several works that considers some of the aforementioned characteristics, none of them provides a fully integrated solution. To overcome this limitation, we have developed a software tool that combines geometry processing methods with 3D computational fluid dynamics (CFD), allowing us to simulate in a realistic way the effects of bronchoconstriction in the dynamics of the air flow in the airways of the lung. The developed tool is expected to provide useful information regarding the way that either drug or other harmful particles are being dispersed inside the lungs during different levels of inflammation.

Keywords: Computational models · Computational fluid dynamics · Geometry processing

1 Introduction

Lung diseases (e.g. asthma & COPD) are life-long chronic inflammatory diseases of the airways, affecting over 500 million people worldwide with related costs exceeding 56 billion Euros per year in the European Union [1]. Their main characteristic is the narrowing of the lung airways, a condition known as bronchoconstriction, which alters the geometry and the mechanical properties of the airways and reduces the airflow that reaches the oxygen exchanging areas.

The diagnosis and severity classification of these diseases are largely based on global lung measurements from pulmonary function tests (PFTs). However, these measures have been proven to be poor predictors of patient outcomes for individuals. Therefore, patient specific computational models of the lung, that

© Springer International Publishing Switzerland 2016
V.G. Duffy (Ed.): DHM 2016, LNCS 9745, pp. 100–109, 2016.
DOI: 10.1007/978-3-319-40247-5_11

will provide more sensitive measures of the pulmonary function are required. The knowledge and understanding of the pathophysiology behind the obstructive lung diseases could lead to improved diagnosis and assessment, through the development of novel computational models that take into account details related to (i) the lung geometry deformations, (ii) different lung mechanical features and (iii) the changes of the airflow inside the lung airways.

There are several state of the art approaches related to computational modeling of the lung and other parts of the human body that use 3D computational fluid dynamics, utilizing generic 3D representations of the structure [4,9,14] Although, both experimental and simulation studies have demonstrated the influence of geometric structure on functional outcomes none of the SoA approaches considers fully patient specific structures, represented by high-resolution computational meshes of the central airways that are deformed appropriately in order to simulate bronchoconstriction effects. To overcome these limitations and allow the processing of the patient specific lung geometry, we provide a toolset allowing to view and deform lung 3D structures in order to be used for computational fluid dynamics, allowing the visualization of the airflow for different kinds of geometry. The output of the CFD simulation is essential for predicting particle deposition upon the inner part of the airway walls, allowing: (i) the clinician to study the way the drug or other harmful particles that cause inflammation are dispersed inside the lungs for different stages of a crisis and for different levels of inflammation (ii) the user to determine the effectiveness of a delivery system upon inflamed airways [7,9] and use the results as input for assessing which parts of the patient's lung are more easily affected and predicting an obstruction of a specific airway.

The rest of the paper is organized as follows: The second section presents the related work on computational models. The third focuses on the developed geometry processing approaches that allow the user to simulate realistic bronchoconstriction that occur during exacerbation episodes. In section four, we analyze the adopted 3D computational fluid dynamics methodology. The fifth section deals with the demonstration of the tool interface and the presentation of the simulation results. Finally, the sixth section is dedicated to discussion related to the strengths, weaknesses and future directions of the presented work.

Notation: Lower- and upper-case boldface letters are used to denote column vectors and matrices, respectively; calligraphic letters are used to denote sets; The entry in the i-th row and j-th column of a matrix $\mathbf{A}$ is denoted by $\mathbf{A}_{(i,j)}$, while the i-th row and j-th column is denoted by $\mathbf{A}_{(i,:)}$, $\mathbf{A}_{(:,j)}$ respectively. $(\cdot)^T$ denotes transposition;

2   Related Work

There are several studies related to computational modeling of different aspects of the pulmonary function. These include aspects related to airflow analysis and ventilation [4,8,12,14], particle transportation and deposition [3,7,9] and mechanical properties of the lung airways tissue [10,13]. However, their major drawback is that they refer to healthy lungs without taking into account structural alterations present in obstructive lung diseases.

In addition to the aforementioned models there are applications that focus on the lung geometry allowing either to reconstruct the 3D lung model from CT scans or to view and study the lung geometry [11] without proving the ability to perform alterations appropriate for applying computational fluid dynamics simulation. Thus, their major drawback is that they do not combine the ability to simulate geometry alterations present in obstructive lung diseases with computational fluid dynamics simulations. To cope with the aforementioned issues and allow the processing of patient specific lung airways geometry we propose a method that combines the deformation of the geometry in a manner that simulates bronchoconstriction with computational fluid dynamics models. The output of the simulation can be used for predicting particle transfer and deposition to the lung airways walls allowing the researcher or the clinician to study how drug particles or harmful particles travel inside the airways for different levels of airways obstruction.

3   Structural Modeling of the Lung, Parametrization and Deformation

In this section, we present the developed geometry processing approaches, that allow the user to simulate the effects of the obstructive diseases in the 3D lung structure, and study their impact on airflow in the lung, by using a 3D CFD simulation. The proposed approaches are executed directly on already available 3D models of the lung, extracted from CT scans, by using conventional SoA methods. The user interface allow the user to select the area of interest, e.g. either a specific branch, or all the branches of the i-th generation, or the whole model itself and perform narrowing by executing a Laplacian mesh contraction approach. The surface of the given object is iteratively contracted either in the direction of the inward normal or according to a customized function that deforms the mesh in a user selected manner. A skeleton extraction technique has been also developed for converting the 3D object into a 1D curve skeleton that is essential for airway segmentation, for personalization and for predicting the structure of airways in models that include more than 9 generations of branching.

3.1   Lung Geometry Contraction in the Direction of the Inward Normals

In order to apply mesh contraction we employ the Laplacian mesh processing scheme presented in [2]. For the shake of self-completeness, we provide a short overview of the method. A lung 3D model is described by a mesh $G = (V, E)$ with vertices V and edges E. Using cotangent weighting the Laplacian coordinates approximate the curvature-flow inward normal. Thus solving iteratively the discrete Laplacian equation $\mathbf{L}\mathbf{v} = 0$ we can achieve mesh contraction and reduce the 3D model to an 1D shape. Let $\mathbf{L}$ be the Laplacian operator and $\mathbf{v}'$ the vertices final position, then we have:

$$\mathbf{L}_{i,j} = \begin{cases} \omega_{i,j} = \cot a_{ij} + \cot b_{ij} \\ \sum_{i,k \in E}^{k} -\omega_{ik} \\ 0 \end{cases} \tag{1}$$

Since $\mathbf{L}$ is singular, further constrains need to be used in order to ensure a unique solution for $\mathbf{v}'$. Thus we focus on solving the equations:

$$\begin{bmatrix} \mathbf{W}_L \mathbf{L} \\ \mathbf{W}_H \end{bmatrix} \mathbf{v}' = \begin{bmatrix} 0 \\ \mathbf{W}_H \mathbf{V} \end{bmatrix} \tag{2}$$

where $\mathbf{W}_L$ and $\mathbf{W}_H$ are the diagonal matrices. These matrices represent a contraction and an attraction force correspondingly. However by experimentation on can easily observe that the solution of (2) does not converge to an 1D shape and thus an iterative scheme need to be used as the one described below:

---

1. Initialize W_L and W_H in the following manner:

$$W_L = k \cdot \sqrt{A} \tag{3}$$
$$W_H = I \tag{4}$$

where I is a unitary matrix, k a double constant and A the average face area of the model.
2. Solve (2) for V'.
3. Update W_L and W_H so that

$$W_L^{t+1} = s_L \cdot W_L^t \tag{5}$$
$$W_{H,i}^{t+1} = W_{H,i}^0 \cdot \sqrt{A_i^0 / A_i^t} \tag{6}$$

where t denotes the iteration index.
4. Recompute L.
5. Repeat steps 2 to 4 for a given number of iterations.

Based on the aforementioned scheme we can also apply mesh contraction at a selected part of the mesh in order to simulate narrowing by using stopping criteria related to the difference between the updated and the initial position. The part can be any type of airway of the 3D mesh under investigation. After the user has selected the branch by using the available interface, the branch is segmented for more efficient processing and mesh contraction is achieved. For this procedure we choose the same attraction weight and a different contraction weight for every node. However, as the processed part is reconnected with the rest of the mesh discontinuities may appear. In order to cope with this fact, we gradually reduce the weight of points of the stable regions of the mesh based on geodesic distance between each processed point and the edge points (anchor points) of the stable region of the mesh (Fig. 1).

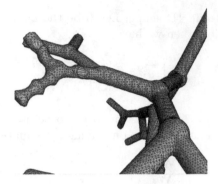

Fig. 1. Airway narrowing based on mesh contraction augmented by a custom function

3.2 Custom Function Based Mesh Contraction and Skeletonization

The aforementioned method of mesh contraction will generate a contracted mesh meaning that the airway diameter will be smaller for the contracted parts. In order to augment the mesh contraction process so as to simulate the surface abnormalities during bronchoconstriction we propose the application of different levels of deformation across the airways as a function of distance. Thus we propose a new W_L^0 weighting diagonal matrix using the following formulation:

$$\mathbf{W}_L^0 = W_L^0 \cdot W_V \tag{7}$$

where W_V is a diagonal weighting matrix. For W_V we can use a customized function:

$$\mathbf{W}_V = f(d) \tag{8}$$

where d is the geodesic distance of a point of the mesh from an anchor point. In this study and for demonstration purposes only we used a sinusoidal function. The function can be defined by the user on a case-by-case basis. Thus a weighting parameter is set for each vertex equal to:

$$\mathbf{W}_V(i) = r_0 + \frac{1 - r_0}{2} sind \tag{9}$$

where r_0 is the minimum allowable radius as percentage of the initial radius of the airways cylindrical like shape. The result of this method is shown in the following section.

The aforementioned scheme can be used in order to extract the 1D skeleton. This can be achieved by repeating the iterative process until any face area of the model is smaller than 10^{-7}. In Fig. 3 we present the result of curve skeleton extraction by applying the iterative mesh contraction process.

4   Computational Fluid Dynamics

The resulting mesh is used for computational fluid dynamics simulation. The CFD simulation is based on the integration of open source fluid dynamics libraries [6]. The volume inside the surface mesh is assumed to be the fluid domain consisting only of air. The flow is assumed to be incompressible and the fluid to be Newtonian. The used scheme is the solving the Reynolds Averaged Navier-Stokes equation allowing the simulation of turbulence written as:

$$\rho \left[\frac{\partial \tilde{u}_i}{\partial t} + \tilde{u}_j \frac{\partial \tilde{u}_i}{\partial x_j} \right] = -\frac{\partial \tilde{p}}{\partial x_i} + \frac{\partial \tilde{T}_{ij}^{(v)}}{\partial x_j} \tag{10}$$

$$\left[\frac{\partial \tilde{\rho}}{\partial t} + \tilde{u}_j \frac{\partial \tilde{\rho}}{\partial x_j} \right] + \rho \frac{\partial \tilde{u}_j}{\partial x_j} = 0 \tag{11}$$

where $\tilde{u}_i(\boldsymbol{x}, t)$ represents the i-the component of the fluid velocity at a point in space, $[\boldsymbol{x}]_i = x_i$, and time, t. Also $\tilde{p}(\boldsymbol{x}, t)$ represents the static pressure, $\tilde{T}_{ij}^{(v)}(\boldsymbol{x}, t)$, the viscous(or deviatoric) stresses, and $\tilde{\rho}$ the fluid density. The tilde over the symbol indicates that an instantaneous quantity is being considered. Also the einstein summation convention has been employed. In Eq. (10), the subscript i is a free index which can take on the values 1, 2 and 3. Thus Eq. (10) is three separate equations. These equations represent the Newton's second law written for a continuum in a spatial(or Eulerian) reference frame. Together they relate the rate of change of momentum per unit mass (ρu_i) which is a vector quantity, to the contact and body forces. Equation (11) is the equation for mass conservation in the absence of sources(or sinks) of mass. Incompressible flow implies that derivative of the fluid density is zero. Thus for incompressible flows, the mass conservation equation reduces to:

$$\frac{D\rho}{Dt} = \frac{\partial \tilde{\rho}}{\partial t} + \tilde{u}_j \frac{\partial \tilde{\rho}}{\partial x_j} = 0 \tag{12}$$

The solution scheme is the Semi-Implicit Method for Pressure Linked Equations algorithm (SIMPLE) [5]. Regarding the boundary conditions, the input and the outputs are manually selected by the user through ray tracing technique via the user interface. The initial conditions, the velocity and pressure input is selected by the user.

5   Simulation Studies

This section presents the simulation setup and the user interface implemented in c++ for illustrating the output of the simulation. The input required by the proposed method is a 3D bronchial tree model. The aforementioned model can either be synthetic or originate from available CT scans [7]. After the model is loaded the implemented tool allows the user to pan, rotate zoom in or out the object. The figure below presents a screenshot of the interface after having loaded a synthetic 3D lung model (Fig. 2).

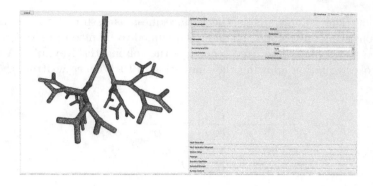

Fig. 2. User interface snapshot

5.1   Interface

The interface includes a geometry processing module and a fluid dynamics module. The first includes an analysis, a skeletonization and a narrowing functional module. The analysis module presents data to the user regarding the number of vertices, the number of faces, minimum and maximum bounds of the object in the 3d space. Additionally, it segments the mesh in selectable parts. The skeletonization converts the 3D Mesh to a curve skeleton allowing the 1D representation providing morphological information to the user. The narrowing part includes a selection functionality, allowing the user to select parts of the mesh and specify the reduction percentage and the custom narrowing function.

The fluid dynamics module includes a simplistic interface setup and an interface setup for the user that is familiar with CFD. The first includes a mesh generation tab, a boundary conditions tab and a runtime tab leaving out details. The mesh generation part includes a functionality that creates the tetrahedral mesh

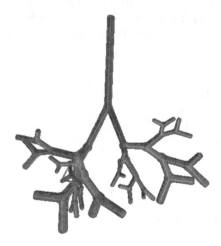

Fig. 3. Curve skeleton for a certain bronchial tree mesh

from the processed surface mesh and a functionality that checks the integrity of the final mesh. The boundary conditions tab allows the user to set the input velocity and pressure and select the inputs and the outputs for the fluid dynamics simulation. Finally, the runtime part allows the user to set the time duration for the simulation to run and start the simulation. After the simulation completion the user can see the results. The advanced user interface part includes specific details relevant to the simulation.

5.2   Results

This section presents results of the execution of the geometry processing module and the fluid dynamics simulation module illustrating all the output of all the

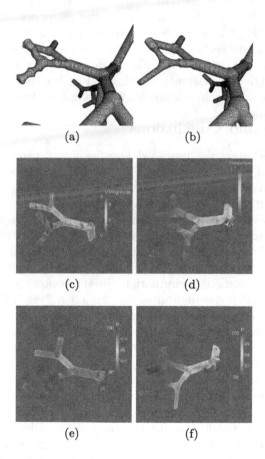

Fig. 4. (a), (b): Bronchoconstriction simulation. The left image shows a uniformly narrowed airway and the right the narrowing of another airway based on a sinusoidal function. (c), (d): Fluid dynamics simulation depicting the air velocity distribution in contracted airways. (e), (f): Fluid dynamics simulation depicting the pressure drop in contracted airways.

supported functionalities that were described in sections three and four. By inspecting Fig. 3 it can be easily seen that the skeletonization process produces a 1D curve skeleton providing a simple morphological representation of the input mesh.

The mesh contraction process either uniform or based on a custom function deforms the selected airway, simulating bronchoconstriction. The results of this method are shown in the following figures. In Fig. 4a we present a branch narrowed by applying a custom(e.g. sinusoidal) function to the lung part selected by the user presented while in Fig. 4b we illustrate the branch contracted in a uniform manner.

Finally, the results of the CFD simulation are presented in Fig. 4. as they were generated by our interface. Figure 4c shows the output of the fluid dynamics simulation depicting velocity distribution. It is obvious that air velocity has decreased in the contracted part in relevance to the non-contracted branch. Within the contracted branch by inspecting the figure we can also see that air velocity is slightly greater in most contracted parts. Similarly, Fig. 4e shows a fluid dynamics simulation showing the pressure drop in the contracted part. Correspondingly, for the uniform case, Fig. 4d shows air velocity distribution verifying the aforementioned observations. Finally Fig. 4f shows clearly a pressure drop in the contracted part in relevance with the non-contracted one.

6   Discussion and Conclusions

The benefits of including the proposed lung geometry processing approaches to a computational model are twofold. The first is that these approaches are essential for creating patient specific 3d models, corresponding to different levels of airway narrowing related to different levels of inflammation, from existing 3D models that have been constructed from available CT/MRI scans. Thus, the user can study the changes in airflow during bronchoconstriction by inspecting the outcome of the CFD simulations. In addition, they could be also applied in cases that these scans are not available. This can be achieved by performing iteratively the aforementioned geometry deformations in the context of an optimization approach so as to match specific Pulmonary Function Test (PFT) metrics that assess and quantify airflow limitation. These metrics include forced vital capacity (FVC), i.e. the amount of air a person can exhale with force after inhaling as deeply as possible and forced expiratory volume (FEV) i.e. the amount of air a person can exhale with force in one breath.

Regarding our limitations, in order to be able to provide validation of the bronchoconstriction appearing in obstructive lung diseases during crisis such as asthma or permanently COPD, are needed CT scans from patients with the aforementioned diseases. Additionally, we would like to point out that the definition of a custom function that simulates appropriately the surface abnormalities during bronchoconstriction is a crucial task that we are currently investigating.

Acknowledgments. This work has been funded by the H2020-PHC-2014-2015 Project MyAirCoach (Grant Agreement No. 643607).

References

1. World health organization: World Health Statistics Geneva, Switzerland (2008)
2. Au, O.K.C., Tai, C.L., Chu, H.K., Cohen-Or, D., Lee, T.Y.: Skeleton extraction by mesh contraction. In: ACM Transactions on Graphics (TOG), vol. 27, p. 44. ACM (2008)
3. Darquenne, C., van Ertbruggen, C., Prisk, G.K.: Convective flow dominates aerosol delivery to the lung segments. J. Appl. Physiol. **111**(1), 48–54 (2011)
4. De Backer, J., Vos, W., Gorle, C., Germonpré, P., Partoens, B., Wuyts, F., Parizel, P.M., De Backer, W.: Flow analyses in the lower airways: patient-specific model and boundary conditions. Med. Eng. Phys. **30**(7), 872–879 (2008)
5. Ferziger, J.H., Peric, M.: Computational Methods for Fluid Dynamics. Springer, Heidelberg (2012)
6. Jasak, H., Jemcov, A., Tukovic, Z.: Openfoam: A C++ library for complex physics simulations. In: International Workshop on Coupled Methods in Numerical Dynamics, vol. 1000, pp. 1–20 (2007)
7. Lambert, A.R., O'shaughnessy, P.T., Tawhai, M.H., Hoffman, E.A., Lin, C.L.: Regional deposition of particles in an image-based airway model: large-eddy simulation and left-right lung ventilation asymmetry. Aerosol Sci. Technol. **45**(1), 11–25 (2011)
8. Lambert, R.K., Wilson, T.A., Hyatt, R.E., Rodarte, J.R.: A computational model for expiratory flow. J. Appl. Physiol. **52**(1), 44–56 (1982)
9. Lin, C.L., Tawhai, M.H., Hoffman, E.A.: Multiscale image-based modeling and simulation of gas flow and particle transport in the human lungs. Wiley Interdisc. Rev. Syst. Biol. Med. **5**(5), 643–655 (2013)
10. Rausch, S., Martin, C., Bornemann, P., Uhlig, S., Wall, W.: Material model of lung parenchyma based on living precision-cut lung slice testing. J. Mech. Behav. Biomed. Mater. **4**(4), 583–592 (2011)
11. Schmidt, A., Zidowitz, S., Kriete, A., Denhard, T., Krass, S., Peitgen, H.O.: A digital reference model of the human bronchial tree. Comput. Med. Imaging Graph. **28**(4), 203–211 (2004)
12. Swan, A.J., Clark, A.R., Tawhai, M.H.: A computational model of the topographic distribution of ventilation in healthy human lungs. J. Theor. Biol. **300**, 222–231 (2012)
13. Tawhai, M.H., Nash, M.P., Lin, C.L., Hoffman, E.A.: Supine and prone differences in regional lung density and pleural pressure gradients in the human lung with constant shape. J. Appl. Physiol. **107**(3), 912–920 (2009)
14. Yin, Y., Choi, J., Hoffman, E.A., Tawhai, M.H., Lin, C.L.: A multiscale MDCT image-based breathing lung model with time-varying regional ventilation. J. Comput. Phys. **244**, 168–192 (2013)

Bone Structure Monitoring Systems Applied to Physiotherapy of Children with Cerebral Palsy

Danilo Saravia[1] and Victor M. Gonzalez[2(✉)]

[1] Universidad del Azuay, Cuenca, Ecuador
danilosaravia@hotmail.com
[2] Instituto Tecnologico Autonomo de Mexico, Mexico, Mexico
victor.gonzalez@itam.mx

Abstract. The cerebral palsy (CP) is an irreversible disorder that affects the human brain and causes problems with mobility and communication. This paper presents the results of designing, implementing and evaluating an easy-to-use and low-cost equipment that seeks to increase the motivation and effort of the children with cerebral palsy while they do their physical therapies. Through a validation process with the help of patients and physiotherapists, we designed a set of multi-media applications that were evaluated with children with cerebral palsy while doing their therapies. Our emphasis was on providing support for the distension muscle exercises as they are identified as the most painful activities that take place in a physical therapy session. The application was based on a Wiimote control, connected to a personal computer via Bluetooth, as a receptor of the infrared light emitted by a simple control made of an infrared led, an interrupter and a battery.

Keywords: Assistive environments · Cerebral palsy · Bone movement-tracking

1 Introduction

Many applications have been built around devices emitting and receiving signals of infrared light. In 2008, Johnny Chung Lee showed the potential of using the Nintendo Wiimote control, a receiver of infrared light, for the purposes of creating a low-cost interactive whiteboard [1]. Similarly, Joa Ebert and Thibault Imbert developed a programming library called Action Script 3 Wiiflash, which allows connecting the Wiimote to the computer to generate applications or control movements based games [2]. These achievements have enabled low-cost body-computer interaction scenarios, where the movement of a person is transformed into a computer action. Such applications can clearly be extended beyond entertainment and support other goals such as physical therapies based on motivating body movements.

Physiotherapy is a resource that is used in the treatment of children with cerebral palsy (CP), in order to maintain or improve their capacity of movement; thus depending on the particular scenario presented by a child with this type of brain disorder, a physiotherapist might apply different physical exercises. Regardless of the mental-physical situation held by the patient, all exercises involve muscle strain. The exercises of muscle strain are activities requiring great physical effort and often causing pain and discomfort

© Springer International Publishing Switzerland 2016
V.G. Duffy (Ed.): DHM 2016, LNCS 9745, pp. 110–119, 2016.
DOI: 10.1007/978-3-319-40247-5_12

in children; and by being a repetitive activity, they may produce boredom. The pain, discomfort and the boredom related to practicing these exercises become factors that cause children to seek to leave such therapies.

This paper presents the results of designing, implementing and evaluating a bone movement-tracking computer application for supporting muscle strain therapies by children with CP, which is both inexpensive and easy to use. Our design is based on the use of a Wiimote control and an infrared signal, which is emitted by a secondary control, which moves and produces an action on the computer screen. Based on our results we can argue that the usefulness of this basic interaction is likely to increase motivation and the effort made by children with cerebral palsy, while performing muscle strain exercises during physical therapies.

2 The Concept

One challenge commonly encountered in the work with children with cerebral palsy is to capture and hold their attention while performing any activity. However, this lack of attention does not always occur when interacting with a computer. Thus, a good alternative to work with these children is to try to include activities based on computer devices that attract their attention as a result of the interaction [3].

Furthermore, considering that pain, physical exertion and boredom are the components that produce nuisance and abandonment of physical therapies by children, the main idea of this project was to create a playful multimedia system, which provides physical therapists with a tool that allows them to apply muscle strain exercises in a nice and simple way. The implicit goal of our design is to get the child to play while doing physical therapy. Likewise, our system was designed to be adapted to different levels of patients' motor skills as there is variation on them.

Finally, our design considers that the use of multimedia elements within therapies could generate a "biofeedback" where the children with cerebral palsy associate the movement of their body with possible events that are raised on a screen [4].

3 Materials

3.1 Wiimote and Wiiflash

For this project we used the Nintendo Wiimote control, which has a receiver of infrared light to detect up to four lights of this type, and based on that determining its position on a screen. With respect to programming the applications, this was done using a library of Action Script 3 Wiiflash. We also used the Wiiflash server program that allows the connection between the computer and Wiimote [2].

3.2 Controls

Given that the level of spasticity in children with cerebral palsy is not always the same, the control system that we designed avoids the use of buttons and complex gestures.

Moreover, given its size, it allows to be placed in different parts of the body to facilitate its use.

The controls that we developed are based on a simple circuit where a 1.5-volt battery uses a pulsing switch to turn an infrared LED. Based on this principle two designs for the control device were defined and are described in the following lines (Fig. 1).

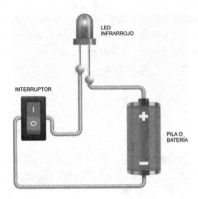

Fig. 1. Basic operation of the control circuit

Control Type One. For this model of control, the idea was to produce a rectangular shape that has a minimum size, which allows it to be placed in different parts of the body by means of Velcro straps, handles or headbands. The materials used in this control are a piece of plastic (box), 2 cm by 4 cm and 1.5 cm thick, which served as a box in which it is installed an infrared LED connected to a watch battery of 1.5 volts and a switch (Fig. 2).

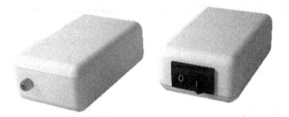

Fig. 2. Image of control type one

Control Type Two. For the form of this control the idea was to think on an exercise based on riding a bicycles and how it can be achieved. The idea and motivation for designing this type of control is because existing machines on the market have a high cost. With regard to the materials used to manufacture this control, we used wood (mdf) 15 mm to generate the case and in this where an axis passing through a bearing with smaller pivots. The movement generates a pulse that in once turned on the light generating interaction with the application on the screen (Fig. 3).

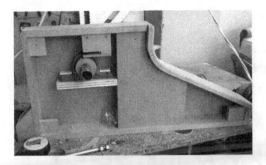
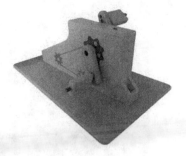

Fig. 3. Control type two mechanism

4 Applications

The applications we designed were defined from our analysis of the basic muscle strain exercises that we observed being applied in physical therapies. Thus it has sought to take into account the three body parts that generate most of the movements: the head, arms and legs.

4.1 Application 1 – Shooting Game

The exercise of distended arms for children with CP comprises an activity of flexion and extension that seeks to relax the muscles of the limb. Thus we created a target shooting game where the child must perform this exercise (flexion and extension of arm) to achieve shooting an arrow into a target displayed on screen (Fig. 4).

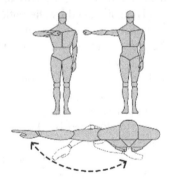

Fig. 4. Arm distension exercise

Application Operation. The application is controlled by two main components of interface where in the first instance, the therapist is the one who controls and defines the complexity of the exercise through activation buttons (G) for accelerating the speed at which the target moves. The physical therapist can restart the game at any time by pulsing a button (H). The therapist interacts with the application via the computer mouse (Fig. 5).

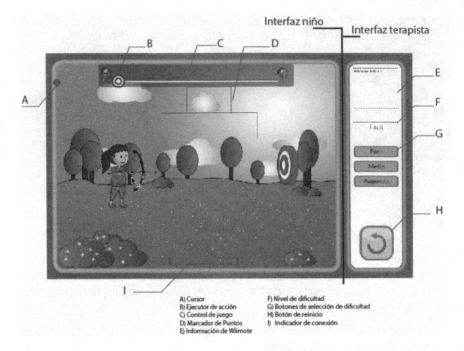

Fig. 5. Shooting game interface: (A) Cursor, (B) Executor of action, (C) Game control, (D) Score, (E) Wiimote info, (F) Level of difficulty, (G) Selection of difficulty, (H) Restart button, (I) Connection indicator.

In the second interface (main area depicting a kid with an arch), the cursor (A) is controlled by the IR remote that is manipulated by the patient. The patient attempts to drag the cursor to the executor of action (B) for this to move up to a distance limit from where the action of shooting the arrow at a fixed target or a target that is moving will be done.

The use of such controls and tracking system of bone structure allows the exercise to change in complexity and how it is performed depends on the location and rotation of the Wii control with respect to infrared control.

In Fig. 6, the moving distance (y) achieved by the patient is a function of (x) the distance between the Wiimote and the patient.

If the control is rotated, the arrangement or interaction of the exercise changes since it depends on its rotation. Consequently, exercises can be done from left to right, right to left, top-down or bottom-up. This allows the same application to change the way in which it runs in a simple way providing so much flexibility for applications requiring it (Fig. 7).

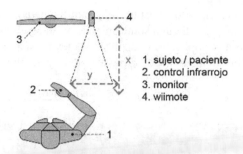

Fig. 6. Interaction of the controls (1. Patient, 2. Infrared control, 3. Screen, 4. Wiimote)

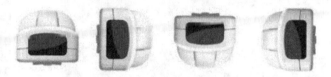

Fig. 7. Wiimote control rotation

4.2 Application 2 – Bicycle Simulation

In muscle strain exercises, the therapists apply leg flexion and extension, where the work done simulates the action of pedaling, but in a horizontal position (the patient laying on a surface) (Fig. 8).

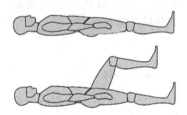

Fig. 8. Legs distension exercise

Application Operation. This application simulates a bicycle race to motivate the child with CP to perform an exercise where stretching and contraction of legs is achieved within the context of a leg pedaling action on a bicycle. The interface of this game is controlled by two users: the child and the physiotherapist. Thus the physiotherapist is who can control the level of difficulty application (F), while they can also determine when the game starts or restarts using the button (G). The child, once the game has started, should start pedaling so the figure on the screen (A) starts to move up to the checkered flag. The control that we designed for this game has a base with pedals that allows the exercise to be conducted from a chair or wheel chair depending on the case.

This control also has the facility to adjust the length of the pedal lever to adjust it to the length of the children's legs. Although some children with cerebral palsy cannot move their legs, this stretch is also applicable to them since they must avoid muscle spasticity. If this were the case, this application could run assisted by the therapist (Fig. 9).

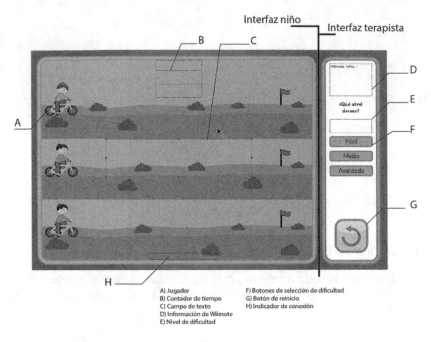

Fig. 9. Bicycle simulation game interface: (A) Player, (B) Time counter, (C) Text field, (D) Wiimote info, (E) Difficulty level, (F) Selection of difficulty, (G) Restart button, (H) Connection Indicator.

4.3   Application 3 – Pick a Color Game

Although the head is not considered an extremity (tip), it is a joint body part, which in the treatment of cerebral palsy should be exercised to avoid having bad posture, which might result on other problems. That is why we designed an application in which there is a dynamic movement of the head as the main mechanism of interaction (Fig. 10).

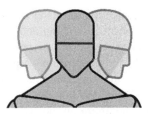

Fig. 10. Head movement

Application operation This application (Fig. 11) seeks to exercise the head with an associative game of shapes and colors where the child can indicate the color of a fruit by moving his head; the game can also be controlled by using the arms. The interface requires the physiotherapist to use the selector (E) to define a fruit that appears on the board (C) and thus the child moves the cursor (A) to set the color of the fruit selected.

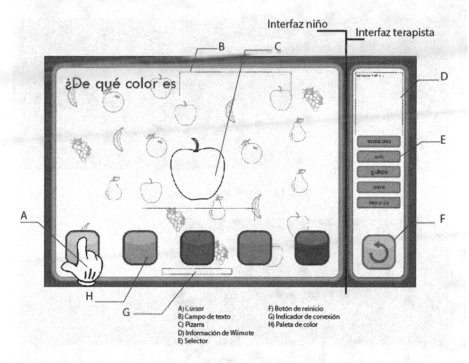

Fig. 11. Pick a color game interface. (A) Cursor, (B) Text field, (C) Whiteboard, (D) Wiimote info, (E) Selector, (F) Restart button, (G) Connection indicator, (H) Color Palette (Color figure online).

5   Results

The results of this research have been satisfactory since it has been possible to see the benefits of a therapy based in the implementation of a bone movement-tracking system as the Wiimote. Through a series of tests with twelve children (9 with limited CP and 3 with high CP) at the Instituto Stephen Hawking in Cuenca, Ecuador, we noticed that running a therapy for a child with CP based on a fun application, helped them to perform better their exercises of muscle strain, kept them motivated and they began to lose their fear of this type of therapy. Figures 12 and 13 shows pictures of one of the children performing the activities.

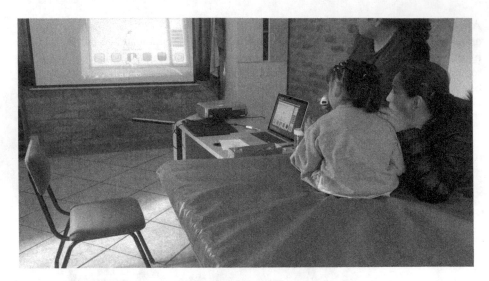

Fig. 12. Application testing

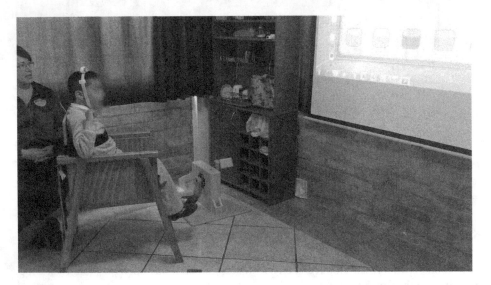

Fig. 13. Application testing

Similarly, the simple and friendly interaction that is created between the child and the application allows a reaction from the brain where it can learn how to make a body part to react for a certain activity.

The possibility that this bone movement-tracking system could be adapted to different degrees of motor skills gives our design flexibility to support different types of applications that pursue other learning or communication purposes.

One point that should be made clear, is that the application of this technology within physiotherapy of children with CP, does not seek to displace or replace the activity of the physical therapists, but rather, one should consider that this technology is a tool to support their work.

6 Conclusions

For the treatment of cerebral palsy there are several therapies, where it is intended that the child with a brain affected, depending on the degree of affection they have, can learn to perform certain activities based on perception and motor development. Because of this, the motivation that a child may have plays a very important role in the rehabilitation; thus games can become a necessary tool and ally for the creation of effective therapeutic activities.

This research project has revealed that the implementation of a Bone movement-tracking system, as is the Wiimote, within the physiotherapy which applies to children with cerebral palsy, can be effective because beyond the benefit of providing a fun method for exercises which usually (in the traditional way) can be annoying or boring, you can generate a neuro-perception based on where the brain learns and relates a movement with a learning event.

The applications that we designed for this research have shown a good level of effectiveness, because during the tests we performed it has been noted an increase in motivation and effort put by children to perform relaxation exercises.

In addition, we can see that the cost to build the controls that are required for the applications is low compared to the others machines and tools used in physical therapy. An advantage that has been found in the creation of these applications is that infrared controls that are used to detect the movement can be of any shape while an infrared light is lit and can be detected by the Wiimote.

The use of this type of controls and intuitive interfaces, allows the development of applications that can be adapted to different cases or levels of motor skills experienced by children with cerebral palsy. This becomes an advantage in comparison to other solutions that are usually designed and defined from fixed anthropometric and ergonomic requirements.

Acknowledgment. We would like to take all participants and physiotherapists that help us to inform our study, and evaluate our design. We thank the Instituto Stephen Hawking de Cuenca, Ecuador for their support. We would like to thank the support for the second author from Association Mexicana de la Cultura, A.C.

References

1. Raya, R., Ceres, R., Rocon, E., Frizera, A., Pons, J.L.: Comunicador inercial para potenciar la autonomía de niños con parálisis cerebral en el uso del computador (2009)
2. Lee, J.C.: Hacking the Nintendo Wii remote. Pervasive Comput. **7**(3), 39–45 (2008)
3. Ebert, J., Imbert, T.: 21 Octubre 2015. wiiflash.bytearray.org. Retrieved from WiiFlash. http://wiiflash.bytearray.org/?page_id=2
4. Rosas, R., Perez, C., Olguin, P.: Pizarra interactivas para un aprendizaje motivado en niños con paralisis cerebral (2010)

Motion Prediction and Recognition

Exploring Rhythmic Patterns in Dance Movements by Video Analysis

Camilo Argüello and Marcela Iregui[✉]

Universidad Militar Nueva Granada, Bogotá, Colombia
{u1201244,hilda.iregui}@unimilitar.edu.co

Abstract. Treatments of coordination disorders may be benefit from modern assistive technologies by achieving effective feedback that improves the rehabilitation protocols. In this paper, a method to identify movement patterns from video sequences is presented, providing acoustic stimuli by means of sounds generated from motion analysis. The method explores rhythmic patterns in movements, through fundamental concepts as: motion detection and analysis, Principal Component Analysis (PCA) and frequency analysis. The proposed method was evaluated by using four (4) dance steps, used typically in Latin music, showing good performance in detecting and reproducing acoustic beats.

1 Introduction

The rhythm has an important role in human life by enhancing perceptive functions and sensitivity. Especially, corporal rhythm contributes to the improve motor, visual and auditory skills [1] and hence the physical and social-emotional development.

Previous researches have demonstrated that rhythm is typically developed between 4 and 8 years of age [4]. To be able to keep musical rhythm with body motion means perceiving changes in the cadence or sound type. However, some people have limitations to coordinate any movement, because their cognitive, psychological and motor processes are not developed. In children this is known as Developmental Coordination Disorder (DCD), which includes limitations in the three process mentioned previously [5]. This trouble makes it difficult to perform the required corporal expression on some activities such as dance where it means be able to perceive changes in speed and sound types. The objective of this work is to bring support to people who have some coordination troubles in dance, especially keeping the musical rhythm with their body, by means of a feedback i.e. to give the possibility for people to listen their sound pattern based on their movements, through computer technology by using interaction techniques based on computer vision algorithms, signal processing and audio synthesis.

This paper is organized as follows. The Sect. 2 displays the related work in musical applications interaction. The Sect. 3 focuses on the explanation of the proposed method. In Sect. 4, a results and evaluations are presented. The Sect. 5

© Springer International Publishing Switzerland 2016
V.G. Duffy (Ed.): DHM 2016, LNCS 9745, pp. 123–131, 2016.
DOI: 10.1007/978-3-319-40247-5_13

shows a discussion of experimental results. The Sect. 6 contains the conclusions as well as the future work directions. Finally, acknowledgements section displays the Acknowledgements.

2   Related Work

Researches have pursed different approaches regarding musical applications that use the human-computer interaction and specifically corporal motion and audio synthesis. One of those which was development by Chattopadhay [11], taking available technologies as Microsoft Xbox Kinect to label some body positions in musical notes through tracking in real time of human skeleton. Another research made by Shiratori [13] which the main target is to realize an audio synthesis based on a dance perform video, using relationships between corporal motion and musical rhythm and comparing speed of both respectively. Also, several works have been analysing the human being motion, specially approached to aspects like a treatments for gait rehabilitation in Parkinson's Disease [12] analysing the gait patterns of a person with Parkinson's disease and another person without this disease.

In this paper, It's presented a method that makes an approach for analysis of rhythmic patterns in dance movements based on segmented video input. Unlike most previous methods where to the problem of rhythmic stimulation was included using available technologies or computer vision techniques without auditory response, this approach generates an audio response which perform as rhythmic auditory feedback, from input parameters extracted of motion periodic patterns.

3   Proposed Method

Interaction process starts by recording a video of an individual dancing a specific latin music step. Sequences of periodic movements of both lower limbs in the video are analysed to find motion patterns and finally produce a rhythmic sound using the workflow, Fig. 1. Next, the process that shows the hypothesis, is presented with its corresponding description.

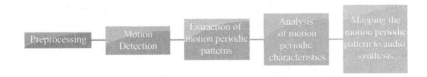

Fig. 1. Work flow proposed method

3.1   Preprocessing

Starting from a video input, the first step corresponds to filtering and color transformation. The video is transformed to grayscale using RGB to YUV transform. Additionally, a Median filter is set to reduce the noise in the video.

3.2   Motion Detection

In order to segment the video by extracting the background. The Sigma Delta proposed by Manzanera [6], algorithm was used. For the initialization, the method reads the video frame by frame, each one represented as $I_t(x)$ and the initialization it's matched with estimated background value, described as $M_t(x)$. The same way, the algorithm update the estimate using the sign function Eq. 2, which returns three values depending the input value, and the estimate varies a bit. So, each frame, the estimate is simply incremented by one if it's smaller than the sample, or decremented by one if it's greater than the sample.

$$sign(n) = \begin{cases} -1 & \text{if } n < 0 \\ 1 & \text{if } n > 0 \\ 0 & \text{if } n = 0 \end{cases} \tag{2}$$

Once the background is estimated, the next step is to calculate differences between consecutive frames with the background. Finally, the algorithm considers a thresholding process for rendering the detection. Algorithm 1

The result, as shown in Fig. 2, presents motion detection of the lower limbs.

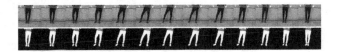

Fig. 2. Motion Detection results with an image sequence making

3.3   Extraction of Motion Periodic Patterns

After the pattern is determined, and the characteristic that define the motion type is obtained, the method consists in analyzing the video to find profiles for the X and Y directions, Fig. 3. The goal is to determine the motion in each specific direction. A normalized image is created with the profile values for each axis. As an example, Fig. 4 shows the patterns for a step side by side. Colors represent intensity values of the frequency of movements, i.e. if the colors tend to red there is many motion times.

Algorithm 1. The $\Sigma - \Delta$ background estimation

Initialization
for each pixel x **do**
    $M_0(x) = I_0(x)$
end for
For each frame t
for each pixel x **do**
    $M_t(x) = M_{t-1}(x) + sign(I_t(x) - M_{t-1}(x))$
end for
For each frame t
for each pixel x **do**
    $\Delta_t(x) = |M_t(x) = I_t(x)|$
end for
For each frame t
for each pixel x
if $I_t(x) < \Delta_t(x)$ **then**
    $D_t(x) = 0$
else
    $D_t(x) = 1$
end if

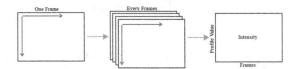

Fig. 3. Representation of profile sum for each frame

3.4   Analysis of Motion Periodic Characteristic

To extract periodicity information in figure a dimensionality reduction is performed using the Principal Component Analysis (PCA) method [7,9], which projects data in a new subspace Fig. 5. The most powerful ingredient that has PCA is to keep the same relationship in the new data set. One side maximizes the variance of projection data for each component and another side reduces the error rate of reconstruction.

For example, given a data set belonging to $\mathbb{R}^p$ space:

$$x_1, x_2, \ldots, x_n \in \mathbb{R}^p \tag{1}$$

PCA defines data reconstruction in $\mathbb{R}^q$ to $\mathbb{R}^p$ as

$$f(\lambda) = \mu + v_q \lambda \tag{2}$$

Being $\mu \in \mathbb{R}^p$ and v_q a $p \times q$ matrix taking q as orthogonal unit vectors. Also, $\lambda \in \mathbb{R}^q$ is new data of projected dimensionality. An important factor making process of dimensionality reduction is to minimize the reconstruction error shown in Eq. 3.

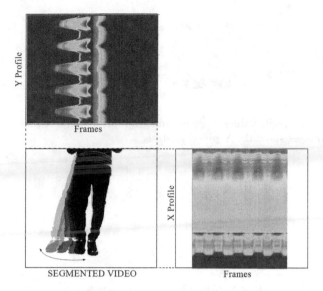

Fig. 4. Representation of a extraction of motion periodic patterns. The lower left box displays the segmented video with the dance movement. The upper left box shows the profile extracted from video for Y pixels and the lower right box shows the profile for X pixels. The upper right box displays 3D image taking the intensity value.

$$\min_{\mu_1 \lambda_1 \dots N v_q} \sum_{n=1}^{N} \| X_n - \mu - v_q \lambda_n \| \tag{3}$$

For this case μ is intersection point between subspace and original space. The above defines a $\mathbb{R}^p$ using μ and v_q as is shown in Fig. 5.

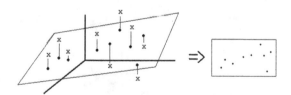

Fig. 5. Data projection with PCA, projecting $\mathbb{R}^3$ data to $\mathbb{R}^2$, made by Blei [9]

The Fig. 6 has three parameters (x, y, z), which represent frame number, profile value and pixel intensity respectively, i.e. data set $(x, y, z) \in \mathbb{R}^3$. When the dimensionality reduction is made, the result is a signal, i.e. data set $(x, y, z) \in \mathbb{R}^2$ with the same periodic pattern like the image created.

To determine the periodicity value, a frequency analysis of the resulting signal is performed, in order to find the fundamental frequency (Fig. 7).

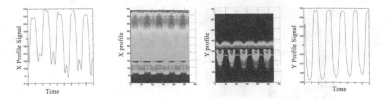

Fig. 6. Image with profile values. Two left images represent the X pixels analysis, and the two right images show the Y pixels analysis

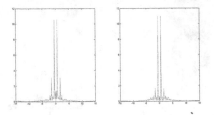

Fig. 7. Signal in frequency domain

3.5   Mapping the Motion Periodic Pattern to Audio Synthesis

Once obtained the results of frequency analysis, The feedback audio is produced to create a beat which reflects the periodic pattern according to video input parameters at the cadence of the dance steps. Thus, audio produced offers the possibility to the person of listening with how often the the movement is realized, which it's a feedback that makes understand the speed of dance movement in progress (Fig. 8).

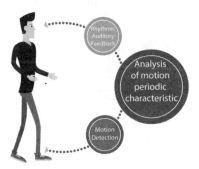

Fig. 8. System structure

4   Results and Evaluations

The method effectiveness was assessed by determining variations between control and the automated groups. The performed evaluation aims to verify that

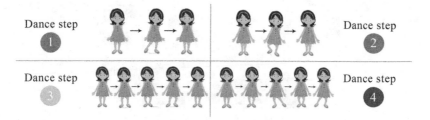

Fig. 9. The basics 4 dance steps established. 1 shows the first step, which it's charac terized to carry the right or left foot to the side, then return it to the starting position and repeat the process. 2 the movement is to raise the left or right foot. 3 the person must move from side to side to make the step correctly. 4 provides the ability to perform it with more rhythmic expression because it contains two times; the first is to alternate between right and left foot and the second is the kick.

the produced sound is consistent with the motion. Forty-eight (48) videos were used for testing, recorded from twelve (12) persons, each with four (4) dancing steps (Fig. 9). From each video, the beat is extracted and compared with reference values manually selected by an expert. The objective is to measure the misalignment between periods in both signals in milliseconds. Table 1 shows the results value and the Fig. 10, shows that results measuring each person and the difference range in miliseconds.

Table 1. Table of difference value between method and control values on milliseconds (ms). The control values were established based on expected data for each dance step, in this case the expected data were defined taking information of one person who doesn't have troubles keeping time of the rhythm. If the difference among Control Value and Result tends to zero, the method is most accurate.

User	Step 1	Step 2	Step 3	Step 4
1	0.177	0.057	0.005	0.612
2	0.095	0.323	0.152	0.211
3	0.118	0.296	0.005	0.612
4	0.019	0.091	0.188	0.410
5	0.073	0.295	0.071	0.143
6	0.004	0.043	0.118	0.217
7	0.019	0.081	0.066	0.457
8	0.011	0.096	0.112	0.746
9	0.113	0.032	0.081	0.621
10	0.007	0.103	0.045	0.132
11	0.012	0.067	0.184	0.383
12	0.080	0.096	0.055	0.486

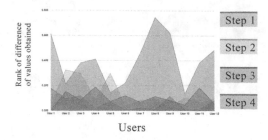

Fig. 10. Graph of difference value between method and control values, it based on table presented in Table 1

5   Discussion

Analyzing the obtained results, the method works correctly when simple movements are performed. The first three steps show among 58 % and 75 % of accuracy, i.e. the margin of difference is lower than 0.100ms. However, for complex steps (4), the method precision is lower. (Fig. 11)

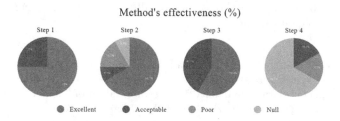

Fig. 11. Percentage of Method's effectiveness for each dance step. The blue colors represent higher accuracy and the yellow colors represent lower accuracy. (Color figure online)

When each movement was analysed, it was checked the pattern that defines the characteristic of the motion came from Y profile image. Also, it was proved that the most dance movements created an sinusoidal waveform, because the movement is constantly repeated.

6   Conclusions and Future Work

This work presents a method that determines, from a video sequence, the beat associated to the body motion. The proposed method is useful at identifying periodic patterns in actual motion. This study marks a starting point with the proposed motion analysis in dance steps. However, for complex movements it is necessary to improve the method.

The study of human movement will always require more optimization in terms of processing, systems interaction, etc. The proposed method is made available to be used in more aspects of people's life, not only for entertainment purposes. It can also be used for patients who suffer diseases such as Parkinson, supporting treatments related to gait analysis.

Acknowledgements. We appreciate the anonymous reviewers for their helpful comments provided during the development of this work. Also, we are grateful to Acceder Research group and its members.

References

1. Perez, M · Rhythm and Musical Orientation. Universidad del Atlantico, Barranquilla (2012)
2. Phillips-Silver, J., Trainor, L.J.: Feeling the beat: movement influences infant rhythm perception. Science **308**, 1430 (2005). sciencemag.org
3. Thaut, M., Abiru, M.: Rhythmic Auditory Stimulation in Rehabilitation of Movement Disorders: A Review of Current Research. Colorado State University, Kyoto University, Kyoto (2009)
4. Zentner, M., Eerola, T.: Rhythmic engagement with music in infancy. Proc. Natl. Acad. Sci. U S A **107**(13), 576–873 (2010). doi:10.1073/pnas.1000121107. Department of Psychology, University of York. United Kingdom
5. Missiuna, C., Rivard, L., Pollock, N.: Children with Developmental Coordination Disorder: at home, at School and in the Community. Mc Master University, Hamilton (2011). School of rehabilitation science
6. Manzanera, A., Richefeu, J.: A new motion detection algorithm based on - background estimation. Ecole Nationale Suprieure de Techinques Avances (ENSTA), Laboratoire dElectronique de Informatique (LEI), Paris, France (2006)
7. Jolliffe, I.: Principal Component Analysis, 2nd edn. University of Aberdeen, Aberdeen (2002). Department of Mathematical Sciences
8. Gomez, E.: Introduction to Sound Synthesis. Escola Superior de Musica de Catalunya, Barcelona (2009). Departament of Sonologia
9. Blei, D.: Cos 424: Interacting with Data. Scribe by: CJ Bell and Ana Pop
10. Ortega, M.: Lecciones de Fisica Mecnica 2. Universidad de Cordoba, Cordoba (2006). Departamento de Fisica Aplicada
11. Berg, T., Chattopadhyay, D., Schedel, M., Vallier, T.: Human Motion Initiated Music Generation using Skeletal Traking by Kinect (2011)
12. Cho, C.W., Chao, W.H., Lin, S.H., Chen, Y.Y.: A vision-based analysis system for gait recognition in patients with Parinsons disease. Department of Electrical and control engineering, National Chiao University. Department of Biomedical Engineering, Yuanpe University. Department of neurology, Tzu Chi General Hospital, Taiwan (2009)
13. Shiratori, T.: Synthesis of Dance Performance Based on Analyses of Human Motion and Music. University of Tokyo, Tokyo (2006)
14. de Rossi, I., Gallo, F., Gonzales, D.: Prctico de la Salsa. Prof. Alexis Frutos (2010)

Study on Braiding Skills by Comparing Between Expert and Non-experts with Eye's Movement Measurement

Tadashi Uozumi[1], Shuhei Yasuda[2], Kontawat Chottikampon[2(✉)],
Suchalinee Mathurosemontri[2], Akihiko Goto[3], and Hiroyuki Hamada[2]

[1] Gifu University, 1-1 Yanagido, Gifu City, 501-1193, Japan
[2] Kyoto Institute of Technology, Matsugasaki, Sakyo-ku, Kyoto 606-8585, Japan
ruklongtime@hotmail.com
[3] Osaka Sangyo University, 3-1-1 Nakagaito, Daito, Osaka 574-8530, Japan

Abstract. A braiding rope is the Japanese traditional rope that a quality and beauty of them have depended on the skill and experience of a braider. In this research, the skill of an expert and two non-experts who practice the braiding every day and every week, respectively were measured and compared through the eye's movement measurement and observed the braiding rope quality. The measurement was carried out every month for three times. It was found that the expert showed the constant of eye's focus at the center of a marudai plate and revealed a complete pattern of braiding rope. For two non-experts, their eye's movement wobbled around the marudai plate for all trials. Furthermore, expert's skill was investigated focusing on how to keep location of braid rope at the center of marudai plate during braiding process. We clarified the way how the strands were moved above the marudai plate to make good braid rope.

Keywords: Braiding · Kumihimo · Eye's movement measurement · Braiding skill

1 Introduction

Kumihimo is a traditional Japanese braiding technique that is used for making of long decorative rope. In that past, kimihimo is the important accessories for Japanese kimono and samurai armor. The styles and uses for the braids have changed over time. Nowadays, these braiding ropes are used in a variety of decorative ways. Some people wear them as bracelets or necklaces. In general silk was used as a braiding material due to its beauty and strength. However, many types of fiber can be used to braid kumihimo such as cotton floss or pearl cotton even metallic thread is used also. The beauty of the braid is accomplished by the color of threads. For the processing, the Japanese braiding technique is braided by specialized stands. The most common pattern of kumihimo is carried out on the marudai, which means a round stand. The braiding is done on the top of the marudai plate and the finished braid goes down at the center of the plate. The sequence of moving the treads creates the shape. The initial placement of the colors will create a repeating pattern. The shape is usually round. However, there are many shapes that can be created from the different specialized stand such as a square shape, which is braided

© Springer International Publishing Switzerland 2016
V.G. Duffy (Ed.): DHM 2016, LNCS 9745, pp. 132–139, 2016.
DOI: 10.1007/978-3-319-40247-5_14

from kakudai or square stand [1, 2]. We have researched braiding skill by analysis of maker's motion and eye's movement comparing between expert and non-expert [3]. These results indicated that one of important points to making "good braiding ropes" was to keep braiding rope position at the center of a marudai plate during braiding process. "Good braiding ropes" means that braid pattern was aligned longitudinally.

In this study, new measurement method was developed in order to evaluate linearity of braid pattern. The measurement results were compared between expert and non-experts. Furthermore, expert's skill was investigated focusing on how to keep location of braid rope at the center of marudai plate during braiding process. We investigated especially the way how the strands were moved above the marudai plate.

2   Braiding Method

The cotton strands and the marudai stand were prepared for braiding experiment. The first braiding step starts by gathering all eight strands and ties a knot at one end as shown in Fig. 1(a). Then drop the knotted end into the center of a hole of the marudai in Fig. 1(b). Next separate the strands out into four groups with two strands each and lay them over the marudai as in Fig. 1(c). After that reel strands around the bobbins tightly as presented in Fig. 1(d).

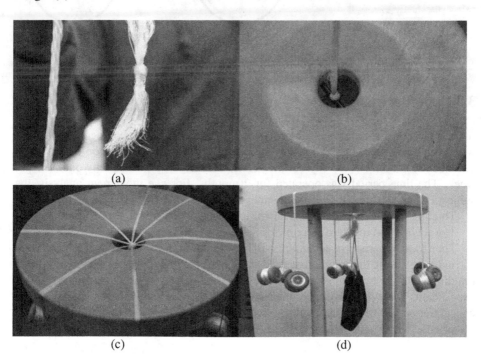

(a)   (b)

(c)   (d)

Fig. 1. Strand and marudai stand preparation

The braiding method is shown in Fig. 2. Firstly, to start by moving the strand A across strand B and strand E across strand F. After that move strand C across strand D and strand G across strand H. Next the strands are braided anticlockwise. To start by moving the strand F across strand C and strand B across strand G. Finally move strand D across strand A and strand H across strand E. Continue the braiding from first step until finish.

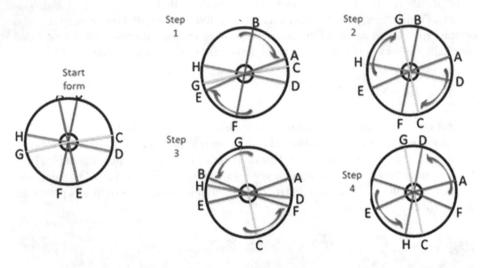

Fig. 2. Braiding method

3   Experimental

In this research, there are three subjects of the expert and two of non-experts. The expert will teach both of the non-experts how to fabricate kumihimo. Firstle, non-expert has to practice the braiding every day but the second non-expert practices only one time per week. The time period was operated for 2 months. For eye movement analysis, the subjects were measured their eye movement for three times as tabulated in Table 1.

The first started after the expert taught two non-experts how to braid kumihimo.

The second and the third were measured after 1 and 2 month later.

Then the comparison of a braiding skill between the expert and two non-experts were carried out by using the common method as the marudai plate. In order to study the basic braiding skill, the braiding speed was the first parameter that was investigated in this experiment. The eye's movement measurement was selected to study and explain the concentration position of braider's eyes during the process. The braiding ropes were observed and measured the diameter to evaluate the quality of ropes.

Table 1. Summary of the experimental

Sample	Braiding practiced time	Eyes movement testing
Expert	X	1st
Non-Expert 1	Everyday	1st, 2nd and 3rd
Non-Expert 2	1 time/week	
1st	2nd	3rd
First day	After 1 month	After 2 month

4   Comparison of Braiding Rope Quality

A quality and a beauty of the braiding rope of the expert and non-experts were observed. Figure 3 shows photographs of braiding ropes. The braiding rope of the expert revealed the complete braiding pattern along the rope. The quality of braiding ropes that were fabricated by both of non-experts at the first trial showed the defects due to the incorrect pattern. However, the everyday practice of braiding for one month of the non-expert 1 led to the development of braiding speed and the beauty of the braiding rope. There was no the defects of the incorrect pattern both of trial 2 and 3. For the braiding rope quality of the non-expert 2, they were also no defect in the braiding ropes in trial 2 and 3.

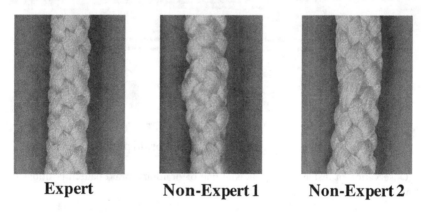

Expert   **Non-Expert 1**   **Non-Expert 2**

Fig. 3. Photographs of kumihimo ropes from the expert and two non-experts.

Because expert is always process at the middle of the marudai, she can control the angle of the braided rope, which was better than both non-experts. Figure 4 shows photographs of the ropes with distance between axial lines of the braid and braid pattern positions. The expert rope line showed a straight line over the non-experts. Figure 4(c) presents the distance from the center to the rope that the expert has less distance for making the straight line, which looks beautiful when compared to the non-experts.

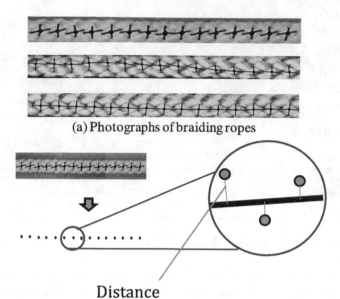

(a) Photographs of braiding ropes

Distance

(b) Distance between axial line of braid and braid pattern positions measurement

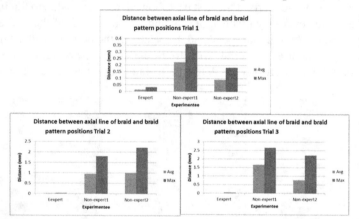

(c) Distance between axial line of braid and braid pattern positions

Fig. 4. Observation of distance between axial line of braid and braid pattern positions (Color figure online)

5   Eye's Movement Analysis

Figure 5 shows the eye's movement position of 1st, 2nd, 3rd and 4th process. These figures present the position of eyes in 4 braiding process. In trial 1, the expert revealed the position in the middle of the marudai from starting to ended process. On the contrary, both of non-experts are more distribution when compared with expert.

Left eye   **Right eye**

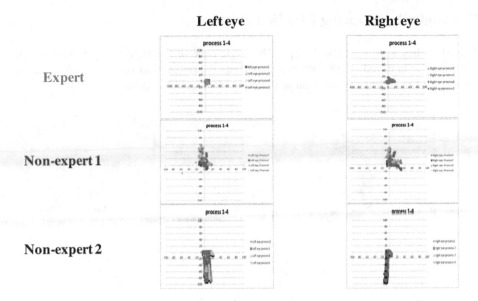

Fig. 5. Eye's movement of the expert and non-experts during the braiding process.

6 Braiding Rope Position

Figure 6 depicts the position of the braided rope during braiding process. The position of the rope was directly influenced by the tension of each thread. The braided rope positions of an expert scatter around the center of the marudai while the non-experts show the unsymmetrical scattering of the rope positions. The unsymmetrical distribution of the rope position is caused by the instability of the tension of the thread during braiding process.

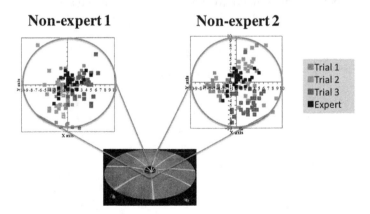

Fig. 6. Brading position of the expert and non-experts around the marudai. (Color figure online)

7   Angle Rope During Braiding Process

Figure 7 illustrates the angle of rope. The angle rope of the expert has in the range of
170°–180°. On the other hand, the non-expert has the range from 160°–180°. As a result,
the expert can control the position of the rope while braiding process.

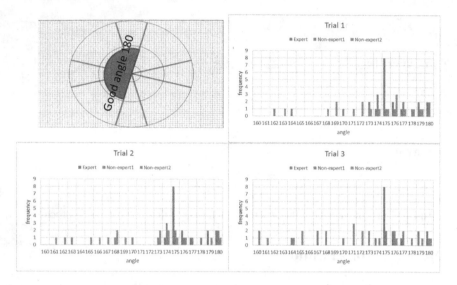

Fig. 7.   Measurement of the angle of the rope around the marudai. (Color figure online)

8   Distance Raising Rope During Braiding Process

Figure 8 presents the distance of rasing rope during the braiding process. As the comparison, it can be seen that the rasing of rope of the expert exhibited constantly while both

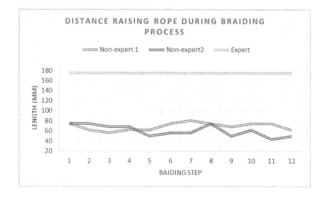

Fig. 8.   The distance of raising rope during the braiding process. (Color figure online)

of non-experts rose up the rope uncertainty during the braiding process. Therefore, the skill of braiding led the beneficial on the quality and the beauty of the braiding.

9   Conclusion

The expert showed the high performance and constant of braiding skill. Her eye's movement focused at the center of the marudai plate that according with the braiding rope position. The expert can balance the rope tension during the braiding process well. On the other hand, the eye's movement of non-experts did not relate with the braiding rope position. Furthermore, expert's skill was investigated focusing on how to keep location of braid rope at the center of marudai plate during braiding process. We investigated especially the way how the strands were moved above the marudai plate. The skills were clarified as follows,

- The moved strands of the expert has in the range of 170°–180°. On the other hand, those of the non-expert has the range from 160°–180°,
- Expert raised up strands higher than non-experts.

References

1. Martin, C.: Kumihimo: Japanese Silk Braiding Techniques. Old Hall, Leeds U.K. (1986)
2. Sahashi, K.: Exquisite: the World of Japanese Kumihimo Braiding. Kodansha Amer Inc., New York (1988)
3. Chottikampon, K., Mathurosemontri, S. Marui, H., Sirisuwan, P., Goto, A., Uosumi, T., Inoda, M., Tada, M., Nishimoto, H., Hamada, H.: Comparison of braiding skills between expert and non-experts by eye's movement measurement. In: Duffy, V.G. (ed.) DHM 2015. LNCS, vol. 9184, pp. 14–23. Springer, Heidelberg (2015)

Visual Representation of Dynamic Pressure Map on the Digital Human Model of Patient with a Lower Limb Prosthesis

Giorgio Colombo[1], Claudio Comotti[2], Daniele Regazzoni[2(✉)], Caterina Rizzi[2], and Andrea Vitali[2]

[1] Department of Mechanical Engineering, Polytechnic of Milan, Milan, Italy
giorgio.colombo@polimi.it
[2] Department of Management, Information and Production Engineering,
University of Bergamo (BG), Dalmine, Italy
{claudio.comotti,daniele.regazzoni,caterina.rizzi,
andrea.vitali1}@unibg.it

Abstract. The socket for lower limb prosthesis is the central element of artificial leg that needs to be optimize with the aim to increase comfort and reduce pain. Nowadays, the modeling of this part is completely manual and based on prosthetist skills. The key parameter determining if the socket is properly designed is the pressure distribution in the interface between the skin of residual limb and the internal surface of the socket. In this paper, we expose a method to measure this pressure thought resistive pressure sensors and we illustrate a case study of a transfemoral amputee patient. A visualization tool has been developed to dynamically show pressure data on the 3D model of the residual limb during topic moments of the gait by a color scale. Achieved results and future work will be discussed in the paper.

Keywords: Lower limb prosthesis · Pressure mapping · Gait

1   Introduction

Lower limb prostheses represent the solution to restore patient autonomy in all moments of his/her life such as walking, standing up and working. Nowadays, lower limb prostheses are a mix of mechanic and electronic technologies based on medical knowledge. Their features allow patients to live a normal life, but existing solutions are still influenced by some disadvantages and issues. Beyond eventual psychological problems, the adaptation process of the patient to the prosthesis is one of the leading causes of people to reject the artificial leg. If this process fails, actually, patient condition will get worse and maybe s/he will give up and lose the chance to walk again. The socket represents the interface between patient and prosthesis through which all forces are transmitted and, for this reason, it carries out the most relevant role, together with the mechanical joints of the leg. Patients may be asked to evaluate the discomfort or pain due to the contact between skin and socket, but this is too subjective to be used as a measure to evaluate socket design, especially for the patients at their first prosthesis. By the way, a

© Springer International Publishing Switzerland 2016
V.G. Duffy (Ed.): DHM 2016, LNCS 9745, pp. 140–149, 2016.
DOI: 10.1007/978-3-319-40247-5_15

bad design or a bad size may cause acute pain, skin lacerations and ulcers due to friction with prosthetic socket. This frequently do not permit to use it all day long, introducing an important limit.

2 State of Art

This paragraph shows a literature overview on lower limb prostheses for transfemoral (above knee amputation) patients. The most diffused process for creating a socket is still completely manual and realized by skilled craft workers [1]. The complexity to reproduce the three-dimensional shape and to adapt it to lower residual limb of the patient represent the reason to make it by hands. In addition, the large anatomical variability of the residual limb (e.g., length, bone protuberances, soft tissues thickness) prevent orthopaedics from standardizing the morphology of prosthetic socket. The orthopaedic technician creates the socket following several operations based only on his/her experience. In some rare cases, the process is partially based on CAD/CAM systems.

- The first phase is to create the negative moulding of the residual limb with the usage of soft chalk wraps.
- After obtaining a positive model, three main operations have to be executed: initial plaster circumference reduction, identification of load and off-load zones and critical zones manipulation by adding/removing chalk.
- Afterwards, technicians can make a prototypal thermoformed socket that is manufactured directly on the modified positive model with a thermo-deformable layer of plastic material.
- After some modifications, the technician realizes the final socket, assemble it on the prosthesis and performed the necessary adjustments.

All this operations rely on the manual skill and the knowledge of the technician and they do not offer quantitative parameters to optimize the process or to make a check. The orthopaedic technician have to identify tissues of residual limb such as skin tissue, scars, thickness of adipose tissue, bones, muscles and nerve terminals positions to model the correct shape guaranteeing maximum comfort.

The main parameter driving the information about the good fit of the prosthesis is the pressure in the contact zone between the residual limb and the socket that in traditional approach is only qualitatively assessed by the patient him/herself.

If the contact between residual limb skin and socket surface is not optimal, the patient will incur in chronic pain and skin pressure. The main causes of pain are an excessive compression and shear stress. The shear stress, due to the local sliding of two surfaces, is the main cause of skin lesions according to work of Zhang et al. [2]. By the way, the socket must transmit a considerable load due to patient's weight and to forces and moments characterizing the gait. A well-designed socket has the goal to provide the best distribution of loads to avoid stress peaks while guaranteeing a safe use. Literature presents some research works that show ways to measure pressure with several systems. Direct mode consists in the displacement of sensors in the internal surface of the socket. The authors in [3] used hydraulic sensors that measure changes in pressure of the fluid they contain. In some others research works [4–6] have been used small load cells able to provide localized pressure values. More recent studies [7–9] presented methods that use thin film of resistive material between two plastic films.

It is possible to acquire pressure data also in an indirect way measuring external properties of the socket. Extensometers or load cells fixed on the external surface of the socket can provide data concerning deformation useful to extract pressure information. An alternative method presented by authors in [10] is based on inverse dynamic of the prosthetic leg that allows obtaining forces and moments by starting from motion of joints, such as knee, ankle and hip.

In this research paper, we used four Tekscan sensors 9811E that are resistive sensors made of silver filaments covered between two layers of plastic material. These devices provide a matrix of 6 × 16 cells, called *sensels*, and each sensel provides a value of localized pressure. The software used to acquire data was Research Foot 6.70 by Tekscan [11].

3   New Proposed Approach

This paper shows a novel opportunity to design the socket by means of a digital solution that replicate traditional process and exploits low cost technologies for 3D scanning and Motion Capture.

3.1   3D Scanning

Nowadays, scanners allow acquiring a 3D shape and convert it in a meshed virtual model that reproduce the real one with desired precision. A variety of industrial scanner are available on the market with different prices, but the most interesting one is the MS Kinect derived from the video-gaming world and available on the market for 150 USD. The first version of this optical device permits to acquire a 3D geometry exploiting the projection of a pattern of IR beams and the triangulation principle. Surely, the precision it ensures is worse of that of more expensive laser scanners; the main differences concern small details, but for this research, we need only global shape to be reproduced and this can be done properly. For this application, we use in combination with MS Kinect, the Skanect software that, after a preliminary phase of setup of bounding box size, enables to make scan by moving the sensor around the object. In our case, the user has to move the Kinect around patient following, where possible, a circular path. S/He has to pay attention to the zone between legs and, eventually, around scars. In real time, Skanect software create a virtual model of the limb scanned: through colors (green/red) it provides a direct evaluation of which zones are successfully scanned and vice versa. In this phase, it is also possible to apply filters or reduce numbers of points mapped to simplify mesh geometry.

This type of acquisition is low cost and easy to be used. Moreover, it allows acquiring the geometry of the residual limb in a vertical position that is hardly obtainable with other scanning solutions.

3.2   SMA and Pressure Analysis

A virtual environment to design sockets [12], called SMA (Socket Modelling Assistant) has been developed by VK research group of the University of Bergamo in the last decade and it is an ad-hoc knowledge-guided CAD system which offers a kit of tools useful to emulate technician operations, but having a quantitative feedback.

Socket Modelling Assistant (SMA) starts from the digital model of the residual limb acquired by either Magnetic Resonance Imaging (MRI) or using a low cost RGB-D depth sensor. The prosthetist is guided step-by-step by the system that applies in automatic or semi-automatic way the rules and the modelling procedures. Actually, it embeds a set of design rules and procedures (e.g., where and how to modify the socket shape) and makes available a set of interactive virtual tools to manipulate the socket shape according to traditional procedures. Beyond the technical challenge of creating such a complex ICT tool, the relevance of this part is mainly due to the inner connection it has with the medical application. The module has been built exploiting orthopaedic knowledge extracted from physicians' interviews and best cases, coded and embedded into the system. Moreover, the real applicative condition in a prosthetic lab has been kept in high consideration while designing the process and the user's interface. This should ease the transition to a digital way of designing the socket. In this application, besides taking precise measurement on the 3D scanned model, we should also compute a FE analysis to evaluate the compression value and to identify load and off-load zones. We simulated the real condition of pressure on a single patient using Tekscan system to extract the load distribution in static conditions and during a gait phase. These tests are useful to calibrate the FE model to simulate in the best way the real residual limb behaviour. Pressure sensors give us a load map to be compared with FE results in order to tune the simulation model.

3.3   Motion Capture

Another important set of data comes from the Motion Capture system based on two MS Kinect that provides the tracking of each of the 27 joints in the digital human model. Such data offer a way to analyse gait features and eventually to detect some gait abnormalities [13]. The second generation of Kinect sensors offers a high-resolution camera (1080p) and it exploits the Time of Flight (TOF) principle to create the depth map of the environment. This new technology is be more precise and it solves the interpretation errors in the use of multiple Kinect v2 for the same scene. The amount of information required by Kinect v2 is very considerable and it needs a USB 3.0 port to communicate with PC (instead of the USB 2.0 required by the first version). The most important problem, in this case, is that the PC needs to have a USB 3.0 controller and one sensor requires a large part of the bandwidth. This problem has been solved, for the moment, by synchronizing information coming from two different devices connected to two different computers and merging them. Exploiting iPisoft software, we are able to acquire the point cloud of each movement and to export data of positions and rotations of each human joint.

Figure 1 shows the adopted disposition of Kinects to track the scene where patients walk on a straight path.

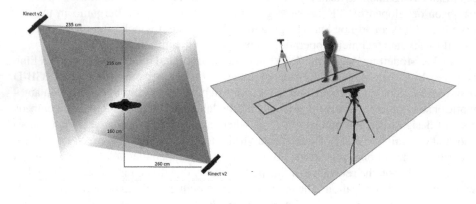

Fig. 1. Disposition of Microsoft Kinect for motion capture

3.4   3D Visualization Tool

We introduce a visual representation that combine all data acquired with 3D scanner, pressure sensors and motion sensors. A software application has been developed in-house in order to permit the merging of data acquired by scanning and pressure acquisition systems.

Input file are the CSV files coming from Tekscan acquisition. The structure of CSV file is made of 16 rows in each of them 6 values of pressure, separated by a comma, are contained, basing on the structure of Tekscan 9811E sensor. To map the pressure 4 CSV file are needed, one for each sensor, frame by frame. The application is configured to work with frame-rate of 30 FPS. The reason of this choice comes from the need for synchronizing motion capture system with pressure sensors. Using the same frame rate permits to synchronize pressure data and gait animation in an easy way.

The application visualizes the 3D model of the residual limb, which is acquired with 3D scanning previously described. The 3D model is imported in OBJ format in which the vertex color data has been added with the exporting module of Skanect.

Exploiting the texture applied on the scanned model of the residual limb, we can identify the position of each sensor stripe on the 3D model of the residual limb. This process is called sensor mapping and by marking each sensor with a color we select points of mesh relative to it on the virtual thigh.

Then, a 3D plane has been used to parameterize each marked point clouds. Each point of the parametric plane has coordinate values (u, v) between 0 and 1. The parametrization permits the association of a point on the mesh with a position on the surface of sensor and with the relative value of pressure.

After the mapping has been done the visualization of pressure data is easily understood and the final step consists in the dynamic update of pressure data on the limb during gait frame by frame.

4   Case Study

The proposed solution has been applied on the case study of a patient with a trans-femoral amputation on the left lower limb. This paragraph shows all testing procedures and data acquired, the resulting 3D model of residual limb and, finally, the animated distribution map of pressure.

The first step is the scanning phase to reconstruct the residual limb geometry. We executed it by using Microsoft Kinect in the first version. In the Fig. 2a and b it is possible to see the differences between reconstructed 3D model and the real model of the residual limb. The resolution of this device surely is not comparable to laser scanners one, but as we can note, global geometry reflects the real model by following curvatures and measures. The model that come from Skanect software needs to be cleaned and remeshed. By using software for mesh manipulation (e.g., Netfabb, Meshmixer or Meshlab) we could solve problems of scanned mesh like holes, degenerated triangles and overlapped faces. For this research work, it was useful also to acquire 3D geometry with sensors already on the residual limb in order to obtain the texturized model (Fig. 2c). This allows identifying sensors disposition for the following application.

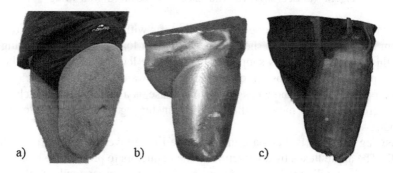

Fig. 2. (a) Real residual limb model (b) 3D scanned model (c) texturized model with pressure sensors applied

The combined acquisition of gait motion and pressure at the interface between socket and residual limb require the use of two systems at the same time.

Taking into account the pressure acquisition, we use the Tekscan system exposed in Sect. 2. We evaluated which is the best disposition of sensors to avoid creases and undesired movements, thus we put sensors directly on the residual limb of the patient covering them with an extra thin plastic film. In this way, sensors follow the curvatures of the limb and they eased the donning of the socket.

Motion capture system has been performed as described in Sect. 3.3 and it allows acquiring data for some steps of the patient's gait.

The combination of these two types of data has been possible thanks to an ad-hoc application developed in house that allows visualizing frame-by-frame pressure data on the 3D model of the residual limb. The planar data of pressure of each sensor was parametrized and adapted to 3D geometry of the residual limb acquired with Kinect scanner.

For each gait acquisition we can visualize dynamic changing of pressures and according to video/depth image acquisition, it is possible to identify loads in particular moments of step. Basing on literature of gait analysis, we chose four main instants characterizing step. Heel strike, mid stance, toe off and mid swing are these key frames in which it is useful to acquire pressure to understand the behavior and the contact areas of the residual limb in each moment.

Heel strike (Fig. 3a), also known as initial contact, is the period between the first contact of heel with the ground and the first phase of double support. 30° flexion of the hip and full extension in the knee is observed. The ankle moves from a neutral position into plantar flexion. After this, knee flexion (5°) begins and increases, just as the plantar flexion of the heel increased.

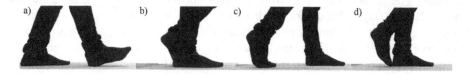

Fig. 3. (a) Heel strike (b) Mid stance (c) Toe off (d) Mid swing

Midstance (Fig. 3b) is the longest phase. It starts with the detachment of the other foot from the ground and it finishes when full weight load is on the supporting foot. During this phase, the body is supported by only one leg. At this moment, the body begins to move from force absorption at impact to forward force propulsion.

Toe off (Fig. 3c), also known as Pre-Swing phase, is a gait phase in which the toes leave the ground. In this moment there is the transferring forward of the load on the other foot.

Midswing (Fig. 3d) is the phase in which the limb moves in a forward position to the trunk. The ankle flexes by contraction of the adductors to prepare the next support. It ends when the oscillating limb advances and the tibia is perpendicular to the ground.

After a synchronization process between the two systems, we were able to visualize data of pressure on the 3D shape of residual limb. Figure 4 shows the results for each gait moment of a single step. Pressure of each sensel is provided into a colored scale with a maximum value of 40 kPa (red).

Outcomes highlights the behavior of the residual limb in the socket during gait. In "heel strike", we can see how the socket push on the residual limb in the high frontal zone and low back zone due to contact with the ground. It is possible to imagine the coupling of socket-residuum like a powered lever in a friction contact with a cylindrical link. By moving the lever, the link follows the rotation of the lever, but it should present a relative rotation due to its inertia. The same phenomenon appears on the prosthetic leg. When the patient puts the prosthetic heel on the ground, the socket over rotate causing the concentration of pressure in the zones previously described.

In the next phase, conversely, the distribution of pressures on the whole surface of the residual limb is more homogeneous and there are no peaks. The contact of the limb in mid stance phase happens in a large areas and this contributes to reduce peaks and to increase the homogeneity of the average pressure value (about 20 kPa).

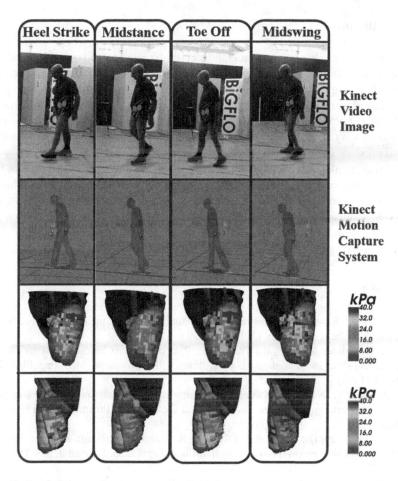

Fig. 4. Visualization of video frame, animation reproduction and pressure mapping on the limb in four topic moments of gait (Color figure online).

The instant of toe off highlights the contraction of rectus femoris muscle that is visible in the frontal view with the increasing of pressure. Here pressures have high peaks on a diagonal path that is very similar to quadriceps disposition.

Mid swing phase needs the contraction of whole quadriceps and of hamstrings muscle. In this phase, pressure sensors show high values on most of the surface of the residual limb.

According to these results, in some areas swing phase results to be the most demanding one due to an uneven pressure distribution; in addition to rotational moments, the whole weight of the prosthesis burdens on the residual limb. Taking into account the patient executing the tests, he does not wear a liner because his prosthesis is a full contact one. Thus, in these tests, the coupling with the prosthetic leg is made through friction between skin of residual limb and internal surface of the socket. Measured stress are only the normal contribution, but there is also a shear stress that is more difficult to evaluate.

5   Conclusions

In this research work, we present a method to visualize and to understand the behavior of the residual limb in the prosthetic socket. It is based on different phases: scanning phase, pressure acquisition and motion capture, and dynamic pressure mapping. The results obtained and analyzed in four topic moments of a gait of a transfemoral amputee patient highlight how load zones change according to motion executed. In this way it is possible to identify zones in which the load have continuous peaks and zones in which measured pressure maintain low values during all gait phases.

This experimental approach allows us to acquire reference values of pressure in the most crucial zone of the prosthesis. This permits to set up a FE analysis in which we will fix material properties and to simulate loads during gait. The final aim is to avoid the pressure acquisition, on the base of correct pressure data coming out from a finite element simulation. Future works will be focused on the optimization of socket shape also in function of gait dynamics.

References

1. Agarwal, A.K.: Essentials of Prosthesis and Orthotics, chap. 11, pp. 86–90. Jaypee Brothers Medical Publishers, New Delhi (2013)
2. Zhang, M., Turner-Smith, A.R., Tanner, A., Roberts, V.C.: Clinical investigation of the pressure and shear stress on the trans-tibial stump with a prosthesis. Med. Eng. Phys. 20(3), 188–198 (1998)
3. Van Pijkeren, T., Naeff, M., Kwee, H.H.: A new method for the measurement of normal pressure between amputation residual limb and socket. Bull. Prosthet. Res. 17(1), 31–34 (1980)
4. Sanders, J.E., Lam, D., Dralle, A.J., Okumura, R.: Interface pressures and shear stresses at thirteen socket sites on two persons with transtibial amputation. J. Rehabil. Res. Dev. 34(1), 19–43 (1997)
5. Goh, J.C.H., Lee, P.V.S., Chong, S.Y.: Stump/socket pressure profiles of the pressure cast prosthetic socket. Clin. Biomech. 18(3), 237–243 (2003)
6. Lee, V.S., Solomonidis, S.E., Spence, W.D.: Stump-socket interface pressure as an aid to socket design in prostheses for trans-femoral amputees–a preliminary study. Proc. Inst. Mech. Eng. H 211(2), 167–180 (1997)
7. Dou, P., Jia, X., Suo, S., Wang, R., Zhang, M.: Pressure distribution at the stump/socket interface in transtibial amputees during walking on stairs, slope and non-flat road. Clin. Biomech. 21(10), 1067–1073 (2006)
8. Dumbleton, T., Buis, A.W.P., McFadyen, A., McHugh, B.F., McKay, G., Murray, K.D., Sexton, S.: Dynamic interface pressure distributions of two transtibial prosthetic socket concepts. J. Rehabil. Res. Dev. 46(3), 405–415 (2009)
9. Pirouzi, G., Osman, N.A.A., Eshraghi, A., Ali, S., Gholizadeh, H., Abas, W.A.B.W.: Review of the socket design and interface pressure measurement for transtibial prosthesis. Sci. World J. 2014, 1–9 (2014)
10. Dumas, R., Cheze, L., Frossard, L.: Loading applied on prosthetic knee of transfemoral amputee: comparison of inverse dynamics and direct measurements. Gait Posture 30(4), 560–562 (2009)
11. Tekscan: Pressure Mapping, Force Measurement and Tactile Sensors. www.tekscan.com

12. Rizzi, C., Colombo, G., Facoetti, G., Vitali, A.: Socket virtual design based on low cost hand tracking and haptic devices. In: VRCAI 2013 Proceedings of the 12th ACM SIGGRAPH International Conference on Virtual-Reality Continuum and Its Applications in Industry, Hong Kong (2013)
13. Regazzoni, D., Rizzi, C., Comotti, C., Massa, F.: Towards automatic gait assessment by means of RGB-D mocap. In: ASME International Design Engineering Technical Conferences and Computers and Information in Engineering Conference IDETC/CIE 2015, Boston, Massachusetts, USA (2015)

Research on the Motion Technique of Japanese Tea Ceremony

Soutatsu Kanazawa[1], Zelong Wang[2(✉)], Yuka Takai[3], Akihiko Goto[3],
Tomoko Ota[4], and Hiroyuki Hamada[1]

[1] Urasenke Konnichian, Kyoto, Japan
kanazawa.kuromon.1352.gentatsu@docomo.ne.jp
[2] Advanced Fibro-Science, Kyoto Institute of Technology, Kyoto, Japan
simon.zelongwang@gmail.com
[3] Department of Information Systems Engineering, Osaka Sangyo University, Daito, Japan
gotoh@ise.osaka-sandai.ac.jp
[4] Chuo Business Group, Osaka, Japan
Tomoko.ota@k.vodafone.ne.jp

Abstract. In this paper, the tea making of motion skill by tea master of "The way of tea" was investigated by High speed camera. The most important process at beginning of tea making, which using tea whisk to mix the hot water and tea powder with high speed, was focused and recorded. The tea master's motion track of tea whisk was clarified and analyzed by software. The final tea also was recorded by camera. The surface of bubbles was measured by numerical method. The expert regular move up and down tea whisk was considered the important Characteristics for the tea making motion.

Keywords: Motion technique · Japanese tea ceremony · The way of tea · Tea making skill

1 Introduction

"The Way of Tea" ("Chado") is one of traditional artistic activities accumulating long Japanese ancient culture. Japanese tea ceremony is developed based on "daily after-meal". "The Way of Tea", also called the "Japanese tea ceremony", is a special ceremonial art preparation and presentation of "matcha" (a kind of green tea powder) to entertain the guests, through the tea ceremony people will achieve temperament, improve the cultural quality and aesthetic view. The essence of "The Way of Tea" is meant to demonstrate reverence and respect between host and guest, both of them can truly experience the artistic conception and taste the most primitive taste of green tea during tea-tasting activity and service process with the tallest state of the etiquette.

"The way of tea" is a special art performance to entertain the guests, through the tea ceremony people will achieve temperament, improve the cultural quality and aesthetic view, which consisted of many specific and strict procedures, whose basic skill just only handed over by oral instructions by expert. However, until now the scientific explanation for the detail process skill is limited. Therefore, it is valuable to conduct some scientific

© Springer International Publishing Switzerland 2016
V.G. Duffy (Ed.): DHM 2016, LNCS 9745, pp. 150–158, 2016.
DOI: 10.1007/978-3-319-40247-5_16

comparison and motion analysis to keep this country cultural treasure and inherit to the next generation effectively.

In previous research, the cluster of small bubbles in the surface and suitable temperature was considered to be an important symbol of a bowl of delicious and aesthetic Japanese tea ("The way of tea").

The experience factors influence on motion technique of "The way of tea" was clarified by numerical method. During tea ceremony process, each process's point of degree of mixing and bubble distribution were focused, relationship between timeliness and different tea whisks were extracted and analyzed according to four stages, 100 %, 80 %, 50 % and 30 % of tea making finishing time. And the whole tea making process was recorded by high-speed camera. Finally, both the relationship between the bubble distribution and stirring frequency was clarified.

It was presented that the expert stirred hot water and tea powder by tea whisk with quickly motion in the first period so that produced the most widespread bubbles quickly at the beginning of tea making. Afterwards, use slowly motion to mix tea to break large bubbles to become small bubbles until the final tea finishing.

Therefore, it was considered that stirring hot water and powder at beginning was one of most important key motion for tea making. The expert was able to perform high stirring speed during the first process in order to agitate the tea powder in hot water quickly.

In this research stirring action influence on bubble formation at beginning of tea making process was paid attention.

A tea master was employed as the behavior subject, who has more than 20 year experiences, who was called as expert in Kyoto. The subject was required to make a tea, mixing tea powder and hot water until she was satisfied for it. The motion and trace of the subject at beginning of tea making process (14 s) was captured by high-speed camera. The bubble of tested tea was recorded by camera. The photo was processed by numerical method in order to measure the bubble size and summary distribution in this study. The mixing frequency and amplitude of stirrings were calculated by software. The features of bubble distribution and motion characteristics were comprehensive analyzed and compared in the end.

Furthermore, the key motion characteristics was found out and discussed. The conclusion was able to provide a reference for learners.

In a word, this study through clarified the tea master's movement during the most important production process of the way of tea in order to find the effective mixing method and obtain the excellent finished tea finally.

2 Experiment

2.1 Participants and Subjects

One Japanese tea master from Kyoto were employed as a participant, who had more than 20 years experiences in "The way of tea", which was called as tea master in this paper. One classical type of Japanese tea whisks was selected for proceeding the experiment called as "Kankyuan" as shown in Fig. 1, whose number of brush was 62.

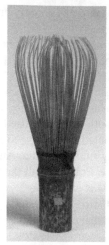

"Kankyuan"

Fig. 1. Japanese tea whisks

2.2 Experimental Process

The participants were required to whisk together green tea powder and hot water. 1.5 g of "Matcha" tea power and approximate 56 g of hot water were dumped into the bowl, and the moisture content of tea was controlled at approximately 97 % steadily. The first 14 s of whole tea making finishing time were clearly recorded by a high-speed camera (FASTCAM SA4 Photron Co. Ltd) as shown in Fig. 2. The shutter speed was 3600 frames per-second.

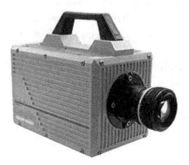

Fig. 2. High-speed camera system

2.3 Processing Analysis

The two marks were affixed to the participant's hand with different colors, the other one mark was affixed to the tea whisk as shown in Fig. 5. The coordinates of three marks in the x or y direction was captured and analyzed by TEMA 3.5 software (Photron Co. Ltd) as shown in Fig. 3.

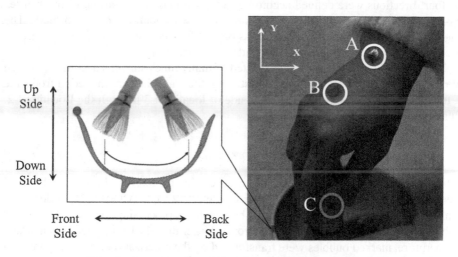

Fig. 3. Location of record markers (Color figure online)

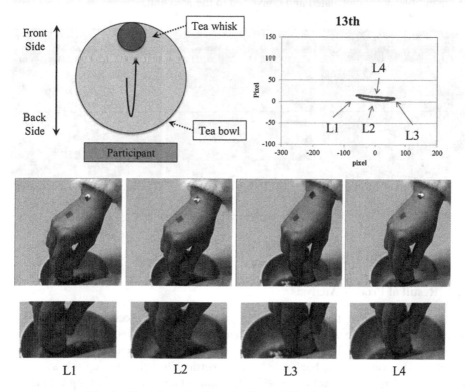

Fig. 4. The schematic diagram of tea whisk stirring process

The first fourteen seconds of tea master's movement was counted and summarized by watching the High-speed video. In order to make the further analysis by software, the four directions were defined according to the tea master's location. In front of tea master's location was defined as front side, which was identified by green mark. The side of closed to tea master was defined as back side. And the up and down in vertical direction were called up side and down side as shown in Fig. 3.

The tea mixing movement was consisted of many times stirrings according to each vibration as shown in Fig. 4. During one stirring, the tea whisk was moved in front side of tea blow (L1), then move to the back side of location L3 through the Location L2. Finally, return to center of tea bowl (L4).

2.4 Image Processing

In this research, the surface of final tea was recorded by camera, the size of the bowl was selected as a reference for calculation, diameter: 12.6 cm. Afterwards, circle region of all bowl were analyzed and transferred by numerical processing from Fig. 5(a) to (b). It should be mentioned that only bubble forms larger than 0.01 mm^2 area was marked. Furthermore, marked bubbles were transformed by the binarization processing method into a white and black two colors as shown in Fig. 5(c). The outlines of bubble form and bubbles' distribution state were also sketched on the processed image. Finally, the areas of the bubbles were calculated and converted to the area unit.

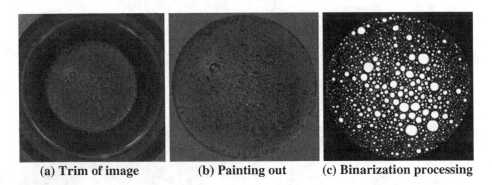

(a) Trim of image   (b) Painting out   (c) Binarization processing

Fig. 5. Procedure of image processing

3   Results and Discussions

3.1   Result of Process Analysis

As the mention above, first fourteen seconds of tea making process was recorded by high speed camera. The movement track of tea whisk was illustrated in Fig. 6. According to Fig. 6, the horizontal direction was working time of fourteen seconds. The depth direction was front side and back side. And the vertical direction was up side and down side. It is easy to found that the tea whisk was moved up and down during tea making process, which was considered as a periodic cycle of mixing movement. During first fourteen seconds, nine cycles were separated each periodic movement.

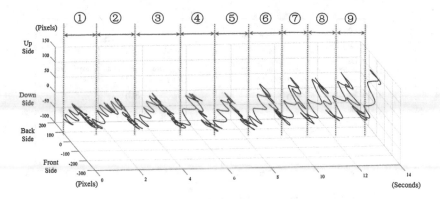

Fig. 6. Movement track of tea whisk

The first periodic cycle was extracted and illustrated in Figs. 7 and 8. The first cycle was consisted of eight stirrings. The all stirring track of tea whisk was shown a slight concave trajectory during moving to back side (from L1 to L3), which was considered that more conform to the shape of the bowl. The track of tea whisk was shown a slight lift when tea whisk return to the center from back side (L3 to L4).

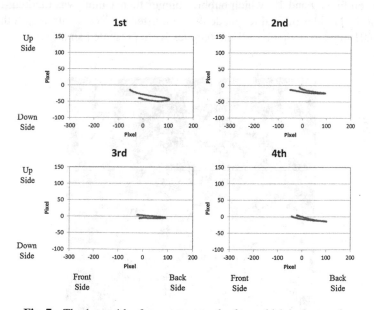

Fig. 7. The 1st to 4th of movement track of tea whisk in first cycle

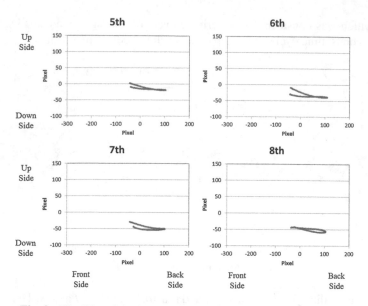

Fig. 8. The 5th to 8th of movement track of tea whisk in first cycle.

3.2   Result of Image Analysis

The final proceeded product by tea master after image process and distribution were illustrated on Figs. 9 and 10, which bubbles bigger than 1 mm^2 was marked. It is can found that the bubbles of final tea made by tea master were concentrated on the range of from 0.01 mm^2 to 0.9 mm^2. All the bubbles were presented small sizes, which had

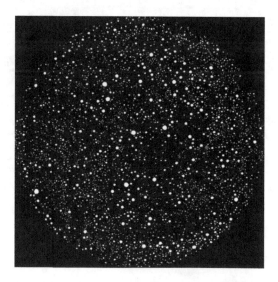

Fig. 9. The proceeded photo of tea surface

more bubble's size closed to the range of 0.01 mm²~0.9 mm². There was few bubbles was bigger than 0.9 mm², which located at the range of 1 mm²~9.9 mm². Comparing the previous research, the tea masters' bubble was shown a very ideal distribution.

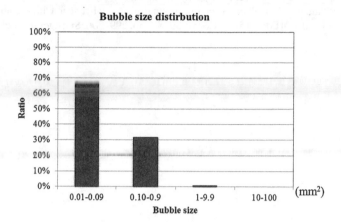

Fig. 10. The bubble distribution of bubble on surface of tea

4   Conclusions

In a word, the tea master was shown regular move up and down during tea making during high speed stirring process. And the tea whisk of each stirring was also presented stable movement. The bubble distribution of final tea was concentrated on the range of small size. It can be considered that, tea masker's motion can achieve a good tea.

References

1. Tujimoto, N., Ichihashi,Y., Iue, M., Ota, T., Hamasaki, K., Nakai, A., Goto, A.: Comparison of bubble forming in a bowl of thin tea between expert and non-expert. In: Proceeding of 11th Japan International SAMPE Symposium and Exhibition (2009)
2. Goto, A., Endo, A., Narita, C., Takai, Y., Shimodeand, Y., Hamada, H.: Comparison of painting technique of Urushi products between expert and non-expert. In: Advances in Ergonomics in Manufacturing, pp. 160–167 (2012). ISBN: 978-1-4398-7039-6
3. Aiba, E., Kanazawa, S., Ota, T., Kuroda, K., Takai, Y., Goto, A., Hamada, H.: Developing a system to assess the skills of Japanese way of tea by analyzing the forming sound: a case study. In: Human Factors and Ergonomics Society International Meeting (2013)
4. Kanazawa, S., Ota, T., Wang, Z., Wiranpaht, T., Takai, Y., Goto, A., Hamada, H.: Experience factors influence on motion technique of "the way of tea" by motion analysis. In: Duffy, V.G. (ed.) DHM 2015. LNCS, vol. 9185, pp. 155–163. Springer, Heidelberg (2015)

5. Kanazawa, S., Ota, T., Wang, Z., Tada, A., Takai, Y., Goto, A., Hamada, H.: Research on the performance of three tea whisks of "the way of tea" with different experience. In: Duffy, V.G. (ed.) DHM 2015. LNCS, vol. 9184, pp. 95–103. Springer, Heidelberg (2015)
6. Kanazawa, S., Ota, T., Wang, Z., Wongpajan, R., Takai, Y., Goto, A., Hamada, H.: Visual evaluation of "the way of tea" based on questionnaire survey between Chinese and Japanese. In: Duffy, V.G. (ed.) DHM 2015. LNCS, vol. 9184, pp. 299–306. Springer, Heidelberg (2015)

Performance Analysis of Professional Sewing Scissors Using the "So-Hizukuri" Forging Process

Yasuko Kitajima[1(✉)], Akihiko Goto[2], and Hiroyuki Hamada[3]

[1] Faculty of Nursing, Tokyo Ariake University of Medical and Health Sciences,
2-9-1 Ariake, Koto-ku, Tokyo, 135-0063, Japan
kitajima@tau.ac.jp

[2] Faculty of Design Technology, Osaka Sangyo University, 3-1-1 Nakagaito, Daito,
Osaka 574-8530, Japan
gotoh@ise.osaka-sandai.ac.jp

[3] Department of Advanced Fibro-Science, Kyoto Institute of Technology, Matsugasaki,
Sakyo-ku, Kyoto 606-8585, Japan
hhamada@kit.ac.jp

Abstract. Scissors have been around since the ancient times as a useful tool. They come in many varieties and serve just as many purposes. This team of researchers completed an earlier study, investigating the secret to the sharpness of Japanese sewing scissors. Japanese sewing scissors can be traced back 160 years ago to the time Commodore Perry arrived in Uraga, Japan, then perfected over time by the grandfather of Japanese scissors, Yakichi Yoshida, to fit Japanese hands. This forging process came to be known as "so-hizukuri." Today, this traditional technology is known and handed down to just a handful of craftsmen.

Our research team wanted to know why this process created scissors that were so sharp, so we began measuring each ridge in the blades of the scissors. Results showed that scissors forged under the so-hizukuri process had blades that curved between 0–150 micrometers in width. When, in use on a fabric, the two blades intersect along the curve, generating greater friction that translates into sharper blades. We also learned that when the two blades intersect, other parts of the blades do not touch each other.

In this study, we looked at what happens to the user of the scissors and the fabric at the very moment the sharp blades of so-hizukuri forged scissors cut into the fabric. We armed a tailor – someone who is an expert scissor handler – with two different pairs of scissors: one that's so-hizukuri forged, and another that's cheap and sold in discount stores. We then had the tailor cut the same fabric using the same method but with two different scissors and recorded the process using a high-speed camera. We analyzed the footage. Additionally, we observed the surface of the fabric cut by the two scissors under an optical microscope. We found clear differences in the user's movements and the scissors' effects on the fabric, which shall be elaborated upon here.

Keywords: Sewing scissors · Forging process · High-speed camera · Optical microscope

© Springer International Publishing Switzerland 2016
V.G. Duffy (Ed.): DHM 2016, LNCS 9745, pp. 159–169, 2016.
DOI: 10.1007/978-3-319-40247-5_17

1 Introduction

There are numerous types of scissors in the world that serve a variety of purposes. And sewing scissors are among those that evolved in a uniquely Japanese way. The mainstream scissors we see today that's shaped like the letter "X" were introduced by Commodore Perry some 160 years ago in the Edo period when his Black Ship docked in at Uraga. Referred to as "Meriken" scissors at the time, they weighed about 1 kg and measured 330–360 mm in length. They were heavy duty scissors used to cut through thick fabric like coarse Rasha and were in no way suited for the hands of the more diminutive Japanese of the time. Yakichi Yoshida was responsible for modifying them to better fit Japanese hands [1]. His proprietary method of forging was called so-hizukuri and has been handed down largely nonverbally from master to apprentice. His forging technique was passed on far and wide, bringing the total number of houses with craftsmen trained in the Yoshida technique to 23. Today, however, very few can say they are able to make scissors using the so-hizukuri method. One of them continues to make sewing scissors that are well respected by high-end apparel tailors.

This team of researchers has studied the secret of scissors forged in the so-hizukuri process. What makes fabric-cutting possible in the first place is the reduction of the two blades' intersection point to the smallest possible width. When we researched why the so-hizukuri scissors are so sharp, we found that they were designed to concentrate the blades' stress point down to the point where the blades intersect. It would not be an exaggeration to say that the size of these points determines the performance of the scissors. We measured the two blades forged in so-hizukuri using a three-dimensional measuring device. The result: with the inner part of the blade as a 0, the deepest part registered a 150 µm curve along the surface. The curve on the inside of the blades catches the fabric as the blades come together. And when the blades meet, the part of the blades that were not touching could be visually confirmed. When light is flashed from behind the scissors, light leaks through the space between the blades and as the blades slide together when the scissor handles are squeezed, one can visually detect a shadow reduced to a black dot rising all the way up from the base of the blades to the tip of the scissors. We realized that the scissor's sharpness was due to this design of concentrating the force of the blades into this one point where it meets the fabric. The inner curve of the blade appears to have been a calculated one made by a precision machine. However, so-hizukuri craftsmen don't rely on machinery, but on their own intuition when they wield their hammer and strike at the metal to pound out a 0–150 µm curve on the blades [2].

In this study, we looked at what effect sharp, so-hizukuri forged scissors had on the user and the fabric the moment the sharp blades cut into the fabric. There are virtually no differences between a pair of craftsman- made sewing scissors and a pair purchased at a 100-yen shop if the issue was simply about dissecting fabric. We had an expert who uses scissors in his profession to use each type of scissors to cut fabric and recorded the action. We then studied the amount of time the cutting action took and analyzed results from the footage obtained on a high speed video camera. The results pointed to a big difference in the cutting process of the two scissors. We also studied the cross section images of the cut fabric under a microscope and detected differences there too. The results will be presented along with an interview with the expert. Through this study, we will discuss the value sharp so-hizukuri scissors add to the cutting process.

2   Methods

2.1   Test Subject

A tailor with more than 45 years of experience in high-end apparel.

2.2   Procedures

We asked the tailor to cut wool fabric using pairs of so-hizukuri forged scissors (Fig. 1), and pairs purchased from a 100-yen shop (Fig. 2). The tailor was asked to cut across the grain, along the grain and on the bias. The tailor used the workstation he usually uses for his work.

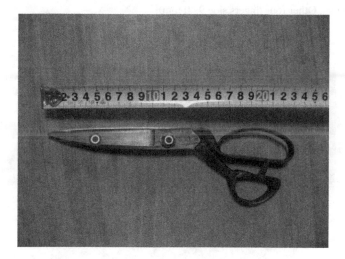

Fig. 1. Pairs of so-hizukuri forged scissors (The length of the blade: Thumb finger ring side 99.0 mm, Other four fingers side 100.0 mm).

A high-speed camera, Photron© FASTCAM SA4, was set up in front of the workstation. Markings were made on two points along the blade: Point 1, about a third of the way below the tip of the blade, and Point 2, at the base by the screw. The cutting process was filmed in its entirety and analyzed. Another marking was made on the fabric to indicate the end so that each cutting test would cover the same distance. The motions of the scissors through Points 1 and 2 recorded on the high speed video camera were entered in as data on the x axis, y axis, xy synthesis, then calculated the marker points, speed and acceleration (Fig. 3). Then the dissected fabric was observed under an optical microscope, KEYENCE CORPORATION VHX-900F Series.

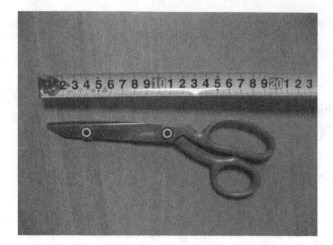

Fig. 2. Pairs of purchased from a 100-yen shop scissors (The length of the blade: Thumb finger ring side 85.0 mm, Other four fingers side 99.0 mm).

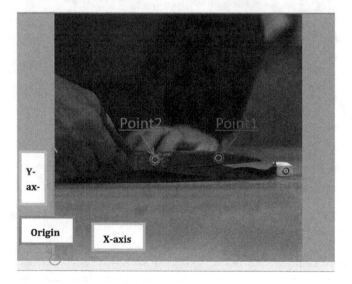

Fig. 3. The position of the markers.

3   Results and Discussion

Figure 4 shows the Point 1 position of so-hizukuri scissors on the X-axis and Fig. 5 shows the Point 1 position of so-hizukuri scissors on the Y-axis. Figure 6 shows the Point 1 speed of so-hizukuri scissors on the X-axis and Fig. 7 shows the Point 1 speed of so-hizukuri scissors on the Y-axis. Figure 8 shows the Point 1 position of 100-yen scissors on the X-axis and Fig. 9 shows the Point 1 position of 100-yen scissors on the Y-axis. Figure 10 shows the Point 1 speed of 100-yen scissors on the X-axis and Fig. 11 shows the Point 1 speed of 100-yen scissors on the Y-axis. The wool fabrics used for the evaluation of the figures from 4 to 11 were cut across the grain.

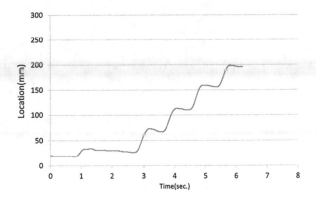

Fig. 4. The Point 1 position of so-hizukuri scissors on the X-axis, when cut across the grain on the wool fabric.

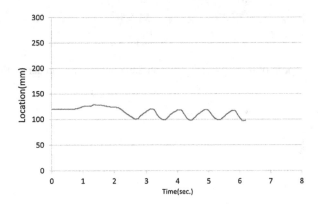

Fig. 5. The Point 1 position of so-hizukuri scissors on the Y-axis, when cut across the grain on the wool fabric.

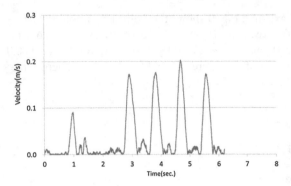

Fig. 6. The Point 1 speed of so-hizukuri scissors on the X-axis, when cut across the grain on the wool fabric.

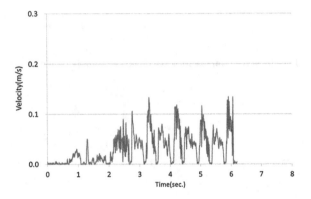

Fig. 7. The Point 1 speed of so-hizukuri scissors on the Y-axis, when cut across the grain on the wool fabric.

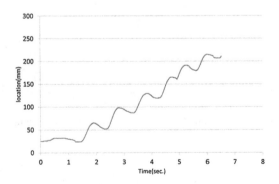

Fig. 8. The Point 1 position of 100-yen scissors on the X-axis, when cut across the grain on the wool fabric.

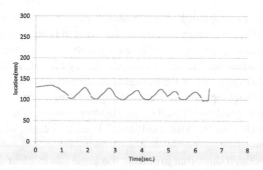

Fig. 9. The Point 1 position of 100-yen scissors on the Y-axis, when cut across the grain on the wool fabric.

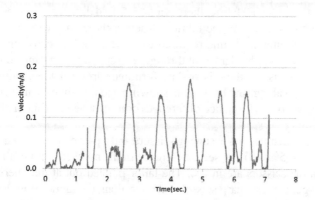

Fig. 10. The Point 1 speed of 100-yen scissors on the X-axis, when cut across the grain on the wool fabric.

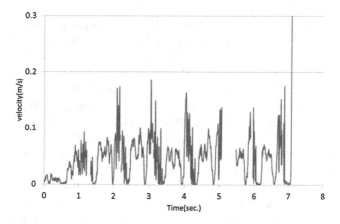

Fig. 11. The Point 1 speed of 100-yen scissors on the Y-axis, when cut across the grain on the wool fabric.

When comparing, Figs. 4 and 8, Figs. 5 and 9, Figs. 6 and 10, Figs. 7 and 11, the amount of the time used for cutting are almost the same in both so-hizukuri scissors and 100-yen scissors, however, there were differences in the movements. It took 3 s for the so-hizukuri-scissors when the blades opened until they closed, while for the 100-yen scissors, it took a little over 1 s when the blades opened until they closed. When observing the number of the blades opened and closed through the entire cutting process, the number of the blades opened and closed of the 100-yen scissors was 1.5 times more than that of the so-hizukuri scissors. Also the blades' open and close width of the 100-yen scissors was irregular.

Results of this research show that in cutting the same fabric, clear differences emerge in the way the tailor moves the scissors and the amount of time he spends cutting the fabric depending on the scissors and in which direction relative to the weave. We will study these results along with an interview with the tailor. When comparing longitudinal and lateral directions of wool fabric, there is a 1-, 1.5-fold difference in speed. This stems from the strength of the yarn in the fabric – whether the yarn is easy to cut through or not determines the amount of time required to dissect the fabric. When we asked the tailor which direction was harder to cut through, he replied that cutting across the fabric was harder. This means that the scissors' performance dropped when cutting across the grain compared with along, and backs data showing a longer time spent on cutting. Even with the same scissors, performance differences emerge when cutting in different directions.

In comparing craftsman- made sewing scissors and a pair purchased at a 100-yen shop (Figs. 4 and 8, Figs. 5 and 9), we see a difference in the number of times the blades open and close when the scissors are in use. The tailor pointed out at the interview that one squeeze did not get the less sharp scissors very far along the fabric. With less sharp scissors, one must tug the scissors back a little on the fabric because pushing them forward only makes the fabric bunch up into the blades. This naturally shortens the distance of each cutting. In this way, dull scissors and sharp scissors end up requiring a different number of strokes to cover the same distance.

When comparing craftsman- made sewing scissors and a pair purchased at a 100-yen shop (Figs. 6 and 10, Figs. 7 and 11), one can see differences in the angle of the blades for sharp vs dull scissors. The tailor said at the interview that he had to open the scissors wide when using the dull pair to cut the fabric. This indicates that the 100-yen scissors are dull, and because the fabric was to be cut crosswise, the scissors under performed.

The cross-section view of the fabric as seen under a microscope is visual evidence of the 100-yen scissors' inadequate severing ability (Figs. 12, 13, 14 and 15). The fabric did not yield properly to the cheap scissors and its surface had flattened. Furthermore, the length of the fabric is also inconsistent (Figs. 13 and 15). With the so-hizukuri forged scissors, on the other hand, there's no fabric flattening and the cut edges are uniform and even (Figs. 12 and 14). Judging from these images, one could conclude that 100-yen scissors, which cause flattening in the fabric, force the users to expend more energy. The pictures show that the fabric was squished and cut. In the interview with the tailor, we were informed that the 100-yen scissors were the hardest to handle. Images from the microscope, the speed with which it took for those scissors to cut, the number of times the blades had to move and how wide they had to open – all back up the tailor's assessment.

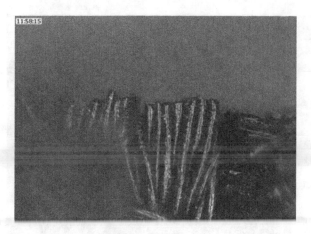

Fig. 12. The cross-section view of the fabric of so-hizukuri scissors (lateral directions of wool fabric, 500 magnifications, 3D).

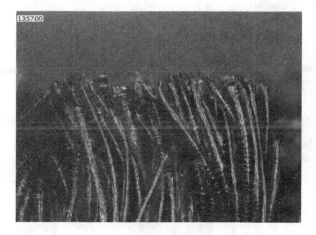

Fig. 13. The cross-section view of the fabric of 100-yen scissors (lateral directions of wool fabric, 500 magnifications, 3D).

On the other hand, regardless of the scissors, and even with fabric that's famous for being difficult to cut like wool, the naked eye was unable to observe a clear difference in the tailor's movements. However, the high speed camera and the optical microscopic observation revealed that there was a large difference. When asked about that the tailor replied that when a craftsman approaches a piece of fabric he subconsciously begins assessing the characteristics of the fabric and how best to move the scissors well before he starts to cut. The consideration that the tailor puts into cutting fabric that's tough or with dull scissors is what makes it difficult for any third person to notice the difference. However, it was not possible to describe in words how the tailor used his scissors. The moment his scissors touch the fabric, the tailor subconsciously selects the best possible

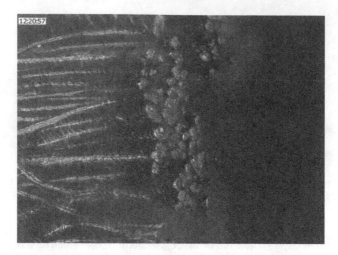

Fig. 14. The cross-section view of the fabric of so-hizukuri scissors (lateral directions of wool fabric, 500 magnifications, 3D, angle of 30 degrees).

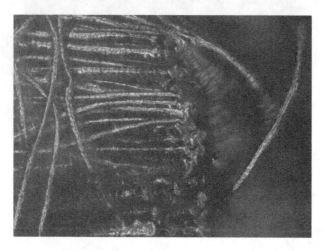

Fig. 15. The cross-section view of the fabric of 100-yen scissors (lateral directions of wool fabric, 500 magnifications, 3D, angle of 30 degrees).

way to handle the scissors to improve its performance. This, we learned, was what is often referred to as the craftsman's technique.

4   Conclusion

Scissors have become such an integral part of our daily lives that we may not even think about their existence. One can say that if their only purpose was to cut paper or fabric in two there are plenty of scissors out there that satisfy those conditions. The act of cutting something in two may appear identical for any pair of scissors, but as the terms "sharp scissors" and "dull scissors" imply, outside of simply dissecting things in two, not all scissors are created equal. For this research, we turned a spotlight on the highly evolved sewing scissors, and investigated the ancient forging process, so-hizukuri, to uncover their secret in producing sharp scissors. We studied what, if any, effect well-performing scissors forged in that process have on the user's movements and the fabric itself. We solicited the help of an expert scissor-handler, a tailor, for this research.

The differences between a dull and sharp pair of scissors are extensive and become apparent in the hands of the users. The characteristics of the scissors affect the speed with which the user can dissect fabric, the way the user moves the scissors, the number of times the blades open and close, among others. The same could be said about fabric alone. The longitudinal yarn in a weave is stronger than the transverse one. It is thereby harder to cut crosswise through the longitudinal thread than the other way around. We found that the direction of the scissors – cutting lengthwise or crosswise – reveals their performance, regardless of the scissors.

Sharp, well-performing scissors rhythmically dissect fabrics without burdening the tailor. We also observed a quantifiable difference in the post-cutting appearance of the fabric. The fabric that was cut by dull scissors was ground down at the edge, creating an uneven and flat appearance to the fabric's weave. This would only serve to lower the quality of tailor made clothes. The purpose of sharp scissors is not limited to simply dissecting fabric in two; they become indispensable tools for scissor-using experts in dramatically raising productivity, bringing out one's abilities and even ensuring a quality finish to tailored outfits.

References

1. Okamoto, M.: Scissors, pp. 233–255. Ekuran-sha, Tokyo (1959)
2. Kitajima, Y., Kito, K., Migaki, M., Matsumuro, K., Murata, Y., Hamada, H.: Process analysis of manufacturing of sewing scissors by all forging process and understanding of its sharpness. In: Duffy, V.G. (ed.) DHM 2015. LNCS, vol. 9184, pp. 124–132. Springer, Heidelberg (2015)

Synaesthesia Design Research of Motion Game in Order to Cure the White-Collar's Cervical Spondylosis

Yuan Liu[✉], Shiguo Li, and Baisong Liu

School of Design, Jiangnan University, Wuxi City, Jiangsu Province, China
Yuanliu19911106@gmail.com, shiguo_edu@qq.com,
Baibainquit@gmail.com

Abstract. Cervical vertebra disease has become another defining characteristic of the White-collars, following with good benefits and high income. Cervical spondylosis usually occured due to long-term working and lack of exercise, and can be very hard to recover from. Yet in the early stage of the disease it can be relieved by frequently doing a kind of cervical gymnastic and developing good exercise habits. In recent years, young people's neck-shoulder problem has become ever more serious, but they haven't pay enough attention, and did not take the corresponding action to the situation. In the mean time, crossing over both sports and entertainment, motion games are getting more popular among White-collars, allowing them to exercise after stressful works, but yet has not yet successfully realized it's potential in medical field. In this paper, we will discuss this newer area of HCI, that is using motion game as a media, summarize and modularize the method of working out shoulder and neck. Also by using the knowledge of synaesthesia design, finally we acquire the design method and game model, that shows how to use synaesthesia design in motion game to achieve the desired effect.

Keywords: Motion game · Cervical spondylosis · Synaesthesia design

1 Health Condition of the White-Collars

The term "Sub-healthy" indicates a kind of condition where the body is either healthy or sick, organs are still technically healthy but function not as well as before. At this point, how to treat the body decides how the health condition will be. The white-collar class is one crowd where this condition is mostly seen, and lacking of physical exercise is the most important reason to that. The lifestyle of a white-collar usually consists commuting by car, constant sitting down and working overtime, leaving them no time to exercise. Over time, problems in cardiovascular system, digest system, immune system and neck malfunction would occur [1].

Among all the diseases, neck is a mostly affected area. Cervical spondylosis is also called cervical vertebra syndrome, which includes cervical vertebra osteoarthritis, hyperplasia of cervical spine, syndrome of cervical nerve root and cervical intervertebral disc herniation, is a disease on the bases of degeneration. If the patient have the conscious to keep doing proper neck exercise during its' early stage, the condition can be prevented,

© Springer International Publishing Switzerland 2016
V.G. Duffy (Ed.): DHM 2016, LNCS 9745, pp. 170–178, 2016.
DOI: 10.1007/978-3-319-40247-5_18

and the pain can be effectively relieved or even eliminated before any irreversible damage happen.

2   The Possible Solution of Cervical Spondylosis

2.1   Damage of Cervical Spondylosis

Cervical spondylosis hurts people in many ways. It will endanger digest system, causing loss of appetite, nausea, vomiting, constipation, weight loss, etc., so the modern medical has the second name for cervical spondylosis as "cervical stomach syndrome". Cervical spondylosis can make it hard to swallow, and some of the cervical spondylosis patients often feel sick when eating hard food, they may feel a burning and stabbing pain in breasthone; Cervical spondylosis can also be bad for the heart, that also affects writing and eyesight; Cervical spondylosis can cause abnormal blood pressure and so on [1].

Once cervical spondylosis attacks, it will bring incalculable damage to work and life. Early prevention and treatment of cervical spondylosis in today's society is of great significance and has much research to do in the future.

2.2   Prevention and Cure of Cervical Spondylosis

In modern medical science, it is difficult to completely cure advanced cervical spondylosis, due to the needing of regular hospital consultation and medical treatment. But patients in the early stage, or people did not evolve into the disease but just have pain in the shoulder, cervical gymnastic is a good choice for the prevention and treatment of cervical spondylosis. It is not only easy to operate, but also not limited by time and environment. Twice a day by scientifically moving the neck, can keep the neck pain away from you.

3   Synesthetic Design

3.1   The Concept of Synesthetic Design

In our subconscious, the taste of sweet is always represented by red, the taste of acid is represented by yellow-green or lemon yellow. And when we say we feel "blue" today, It's a subconscious association to combine color and feelings together.

People explore their surroundings with by their senses, as a person's main sensory organs,— eye, ear, tongue and nose, each has a clear division of responsibilities. This phenomenon not only take place between two different senses of feeling, but also can appear among variety of senses. Although these senses have different functions and range of activities, they combined together sometimes and has mutual expressions with each other. For example, in the field of visual food advertising, visual feelings can cause reaction in the sense of taste, red for sweet and yellow for acid. The so-called "color, aroma and taste", is the emphasis on the combination of vision, smell and taste all together. "Color" for the vision, "sweet" for the taste, they are set to stimulate taste

. reaction therefore to generate appetite. That is why food packaging and advertising is always set to the pursuit of better taste association.

As demonstrated, synaesthesia is a common psychological phenomenon in our daily life, a corresponding psychological reaction due to the external things act on human's senses, causing the synergy of one or more other feeling [2].

3.2   The Synesthetic Interchange in Synaesthesia Design

In the field of synesthetic design, many experiments have already been carried out to discuss how the senses of human work together and how they use themselves to express other feelings. In the research below, two professor from Politecnico di Milano, G. Anceschi and D. Riccò,designed some experiments to see the relationship between vision and gustative sensations—visual restitution of one of the three gustative sensations: sweet, bitter and acid.

As in the image they give, we can see gustative sensations can be easily transformed into colors with shapes, consists with point, line and surface [3].

– sweet sensation is mostly represented with round lines and circle shapes;
– acid and salad sensations is with fragmented lines and angular shapes;
– bitter sensation is with irregular lines and shapes (Fig. 1).

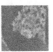

Fig. 1.   Examples of exercises on gustative and chromatic sensations

4   Motion Sensing Game

4.1   Relevant Concepts

Motion-sensing game is a kind of recreation which uses our body as instruments to control and interact with games. Different from using game stick, keyboard, mouse to control the game, the recognition of human motion input introduces a variety of sensing equipment instead of the traditional controllers. It emphasized the interaction both between games and players, players and players, thus to make the players feel they were better immersed in the game; When it comes to entertainment, all kinds of sports and athletic games are the first choice for motion-sensing games. It is not subject to sports facilities, time, space, and climate, that gives the most important advantage to motion game—you can play it at anytime, anywhere. The player would just feel like they were at the gym with a connect on the gamebox. And also can get the same amount of exercise as real.

4.2 Why Choose Motion Games to Cure Cervical Spondylosis

- Portability
  Daily life of the White-collars are quite busy, they do not necessarily have a lot of time for outdoors activity. Motion-sensing game provides a chance for them to do sports indoor, no restriction from space, environment and climate. Even after work or in the spare time between working, you can get enough training and exercise.
- Entertaining
  Motion sensing games is fun to play as most of the games are, they also make it more fun with changing the interface scenes and giving different themes to the game. White-collars are a group of people with high consumption and high aesthetic, it's easy to get their attention, but also easy to lose it. Motion game has higher adaptability, with different kinds of competitive sports games like boxing, swimming, ball games and so on. It is not easy to get bored, and it can be strengthened by means of online interaction with family and friends, which meets to social needs of white-collars.
- The same intensity of an actual workout
  During the process of the game, it provides users of a certain intensity of exercise. The game needs to be controlled by extremity movement, makes the users' body movements become inevitable in the process of the game, and due to the way the software is programed, you need to follow certain rules in the process of operation to complete the actions, which is a great interpretation of the most basic physical properties of keeping fit.

  John Porcari, Ph.D. at the University of Wisconsin, United States, conducted a new study shows that "EA Sports activity" and "EA Sports vitality: six weeks to build good figure," these two Wii Sports game product can be defined as effective workout according to the standard set by the American College of Sports Medicine. This study measured the two "EA sports vitality" default fitness activities (" Afterburner "and" Legs and Lungs ") about the relative motion intensity and calorie consumption, participants are energetic adults aged 16 between 25 and 45 years old. According to the results, by taking a healthy active lifestyle and regularly use the "EA sports activity", players not only can improve the activity of aerobic exercise, but also can positively affect physical condition [4].
- Accurate motion correction.
  The motion capture technology in the game can identify player's bones and actions very accurately, by guiding their movements with the conduct on the game screen, to make the training more efficient, just like having a family fitness coach to teach you one-on-one. Kinect is a well-accepted motion capture technology globally, capture people's actions by laser camera, and identify the bone position, so as to identify the movement of the body. For activities that acquire accurate motions like dance and yoga, exercise with the games will be more effective than trying by oneself at home (Fig. 2).

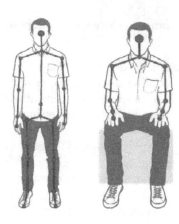

Fig. 2. Kinectbone identifying technology

4.3 Medical Field Application

The medical area already had some achievements in related fields since the import of motion games. Early in 2008, Kentucky, USA, Fort Campbell tried to use the Wii motion game to help 400 soldiers of America's 101st airborne division to recover from brain injury, and to discuss whether they would be able to return. Tests using a variety of odd Wii game (such as "quickly recognize letters game") to test the soldiers of the cognitive ability, coordinating ability and response speed, etc., and every soldier entered war in the previous year must take part in other different types of games except Wii game for brain damage detection. Southern Illinois, a herring hospital rehabilitation center has a Wii gaming platform being used in the rehabilitation training of patients, and in the west of Chicago, some rehabilitation hospitals will also use Wii rehabilitation treatment for spinal injury.

Banner Good Samaritan Medical Center in Arizona clinic uses Wii to enhance the level of surgical operation. Eight internship surgeons play Wii games for an hour before laparoscopic surgery. Results show that with the Wii warm-up, speed and accuracy of the operation have promoted by 48 %.

In the field of archaeological research, the university of California try to use Kinect more suited for archaeological working environment, replacing the expensive, complex professional equipment, such as LIDAR, in order to obtain higher accuracy of 3D scanning positioning information [5].

The above materials certificate, motions games has been used and achieved effective feedback in medical field, it has the possibility to get good curative effect in cervical spondylosis curing.

4.4 Synaesthesia Design in Motion Sensing Game

Because of the leading role body movements played in motion game, sound and visual senses are more important as a guiding media. Motion game often uses sound to guide vision or the other way around. For example, in the boxing module of the game "Kinect Sports", the player controls the movement by their arm movements, and the actions been used in the game is divided into the uppercut, lower hook, straight, quick thrusts, and defense, mainly uses one's shoulder and neck. When you use quick thrusts to attack the enemy, player's constant struck of opponents get him an extra score, then the screen shows a special effect of flame burning, prompt players to continue the hitting, accompanied by increases sound effects, indicates player to attack harder. Also, when the opponent who are going to be knocked out soon, the system will count down to remind the lose. These two phenomenon are the typical examples of how synaesthesia design been used in game interface, with the combination of vision and hearing, gamers can focus on the game instead of reading game instructions (Fig. 3).

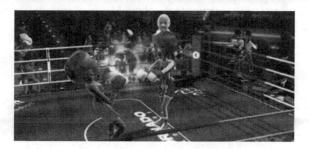

Fig. 3. Player's constant struck with fire effect

Similarly, in the opening interface of motion game, players can use gestures to select columns or resume the game. When move the hand to the corresponding option, with the palm suspended in the air and maintain for a few seconds, there will be a prompt system getting louder to indicate that you are about to enter the next level of the interface, using sound changes from low to high to indicates the page forwarding (Fig. 4).

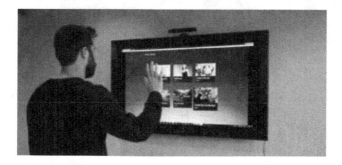

Fig. 4. The opening interface of motion game

5   Experiments

According to the research about cervical spondylosis and motion game, a experiment need to be down in order to test how the motion game effect on human's cervical vertebra. Two motion games based on the movement of neck and shoulder, both from the game ≪Kinect Sports≫, have been chosen as the experimental materials.

Location: HUAWEI UCD Center

Target Group: Designers, Programmers, totally 20 people.

Experimental material: XBOX, Kinect, ≪Kinect Sports≫ motion games

Research Method: comparison method, observation method.

Proceeding: Choose two motion games basically using shoulder and neck— "boxing" and "Beach Volleyball" as the tester, set the timer to 5 min for each game, let the gamers play by the leading on the screen, each game for 5 min. When finished, let them compare the effects of two games to the shoulder-neck area, and which action they prefer the most (Fig. 5).

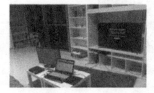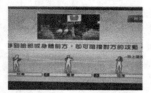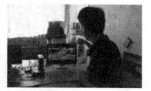

Fig. 5.   Test scenario in HUAWEI UCD

Research Result: Experiment results show that 16 of 20 people prefer boxing, the angle of moving arms is suitable, compared with intense and fast action, smooth shoulder movement is more conducive to the relaxation of muscles. Arm and shoulder movements should follow definite frequency, not too hard nor to weak (Fig. 6).

Game	Shoulder			Neck	
	Movement	Angle	Lasting Time	Movement	Lasting Time
Boxing	uppercut,uppercut quick thrusts, straight punch, defense	90°~135°	0.5s~3s	dodge	0.5s~1s
Beach Volleyball	serving, smashing	90°~180°	0.5s~1s	dodge	0.5s~1s

Fig. 6.   Details of movements in the two games

5.1 Designed Game Model

"Chan" is a motion-based music game designed to alleviate neck pain and provide the prevention for cervical spondylosis. The game process lasts for 5 min, according to the time and operation method of cervical vertebra gymnastics. Gamers are asked to move their head and shoulder by the leading on the screen, if speed and action are standard, the music will continue smoothly without noise, if not, the game will remind you by the changing of color and sound until you reach the standard. With all the perfect motion, you can play out a wonderful music and get the perfect trophy.

In-game actions:

- Head tilt to the left, hold for 5 s, to the right, hold for 5 s. Repeat three times.
- Head stretch to the front, hold for 5 s, tilt back, hold for 5 s. Repeat three times.
- Both hands on the shoulder, rotate forward and backward 20 times respectively.
- Rotate head both direction for three times.
- Hand over head, fingers crossed, head up, hold for 10 s. Repeat three times.
- Reorganization movements (Fig. 7).

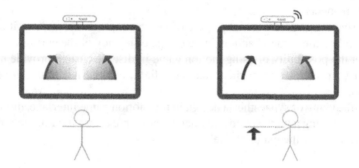

Fig. 7. Schematic diagram of the module

5.2 Simulation Test

Location: Interaction Lab, School of design, Jiangnan University.

Target Group: Designers, in total 6 people.

Test equipment: PC, Music player, Mobile phone

Test method: Simulate the progress of "chan" by the exercise of cervical vertebra set in soothing music, lasts for five minutes in total. In order to ensure the accuracy of the action, when conductors of the experiment found out some wrong actions, they use a mobile phone to play error suggested sounds, thus to remind the subject to correct their movements.

Test Result: Subjects' feedback showed an improvement of their necks condition. Comparing to exercise on oneself, the visual reminder and sounds of the game helps them to do the exercise correctly, and help to adjust the pace of the movements.

6   Summary Methods of the Motion Game Designed for the Treatment of Cervical Spondylosis

- Smooth limb stretching is more conducive to the relaxation of the cervical spine, one single movement should last for more then 2 s, and the total playing time is better for around 5 min.
- Using fluctuation of music to remind the accuracy of the action, can let gamers' attention focus on the exercise, instead of always staring at the screen like the other games.
- Slow type of music like piano and light music is more conducive to the user's relaxing, so does clean interface design and concise game guidance.

7   Significance

- Provide a new way for the white-collars to ease the cervical spondylosis, explore the development prospects of motion game in the field of health and its' future development prospects.
- Motion-sensing game has a high degree of motion capture recognition, it can effectively regulate the gamers' action, increase the efficiency of the curing.
- Consider the possibility of using motion game in disease curing, provide new ideas for the HCI principles in medical treatment field, explore its' future development direction.
- Explore the using of synaesthesia design in the motion game interface, discover new uses of combining action, sound and image together, explore it's function of guiding the gamers during the game progress.

References

1. Editorial Department of China's New Era: Investigation and Analysis on the Health Status of White-collars. China's New Era (2014) (in Chinese)
2. Jin, X., Xinhua, C.: Study of synaesthesia in visual communication design. Jiangnan University, pp. 23–40 (2008) (in Chinese)
3. Dina, R., Silvia, G., Design Research Unit GaMS., Giovanni, A.: Synesthetic Design-The Laboratory of Basic Design as Place of Experimentation on the Intersensory Correspondences. In: International Multisensory Research Forum, 3rd Annual Meeting, Geneva, Switzerland (2002)
4. Sina News. http://news.sina.com.cn/w/2007-07-22/123912250060s.shtml (in Chinese)
5. Fang, L., Guosheng, S.: Research on the Sports Value of the Electronic Somatosensory Game. Nanjing Sport Institute (2013) (in Chinese)

Introducing a Language
for Human Stance Description

António C. Mabiala[1], Antonio W. Sousa[2], Norton T. Roman[1(✉)],
João L. Bernardes Jr.[1], Marcelo M. Antunes[3], Enrique M. Ortega[3],
Luciano A. Digiampietri[1], Luis M. del Val Cura[4], Valdinei F. da Silva[1],
and Clodoaldo A.M. Lima[1]

[1] University of São Paulo, São Paulo, Brazil
norton@usp.br
[2] São Paulo Faculty of Technology, São Paulo, Brazil
[3] Central Kung Fu Academy, Campinas, Brazil
[4] Campo Limpo Paulista Faculty, Campo Limpo Paulista, Brazil

Abstract. The ability to automatically determine a human body's
sequence of postures during movement has many practical applications,
from the evaluation of the performance of physical activity practitioners
to the evaluation and design of the user experience in certain systems.
Current representations for such postures, however useful, are not capable of capturing all necessary features for a complete description of a
human stance, such as the relationship between non-directly connected
body parts. In this article, we introduce a mark-up language for body
stance and movement description, designed to allow for the unambiguous representation of movement as well as the extraction of relationships
between directly and non-directly connected body parts. Along with the
language, we also present a computer program, developed to help end
users in codifying stance and movement without having to know the
language in detail.

1 Introduction

The ability to automatically determine a human body's sequence of postures
during movement has many practical applications, from the evaluation of the
performance of physical activity practitioners (e.g. [1]) to patients' physical rehabilitation (e.g. [3,4]), posture assessment (e.g. [6]), aiding in learning (e.g. [16])
or in exercising (e.g. [5]) and even for the evaluation and design of the User
Experience in certain systems (e.g. [2]). Such tasks, however, depend not only
on some existing apparatus for capturing and tracking the position of body parts
(such as Microsoft Kinect, for example), but also on some form of representation suitable for future inspection, comparison or specification of detected and
recorded postures.

© Springer International Publishing Switzerland 2016
V.G. Duffy (Ed.): DHM 2016, LNCS 9745, pp. 179–190, 2016.
DOI: 10.1007/978-3-319-40247-5_19

Current representations, such as the Human Mark-up Language[1] and the Human Performance Mark-up Language[2], for instance, however useful, are not capable of capturing all necessary features for a complete description of a human stance. More specifically, they have no straightforward way to determine the relationship between non-directly connected body parts, such as the position of the left hand related to the right foot, for example, which is paramount to describe some physical activities, such as dancing and practising martial arts.

In this article, we try to fill in this gap, by introducing a mark-up language for the description of human postures, taking into account not only the relationship between directly connected body parts, but also between indirectly connected ones, along with some symmetry relations. This effort is taken as part of a bigger project, called *Education and monitoring of physical activities through artificial intelligence techniques*[3], which aims at the teaching and monitoring of physical activities, specially within the practice of martial arts.

Within this scope, this research aims to define requirements for body posture descriptions in an unambiguous way, allowing different descriptions to be evaluated and compared. We then introduce a language designed to fulfil all these requirements. Formatted as an XML file, the language offers both a reference system in conformance to the ISO/IEC FCD 19774:200x Humanoid animation H-Anim standard, and a description based on the identification of different angles between connected parts. Both descriptions co-exist in the XML: while the former is mainly used to unambiguously describe the stances, the later is meant to be used by the end user, given its more intuitive nature.

Along with the language specification, we also developed a computer program to help users describe postures through a graphical interface, where relationships between body parts can be described by selecting the type of relationship from a previously defined list, along with possible angles between connected parts[4]. With this software, we intend both to reduce the cognitive load on the user, by moving the description details away from the user's attention, and to reduce the possibility of errors in the codification of the posture.

Finally, all produced materials, such as the language documentation and end-user software (along with its source code), will be freely available to the community under a creative commons license. The rest of this article is organized as follows. Section 2 introduces some of current movement notation systems, along with a brief discussion about computational models that use them. In the sequence, Sect. 3 describes some related work on mark-up languages for human postures. Section 4, in turn, presents the specification of the language we

---

[1] https://www.oasis-open.org/committees/download.php/60/HM.
Primary-Base-Spec-1.0.html.

[2] http://www.sisostds.org/StandardsActivities/StudyGroups/
HPMLSGHumanPerformanceMarkupLanguage.aspx.

[3] Process N°: 14.1.00923.86.4.

[4] Notice that the definition of a sequence of connected angles would eventually lead to the definition of an angle between non-directly connected parts.

developed, whose working model is presented in Sect. 5. Finally, Sects. 6 and 7 present our results and a conclusion to this research.

2   Movement Notation Systems

Created by Joan and Rudolph Benesh to record the movements of classical ballet, the Benesh System [14] is committed to the line of execution and the visual result of the movement. Based on a body position that resembles the T-stance, commonly used by game developers and 3D characters animators, the system uses a set of symbols to show the position of the dancer and the posture being performed, along with five parallel lines to determining the height of body parts positions. Within the same framework, Laban's Movement and Dance Notation [8] uses a finite model of space, where the body moves immersed in a sphere, separated by three perpendicular planes, to record any type of human movement. The system then uses distinct symbols do represent body parts and movement directions, taking into account the sphere in which the model is fit.

Alternatively, the Eshkol-Wachman Notation [14] divide the space with planes, using pair of numbers to represent important points. Also relying on a set of symbols to represent body parts and movement directions, the system was used in computer graphics, architecture and work related to animal behaviour, being also used to describe the Israeli Sign Language and to evaluate the movements of the Tai Chi Chuan Chinese martial art [7]. Within this notation, the body is represented as a "stick-figure", with segments and points. The segments connect pairs of joints or points, so that every part of the body has a representation in a manuscript defined by five parallel lines. As in the Laban Notation, Eshkol-Wachman also uses a spherical reference system, but with pairs of numbers representing specific positions in space, as opposed to symbols.

Finally, the HamNoSys – Hamburg Notation System [9] – is a notation system designed to support avatar-independent sign language transcriptions, recording only the relevant aspects of language for the correct execution of gestures. The system defines a spacial volume where gestures are performed, taking into account just hand and arm movements, thereby considering the rest of the body as static. This notation has, in turn, served as the basis for SiGML (Signing Gesture Mark-up Language) [13], a mark-up language used to record gestures in sign languages, also being avatar-independent.

Existing computational models usually rely on some of these notations, such as the one presented in [15] which, based in Laban's Kinesiography, deals with gesture acquisition and synthesis. However interesting, such models usually need some previous knowledge and preparation from the person performing the movements, also needing a controlled environment. Additionally, despite the fact that notation systems try to make easier the record and the understanding of gestures by people with proper training, they are still not suitable for non-specialist in the system. Another noteworthy point about them is that they are not interoperable, being necessary some sort of adaptation or conversion from one system to another.

3   Related Work

The proposal of a mark-up language for human postures and expressions is not something new, with many alternatives being proposed over the last few years, each of them with different objectives and scopes. One such example is VHML – Virtual Human Mark-up Language[5] – which was designed to encompass various aspects of Human-Computer Interaction. Acting like a super-set of languages, VHML paved the way to other more specific languages, such as EML – Emotion Markup Language, FAML – Facial Animation Markup Language and BAML – Body Animation Markup Language, amongst others. However also designed to be expansible and generic, VHML was primarily created to make easier the communication between humans and avatars.

Others languages, such as Human Markup Language [16], for example, propose to encompass cultural aspects and its specification, since high-level languages can show some problems when defining concepts like angry or happy. Just like VHML, HumanML is a high-level language, being used to record the behaviour and expression of virtual agents, especially in their interaction with the user. A different proposal, but with a similar goal, is XSTEP [11], a mark-up language based on the STEP [10] script language. As a language, XSTEP has the interesting feature of allowing other languages to be embedded in it.

Our research differs from these in that we move away from the goal of describing a human being, be it virtual or not, in its entirety, thereby setting aside aspects such as culture and emotion, or the possibility of having them added to the language. Instead, we focus on how to represent body stances and movements, specially for the use in the realm of martial arts. Hence, and as it will be made clearer in the forthcoming sections, we try to fulfil some requirements specific to this task, being able to describe relations between both connected and non-directly connected body parts (which, in our model, can be described as sequences of positions and angles between all connected body parts along the way from one unconnected part to the other).

4   Language Specification

In order for the language to be computationally useful, it should [12]:

1. Be convenient, in that posture specifications should hide geometrical details away from the user, thereby allowing it to be used in the most natural way possible by domain experts; and
2. Possess a compositional semantics, thereby allowing for complex descriptions to come out as relationships between simpler component descriptions.

Additionally, in our interactions with martial arts experts, we set up a list of further requirements for the language, according to which it should also be able to represent:

---

[5] http://www.vhml.org/.

1. The relationship between body parts in symmetry and asymmetry;
2. The relationship between upper body parts and between upper and lower parts, both in the same side and opposite sides of the body;
3. The relationship between the head and the transversal body line (the line crossing the so called Dantian[6]);
4. The relationship between the position of the head in relation to the body balance area, as determined by the position of the feet;
5. The relationship between the head and the body gravity centre; and
6. The relationship between gaze and the direction of subsequent movements.

To comply with these requirements, we begin by defining the starting position of any description, which corresponds to a body standing along the y axis (Fig. 1(a)), with the x axis going from left to right and the z axis moving in the front to back direction. The origin point $(0, 0, 0)$ is located at the ground level, between the feet. The arms are straight and parallel to the sides of the body, with the palms facing inward towards the thighs. The reference system is builds on these three dimensions. Figure 1(b)[7] illustrates some combinations based on these three dimensions.

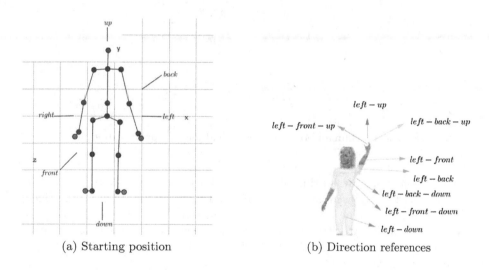

(a) Starting position   (b) Direction references

Fig. 1. Starting position and direction of reference of body parts.

Additionally, the *ISO/IECFCD19774:200x Humanoid animation H-Anim17* specification also contains a set of nodes that are arranged to form a hierarchy. Each node contains other nodes and a number of nodes that specify which vertices correspond to a particular characteristic or configuration.

---

[6] Energy centers in Chinese martial arts.

[7] Adapted from [11].

5   Working Model

The articulated design model consists of points, called elements, which represent different parts of the human body. Based on this representation it is possible to extract angles and establish relationships between them. Figure 2 illustrates the representation parts to be considered in our model, while Fig. 3 shows the working model associated with them. The language, however, was designed to accommodate several elements of human body, not only those described in the working model.

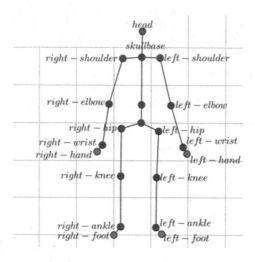

Fig. 2. The human body and its typical joints representation

Since the language was primarily designed for the use in a martial arts context, body parts may assume some pre-defined descriptions, such as the tiger, snake, panther and crane kung-fu stances, for instance. These description apply both to the whole body or to specific body parts, such as the hands, for example. Other elements, not mentioned in the working model, along with other language features, are described in the language documentation[8].

Following the pivot points described in Fig. 3, base input parameters can be provided to represent stances, thereby ensuring that each of them will have a unique description that can be extracted from the angles of their hinged parts and the relations of symmetry and asymmetry between them. Also, and to ensure more consistency between the elements, we defined a hierarchy between the various body parts, as shown in Fig. 4. Following the hierarchy, in order to describe the angles between the joints of the upper limbs, one has to start from the skull. Similarly, for the angles between the joints of the lower limbs, the hips are the starting point.

---

[8] http://1-dot-term-paper-1121.appspot.com/pack/documentation/index.html.

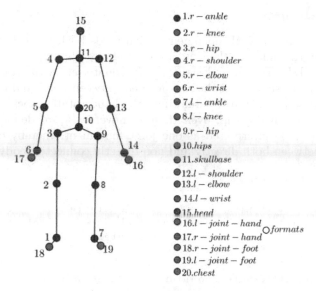

Fig. 3. The working model and its elements.

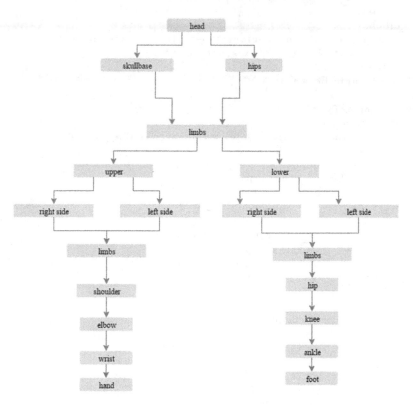

Fig. 4. Elements' hierarchy in our model.

5.1 XML Scheme

The scheme rests in an XML document which holds both the rules for encoding and the way the different elements are related to each other. As an example, consider the XML below, which describes a 30° counter-clockwise rotation of the hand, shaped as a fist, around the axis formed between hand and elbow, measured at the wrist joint. At the same time, the hand rotates clockwise, around the elbow. Within this set-up, even though movements are defined independently, they must be interpreted as one joint movement, thereby establishing relationships between both directly and non-directly connected body parts.

```
1  <node1_angle_between>
2    <hand>
3      <format_attributes>fist</format_attributes>
4        <min_rot_attributs>counter_clockwise</min_rot_attributs>
5        <axis_attributes>x</axis_attributes>
6    </hand>
7    <wrist>
8        <min_rot_attributes>counter_clockwise</min_rot_attributes>
9        <axis_attributes>y</axis_attributes>
10       <angle_attributes>30</angle_attributes>
11   </wrist>
12   <elbow>
13       <min_rot_attributes>clockwise</min_rot_attributes>
14       <axis_attributes>y</axis_attributes>
15   </elbow>
16 </node1_angle_between>
17 . . .
18 <xs: complexType>
19   <xs: sequence>
20     <xs: element name=''node1_angle_between''>
21       <xs: complexType>
22         <xs: sequence>
23           <xs: element name=''hand''>
24             <xs: complexType>
25               <xs: sequence>
26                 <xs: group ref=''format''/>
27                 <xs: group ref=''min_rot''/>
28                 <xs: group ref=''axis''/>
29               </xs: sequence>
30             </xs: complexType>
31           </xs: element>
32           <xs: element name=''wrist''>
33             <xs: complexType>
34               <xs: sequence>
35                 <xs: group ref=''min_rot''/>
36                 <xs: group ref=''axis''/>
37                 <xs: group ref=''angle''/>
38               </xs: sequence>
39             </xs: complexType>
40           </xs: element>
```

```
41          <xs: element name=''elbow">
42           <xs: complexType>
43            <xs: sequence>
44              <xs: group ref=''min−rot"/>
45              <xs: group ref=''axis"/>
46            </xs: sequence>
47           </xs: complexType>
48          </xs: element>
49        </xs: sequence>
50       </xs: complexType>
51   .  .  .
```

6 Results

In order to help end users in the task of codifying stances and movements without having to dig too deep into the language idiosyncrasies, we developed a computer program which, through a graphical interface, allows them to select body parts and relationships between them from a list of pre-defined values. With this program, the user describes movements by inserting parameters such as axes and angles between joints and by establishing relations between different elements. The program then generates the XML, showing it to the user, who may choose to export it to an XML file. Figures 5 and 6 illustrate the program's interface. At this point, it is important to notice that the program is still a prototype, available in Portuguese only. New versions are expected soon.

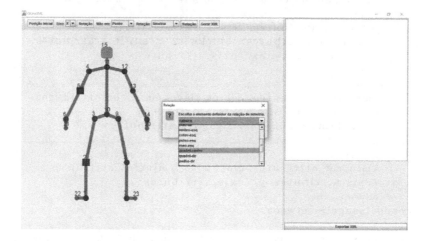

Fig. 5. Program's interface – defining relationships between elements.

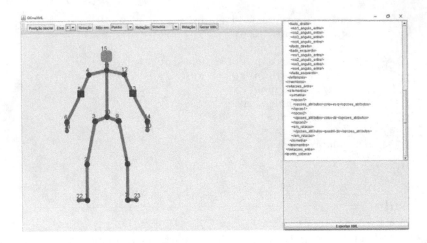

Fig. 6. Program's interface – outputting the XML code.

To test our prototype we carried out some experiments, where one of the researchers would describe the stances and movements, using the program's interface, and then manually verify the generated XML file. Coding samples may be found below[9].

```
 1  <head>
 2    <limb>
 3      <right><!-- angles: upper limbs, right -->
 4      <node1_angule_between> <! --angle in the wrist joint-->
 5        <hand>
 6          <format_attributes> fist</format_attributes>
 7          <min_rot_attributes> clockwise </min_rot_atributes>
 8          <exis_attributes>x</exis_attributes>
 9        </hand>
10        <wrist>
11          <min_rot_attributes> clockwise </min_rot_attributes>
12          <exis_attributes>y</exis_attributes>
13          <angule_attributes>45</angule_attributes>
14        </wrist>
15        <elbow>
16          <min_rot_attributes>clockwise</min_rot_attributes>
17          <exis_attributes>y</exis_attributes>
18        </elbow>
19    </node1_angule_between>
```

In this code snippet, we see the description of the right hand rotated clockwise, by 45°, at the right wrist joint, while taking a fist shape. In the following code, the relation of symmetry between left knee and right knee, relatively to the vertical axis passing through the body centre, is illustrated.

---

[9] Since generated files are too long to be shown here, we present but snippets for illustration purposes only.

```
1  <relationship_between>
2    <limb>
3      < symmetry >
4        <option1>
5          <options_attributes>left_knee</options_attributes>
6        </option1>
7        <options2>
8          <options_attributes>right_knee</otions_attributes>
9        </option2>
10         < regarding>
11           <options_attributes>vertical_exis</options_attributes>
12         </regarding >
13       </symmetry>
14 </relationship _between>
```

7   Conclusion

In this article we proposed a mark-up language for body stance and movement description. Its novelty lies in that it covers many aspects of this subject, from the unambiguous representation of movement to the extraction of relationships between directly and non-directly connected body parts. Along with the language description, we have also developed a computer program to bridge the gap between the end user, that is the person directly dealing with the movements to be codified, and the language details, thereby saving time and reducing the cognitive load imposed by the learning and mastering of the language.

Despite the results we already have, there is still a long road ahead, with much work to be done so as to polish the language, by further testing it and observing its behaviour when dealing with everyday problems in the area. Also, the auxiliary program is still a prototype and, as such, must be tested and further improved, so as to provide the community with a reliable and powerful tool.

References

1. Alexiadis, D.S., Kelly, P., Daras, P., O'Connor, N.E., Boubekeur, T., Moussa, M.B.: Evaluating a dancer's performance using kinect-based skeleton tracking. In: Candan, K.S., Panchanathan, S., Prabhakaran, B., Sundaram, H., Feng, W.C., Sebe, N. (eds.) the 19th ACM International Conference, pp. 659–622 (2011)
2. Bordegoni, M., Camere, S., Caruso, G., Cugini, U.: Body tracking as a generative tool for experience design. In: Duffy, V.G. (ed.) DHM 2015. LNCS, vol. 9185, pp. 122–133. Springer, Heidelberg (2015)
3. Chang, C.Y., Lange, B., Zhang, M., Koenig, S., Rcqucjo, P., Somboon, N., Sawchuk, A., Rizzo, A.: Towards pervasive physical rehabilitation using microsoft kinect. In: Arriaga, R., Matic, A. (eds.) 6th International Conference on Pervasive Computing Technologies for Healthcare (2012)
4. Chang, Y.J., Chen, S.F., Huang, J.D.: A kinect-based system for physical rehabilitation: a pilot study for young adults with motor disabilities. Res. Dev. Disabil. **32**(6), 2566–2570 (2011)

5. Chye, C., Sakamoto, M., Nakajima, T.: An exergame for encouraging martial arts. In: Kurosu, M. (ed.) HCI 2014, Part III. LNCS, vol. 8512, pp. 221–232. Springer, Heidelberg (2014)

6. Clark, R.A., Pua, Y.H., Fortin, K., Ritchie, C., Webster, K.E., Denehy, L., Bryant, A.L.: Validity of the microsoft kinect for assessment of postural control. Gait Posture **36**(3), 372–377 (2012)

7. Eshkol, N., Harries, J.G., Sapir, T., Sella, R., Shoshani, M.: The Quest for Tai Chi Chuan. The Research Center for Movement Notation, Faculty of Visualand Performing Arts, Tel Aviv University (1986)

8. Guest, A.H.: Labanotation: The System of Analyzing and Recording Movement. Taylor & Francis, London (2014)

9. Hanke, T.: Hamnosys - representing sign language data in language resources and language processing contexts. In: Proceedings of the 4th International Conference on Language Resources and Evaluation (LREC 204). Lisbon, Portugal, 26–28 May 2004

10. Huang, Z., Eliëns, A., Visser, C.: Step: a scripting language for embodied agents. In: Proceedings of the Workshop of Lifelike Animated Agents, Tokyo (2002)

11. Huang, Z., Eliëns, A., Visser, C.: XSTEP: An XML-based markup language for embodied agents. In: Proceedings of the 16th International Conference on Computer Animation and Social Agents, (CASA 2003), pp. 105–110 (2003)

12. Huang, Z., Eliëns, A., Visser, C.: Step: a scripting language for embodied agents. In: Gabbay, M., Siekmann, J., Prendinger, H., Ishizuka, M. (eds.) Life-Like Characters. Cognitive Technologies, pp. 87–109. Springer, Heidelberg (2004)

13. Kennaway, R.: Avatar-independent scripting for real-time gesture animation. arXiv preprint (2015). arXiv:1502.02961

14. Kleinman, S.: Movement notation systems: An introduction. Quest **23**(1), 33–34 (1975)

15. Rett, J., Dias, J., Ahuactzin, J.M.: Laban movement analysis using a bayesian model and perspective projections. In: Proceedings of the Brain, Vision and AI (2008)

16. Trajkova, M., Ferati, M.: Usability evaluation of kinect-based system for ballet movements. In: Marcus, A. (ed.) DUXU 2015. LNCS, vol. 9187, pp. 464–472. Springer, Heidelberg (2015)

Process Analysis of Expert and Non-expert Engineers in Quartz Glass Bending Process

Masamichi Suda[1], Toru Takahashi[2], Akio Hattori[2(✉)], Akihiko Goto[3], and Hiroyuki Hamada[4]

[1] Kyoto Institute of Technology, Kyoto, Japan
Masamichi_suda@daico.co.jp
[2] Techno-Eye Corporation, Kyoto, Japan
{takahashi,yoshi_suda}@daico.co.jp
[3] Department of Information Systems Engineering, Faculty of Design Technology,
Osaka Sangyo University, Osaka, Japan
gotoh@ise.osaka-sandai.ac.jp
[4] Advanced Fibro-Science, Kyoto Institute of Technology, Kyoto, Japan
hhamada@kit.ac.jp

Abstract. Quartz glass has a very high purity of silicon, and has heat resistance, chemical resistance, and excellent optical transparency. Therefore, it has been called the king of the glass.

Quartz glass has a superior performance than other glasses. Especially it has been used as a key component of high-performance analytical instruments and scientific instruments and special manufacturing equipment.

Because of its high heat resistance, it is difficult to the processing in a variety of shapes. General borosilicate glass can be mass produced by a hot press processing with precision mold. Quartz glass is difficult to mass-produced by mold because of its high melting point. Therefore, many of the quartz glass product is manufactured by engineer's hand processing for each product.

Therefore, in order to produce high-precision quartz glass product efficiently, engineers training is the most important. Also, engineers with a high processing technology has been aging in recent years. There are situations in which the tradition of technology is not going well. To keep stable supply of high-precision products, to analyze the processing technology of highly skilled engineers, it requires efforts to help education and training.

Keywords: Ergonomics and sustainability · Quartz glass · Process analysis · Fire process · Mechanical property evaluation

1 Introduction

There are several types of the processing of quartz glass. Especially, products used in such analysis equipment, special and complicated shapes are required. Therefore, the heating processing by flame called "Fire-process" is needed.

"Fire-process" is a processing technology that uses a mixed flame of oxygen and hydrogen by heating the quartz glass material to the softening point, to form the softened

V.G. Duffy (Ed.): DHM 2016, LNCS 9745, pp. 191–200, 2016.
DOI: 10.1007/978-3-319-40247-5_20

glass by hand of the engineer. Therefore, to produce high-precision products efficiently it is believed to require special processing technology by many years of experience.

Bending is one of the basic processing technology among fire processing of quartz glass. The bending is a general term for the process of bending at an angle while heating the quartz glass. This technique is used in many products, this technique is essential in the production of complex glass parts used in the analyzer.

In this study, we took up this bending process. This technique is one of the basic processing techniques, it has been made by hand. Also, this process is dependent on the quality and work efficiency by the skill of the engineer. In the current situation, that the low skilled engineers to copy the processing steps have not been able to improve the quality and productivity. On the basis of this situation, the purpose of this study, by the quartz glass bending process analysis under the same conditions by different engineers, is to help the results to the training of future engineers.

2   Experimental Method

This section describes the experimental method of bending.

We chose the engineers of two people with different years of experience as a subject.

Two of the engineers did a bending under the same conditions, and analyzed the process by the video shooting.

The experiment material was normal quartz glass tube with outside diameter: 20 mm, inside diameter: 17 mm, length: 400 mm.

Before bending process, engineers join the glass tube for holding to two ends of quartz glass tube. (Fig. 1).

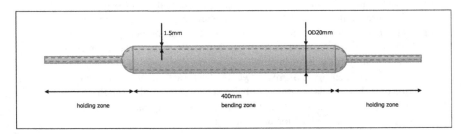

Fig. 1. Quartz glass tube for test, after jointing of hold glass tubes

The status of operator and burner is shown in Fig. 2.

The flame with about 3000 °C which can soften the quartz glass was generated by the combination of hydrogen and oxygen. Operator sat behind the burner and kept sitting posture for processing.

Engineers were directed to perform bending process on quartz glass tube to 90 ° without any other instruction. Meanwhile, each subjects processed one piece of tube at a time and totally 3 times. During process, every experimental subject was controlled in same process environment without distraction. This is so that the subject is not affected

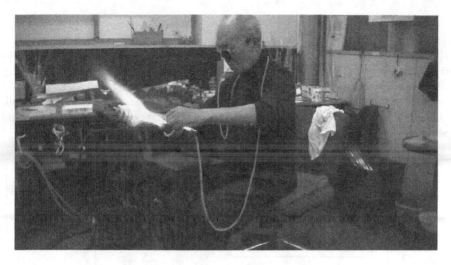

Fig. 2. Processing position of engineer with flame burner

by watching the processing techniques of the other subjects. In order to analyze the detail, the whole process was recorded by digital camera.

3   Engineer's Information

In this study, two different experience engineers were invited as subjects who "Engineer A" has 54 years of experience, "Engineer-B" has 5 years of experience. Two were selected from engineers who works on fire process every day and their experiment of processing was continuous for many years.

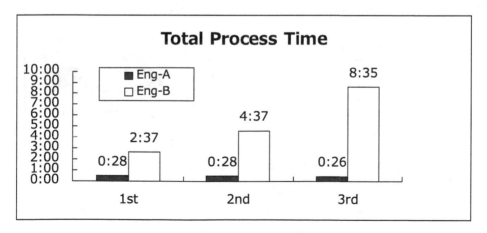

Fig. 3. Total process time

4   Motion Analysis

Firstly, we have analyzed the processing recorded video, were compared for time from start to finish. (Fig. 3).

Firstly, subjects were heated while rotating the quartz glass tube in the axial direction by hand. And After heating, engineer A was bent 90 ° by one of the bending motion. Engineer B was bent 90 ° by the number of times of bending motion. The number of the bending motion is shown in Fig. 4.

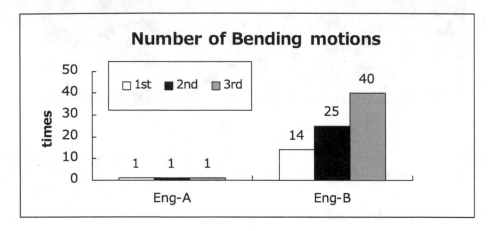

Fig. 4. Number of bending motions

Next, we investigated the difference of heating points and heating time of the glass tube in each subject. The glass tube is divided in four areas (Fig. 5), and measures the heating time by the burners in each area. (Fig. 6).

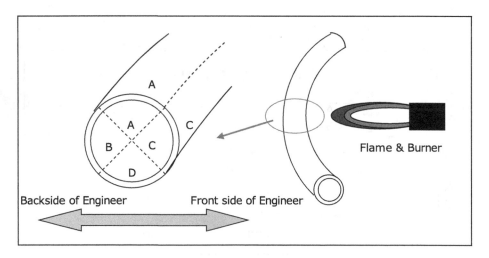

Fig. 5. Area of heating

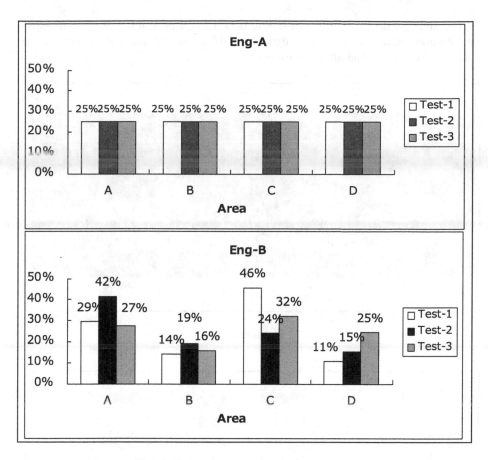

Fig. 6. Ratio of process time by heating area

In the case of Engineer-A, it was processed in a single bending motion. In that case, the glass tube before bending motion had been evenly heated.

In the Engineer-B case, it had been processed in several times of bending motion. In that case, the processing time becomes relatively longer. Addition, it was found that the glass tube is not evenly heated before bending motion.

5   Measurement of Bending Part

Next, we investigated the quality of the quartz glass tube after bending. There are several quality standards for Glass products needs the bending processing. In this study, we measured the outer diameter and wall thickness of the glass tube.

The amount of change before and after processing is the basis for the evaluation of the processing quality.

The image of the quartz glass tube after bending is shown in Fig. 7. Also it shows the measurement points of the outer diameter in Figs. 8 and 9 shows the change in the outer diameter before and after processing.

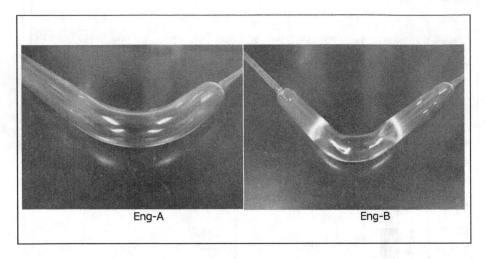

Fig. 7. Sample after bending

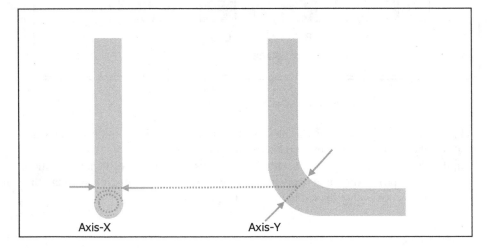

Fig. 8. Measuring point of out diameter

In the case of Engineer-A, the diameter of the glass tube was reduced in the X direction. In the Engineer-B cases, the diameter was expanded. Y direction of the trend was the same as the X direction. In the case of Engineer-A, reduced diameter of the glass tube, in the Engineer-B case, the diameter of the glass tube is expanded. (Fig. 10).

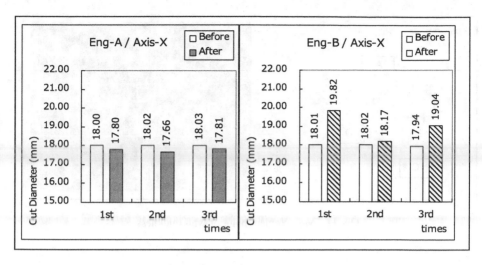

Fig. 9. Changes of axis-X

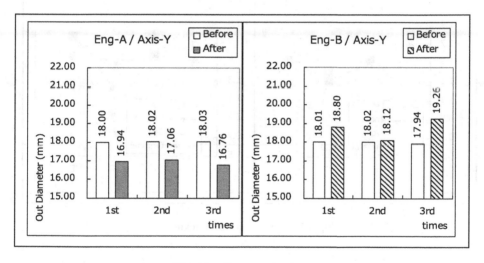

Fig. 10. Changes of axis-Y

The following were the measurement of wall thickness. Figure 11 shows the measurement point. We cut the glass tube, and measured wall thickness with a digital caliper. (Fig. 12).

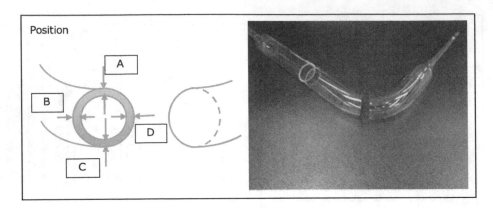

Fig. 11. Measurement point of wall thickness

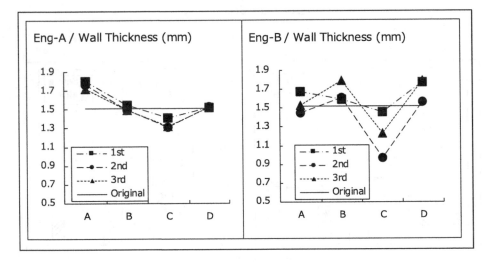

Fig. 12. Changes of wall thickness

In both cases the Engineer-A and -B, the thickness of the C section is thinned in comparison with the wall thickness of the Original. C section had been stretched most at the time of bending. Engineer-A's C section reduction of wall thickness was less.

Addition, Eng-B cross section of the bending is deformed. (Fig. 13) On the other hand, Eng-A's cross-section deformation is small. Eng-A was able to bending with a high roundness.

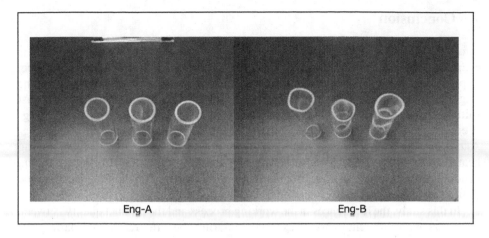

Fig. 13. Cross-section shape of bending part

6   Consideration

In this study, the differences in the working process and the product quality between engineers with different years of experience during the 'fire-process' of quartz glass material were analyzed.

As for product quality, the researches and engineers watched the records after experiment, and engineer-A dictated that the wall thickness, outside diameter of quartz glass tube determined the product quality. Engineer-A told, outside diameter of heated tube will shrink at the beginning of the process. If the tube was heated the outside diameter would shrink and the tube wall would be thicker. Above phenomenon is called 'collect the thickness'. If the tube was stretched the outside diameter would shrink and the tube wall would be thinner, on the contrary, if the tube was compressed to center the outside diameter would expand and the tube wall would be thicker.

In bending process, bending inside part is compressed which cause tube wall thicker, and bending outside part is stretched which cause tube wall thinner. When Eng-A rotate and heat the tube, consciously conducting 'collect the thickness'. Eng-A was able to make a bending products of stable quality because the thickness was conscious control.

In addition, the change in outer diameter of the horizontal (Axis-X of Fig. 8) is generated. (see Fig. 9) Expansion of Axis-X direction, could be confirmed by the glass tube after processing of Eng-B.

By interview, Eng-A had assumed the change. When tube was heated and the outside diameter became smaller, Eng-A promptly bended the tube which can prevent Axis-A&B from expanding and can get approximate circle cross section products.

And researchers also interviewed the Eng-B. Eng-B mainly focused on bending procedure and hardly cared about the collect thickness of tube wall which is very different from Eng-A's operation.

This interview, among engineers, clear differences were found in the knowledge of each process.

7 Conclusion

In order to perform bending with stable quality is to understand that the glass tube is changed by bending motion, and it is important to control the heating of the glass tube. Superficially, it may be seem that the main difference between two engineers is that the Eng-A just conduct one bending movement to process required effect. But it is just suitable for the quartz glass tubes which were used in this study. It's possible that Eng-A conduct more bending-motion for other different size of tube. In this case also, Eng-A told that the most important factor should be concerned is the status of tube during heated and processed. Meanwhile, 'collecting the thickness' is of great concern during bending process, which is useful for determining the process method for specific type of tube and improving product quality.

In this study, the differences in the working process and the product quality between engineers with different years of experience during the fire-process of quartz glass material were analyzed.

The result shows that there was a clear difference in the product quality based on skill maturity.

Eng-A can use 'collecting the thickness' method to control the status of quartz glass tube and expend much less time than Eng-B, which not only improves product quality but also enhance productivity.

In future research, the movement of operator will be as experimental subject with combining the results of this study and the experiment method will be further discussed to improve product quality and the level of production.

References

1. Cibiel, G.: Ultra stable oscillators dedicated for space applications: oscillator and quartz material behaviors vs radiation. In: 2006 IEEE International Frequency Control Symposium and Exposition. IEEE (2006)
2. He, R.: Research on the forming technique and surface treatment process of quartz glass bulbs for arc tubes. In: 2011 Second International Conference on Mechanic Automation and Control Engineering (MACE). IEEE (2011)
3. Cobbold, G.W.N., Underdown, A.E.: Some practical applications of quartz resonators. Inst. Electr. Eng.-Proc. Wirel. Sect. Inst. 3(9), 151–162 (1928)
4. Kaplan, W., Elderstig, H., Veider, C.: A novel fabrication method of capillary tubes on quartz for chemical analysis applications. In: 1994 Proceedings of IEEE Workshop on Micro Electro Mechanical Systems, MEMS 1994. IEEE (1994)
5. Booth, C.F.: The application and use of quartz crystals in telecommunications. J. Inst. Electr. Eng.-Part III: Commun. Eng. 88(2), 97–128 (1941)

Quality and Safety in Healthcare

Assessing the Use of Communication Robots for Recreational Activities at Nursing Homes Based on Dementia Care Mapping (DCM)

Teruko Doi[(✉)], Noriaki Kuwahara, and Kazunari Morimoto

Kyoto Institute of Technology, Kyoto, Japan
mialuna.conme.pino@gmail.com,
{nkuwahar,morix}@kit.ac.jp

Abstract. Using information communication technology (ICT) and communication robots (hereafter referred to as "robots"), we examined a system to assist recreational activities at nursing homes. The system relies on visual content to deliver a variety of recreational activities, from exercises to reminiscence therapy. Robots support those activities by interacting with nursing home residents. These systems are currently being evaluated at various elderly care facilities, where the prototype has been installed. This report will review the recreational contents that are currently under examination and the outline of the assessments, as well as the summery of the data that has been gathered so far and the effectiveness of this service suggested by the summery.

Keywords: Dementia care · Communication robot · Recreation activity

1 Purpose of Study

Recreational activities at elderly care facilities play an essential role in the maintenance of a quality life of residents. Recreation serves more than the purpose of bringing enjoyment to the residents; it also helps with rehabilitation [1, 2]. On occasion, caregivers get stuck in a rut, and the less experienced staff in particular tends to resist taking the lead in livening things up. With regards to managing recreational activities, one of the issues that need addressing is the training of the young staff [3]. Because of this, nursing facilities frequently end up using DVDs or visual aid in leading exercises, singing and other activities. Although healthy elderly possibly enjoy such visual contents, it is difficult to sustain the focus of elderly dementia patients on visual contents. For these people, we developed a prototype of care home recreational service with a moving robot with active body interconnected with the recreational visual contents, and assessed its effectiveness.

Reports indicate that replacing message boards and other static forms of communication with robots that communicate improve the message's reliability. Other reports have shown that when robots facilitated face-to-face communication between two elderly dementia patients through the TV phone, the subjects were more likely to direct

© Springer International Publishing Switzerland 2016
V.G. Duffy (Ed.): DHM 2016, LNCS 9745, pp. 203–211, 2016.
DOI: 10.1007/978-3-319-40247-5_21

their gaze toward the TV monitor and liven up conversations [4, 5]. The presence of robots with active bodies was therefore expected to increase one's gaze and focus on the visual contents. It is anticipated that the addition of robots opens up the usual staff-to-residents communication to a three-way channel that creates more opportunities for communication between the care staff and the residents. As a result, expectations were that the services currently under examination would reduce stress on caregivers who manage recreational activities, and that will in turn bring about positive changes to the entire program.

Nippon Telegraph and Telephone West Corporation (hereafter referred to as "NTT West") and Nippon Telegraph and Telephone East Corporation (hereafter referred to as "NTT East") are currently examining the recreation system in the aforementioned system using ICT and communication robots. In collaboration with two nursing facilities in the Kansai region and two in the Kanto region, assessment of the expected effect mentioned above was conducted.

In this study, we examined how this care recreation service exerts the influence to the care quality provided to care receivers based on an evaluation by Dementia Care Mapping (Hereafter referred to as DCM), and considered the effect provided by this care recreation service.

2   Assessment Method

2.1   System Outline

Figure 1 shows the outline of the system. The hardware used was Hikari BOX$^+$ [7], a set-top box provided by NTT West Japan, and a robot connected to that. We used FLET'S Hikari [8], an Internet service provided by NTT West Japan and NTT East Japan. Nursing home recreational activities (visual contents) will be available as application of Hikari BOX$^+$. Hikari BOX$^+$ and robot are connected via wireless LAN, and the robot will synchronize its actions with the visual content. The robot Sota [9], as seen in the drawing, will appear only as a torso, 30 cm in height and used on a tabletop. Hikari BOX$^+$ is shaped like a box measuring 115 mm × 105 mm × 31.5 mm and operated with remote control buttons. The TV is connected through an HDMI cable. The content will vary from children's stories and exercises, to quizzes (calculations, kanji characters), reminiscing (topics from the past), and an introduction to famous local spots.

The nursing home recreation system can be activated with the mere press of a remote control button on Hikari BOX$^+$. On the other hand, after the remote is used at the time of starting recreation activities or moving on to the next question on a quiz, the robot begins to operate. The robot will then gesticulate and speak words of starting recreations or encouragement.

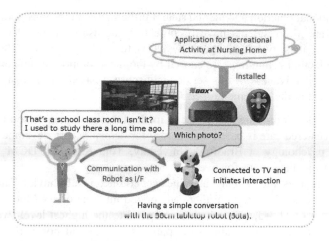

Fig. 1. System outline

2.2   Outline of Assessment Schedule

Care staff were given a 2-week pretrial period to become accustomed to Hikari BOX⁺ and learn how to operate the nursing recreation system. At the same time, contents were narrowed down to those that will undergo the assessment. Afterwards, 3 months trial was conducted. During the trial period, a portion of the usual recreational programs carried out at the facilities incorporated with Hikari BOX⁺ and robot system. Pretrial by NTT West Japan began in mid-June for the Kansai region's assessment, and the 3-month trial began in July. Pretrial by NTT East Japan began in August for the Kanto region's assessment, and the trial was held between August to October.

2.3   Facilities Collaborated with the Assessment

4 facilities in total collaborated with our assessment. In the Kansai Region, Super Court Co., Ltd., Kyoto Shijo Omiya (privately run nursing home, hereafter referred to as SC) and Telwel Nishi Nihon – Care Port Osaka Nishi Suita Center (day care, hereafter referred to as CP). In the Kanto region, Social Welfare Corporation Zenkokai – Butterfly Hill Hosoda (special elderly nursing home, hereafter referred to as BH) and Telwel Higashi Nihon – Setagaya Day Service Center (day care, hereafter referred to as SD).

2.4   Assessment Method

Assessment Outline. The assessment included a survey after the 2-week pretrial period that asked the subjects their impressions and opinions of each recreational activity, and the service improvement in response to that. Then, every two weeks during the 3-month trial period of the improved service, that followed, the GBS scale [10] for rating the severity of dementia and its qualitative differences are being used to measure the subjects' emotional function and mental state. Furthermore, on the third month when the nursing staff and the residents have become fully accustomed to the robot and the recreational activities, two evaluations by DCM took place to assess changes in the quality of the facilities' nursing care caused by the incorporation of the new service. In this paper, the effectiveness of this service is discussed based on the result of 2 DCM assessments held at the aforementioned 4 facilities.

About DCM. Dementia Care Mapping is a method that evaluates person-centered care [11]. Person-centered care is based on a theory for dementia care developed by the late Professor of psychology at Bradford University, Tom Kitwood. DCM is based on observing a dementia patient for over 6 h.

Every five minutes, the patient's activities are codified in a Behavior Category Code; from there, the patient's state is further categorized into one of six Mood Engagement levels (+5, +3, +1, −1, −3, −5), which correspond to the highest level (well-being) to the lowest (ill-being). BCC stratifies the patients' verbal and non-verbal interactions with their surroundings into 24 levels, from A through Z. DCM is carried out by specially certified individuals called mappers. The mapping is typically performed by 2 to 3 such individuals, who after a period of observation, come up with a consensus on BCC and ME values before arriving at a final diagnosis.

Although DCM is commonly carried out with around 6 h observation, we kept the observation time to two hours in order to observe changes in the residents participating in recreational activities, which included group recreation time and the residents' free time. The evaluation was carried out by specially certified mappers. In the Kansai region, it was carried out by 3 mappers, and in the Kanto region it was carried out by 2 mappers, at each facility.

Participants to DCM. Each facility selected 3 people from their users, who became the observation subjects of DCM. The subjects were selected from residents whom the care staff expected to improve their conditions with this service. Table 1 shows the gender, age, nursing level [12], independent life level of participants with dementia and bedridden level [13].

3   Result of DCM Evaluation

3.1   Comparison of ME Value Averages When This Service Is in Use or not

As shown in Fig. 2, transitions of activities and ME values of each participant through time can be obtained through DCM. The series of alphabets recorded below the graph is the BCC corresponding to the activities of the participants assessed every 5 min, and the graph shows the transition of ME value expressing the conditions of participants during this time. Figure 2 shows the result of first DCM of participant G from care facility BH. At BH, DCM observation stated at 10 AM, and care recreation using this service was conducted from 10:10 to 10:40. Moreover, another care recreation using this service was conducted from 11:08 to 11:40. Table 2 shows the codes appeared in Fig. 2.

Table 1. Participants to DCM

Care facility	Participant	Gender	Age	Nursing level	independent life level	Bedridden level
SC	A	Female	91	4	III	Unknown
	B	Female	88	4	IV	Unknown
	C	Female	81	2	IIIa	Unknown
CP	D	Female	84	2	IIb	A
	E	Female	95	3	IIIa	A2
	F	Female	95	4	IIIa	B1
BH	G	Female	90	4	Unknown	B2
	H	Female	89	4	Unknown	B2
	I	Female	82	2	Unknown	A1
SD	J	Female	94	1	Unknown	Unknown
	K	Female	85	1	Unknown	Unknown
	L	Female	78	2	Unknown	Unknown

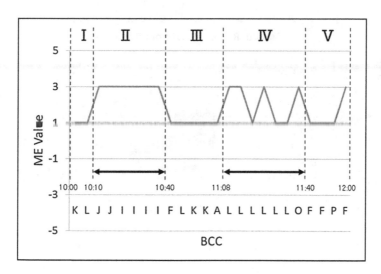

Fig. 2. Transition of activities and ME value following time

As shown in the Fig. 2, when this service is in use, I (mental activity), J (sports), L (leisurely activities) appears often, and F (eating and drinking) and K (moving) appeared often when not in use. In this paper, with the ME value gained through this method, the effectiveness of this service by comparing the conditions of the nursing home residents when they are using this service or not; for instance from Fig. 2 the average value of the area between II and IV, where this service is in use, and the average value between I, III, and V where this service is not being used. When ME value is +1, it is considered that the facility user is in relatively good condition, but this really means that he/she is in neutral state. +3 means he/she is in a good state, +5 means he/she is in exceptionally good state.

Table 2. BCCs and descriptions

BCC	Description
A	Verbal and non-verbal exchange with the surrounding (no other clear activity)
F	Eating and drinking
I	Prioritizing the use of intellectual abilities
J	Exercise or physical sports
K	Independent walking, standing or wheelchair-moving
L	Leisure, fun and recreational activities
O	Displaying attachment to or relating to inanimate objects
P	Receiving practical, physical or personal care

Firstly, the total data time using this service was 1335 min (BCC, ME Value, 267 samples), and the time when the service was not being was 1445 min (BCC, ME Value, 289 samples). Figure 3 shows the result of comparison of the average ME Values of these samples.

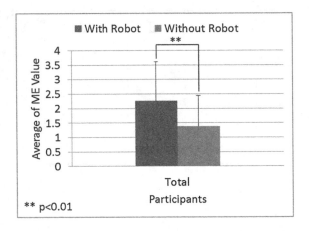

Fig. 3. Comparison of the average of ME values of the total samples

As shown in Fig. 3, when this service was being used, the average of ME value was high number of about 2.3. On the other hand, when this service was not being used, it was 1.8. Moreover, a meaningful difference was acknowledged between these average values. This suggested that using this service was effective to the improvement of the conditions of the nursing home residents.

3.2   Comparison of BCC Frequency When This Service in Use or not

Figure 4 shows the comparison of BCC frequency when this service was in use or not. Figure 4 demonstrates that when this service was in use, E (being involved in expressive or creative activities), G (reminisce or look back on life) or I (activities that mainly use mental faculty) were frequent. This shows that the contents of the care recreation, such as Origami, local photographs or quiz, are being effectively used. When this service was not in use, the frequency of sections such as A (verbal and non-verbal exchange with the surrounding [no other clear activity]), F (eating and drinking) or J (physical activities or sports) was clearly higher. Moreover, the frequency of L (being involved in leisurely activities for enjoyment or change of mood) was about the same in the both situations.

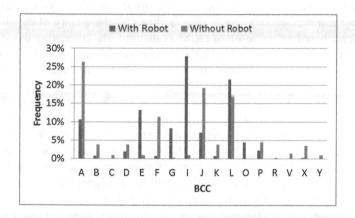

Fig. 4. Comparison of BCC frequency when this service was in use or not

Focusing on A, when comparing the averages of ME value when the service was being used or not, the value of former was 1.10 (SD = 0.62), that of the latter was 1.14 (SD = 1.02), thus meaningful difference was not displayed. On the other hand, the averages of ME value of other sections were 2.42 (SD = 1.29) for E, 3.76 (SD = 1.34) for G and 2.97 (SD = 1.11) for I, uniformly showing exceptionally high number. By using this service, it shows the reduction of a neutral state such as A, where the state of nursing home residents are neither good nor bad. It also triggered the increase of good state such as E, G or I. Therefore, it seems to be considered that this service can contribute to high quality care to the nursing residents.

Moreover, regarding J, though there were not many occasion while using this service, the average of ME value when using this service was 2.90 (SD = 0.77), that of when the service was not being used was 2.42 (SD = 0.77), both showing good states. However, it showed significantly higher number ($p < 0.05$) when the service was in use. Also, regarding L, the average of ME value when this service in use was 1.93 (SD = 1.15), that of when the service was not being used was 1.05 (SD = 0.86), showing meaningfully higher number when this service was in use ($p > 0.01$). It was indicated that the nursing home residents were in better condition when the service was in use.

Finally, though it was not very frequent, regarding O (interact with objects, show emotional attachment/interest to objects) which shows the relationship between the nursing home residents and the robot, the average of ME value when this appeared was 3 (SD = 1.41), indicating that interaction with the robot had positive influence on the nursing home residents.

4 Conclusion

In this paper, we examined the influence brought by the introduction of care recreation service using communication robot to care facilities on the quality of care for nursing home residents based on the result of DCM evaluation. By comparing the averages of ME value when this service is in use and when it is not during the trial at 2 facilities in Kansai region and 2 facilities in Kanto region with 12 participants (nursing home residents), it was demonstrated that ME value was significantly higher when this service was in use. In other words, the nursing home residents were in better state while receiving this service, which means that they received better quality care. The feedback from the care staff included many opinions that using this service gave them more time and mental space. There were also views that by leaving the recreational activities to the robot, the care staff could focus on helping the nursing home residents, leading one to infer that this extra space for the staff resulted in the higher quality care toward the nursing home residents. It is considered that this mental space resulted from the change in communication and relationship caused by the introduction of the robot in the relationship between the staff and the nursing home residents.

From the analysis of the observation results of the nursing home residents' activities, i.e. the analysis of BCC, it shows that by using this service, it triggers higher ME value, such as E (being involved in expressive or creative activities), G (reminisce or look back on life) or I (activities that mainly use mental faculty) more frequently, meaning that good state of the nursing home residents could be maintained. The care staff gave feedback that the activities often involve each person work on Kanji exercise book or other such material in silence. But by the robot of this service taking up the roles of MC and teacher, it enabled the nursing home residents and care staff to be involved in light-hearted intellectual activities together. This is regarded as the effect of the change in communication and relationship caused by the introduction of the robot between the nursing home residents and care staff. Moreover, significantly higher number was gained when this service is use regarding J (physical activities or sports) and L (being involved in leisurely activities for enjoyment or change of mood). This points to the possibility that, in addition to the mental space created among the care staff through the use of this service, it is the effect of the drawing power of the visual contents of the communication robot and concentration it causes. However, this needs further examination.

Finally, though it was not very frequent, regarding O (interact with objects, show emotional attachment/interest to objects) which shows the relationship between the nursing home residents and the robot, the average of ME value when this appeared was 3 (SD = 1.41), indicating the nursing home residents interact with the robot with emotional attachment. If two-way communication is realized in future, it is expected to lead to higher frequency of O, and consequently resulting in better condition of the nursing home residents.

Acknowledgements. In realizing this research, we would like to thank NTT West Japan and NTT East Japan for coordinating the assessment and providing us some of the equipment. We thank Vstone Co., Ltd. for providing the robot, and thank Smile Plus Co., Ltd. for providing us some of the visual contents. We thank Super Court Co., Ltd., Care Port Osaka Nishi Suita Center, Social Welfare Corporation Zenkokai – Butterfly Hill Hosoda and Setagaya Day Service Center for participating in the study. We also would like to thank all DCM mapper for helping us with DCM evaluation. And a part of this study received the assistance of JSPS KANENHI Grant Number 15H01698.

References

1. Doi, T., Kuwahara, N., Morimoto, K.: Effective design of traditional Japanese tea ceremony in a group home for the elderly with dementia. In: Duffy, V.G. (ed.) DHM 2015. LNCS, vol. 9184, pp. 413–422. Springer, Heidelberg (2015). http://link.springer.com/chapter/10.1007/978-3-319-21070-4_41
2. Ikenobo, Y., Mochizuki, Y., Kuwahara, A.: Usefulness of Ikebana a nursing care environment. In: Duffy, V.G. (ed.) DHM 2015. LNCS, vol. 9185, pp. 441–447. Springer, Heidelberg (2015)
3. Yamamoto, A., et al.: The transfer of expertise in conducting a participatory music therapy during a combined rehabilitation-recreational program in an elderly care facility. In: Duffy, V.G. (ed.) DHM 2015. LNCS, vol. 9185, pp. 500–511. Springer, Heidelberg (2015). http://link.springer.com/chapter/10.1007/978-3-319-21070-4_51
4. Yonezawa, T., Yamazoe, H., Utsumi, A., Abe, S.: Attractive, informative, and communicative robot system on guide plate as an attendant with awareness of user's gaze. Paladyn J. Behav. Robot. 4(2), 113–122 (2013)
5. Yonezawa, T., Yamazoe, H., Utsumi, A., Abe, S.: Assisting video communication by an intermediating robot system corresponding to each user's attitude. Hum. Interface Soc. J. 13(3), 5–13 (2011)
6. Fossey, J., Lee, L., Ballard, C.: Dementia care mapping as a research tool for measuring quality of life in care settings: psychometric properties. Int. J. Geriatr. Psychiatry 17(11), 1064–1070 (2002)
7. https://www.ntt-west.co.jp/kiki/hikaribox/spec/ (in Japanese)
8. http://hikari-n.jp/west/service/ (in Japanese)
9. https://www.vstone.co.jp/products/sota/ (in Japanese)
10. Bråne, G.: The GBS-scale – a Geriatric Rating Scale – and its Clinical Application. Gothenburg University, Gothenburg, Sweden (1989)
11. Kitwood, T.: When your heart wants to remember: person-centred dementia care. RCN Nurs. Update, Nurs. Stan. 13, 1–22 (1999)
12. http://www.e-kaigoshien.net/2006/08/post_13.html (in Japanese)
13. http://www.mhlw.go.jp/file/06-Seisakujouhou-12300000-Roukenkyoku/0000077382.pdf (in Japanese)

Improving the Palatability of Nursing Care Food Using a Pseudo-chewing Sound Generated by an EMG Signal

Hiroshi Endo$^{(\boxtimes)}$, Shuichi Ino, and Waka Fujisaki

Human Informatics Research Institute, National Institute of Advanced Industrial
Science and Technology (AIST), Central 6, 1-1 Higashi, Tsukuba, Ibaraki, Japan
{hiroshi-endou,s-ino,w-fujisaki}@aist.go.jp

Abstract. Elderly individuals whose eating functions have declined can only
eat unpleasant foods with very soft textures. If more varied food textures could
be delivered, the pleasure derived from eating could be improved. We tried to
influence the perception of food texture using a pseudo-chewing sound. The
sound was synchronized with mastication using the electromyogram (EMG) of
the masseter. Coincidentally, when the EMG is heard as a sound, it is similar to
the "crunchy" sound emitted by root vegetables. We investigated whether the
perceived texture of nursing care food would change in subjects exposed to the
EMG chewing sound. Elderly participants evaluated the textures of nursing care
foods. When the EMG chewing sound was provided, they were more likely to
evaluate a food as chewy. In addition, several scores related to the pleasure of
eating were also increased. These results demonstrate the possibility of
improving the palatability of texture-modified diets.

Keywords: Texture-modified care food · Chewing sound · Electromyography ·
Elderly · Meal support

1 Introduction

Although we use vision to obtain information about the palatability of dishes, such as
their color and appearance, oral sensation and audition predominate once food is taken
into the mouth. Although we do not usually pay attention to the sounds emitted when
we chew food, these sounds can influence the perception of food texture [1, 2]. Here we
describe the development of a meal support technology for elderly individuals that
exploits these chewing sounds.

With aging, the ability to chew and swallow deteriorates, and the risk of aspiration
becomes higher, potentially leading to asphyxia or pneumonia. Consequently, elderly
individuals whose eating functions have declined can only eat food with very soft
textures. Because food texture makes an important contribution to palatability [3, 4],
unpleasant food texture decreases quality of life (QOL) of the elderly [5, 6]. Hence, if
varied food textures could be delivered to the elderly even when they are only capable
of eating texture-modified diets, the pleasure derived from eating and QOL related to
meals will be improved.

© Springer International Publishing Switzerland 2016
V.G. Duffy (Ed.): DHM 2016, LNCS 9745, pp. 212–220, 2016.
DOI: 10.1007/978-3-319-40247-5_22

However, it is difficult to change the physical properties of food in order to cause people to experience various food textures. Therefore, novel apparatuses have been developed that directly stimulate oral sensation. A "food simulator" has been used to generate virtual chewiness by controlling the biting force of the device [7], and a "straw-like user interface" has been used to generate a virtual drinking sensation by controlling air pressure and vibration [8]. The aim of these apparatuses was to virtually simulate sensations, and they were not intended for use at mealtimes. Importantly, to enhance their effectiveness, these apparatuses provided the corresponding sounds simultaneously.

Changes in chewing sounds influence the perception of food texture. Zampini et al. reported that the perception of the crispness and staleness of potato chips can be altered by varying the loudness and/or frequency composition of the biting sound [9], and these findings were subsequently replicated by other researchers [10]. Thus, food texture is a complex sense that is composed of audition as well as oral sensation. Therefore, it might be possible to make people experience varied food textures by changing chewing sounds, even if the actual texture of a food is dull.

In this study, we tried to influence the perception of food texture by modifying the chewing sound. Previous studies investigated the relationship between biting or chewing sounds and the texture of crispy or crunchy foods. However, the target foods in this study were very soft and barely emitted chewing sounds. Therefore, chewing sounds had to be artificially generated. We developed a technique for presentation of a pseudo-chewing sound generated from the electromyogram (EMG) of the masseter muscle. Using this technique, we investigated whether the perceived textures or impressions of nursing care foods were altered when accompanied by an artificially generated pseudo-chewing sound.

2 Methods

2.1 Generating of Pseudo-chewing Sound

Because texture-modified care foods are very soft and barely emit sounds when chewed, chewing sounds must be provided from an external source that is synchronized with chewing behavior. To achieve this synchrony, we used the EMG of the masseter muscle, an agonist of mastication whose contractions are synchronous with the closing of the mouth. By monitoring the EMG of the masseter, chewing sounds can be provided that are synchronous with chewing behavior. Because the amplitude of the EMG signal correlates with chewing strength, the chewing sound can be provided at an appropriate intensity. Moreover, because the EMG is an electrical waveform, it can be readily interpreted as a sound. Coincidentally, the sound of the myoelectric waveform is similar to the chewing sound emitted by crunchy root vegetables. Therefore, by feeding back the EMG signal as sound, we can provide a "crunchy" chewing sound with high verisimilitude (EMG chewing sound).

The principal frequency range of the surface EMG is up to several hundred Hz [11], and thus does not contain the high-frequency components included in crispy and crunchy sounds [12, 13]. However, based on a principal component analysis of crispy, crunchy, and crackly sounds, the frequency range from 125 Hz to 1250 Hz was extracted as the first principal component of air-conducted chewing sounds [13]. Ultimately, we used the frequency range from 250 Hz to 1 kHz of EMG signal to generate the pseudo-chewing sound. The EMG chewing sound was similar to the crunchy sound of hard moist foods, although it did not contain the frequency components that characterize crispness, crunchiness, and crackliness.

As shown in Fig. 1, the EMG was recorded using surface electrodes. A pair of bipolar Ag/AgCl surface electrodes was attached to the skin overlying the right and left masseters with an inter-electrode distance of 20 mm, while a ground electrode was also attached to the forehead. The EMG signals were amplified (BioAmp FE132, AD Instruments), with a low-pass filter at 5 kHz and a high-pass filter at 10 Hz, then recorded at a sampling rate of 10 kHz (PowerLab8/35, AD Instruments). The masseter with the higher amplitude was used to generate the chewing sound. The analog output voltage of the masseter EMG signal was sent to a mixer/graphic equalizer (ZMX124 FX USB, ALTO Professional). The amplitudes of each frequency bands were adjusted using the function of the graphic equalizer with one-octave resolution. The adjustment was performed by setting the frequency range less than 125 Hz and over 2 kHz to the minimum level (−15 dB) and the frequency range between 250 Hz and 1 kHz to the maximum level (+15 dB). The EMG chewing sound was delivered via headphones. The frequency characteristics of the EMG and the EMG sound during clenching are shown in Fig. 2.

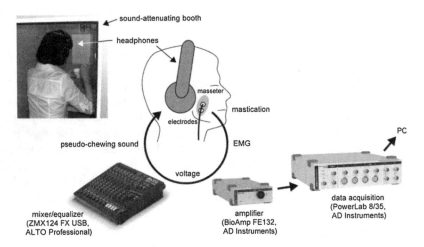

Fig. 1. Experimental setup

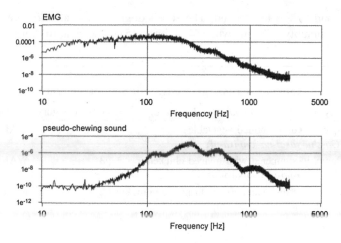

Fig. 2. Frequency characteristics of EMG and pseudo-chewing sound

2.2 Participants and Sample Foods

Ten healthy elderly participants (five male and five female, age range 66–74 years, [70 ± 3 years]) without signs of oromandibular and auditory diseases took part in the experiment. These participants usually ate normal foods, and did not eat texture-modified diets for their daily meals. They gave informed consent after receiving a full explanation of the study. The ethics committee for human experimentation at the National Institute of Advanced Industrial Science and Technology approved the experimental procedures.

Three kinds of commercially available nursing care foods were used as sample foods (Table 1). All of the sample foods contain several kinds of foodstuff that are cut into small particles and cooked until they are very soft. Consequently, they barely emit a chewing sound. They are classified into categories 2 and 3 of UDF (Universal Design Food) category, which are defined by the Japan Care Food Conference based on care recipients' ability to bite and swallow foods. UDF category 2 foods "can be broken up using the gums", whereas foods in category 3 "can be broken up by the tongue" (http://www.udf.jp/).

2.3 Questionnaire

A set of 16 adjective pairs were used for the experiment, most of which were selected by referring to previous literature [14–17]. For convenience, we first divided the adjectives used for material property ratings into three groups. The first group contained adjectives related to taste (Table 2a); the second, adjectives related to food texture (Table 2b); and the third, adjectives related to perceived feelings and other topics (Table 2c).

Participant used seven-point scales to rate how well these words applied to each of the stimuli. In the analysis of material properties, "1" was assigned to the first adjective in each pair, and "7" to the second. The seven degrees of evaluation were: (1) very much, (2) considerably, (3) somewhat, (4) neither, (5) somewhat, (6) considerably, and (7) very much.

Table 1. Nursing care foods used in the experiment

Food No.	Description of food (*Name in Japanese*)	UDF category	Product maker
1	Spicy fried and boiled vegetables (*Go-shu-yasai-no-kinpira-ni*)	3	WAKODO
2	Pumpkin simmered with minced chicken (*Kabocha-no-tori-soboro-ni*)	3	WAKODO
3	Japanese radish simmered with minced chicken (*Daikon-no-tori-soboro-an*)	2	Kewpie

Table 2. Words selected for material property rating

a. Taste
light taste – heavy taste
stale taste – fresh taste
simple taste – complex taste
unpalatable – palatable

b. Food Texture
soft – hard
dry – moist
not chewy – chewy
smooth – rough
fewer ingredients – more ingredients
bad texture – good texture

c. Perceived Feelings
unexciting – exciting
less involved dining experience – more involved dining experience
diminishes appetite – arouses appetite
unable to masticate regularly – able to masticate regularly
unpleasant – pleasant
sound/food combination is unnatural – sound/food combination is natural

Questions were originally presented in Japanese – here translated into English.

The participants evaluated how perception changed in the condition with EMG sound compared with the without-sound condition, and then filled out the questionnaire after the two sound conditions were completed.

2.4   Procedure

The experiments were conducted in a sound-attenuating booth. The sound pressure level depended on the amplitude of the individual EMG signal. Therefore, to adjust the sound pressure level, a mastication evaluation gum (Masticatory Performance Evaluating Gum XYLITOL, Lotte) was used. Each participant was instructed to adjust the sound pressure to a comfortable level while they chewed the gum. In the without-sound condition, no EMG sound was fed back to the participant.

Six trials were carried out (three kinds of sample foods × two sound conditions), and each trial was performed once. The order of sample foods was random. The two sound conditions for each food were carried out sequentially. Half of the participants began in the with-sound condition, and the other half began in the without-sound condition.

In each trial, the participant was informed of the food name and sound condition in advance. Because the purpose of this experiment was to examine the influences of the chewing sound, the participants were instructed to chew more than ten times on the side where the EMG signal was being received. No restriction was imposed on the timing of swallowing, provided that mastication was performed over ten times. The task of participants was to rate the sensations and impressions described in the questionnaire. The participants filled out the questionnaire when the two sound conditions for each food were completed.

3   Results

The results of the subjective evaluation of each food are shown in Fig. 3. Although there were some food-dependent differences, several questionnaire items revealed similar changes regardless of the identity of the food. Figure 4 shows the averaged score of all sample foods. When the EMG chewing sound was provided, participants were more likely to evaluate a food as having the property of chewiness ("not chewy – chewy"). In addition, they were more likely to feel that they were engaged in an actual eating experience ("less involved dining experience – more involved dining experience"). The scores were also higher for several questionnaire items related to the pleasure of eating. Thus, overall, the perceptions of food texture and the subjects' feelings about their eating experience were improved.

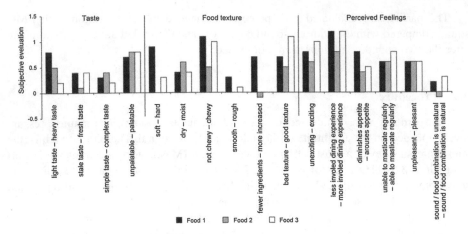

Fig. 3. Results of subjective evaluations of each food

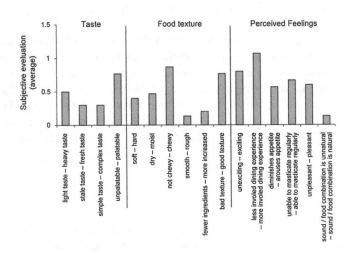

Fig. 4. Averages of subjective evaluations of all foods

4 Discussion

In this study, we found that a "crunchy" pseudo-chewing sound influenced the perceived texture and other properties of food. When the pseudo-chewing sound was provided, participants were more likely to evaluate a food as chewy. Consistent with this, previous work showed that crispy and crunchy food properties can be evaluated based on sound [18, 19]. In addition, perceived crispness is affected by the frequency components and loudness of the sound [9, 10]. Considering the effects inherent to crispy and crunchy sounds, it is plausible that the participants perceived crispness or crunchiness in response to the pseudo-chewing sound even when the sample foods were soft. In addition, several scores related to the pleasure of eating were also increased.

If elderly people who are only capable of eating texture-modified diets could be induced to experience varied food textures associated with positive impressions, then the quality and pleasure of their meals should be improved, potentially increasing their food intake and improving their nutritional condition. In future work, we will continue to investigate the relationship between chewing sounds and perceived food properties.

Sound can be processed in the background without consuming many attentional resources, and the sound presentation in our system is realized by a simple apparatus (Fig. 1) that could easily be miniaturized. Thus, the pseudo-chewing sound is considered to be a useful technique for improving the palatability of texture-modified diets.

References

1. Zampini, M., Spence, C.: Assessing the role of sound in the perception of food and drink. Chemosens. Percept. **3**, 57–67 (2010)
2. Spence, C.: Eating with our ears: assessing the importance of the sounds of consumption on our perception and enjoyment of multisensory flavour experiences. Flavour **4**, 3 (2015)
3. Szczesniak, A.S.: Texture is a sensory property. Food Qual. Prefer. **13**, 215–225 (2002)
4. Delwiche, J.: The impact of perceptual interactions on perceived flavor. Food Qual. Prefer. **15**, 137–146 (2004)
5. Mioche, L., Bourdiol, P., Peyron, M.A.: Influence of age on mastication: effects on eating behavior. Nutr. Res. Rev. **17**, 43–54 (2004)
6. Swan, K., Speyer, R., Heijnen, B.J., Wagg, B., Cordier, R.: Living with oropharyngeal dysphagia: effects of bolus modification on health-related quality of life – a systematic review. Qual. Life Res. **24**, 2447–2456 (2015)
7. Uemura, T., Moriya, T., Yano, H., Iwata, H.: Development of a food simulator. Trans. VRSJ **8**, 399–406 (2003). [in Japanese]
8. Hashimoto, Y., Ohtaki, J., Kojima, M., Nagaya, N., Mitani, T., Miyajima, S., Yamamoto, A., Inami, M.: Straw-like user interface: the display of drinking sensation. Trans. VRSJ **11**, 347–356 (2006). (in Japanese)
9. Zampini, M., Spence, C.: The role of auditory cues in modulating the perceived crispness and staleness of potato chips. J. Sens. Stud. **19**, 347–363 (2004)
10. Demattè, M.L., Pojer, N., Endrizzi, I., Corollaro, M.L., Betta, E., Aprea, E., Charles, M., Biasioli, F., Zampini, M., Gasperi, F.: Effects of the sound of the bite on apple perceived crispness and hardness. Food Qual. Prefer. **38**, 58–64 (2014)
11. Palla, S., Ash Jr., M.M.: Effect of bite force on the power spectrum of the surface electromyogram of human jaw muscles. Arch. Oral Biol. **26**, 287–295 (1981)
12. Seymour, S.K., Hamann, D.D.: Crispness and crunchiness of selected low moisture foods. J. Texture Stud. **19**, 79–95 (1988)
13. Dacremont, C.: Spectral composition of eating sounds generated by crispy, crunchy and crackly foods. J. Texture Stud. **26**, 27–43 (1995)
14. Fillion, L., Kilcast, D.: Consumer perception of crispness and crunchiness in fruits and vegetables. Food Qual. Prefer. **13**, 23–29 (2002)
15. Dijksterhuis, G., Luyten, H., de Wijk, R., Mojet, J.: A new sensory vocabulary for crisp and crunchy dry model foods. Food Qual. Prefer. **18**, 37–50 (2007)
16. Fujisaki, W., Goda, N., Motoyoshi, I., Komatsu, H., Nishida, S.: Audiovisual integration in the human perception of materials. J. Vis. **14**(4), 1–20 (2014)

17. Fujisaki, W., Tokita, M., Kariya, K.: Perception of the material properties of wood based on vision, audition, and touch. Vis. Res. **109**, 185–200 (2015)
18. Duizer, L.: A review of acoustic research for studying the sensory perception of crisp, crunchy and crackly textures. Trends Food Sci. Technol. **12**, 17–24 (2001)
19. Saeleaw, M., Schleining, G.: A review: crispness in dry foods and quality measurements based on acoustic – mechanical destructive techniques. J. Food Eng. **105**, 387–399 (2011)

Setting the Degree of Defocus for Video Images in a Monitoring System

Yukiya Horie[✉] and Nobuji Tetsutani

Tokyo Denki University, Tokyo, Japan
yky567lunatic2bump@yahoo.co.jp, tetsutani@im.dendai.ac.jp

Abstract. We develop a persons-existence extraction system to protect the privacy of a user's image. In this paper, we propose a novel video input method that considers both privacy and security, and we describe the degree of the criteria of the blur with the video input method. In addition, we discuss the problems associated with our previous algorithm, which determines the number of people from blurred images. We improve the algorithm and then evaluate it.

Keywords: Privacy · Security · Defocus image · Persons-existence extraction

1 Introduction

Families often wish to monitor the current situation of other family members who are elderly, living alone, or hospitalized in remote locations. However, elderly people and inpatients monitored by video equipment often do not want to share personal details such as their attire or behavior. In this paper, we propose a novel video input method that considers both privacy and security. The degree of the criteria of the blur with video input method is also described here. In addition, we propose a basic algorithm for determining the number of persons in a living room, as an example to estimate the room circumstances from the blurred image. We evaluate and verify the proposed algorithm.

2 Monitoring Systems and Privacy

In general, monitoring systems do not need to capture information that is as detailed as that required by video surveillance systems; typically, monitoring systems only need to provide an approximation of a situation. Moreover, elderly people living alone or inpatients who are monitored with video cameras usually do not want to share personal details such as their faces, attire, or behavior. Therefore, a monitoring system can provide a sufficient level of detail by capturing the following information: the presence or absence of a person in a room, the number of people, their position and movement, and their approximate actions. The required information is obtained by blurring the video image. In general, video blurring methods use mosaics generated by image processing techniques. However, these methods have a security risk. In other words, because the

© Springer International Publishing Switzerland 2016
V.G. Duffy (Ed.): DHM 2016, LNCS 9745, pp. 221–228, 2016.
DOI: 10.1007/978-3-319-40247-5_23

image is processed after raw data is stored on a PC, there is a risk that information may be stolen before processing. To address this problem, we propose a novel video input method that considers security.

3   Proposed Monitoring System and Results

To reduce the risk of information being stolen prior to image processing, we propose a method for blurring input images. This method employs an image that is blurred by the focus ring of the camera. This eliminates security problems, because even if the video images are stolen, they are already blurred. As for utilization problems, users are unaware of the degree of blurring. When using a simple numerical scale for the degree of blurring, a user cannot understand intuitively; a user interface is not preferable. Thus, it is necessary to establish meaningful blurring criteria. We propose using a checkerboard pattern as the input image, and employing the pattern's standard deviation of concentration to determine the blurring criteria. Furthermore, to understand the standard deviation subjectively, this study examines the correspondence between the standard deviation and eyesight.

3.1   Blurring Degree Criteria

The blur settings rotate the focus ring of the WEB camera from the in-focus state to the close-up state. In the experiment, a one-level blur was performed using a 1/4 rotation of the focus ring. By using the value of the standard deviation, it is no longer dependent on the amount of rotation of the focus ring. Furthermore, even with another WEB camera, it is possible to match the same conditions. Figure 1 shows the checkerboard pattern used in the experiment. The image of the checkered pattern was taken at a distance of 30 cm. The checkered pattern is printed over the entire surface of an A4-size generic sheet size. The checkered pattern printed on the A4 sheet was taken from a range vertical width of 90 % and a left and right width of 70 % of A4 sheet. Table 1 and Fig. 2 show the experimental results for the standard deviation of concentration. Because the standard deviation changes linearly for each blurring level, it can be used for determining the degree of blurring.

Table 1. Standard deviation of concentration for the checkered pattern

	Level 0	Level 1	Level 2	Level 3	Level 4	Level 5	Level 6
Standard deviation	96.0	85.0	74.1	63.7	52.2	42.9	31.2

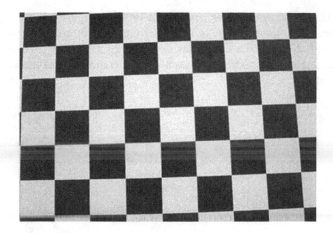

Fig. 1. Checkerboard pattern used in the experiment

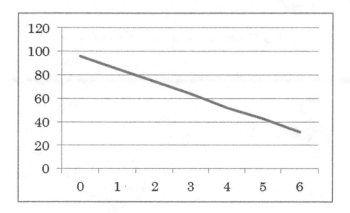

Fig. 2. Graph of the standard deviation of concentration for the checkered pattern

3.2 Correspondence Between the Blurring Level and Eyesight

We conducted experiments to study the correspondence between the blurring level and eyesight. The brightness of the experimental room was 400 lx. The eyesight of the subject was 1.0 or more in corrected visual acuity or naked eye vision. Figure 3 shows the manner in which a Landolt ring is captured. The Landolt ring of an eyesight test was captured at a distance of 30 cm by using a WEB camera. The distance was set to 30 cm to obtain the same blurriness as the checkered pattern. We prepared six images of the Landolt ring, which were captured every 1/4 rotation of the focus ring from the in-focus state to the close-up state. Figure 4 shows an experimental method. The viewing distance is 3 m to an 80-inch monitor. The size of the Landolt ring to be displayed on the monitor is adjusted to be appropriate so as to size at a distance of 3 m. The viewing distance is 3 m, to match the eye chart for 3 m. A display that is large enough to match the size of the Landolt ring to the lower eyesight is required. Thus, an 80-inch display is used in this experiment. The screen resolution is 1920 × 1080 px. Figure 5 shows Landolt rings of blurring level 4 on the monitor. In the experiment, participants viewed images of Rundle rings with different sizes and blurring levels. Subsequently, we measured each participant's eyesight. The experimental results in Fig. 6 show the defocused room image of blurring level 4.

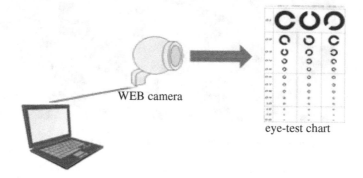

Fig. 3. Landolt ring of acquisition method

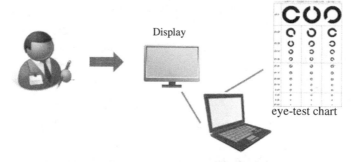

Fig. 4. Experimental method

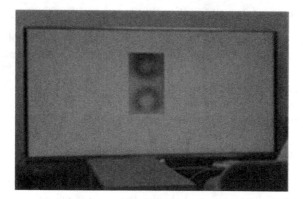

Fig. 5. Landolt rings of blurring level 4 on the monitor

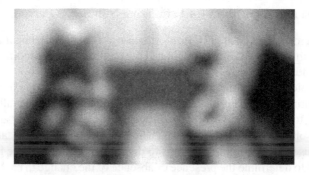

Fig. 6. Defocused room image of blurring level 4

3.3 Experimental Results

Figure 7 shows the experimental results. The vertical axis represents eyesight, and the horizontal axis represents blurring levels. Blurring level 0 is the in-focus state. Level settings from 1 to 4 were found to correspond to eyesight. It was also found that the Rundle ring could not support eyesight levels of 0.01 or less.

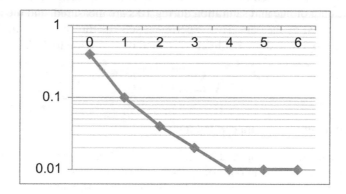

Fig. 7. Experimental results

4 Estimation of Number of Persons Using Blurred Video

We propose a basic algorithm for determining the number of persons in a living room, as an example to estimate the room circumstances from the blurred image. We evaluate and verify the proposed algorithm. We have already studied the algorithm for estimating the number of persons using RGB information. This paper describes an improved algorithm using the HSV color space. We report the results.

4.1   Basic Idea and Algorithms for Estimating Number of Persons

Our previous algorithm [1] using RGB information was poor in terms of accuracy. The first problem is the use of RGB information. If the environmental conditions by shadow and lighting conditions change, it becomes difficult to set the threshold in this method. The second problem is determining the number of persons, depending on the amount of change in the entire image. This method cannot respond to noise and small changes. The first solution is to use the HSV color space which can separate color and brightness. Therefore, the solution is not dependent on changes in the brightness because only color information is used. The second solution is to divide the obtained image into a block of 40×40 px, and to determine the presence or absence of the change in each block. Based on the above details, we implement the algorithm.

4.2   Initial Setting of Hue and Saturation

Hue and saturation are acquired from the room of the image for the determination of a 0 person threshold as the initial value. The hue and saturation value for each block $(40 \times 40$ px) are calculated. The acquired image is in a blurred state. The change values for each block are calculated by the Euclidean distance of the initial value and the measured value for each block. Equation (1) is an expression for the Euclidean distance. The data of hue and saturation during 10 s are measured, and the amount of noise is determined by the data. This experiment sets the threshold for the Euclidean distance of hue to 450 and the Euclidean distance of saturation to 350.

$$d(b,f) = \sqrt{\sum_{i=0}^{n} \left(b_i - f_i\right)^2} \tag{1}$$

4.3   Estimation of the Number of Persons

We detect persons from the blurred images. This proposed algorism uses the labeling by four neighbors and the amount of change measurement technique by the Euclidean distance for each histogram value. We calculate the Euclidean distances of the histogram in the initial state and the current state from the values of hue and saturation in the background image and the current image. bi is the value of the hue or saturation in the background image. fi is the value of the hue or saturation in the current image. The value of n sets the saturation to 359, and hue to 255. The presence or absence of change in each block is determined by comparing the Euclidean distances and thresholds. Next, the labeling by four neighbors technique is performed, and blocks exceeding the threshold are labeled. Using this labeling technique, the number of blocks corresponding to the person-size in the image is determined. In addition, since the size of the captured area of the person by a position standing of a person is different, the weighting of the number of blocks corresponding to the coordinate position of the image is processed. The mean value of the hue of each labeled block is determined. The value of the hue for each labeled block is stored in the array. When the number of persons increases, the number of the newly emerged hue block is calculated. The number of persons is determined, via a comparison between the newly emerged hue block and a threshold number.

4.4 Evaluation and Discussion of the Algorithm

Used video scene (25 s) is that a person enters the living room, is sitting and leaves the living room. Videos for zero person and one and two persons were prepared. Blur is a state as shown in Fig. 8. The room is 20 m^2, and the illuminance is set to 400 lx. The camera installed at a height of 2.3 m at the corner of the room. Table 2 shows the experimental results. The rates for detecting zero persons when using the algorithm are 99 %, 78 %, and 100 %, respectively. On the other hand, the rates for detecting zero persons, one person, and two persons when using the previous algorithm using RGB are 100 %, 86 %, and 50 %, respectively. The proposed algorithm was able to achieve a higher accuracy than the algorithm using RGB. In the future, there will be a need to consider the threshold to improve the detection rate of three or more persons.

Table 2. Experimental results

Determination result Number of people	0 person	1 person	2 persons
0 person	99%	1%	0%
1 person	9%	78%	14%
2 persons	0%	0%	100%

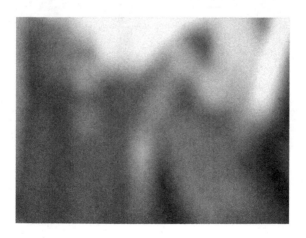

Fig. 8. Blur state image

5   Conclusion

To enhance the effectiveness of monitoring systems, we proposed a novel video input method that considers both privacy and security. By employing a checkerboard pattern and standard deviations to determine blurring criteria, we verified the validity of the image input method in experiments. In particular, we demonstrated the correspondence between the blurring level and eyesight. In addition, we described the problems associated with the algorithm for detecting persons using RGB information, and proposed a method for mitigating the problem. From the experimental results, we showed that a high accuracy in estimating the number of persons was achieved with the quite blurred videos. In the future, we will attempt to estimate a human's behavior patterns from quite blurred videos.

Reference

1. Kikuchi, Y., Kato, K., Inoue, H., Tetsutani, N.: A fundamental study of person recognition in defocused images for privacy protection. In: 2014 International Workshop on Advanced Image Technology, pp. 482–485 (2014)

Qualitative Analysis of the Customer Satisfaction at the Dental Clinics

Yuko Kamagahara[1(✉)], Tomoya Takeda[2], Shanshan Jin[2],
Xiaodan Lu[2], Tomoko Ota[3], Tadayuki Hara[4], and Noriyuki Kida[2]

[1] Andsmile, 1-1-7 Minamishinmachi, Chuo-ku, Osaka 540-0024, Japan
Kamagahara0525@gmail.com
[2] Kyoto Institute of Technology, Matsugasaki,
Sakyo-ku, Kyoto 606-6585, Japan
T.takeda@taste.jp
[3] Chuo Business Group, 1-6-6 Funakoshi-Cho,
Chuo-ku, Osaka 540-0036, Japan
Promot1@gold.ocn.ne.jp
[4] University of Central Florida, Orlando, USA
Tadayuki.hara@ucf.edu

Abstract. The way appropriate manner and speaking for customers is one of the important things for the people who are engaged in the service industry. With the maturity of society and the market, besides the quality of products, improvement of the service extended to customers is one of the important factors to increase the company's turnover and profit. Currently in Japan, due to the upsurge of the dental clinics, the dentistry industry as a whole is suffering from severe and excessive competition. In this study, we focus on the dental clinic management in Japan, where the service quality exerts a great influence to the clinic's outcome. Two dental clinics in Kanto region and three dental clinics in Kansai region were focused and investigated by questionnaire. 1,108 responses were gathered, out of which 898 valid responses, were selected for the analysis, which including 300 male participants and 598 female participants in total. Three categories were investigated by questionnaire, which were basic information, impression evaluation of customer service at each dental clinic, and overall evaluation. The result was showed that a patient who visited a clinic with a fewer times given a higher evaluation of the customer satisfaction level than others respondents. It also was found that recommendation to others by word of mouth can be affected by reception factor, the overall satisfaction level.

Keywords: Qualitative analysis · Customer satisfaction · Dental clinics

1 Introduction

These days, dental clinics in japan have been exposed to a fierce competition. One of the causes of this is the upsurge of dental clinics. There are 102 thousand registered dentists [2] out of 303 thousand, the entire number of registered doctors in the whole country. Moreover, according to the survey report conducted in August 2014, there are

© Springer International Publishing Switzerland 2016
V.G. Duffy (Ed.): DHM 2016, LNCS 9745, pp. 229–242, 2016.
DOI: 10.1007/978-3-319-40247-5_24

68,836 dental clinics in Japan [3]. There are 1.3 times more dental clinics than convenience stores that count 51,367(Japan Franchise Association: JFA Convenience Store Statistics Survey).

Greater competition between dental clinics means more beneficial opportunities for the customers to be able to select the optimal dental services for them. Dental clinics have been trying on the latest equipments, therapeutic methods, and the best materials for treatments. Under this age of over-competition, faced with the growth of the number of dental clinics, as well as repetitive cut-down on the fee, and the decline in the number of the cases of dental caries, some dental clinics are changing their customer gathering methods so that they can meet the needs of the patients who seek dental treatments not covered by the medical care, such as dental prophylaxis, tooth bleaching, and orthodontics.

Since the situation has changed that the customers began to be able to choose which dental clinic to go, medical treatment is now said to have become service industry [1]. The primary service of dental clinics as a service industry is to provide medical treatment to their customers, and the provision of the medical services appropriate for each customer is the most important thing. In other words, the provision of the appropriate therapeutic knowledge and skills is crucial. However, knowing what the customers are seeking is also necessary, not just qualified skills such as dental technique, but also intangible communicative skills to deal with the customers are becoming significant matter [4]. From when a customer comes to a clinic until the treatment is done and he/she leaves, everyone including dentist, dental hygienist, and receptionist is required to have communication and build relationships with the customers for the sake of smooth treatment. This kind of attitude at a dental clinic is assumed to have a possible impact on the customer satisfaction that made them feel as "I made a best choice!"

Like running a goods-selling or service-providing store, retaining repeat customers is necessary for the management of a dental clinic. In order to meet this criterion, it is inevitable to evoke the customers' desire to come back for another service. As a step towards achieving this, some measures have been taken which incorporate the viewpoint of customer service with the aim of raising the customer satisfaction level. For example, For example, at the dental clinic competition, "D1 Grand Prix Dentist Tournament" [5], held by Japan Dental Clinic Competition Association, they are competing the customers' satisfaction level. Some of the higher-ranked clinics at this tournament proclaim Japanese "Omotenashi" hospitality which goes beyond a mere idea of customer service. Those clinics strive to become a central part to contribute to the local community through providing their patients with the world's most cutting-edge treatment and care, to stay aspiring and innovative to build up a system that enables the provision of the best dental care, and to give constant higher-than-expectation support to their patients. Under the banner of this management policy, they have accumulated practical methods to enhance the quality of their customer service which would result in the improvement of the customer satisfaction.

Nevertheless, when it comes to evaluating the quality of customer service at a dental clinic, it is quite hard for a patient to assess the outcome of the highly professional medical treatment. For this reason, evaluation is often conducted from the stand point of assessing the impression of the dentist and the receptionist in service. Because this type of evaluation is usually susceptible to the subjective factors and the difference of the atmosphere at each clinic, it is difficult to carry out an objective evaluation. Considering this problem, this paper primarily aims to invent and introduce a new scale that is suitable to assess impression towards overall customer service felt by the customers at each dental clinic, by referring to the evaluation criteria used in D1 Grand Prix Dentist Tournament.

In addition to that, because there is much ambiguity regarding how much the evaluation of the impression towards overall customer service at a dental clinic can affect customer satisfaction, quantitative evaluation how much customer service given by a receptionist, a dentist, and other medical practitioners can affect the total satisfaction level is set as the second purpose on this paper. Furthermore, taking into account the ever fiercer competition between clinics, it is critical for a dental clinic to retain repeat customers and to have its customers to spread favorable reviews to other prospective customers. Therefore, elucidation of the correlation of overall customer service at a clinic and the total satisfaction level with the customers' desire to come back and their intention to recommend to others is set as the third purpose.

2 Study Methods

2.1 Study Subjects and Methods

This research was conducted at two dental clinics in Kanto region and three dental clinics in Kansai region. These clinics have been in operation for 5 to 32 years (Average: 24.6 years and SD: 10.1 years), and have around 7 to 40 staff (Average: 16.2 years and SD: 12.0 years). Four of them see about 50 patients in average per day, and the other treats about 140 patients a day. Oral or written requests were sent to prospective subjects, and then questionnaire form was sent to the dental clinics that accepted the requests.

The survey was carried out over 19 days from 12th to 30th of November during which period patients who received any type of medical treatment or service were chosen as a target of this survey at the subject clinics. Each clinic was instructed to ask their patients to fill in the questionnaire at the end of their treatment. Request to patients to participate in the survey was made by a staff at each dental clinic. The purpose of this survey was explained to patients, and it was clarified that their personal information and privacy shall be discreetly protected. Those patients who agreed with this condition were asked to answer the questionnaire, and their response was collected on the spot.

1,108 responses were gathered, out of which 898 valid responses, excluding incomplete or false responses, were selected for the analysis. 898 responses comprise 300 male participants (Average age: 52.6 ± 18.1 years old) and 598 female participants (Average age: 48.9 ± 16.6 years old).

2.2 Survey Contents

For this survey, we utilized questionnaire invented originally that is composed of three categories: basic information, impression evaluation of customer service at each dental clinic, and overall evaluation. Basic information includes participants' gender, age, the purpose of visit, the number of years attended, and the motive of visit. The purpose of visit needs to be chosen out of the following four items: "Medical treatment (health insurance)", "Medical treatment (own expense)", "Tooth bleaching", and "Maintenance". Likewise, the number of years attended is to be chosen from: "First time", "Second time", "Third time but less than 1 year", "1 to 3 years", "3 to 5 years", and "More than 5 years". The motive of visit shall be chosen from multiple choices such as "HP", "Referral", and "Reputation".

With respect to impression evaluation of customer service at each dental clinic, original questionnaire was invented based on the undercover inspection conducted by Japan Dental Clinic Competition Association. Five different categories relating to the customer service at each dental clinics were put on the questionnaire, and several questions for each of these five categories were asked. The categories include: "Telephone support before visit", "Reception service at the time of visit", "Service during the consultation and the actual medical treatment", "Facility environment and cleanliness in appearance of staff", and "Medical treatment and communication during the actual practice". Answers for each of these items shall be chosen out of the following choices: "Very pleasant or satisfied (5p)", "Pleasant or satisfied (4p)", "Fair or somewhat satisfied (3p)", "Somewhat unpleasant or dissatisfied (2p)", and "Very unpleasant or dissatisfied (1p)".

As for the actual question items for "Telephone support before visit", the following five questions were asked: "Clinic staff responded clearly with bright tone of voice", "Clinic staff was considerate enough to repeat your name or request", "Clinic staff gave considerate remark like 'Sorry to keep you waiting' when he/she was slow to answer the phone or made you hold on", and "The overall impression of telephone support".

Question items for "Reception service at the time of visit" were the following five: "Receptionist immediately recognized and responded to you", "Receptionist gave you a welcoming eye contact with smile and greet", "Receptionist gave you an appreciation like 'Thank you for coming' or 'We have been waiting for your visit' for your reservation or visit", "Receptionist received your insurance card, ID, or patient's ticket with both hands, and handled them with courtesy", "Receptionist paid attention to and consideration for patients at the waiting room", "Receptionist ushered you to the consultation room with smile and courtesy".

Question items for "Service during the consultation and the actual medical treatment" were the following three: "Inquiry/consultation and treatment started on time, and if there was any delay, they gave you an explanation", "The dentist and other medical staff were easy to talk to with comfort", and "Did you feel like getting medical treatment at this dental clinic?"

Question items for "Facility environment and cleanliness in appearance of staff" were the following three: "The waiting room, the entrance, and the entrance hall were tidy and clean", "Appearances of the dentist and other staff were clean", "Language and behavior of the dentist and other staff were appropriate".

Question items for "Medical treatment and communication during the actual practice" were the following four: "Did you received their thoughtful words or felt their consideration when they reclined the chair or while you were sitting?", "Did you feel their thoughtfulness or consideration from the way they touched the inside of your mouth or when they put medical equipments into it?", "Did you feel they were proactively trying to communicate with you during treatment?", and "Did you feel comfortable about the overall responses and services during consultation and medical treatment?".

The overall evaluation is composed of three categories; The degree of overall satisfaction was measured from the answer to the question "On the whole, you were satisfied with the environment and the service by clinic staff". Similarly, intention to repeat was estimated from the answer to the question "Did you feel like coming back for another service, or would like to repeat in the future?". Intention to recommend to others was evaluated from the question "Did you feel like recommending this clinic to others?". Answers for each of these questions above were to be chosen from: "Very pleasant or satisfied (5p)", "Pleasant or satisfied (4p)", "Fair or somewhat satisfied (3p)", "Somewhat unpleasant or dissatisfied (2p)", and "Very unpleasant or dissatisfied (1p)",

2.3   Analysis Methods

With regard to the question items of the impression evaluation focused on the service at a dental clinic, factor analysis was performed to spot factor structure, and should there be any reliability confirmed, the average of all the question items that constitute each factor was computed. ANOVA for double factors was conducted in order to examine the effect of patients' gender and the number of years attended on the evaluation of the service at a dental clinic and their overall evaluation. In a technical sense, when dealing with the number of years attended, new groups of respondents were made by properly reallocating respondents from the original groups so there would be equally the same number of respondents in each of the new groups. Furthermore, Pearson's correlation coefficient was calculated to examine the correlation between the variables, and multiple regression analyses (Forced entry method) were performed taking the comprehensive evaluations such as the overall satisfaction level, the intention to repeat, and the intention to recommend to others as the dependent variables, and the evaluation of the responses and services at a dental clinic, participants' age, and gender as independent variables. Statistics package software (IBM SPSS22) was used for the statistical processing.

3   Result

3.1   Factor Analysis

Factor analyses (Maximum likelihood estimation and Promax rotation) were conducted as for the 20 question items of the impression evaluation which concerns the responses and services at a dental clinic (Table 1). An item has to have factor loading greater than 0.45 to be valid as a factor. Under this condition, considering the attenuation of eigenvalues at an initial solution and their interpretability, two factors were determined. The first factor was named "Telephone and reception service" factor, which was found to be related to the telephone response and reception service, and was reflected in the questions such as "The overall impression of telephone support" and "Receptionist

Table 1. Result of factor analysis

	F1	F2	Communality
F1(α = .959)			
• "Clinic staff gave considerate remark like 'Sorry to keep you waiting' when he/she was slow to answer the phone or made you hold on"	.935	−.073	.772
• "The overall impression of telephone support"	.926	−.073	.758
• "Clinic staff was considerate enough to repeat your name or request"	.912	−.026	.795
• "Clinic staff responded clearly with bright tone of voice"	.865	−.035	.702
• "Receptionist received your insurance card, ID, or patient's ticket with both hands, and handled them with courtesy"	.718	.168	.731
• "Receptionist gave you an appreciation like 'Thank you for coming' or 'We have been waiting for your visit' for your reservation or visit"	.714	.148	.698
• "Receptionist gave you a welcoming eye contact with smile and greet"	.692	.167	.688
• "Receptionist immediately recognized and responded to you"	.644	.204	.661
• "Receptionist paid attention to and consideration for patients at the waiting room"	.554	.257	.595
• "Receptionist ushered you to the consultation room with smile and courtesy"	.518	.403	.756
F2(α = .956)			
• "You felt comfortable about the overall responses and services during consultation and medical treatment"	−.123	.959	.751
• "You felt they were proactively trying to communicate with you during treatment"	−.073	.905	.722
• "You felt their thoughtfulness or consideration from the way they touched the inside of your mouth or when they put medical equipments into it"	−.017	.900	.786
• "The dentist and other medical staff were easy to talk to with comfort"	.019	.825	.705
• "You felt like getting medical treatment at this dental clinic"	.145	.753	.759
• "You received their thoughtful words or felt their consideration when they reclined the chair or while you were sitting"	.170	.737	.768
• "Appearances of the dentist and other staff were clean"	.295	.586	.701
• "Language and behavior of the dentist and other staff were appropriate"	.320	.572	.715

(*Continued*)

Table 1. (*Continued*)

	F1	F2	Communality
• "The waiting room, the entrance, and the entrance hall were tidy and clean"	.309	.509	.600
• "Inquiry/consultation and treatment started on time, and if there was any delay, they gave you an explanation"	.277	.499	.542
Eigenvalue	13.17	1.04	
Cumulative contribution	65.8	71.2	
Factor correlation		.780	

gave you a welcoming eye contact with smile and greet". The second factor was named "Consultation and treatment service" factor, which was assumed to be associated with the responses and services at the time of medical consultation and treatment, and was reflected in the questions like "Did you feel they were proactively trying to communicate with you during the treatment?" and "Language and behavior of the dentist and other staff were appropriate".

In order to examine the internal consistency, Cronbach's α coefficient was computed from the question items which mainly constitute each of the aforementioned factors. As a result of this examination, α coefficient for both factors were high enough to guarantee the internal consistency ($\alpha = 0.959$ for the 1st factor, and $\alpha = 0.956$ for the 2nd factor). Given these findings, the average score of each item on the first factor was considered as "Telephone and reception service" score, and the average score of each item on the second factor was considered as "Consultation and treatment service" score, and then impression evaluation scale concerning the responses and services of a dentist was determined taking above-mentioned scores as subscales.

3.2 Basic Statistic

Basic statistic including impression evaluation scale regarding the responses and services at a dental clinic, participants' age, the overall satisfaction level, the intention to repeat, and the intention to recommend to others were given, and then influences of gender and the number of years attended were investigated (Table 2). As a result of ANOVA for double factors taking gender (male/female) and the number of years attended (1st time / > 1 year /1 to 5 years / < 5 years) as the factors, no significant interaction effect was spotted between any of the variables. Also none of these variables appeared to have a significant main effect upon participants' gender. The number of years attended was found to exert a significant main effect on the following items: Participants' age, telephone and reception service score, the overall satisfaction level, the intention to repeat, and the intention to recommend to others. As a consequence of multiple comparisons, it was made clear that those participants with the longer history of attending a clinic are generally older than others, while their telephone and reception service score, overall satisfaction level, intention to repeat, and intention to recommend

Table 2. Result of basic statistic

	Male			
	1st time	> 1 year	1 to 5 years	< 5 years
	n=9	n=82	n=90	n=119
Age (years)	49.6 ±13.6	45.6±17.1	50.9 ±16.7	58.7±18.3
Score of telephone and reception service	4.67 ±0.56	4.63±0.48	4.55 ±0.52	4.58±0.51
Score of consultation and treatment service	4.74 ±0.37	4.56±0.52	4.54 ±0.54	4.53±0.54
Score of the overall satisfaction	4.67 ±0.50	4.62±0.57	4.47 ±0.78	4.50±0.80
Score of the intention to repeat	4.67 ±0.50	4.41±0.90	4.49 ±0.65	4.39±0.82
Score of the intention to recommend to others	4.67 ±0.50	4.56±0.65	4.34 ±0.86	4.38±0.82

*,p<.05; *,p<.01

	Female			
	1st time	> 1 year	1 to 5 years	< 5 years
	n=42	n=141	n=205	n=210
Age (years)	48.1 ±18.7	41.8±14.1	46.9 ±15.1	55.8±16.7
Score of telephone and reception service	4.69 ±0.38	4.79±0.35	4.71 ±0.46	4.59±0.54
Score of consultation and treatment service	4.70 ±0.43	4.76±0.46	4.67 ±0.48	4.59±0.53
Score of the overall satisfaction	4.73 ±0.51	4.77±0.56	4.65 ±0.58	4.49±0.77
Score of the intention to repeat	4.73 ±0.45	4.69±0.58	4.56 ±0.74	4.30±0.89
Score of the intention to recommend to others	4.69 ±0.52	4.71±0.61	4.56 ±0.65	4.36±0.80

*,p<.05; *,p<.01

	Main Effect		Interaction Effect	
	Gender	No. of years attended		Gender × No. of years attended
Age (years)	2.80	29.65	**	0.10
Score of telephone and reception service	3.01	2.90	*	1.68
Score of consultation and treatment service	2.56	2.01		1.14

(Continued)

Table 2. (*Continued*)

	Male			
	1st time	> 1 year	1 to 5 years	< 5 years
	n=9	n=82	n=90	n=119
Score of the overall satisfaction	1.77	3.63	*	1.00
Score of the intention to repeat	1.01	4.42	**	2.28
Score of the intention to recommend to others	1.45	5.58	**	1.24

*,p<.05; *,p<.01

to others were inclined to be lower compared to the participants with the shorter history of attending a clinic.

Table 3 shows the correlation coefficients in between each of the following variables: The score of the two factors in the evaluation of the responses and services at a dental clinic, the overall satisfaction level, the intention to repeat, and the intention to recommend to others. Participants' age was found to have a significant and negative correlation with each of the other variables. Similarly, it became clear that the score of the two factors in the evaluation of the responses and services had significant and positive correlations with the overall satisfaction level, the intention to repeat, and the intention to recommend to others.

Table 3. Result of correlation coefficients six items of basic statistic

	1	2		3		4		5		6	
1. Age	–	−.140	**	−.161	**	−.161	**	−.213	**	−.160	**
2. Score of telephone and reception service		–		.818	**	.599	**	.449	**	.614	**
3. Score of consultation and treatment service				–		.653	**	.510	**	.653	**
4. The overall satisfaction						–		.629	**	.836	**
5. The intention to repeat								–		.582	**
6. The intention to recommend to others										–	

**,p < .01

3.3   Multiple Regression Analyses

Next, the influences of the evaluation of the responses and services at a dental clinic on the overall satisfaction level, the intention to repeat, and the intention to recommend to others were studied (Table 4). At this analytic study, for the sake of eliminating the influences of participants' age, gender, and the number of years attended, multiple regression analyses (Forced entry method) were carried out, under whose condition, independent variables were set as follows: The score of the two factors in the evaluation

Table 4. The multiple regression coefficient result of the evaluation of the responses and services at a dental clinic on the overall satisfaction level

	Independent Variables					
	The overall satisfaction		The intention to repeat		The intention to recommend	
β						
Gender (dummy variable)	.007		−.018		.003	
Age	−.062	*	−.142	**	−.038	
The number of years attended	−.052		−.059		−.087	**
Score of telephone and reception service	.146	**	.047		.215	**
Score of consultation and treatment service	.527	**	.459	**	.476	**
R^2	.450	**	.304	**	.470	**
*,p < .05; **,p < .01						

of responses and services, participants' age, gender (Dummy variables), and the number of years attended. Also dependent variables were the following three: The overall satisfaction level, the intention to repeat, and the intention to recommend to others. In consequence, each of the three dependent variables rendered a significant multiple regression coefficient. The values of the adjusted R-square stretched from 0.304 to 0.470.

The overall satisfaction level yielded a significant standardized partial regression coefficient on participants' age, telephone and reception service score, and consultation and treatment service score. The intention to repeat rendered a significant standardized partial regression coefficient on participants' age and consultation and treatment service score. In the same way, the intention to recommend to others showed a significant standardized partial regression coefficient on the number of years attended, telephone and reception service score, and consultation and treatment service score.

After that, in an attempt to eliminate the influences of the overall satisfaction level, concerning the correlation between the intention to repeat and the intention to recommend to others, partial correlation coefficient was calculated taking the overall satisfaction level as the control variable. Although there was a significant and positive correlation (p < .01), the value of partial correlation coefficient was low as r = .145.

4   Result

4.1   Impression Evaluation Scale Concerning the Responses and Services at Dental Clinics

As a result of factor analyses, it turned out that telephone responses and reception services were put together to construct single factor, even though those two items were initially classified in different categories. Similarly, the following three categories were combined to make one factor: Inquiry/consultation, treatment, and the adjustment of the facility environment and appearance of staff. It can be said that telephone responses and reception services have a lot in common because they do not involve physical contact with a patient themselves. Impression evaluation exhibited the same tendency. Conversely, inquiry/consultation, treatment, and the adjustment of the facility environment and appearance of staff are a series of actions from the beginning to the end of the medical services, all of which involve physical contact with a patient. They were treated as an independent factor in the study. In this kind of situation, the responses and services given by the dentist and other medical staff to the patient were supposed to attenuate the patient's nervousness and fear, and thus these responses and services to the patient have great similarity to each other. Behind this is the fact that the patient did not seem to be able to assess precisely the responses and services of the dentist and other medical staff, for he/she was nervous about medical consultation or treatment.

All of the dental clinics that were the subjects of this study marked good evaluations on each and every item. Therefore, it might be possible that five categories were unable to be extracted after factor analyses. Given this, it might be possible to increase the number of factors by inquiring more dental clinics or various types of dental clinics.

4.2   The Influences of Patients' Age, Gender, and the Number of Years Attended

Because there was a significant and negative correlation between patients' age and the impression evaluation concerning the responses and services at a dental clinic as well as between patients' age and the overall satisfaction level, it would be safe to say that older patients tend to have lower impression evaluation towards the responses and services and the lower overall satisfaction level. In an aging society like Japan, dental clinics in general, excluding pediatric dental clinics, are treating older and older patients, so customer service to satisfy elderly patients more is becoming an important factor. Nevertheless, since the number of years attended was found to have a significant correlation with patients' age, it is quite hard to specify which one of the number of years attended or patients' age is the cause of degrading evaluation.

Also, patients who have visited a dental clinic more than others exhibited lower impression evaluation concerning the responses and services at a dental clinic. It is presumably because the more a patient visits a dental clinic, the better he/she comes to realize the details of the actual medical settings, and thus the more a patient visits a dental clinic, the severer his/her evaluation of the medical settings in comparison to his/her initial evaluation. In addition to that, A new patient with a dental disease is usually nervous at the first time of visit, so he/she would feel higher satisfaction if a dentist and other medical staff can make him/her feel comfortable by creating a good atmosphere in a clinic or communicating effectively with an intention to get rid of a patient's nervousness or fear.

As for the impression evaluation concerning the responses and services at a dental clinic, there was no gender difference, which assumably means that gender difference may not especially define the quality of the responses and services. Hereafter, patient's age and the number of years attended were adjusted for the sake of examining the influences of the impression evaluation on the overall satisfaction level and so forth.

4.3   Evaluation of the Responses and Services Affecting the Satisfaction Level

As a result of multiple regression analyses, both telephone and reception service, and consultation and treatment service have a positive impact on the overall satisfaction level. It is believed to be natural that the evaluation of medically functional services provided at a dental clinic ought to be high and it has a tremendous impact on whether to continue medical treatment at the clinic or not. It was noteworthy that services of psychological and emotional aspect like communication with a dentist and other medical staff at the time of consultation and treatment were revealed to have positive effect on the overall satisfaction level. Even though people often distinguish a dental clinic from general service industry, communicative skills for reception service and the general atmosphere at a medical institution are also regarded as important factors.

Fujimura's survey targeting medical service has shown that the outcome of treatment had the greatest impact on the overall satisfaction and then medical staff had the second greatest influence [6]. It seems that relationship between a service provider and a customer which respects their respective humanity is crucial. The outcome of treatment is the quality concerning the outcome of service, and it is an important factor for a customer. Whereas, humane communication is also a meaningful factor especially when the outcome of treatment is up to sufficiently satisfactory standard, or when the outcome of a treatment is hard to evaluate due to its high specialty. This is the fact that implies the importance of human relations at the time of provision of service.

Currently, the oversupply of dental clinics is becoming a social problem, and there are many dental clinics that provide specialized dental care services in an attempt to differentiate themselves from other dental clinics. Unlike other fields of medical care, a lot of dental clinics offer a medical treatment that combines a preventative insurance-covered care with medical care at patient's own expense, a plan of regular medical check-up, and visiting care as a family doctor for the elderly. It is assumed that the impression of the responses and services was added as a factor that can affect the satisfaction level.

4.4   The Intention to Repeat /to Recommend to Others

The intention to repeat and the intention to recommend to others were found to have significant correlation with the overall satisfaction level. Also, the intention to repeat and the intention to recommend to others had a significant and positive correlation ($r = .582$) with each other, but partial correlation coefficient taking the overall satisfaction level as the control variable was as low as $r = .145$, and was barely significant.

First of all, upon examining the intention of repeat, or the desire to attend continuously, it has to be noted that retention of repeater affects greatly on the profitability. Especially, in the case of a dental clinic, they need to retain more repeater seeking tooth bleaching, regular check-up, and maintenance, inclusively. Also, from the standpoint of a dental clinic, in the case of handling a repeater, it would be more cost-effective because they don't need to gather information about patients, their medical history, and the condition of their dental diseases, unlike when they deal with a new customer, so it would be favorable to have more repeaters. Furthermore, as the change of the environment inside people's mouth, the case of dental caries are becoming rare, and more people come to think of switching to a medical treatment including check-up and prevention that combines insurance-covered care with medical care at patient's own expense, so there is another reason which necessitates the retention of repeaters.

The survey displayed that consultation and treatment service score positively affected the intention to repeat, but telephone and reception service score did not make a significant impact on the intention to repeat. Medical practitioners who have a direct contact with a patient take a vital role in motivating more patients to repeat. Although it was out of the scope of this study, the satisfaction level with regard to the expense and medical treatment itself and optional responses or services other than an actual treatment can have a possible influence, and so they are worth further examination in the future.

Next, as for the intention to recommend to others, comparison of different medical services that requires an actual experience incurs a customer costs and risks. It is impossible for a customer to evaluate services before an actual consultation and treatment. In this case, recommendation by word of mouth is greatly reliable. The intention to recommend to others had a positive effect on both telephone and reception service score, and consultation and treatment service score. Not just consultation and treatment service score, but also telephone and reception service score exerted a positive influence. It can be said that not only medical practitioners but other staff are important.

Telephone and reception service did not have an impact on the intention to repeat, but it positively influenced the intention to recommend to others. Being able to listen carefully to a patient to meet each patient's needs and to provide a patient with both psychological and medical care would result in earning patient's trust and consequently getting more repeaters. However, when it comes to recommendation to others by word of mouth, patients seem to tell others about the comprehensive impression of a dental clinic including the impression of reception service.

4.5   Limitation of the Survey and the Prospective Research

Our questionnaire survey was performed only at those dental clinics that consented to it. In order to attain more generality, it is necessary to conduct the survey at many more dental clinics and to continue on further consideration. Not just a questionnaire survey as a form of evaluation method, more integrated manner of survey would be required that takes account of not only the responses and services and an ideal of communication, but also informed-consent and practical consultation and treatment.

5   Conclusion

This study made the following discoveries. A new patient and a patient who has visited a clinic fewer times than others tend to have higher evaluation of the customer satisfaction level. Although it was found that recommendation to others by word of mouth can be affected by reception factor, the overall satisfaction level such as a patient's desire to visit continuously was greatly affected by the responses and services of a dentist and other medical staff at the time of consultation and treatment.

Acknowledgement.   I'd like to express my sincere gratitude to all people who support this research and our questionnaire, Dr. Shinji Arai, Clinic Director of Arai Dental Clinic, Dr. Hideaki Sakai, Administrative Director of Medical Corporation Ikuhokai, Dr. Yasuyuki Shundo, Clinic Director of Medical Corporation Shundo Dental Clinic, Dr. Yasuhiro Hayano, Clinic Director of Hayano Dental Clinic, and all the medical staff who were willing to cooperate this research.

References

1. White Paper for Health and Welfare in 1995, regarding Medical, "Quality, Inforamtion, Selection, and Convincing", the Ministry of Health, Labour and Welfare (1995)
2. White Paper for Information and Communications in Japan, the Outline of the Survey of Doctors, Dental Doctors and Pharmacy Practitioner in (2012)
3. Supply and Demand Problem of Dental Clinics, Background and Opinion, Japan Medical Association, October 2014
4. Kazuko, K.: "Hospitality to ease patients and their families; "Visualization" of the hospitality brought by dental clinics, Karei, Japan Society for Dental Anti-Aging, Number of Issue, 8, 133–136
5. Web site of "D1 Grand Prix Dentist Tournament", Japan Dental Clinic Competition Association. http://dental-1.jp

Movement Analysis of Transfer Assistance Using a Slide Board

Xiaodan Lu[1(✉)], Mengyuan Liao[1], Zelong Wang[1], Yuki Miyamoto[2], Hiroyuki Hamada[1], Tomoko Ota[2], Kengo Yano[3], Yoshihiko Tokumoto[3], Takashi Yoshikawa[4], Yuka Takai[5], and Akihiko Goto[5]

[1] Kyoto Institute of Technology, Kyoto, Japan
luxiaodan0223@gmail.com
[2] Chuou Business Group, Chuou-ku, Japan
promot1@gold.ocn.ne.jp
[3] Tokubetuy ougorouzinhomunanohana, Tokyo, Japan
yano@asokaen.jp
[4] National Institute of Technology, Niihama, College, Niihama, Japan
yosikawa@mec.niihama-nct.ac.jp
[5] Osaka Sangyu University, Daito, Japan
gotoh@ise.osaka-sandai.ac.jp

Abstract. In this study, the transfer process from wheelchair to bed was focused and investigation by comparing expert and non-expert. The 3D motion analysis system was used during transfer process in order to obtain the motion characteristic. The whole transfer was separated into 3 processes to make process analysis. The expert can transfer care-receiver smoothly with a comfortable condition. Using hand support Shoulder bones and hold care-receiver lean forward was considered a current method to adjust care-receiver's position. And the current using method of slide board was also found according to process analysis.

Keywords: Movement analysis · Transfer · Slide board · Process analysis · Expert and non-expert

1 Introduction

Japan has become a super-aged society. In recent years, the importance and demand of care workers are expected to increase. On the other hand, care workers tend to suffer from musculoskeletal disorders such as back pain or cervico-omo-brachial disorder. The Ministry of Health, Labor and Welfare is promoting the measures to prevent these health impairments and the use of slide boards. A slide board is a tool to use when a caregiver transfer a care-receiver from a bed to a wheelchair or a vehicle. Using a slide board, it is not necessary to lift up a care-receiver at the time of transfer assistance. It therefore, reduces the work load of caregivers, which eventually prevent the occurrence of back pains.

However, in order to use a slide board perfectly, practice and time is required. In this study, we focus on transfer assistance work by using a slide board, especially when

© Springer International Publishing Switzerland 2016
V.G. Duffy (Ed.): DHM 2016, LNCS 9745, pp. 243–252, 2016.
DOI: 10.1007/978-3-319-40247-5_25

transferring a care-receiver from a wheelchair to a bed, and then analyze the movements of expert and non-expert to clarify the differences between them.

In order to measure the movement of subjects, 6 MAC3D System cameras were installed (MAC3D System; motion analysis Co. Ltd.). We attached markers on subjects to analyze the movements and obtained the following results.

The whole data was separated into 6 steps and 3 processes. The caregivers' motion was clarified and comparing according to each process. The key points of transfer from wheelchair to bed by using slide board were found by comparing expert and non-expert. Using hand support Shoulder bones and hold care-receiver lean forward was considered in process-1. Insert slide board into space under bottom with a slight angle with bed was considered the basic condition of slide board using method.

2   Experiment

2.1   Participants and Instruments

In this study, two caregivers who had experienced were employed and called expert and non-expert. A man was selected as care-receiver who requiring care.

The caregivers were required transfer care-receiver from wheelchair to bed by using slide board as shown in following (Fig. 1).

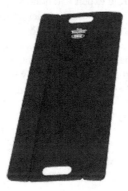

Fig. 1. Slide board

2.2   Motion Analysis

The three-dimensional motion capture system was used for evaluating the motion during the whole transfer process as shown in Fig. 2. (MAC3D System; motion analysis Co. Ltd.) The infrared reflection markers were affixed at the bodies of expert, non-expert and care-receiver. As shown in Fig. 3, 20, 33, 6 points was pasted on the bodies of expert, non-expert and care-receiver in order to analyze motion. And six cameras captured the position of each marker in the three dimensional coordinate system with 100 Hz sampling rate. All markers position data were synchronized and entered into a computer.

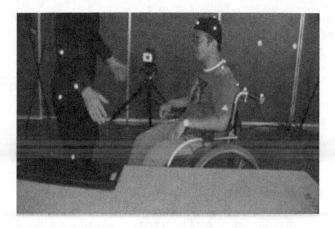

Fig. 2. Experiment setting

Expert   Non-expert   Care-receiver

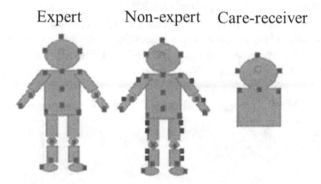

Fig. 3. The Location of infrared reflection markers for expert, non-expert and beginner.

2.3 Working Sequence and Process Analysis

The whole transfer working Sequence was separated into six steps as shown in following:

1. The caregiver stop wheelchair and press wheelchair' brakes before adjust the position of care-receiver's foots and position.
2. Adjust the posture and position of the care-receiver so that obtain a suitable.
3. Put the slide board between the care-receiver's bottom and bed. One side of slide board was inserted into space between bottom and a wheelchair, the other side was put on the bed.
4. The caregiver's right hand was held on care-receiver's back in order to carry care-receiver closing to caregiver's chest. The caregiver's left hand push care-receiver sliding on the board to the bed.
5. Take off the board
6. Adjust care-receiver's position

The first three steps were focused on in this study. And the expert's working time of first three steps was summarized on Table 1.

Table 1. The working time of first three steps (Second)

No.	Process	Expert	Non-expert
1	Adjust care-receiver's position until a suitable location	21	33
2	Put the slide board between the care-receiver's bottom and bed.	11	5
3	Push care-receiver sliding on slide board from wheelchair to the bed	15	21

3   Result and Discussion

The main motion of first three steps for expert and non-expert were illustrated on Fig. 4. As shown in process-1, the expert's hand holding the care-receiver's back, which hand was hugged at the top of the care-receiver's back. However, non-expert's hand was held on the chest of care-receiver. In case of process-2, Experts putted the slide board under care-receiver's bottom had an angle with a wheelchair. The non-expert putted the slide board perpendicular to the wheelchair as shown in Fig. 4. Furthermore, expert was taken crouching posture during process-3. Non-expert was taken standing posture.

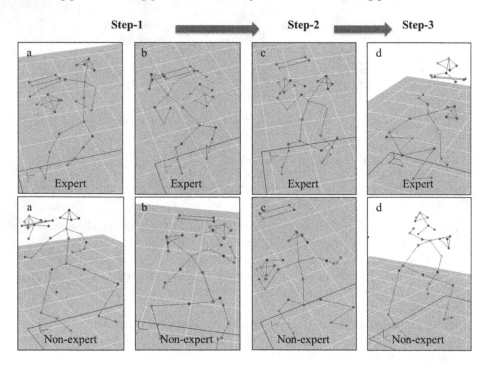

Fig. 4. The main motion of first three steps

Figure 5 was shown the body adjustment by expert and non-expert. As shown in Fig. 5, Experts used one hand support care-receiver's shoulder blade, used other hand pulled care-receiver's body tilted down on him. However, care-receiver's upper body was significantly down to one side during process-1 of non-expert, especially the head.

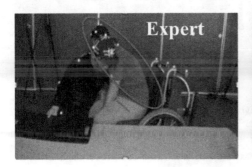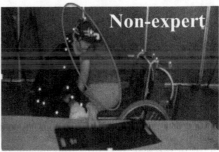

Fig. 5. Body adjustment by expert and non-expert during process-1

The Fig. 6 was the Schematic diagram of distance between care-receiver's shoulder and wheelchair during process-1. The distance change was calculated according to the 3D motion analysis data as shown in Fig. 7. It was can consider that both expert and non-expert was understanding that need lean forward care-receiver's upper body. Comparing with expert, non-expert had to take more often to lean forward care-receiver's upper body.

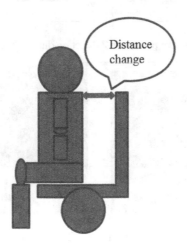

Fig. 6. Schematic diagram of distance between care-receiver's shoulder and wheelchair

The position of care-receiver's left and right shoulder during transfer by expert and non-expert was illustrated in Fig. 8 (Process-1). It is can found that there was a large height difference between left and right shoulder in Z direction when non-expert adjusting care-receiver's position. Comparing with non-expert, it was shown slight

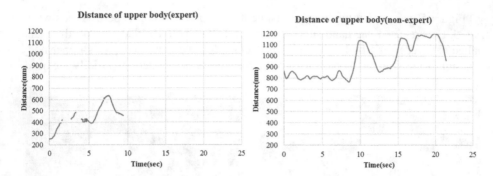

Fig. 7. The Distance change between care-receiver's shoulder and wheelchair for expert and non-expert.

height difference in Z direction, because expert did not raise care-receiver's bottom during adjusting process.

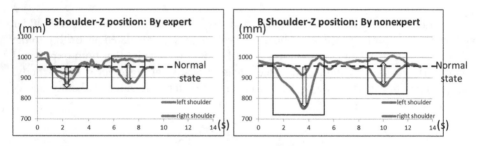

Fig. 8. The care-receiver's shoulder position in Z direction during transfer by expert and non-expert.

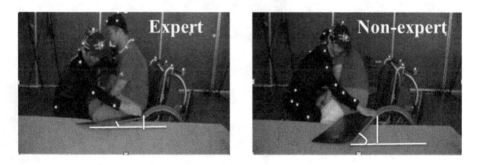

Fig. 9. The slide board insert method of expert and non-expert

As mentioned above, expert and non-expert used the slide board with different methods as shown in Fig. 9 Expert insert slide board had a small angel with bed. Non-expert shown a large angle between slide board and bed when insert board. During this process, expert held care-receiver's body slightly and obtain a space under whole bottom so that easy insert slide board.

The expert and non-expert's left waist joint and left knee angle during the first three processes were shown in Fig. 10, which the first, second, third process were marked by blue, red and green color. As shown in left waist joint angle of process-2, expert can keep the posture because standing work. The non-expert didn't have large angle change, because he working bent waist down. In case of left knee angle, expert shown large change of left knee angle use left angle many time during process-2, which was considered that stable move care-receiver.

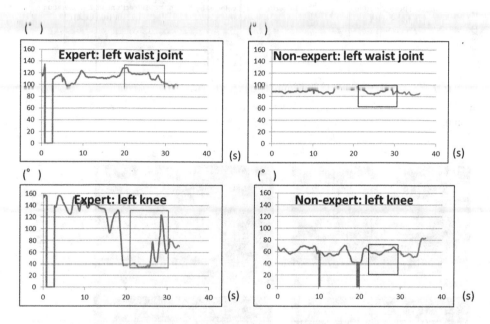

Fig. 10. The left waist joint and left knee angle of expert and non-expert

The position, velocity and acceleration data of care-receiver's head on Z direction was calculated and summarized on Fig. 11, which expert's data was shown on upper side, and non-expert's data was shown on down side. And the process-1, process-2 and process-3 were marked by blue, red and green color.

The head of care-receiver was shown strenuous vibration up and down when non-expert inserted the slide board into space between bottom and bed during process-2. Non-expert's motion was given care-receiver feeling unstable. It was can considered that the care-receiver's head and shoulders were presented small moving range with slight from side to side during expert's process-2.

The Transfer process from wheelchair to bed by expert and non-expert was illustrated in Fig. 12 (Process-3). During the transfer process, expert's hand was hold on care-receiver alar and support his shoulder blade in order to provide a comfortable feeling. Expert can master the transfer technique with current using method of slide board. The non-expert didn't catch the slide board using skill so that have to lift care-receiver and put down again.

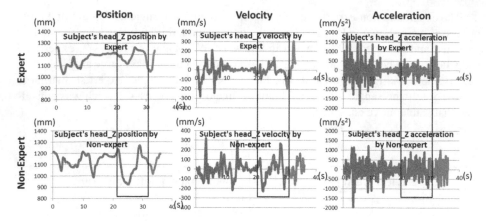

Fig. 11. The position, velocity and acceleration of care-receiver's head on Z direction (Colour fig online)

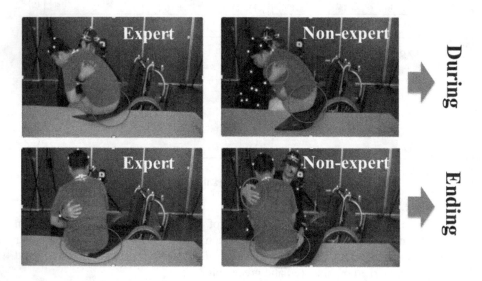

Fig. 12. Transfer process from wheelchair to bed by expert and non-expert

The care-receiver's neck and shoulder position change was shown in Fig. 13 during process-3. As shown in Fig. 13, the working time of process-3 by expert was shorter than non-expert. Care-receiver's neck was displayed a smooth move up and down. The care-receiver's neck was presented a dramatic move up and down during transferring by non-expert, which was same with above mentioned. The shoulder position change had a similar moving characteristic with neck position.

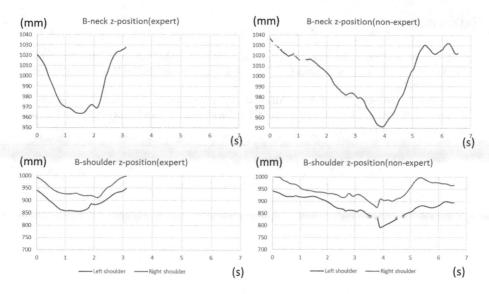

Fig. 13. The care-receiver's neck and shoulder position in Z direction during process-3

4   Conclusions

In a word, the conclusions were summarized as following:

In the case of expert, when adjusting the posture of care-receiver, the expert had the upper-half body of the care-receiver leaned forward slightly and moved him to the right and left in order to move the weight to one leg. While being careful not to lean the care-receiver diagonally forward too much, the expert repeated this movement. Then, the expert secures a wheelchair with his foot to keep the balance of the care-receiver.

The expert had the care-receiver leaned diagonally forward and moved the weight of the care-receiver to one leg. Then, he inserted the slide board between the base of thighs and the ischial bone on the bed side. After securing one end of the slide board on the bed firmly, he adjusted the angle between the slide board and the bed narrower to make the transfer easily.

Then the expert put his arm under the arm of the care-receiver on the bed side to support around his shoulder blade. The expert put his opposite arm around the care-receiver's waist, and had him leaned toward the bed. He transferred him to the bed by pushing the care-receiver's waist to make him slide on the board without lifting. When transferring a care-receiver using a slide board, the angle of the caregiver's back arch changed slightly, and it can be considered to reduce physical burdens of the caregiver. Moreover, a slide board enables the transfer stable, and it helps to minimize uneasiness of care-receivers during transferring.

References

1. Ministry of Health, Labour and Welfare and Central Industrial Accident Pre vention Committee, health and safety measures - low back pain measures · KY activities in social welfare facilities
2. Sakashita, A., Deguchi, T., Honda, A., Matsuda, A., Matsumoto, K., Miyahara, M., Yamamoto, S.: Introduction and utilization - of the work burden of elderly care facility staff - sliding seat and a sliding board (2009)

Health Promotion Community Support for Vitality and Empathy: Visualize Quality of Motion (QoM)

Takuichi Nishimura[1(✉)], Zilu Liang[1], Satoshi Nishimura[1],
Tomoka Nagao[1], Satoko Okubo[1], Yasuyuki Yoshida[2],
Kazuya Imaizumi[3], Hisae Konosu[4], Hiroyasu Miwa[5],
Kanako Nakajima[5], and Ken Fukuda[1]

[1] National Institute of Advanced Industrial Science and Technology,
AI Research Center, Tyoto, Japan
takuichi.nishimura@aist.go.jp
[2] Tokyo Institute of Technology, Graduate School of Decision Science
and Technology, Tokyo, Japan
[3] Faculty of Healthcare, Tokyo Healthcare University, Tokyo, Japan
[4] Japan Dance Sport Federation, Tokyo, Japan
[5] Human Information Research Institute,
National Institute of Advanced Industrial Science and Technology, Tokyo, Japan

Abstract. Nowadays approximately 30 % of the population is suffering from lifestyle-related diseases in Japan. Both individuals and the government are becoming more and more health-conscious and are taking various measures to improve personal health and to prevent lifestyle-related diseases. Among all the measures, improving trunk stability has been given special attention as it is vital for improving physical strength, preventing injury, and extending healthy life span. Many traditional trunk strength evaluation methods were designed to assess core muscle mass. Less emphasis, if any, was given to the stability of the trunk, which could be represented by the smoothness of trunk movement. In this paper, we proposed a new trunk torsion model for the purpose of evaluating two trunk torsion standard movements. We also developed a mobile application named "Axis Visualizer" based on the proposed trunk torsion model, which gives higher score to users who rotate the shoulders or hips smoothly with axis fixed and high frequencies. This application can support trainers and coaches to visualize the smoothness of trunk movement and to increase training outcome, as well as support health promotion community to easily evaluate the effectiveness of group exercise.

Keywords: Health promotion · Community support · Quality of motion

1 Introduction

The rapidly aging population imposes a heavy burden to the social welfare system in Japan. The number of old people reached historical peak 33 million in 2014, which is equivalent to 26.0 % of the whole population [1]. In 2012, the national healthcare cost

© Springer International Publishing Switzerland 2016
V.G. Duffy (Ed.): DHM 2016, LNCS 9745, pp. 253–263, 2016.
DOI: 10.1007/978-3-319-40247-5_26

was more than 39 trillion Japanese Yen, which increased about 627 billion Japanese Yen compared to that in previous year. In addition, long-term care insurance sharply increased to 8 trillion Japanese Yen. Moreover, it is expected that the social welfare for nursing and healthcare will roar in 2025 as the baby boom generation ages beyond 75-year-old. Various efforts have been made, including cooperation between health industry (e.g., private sports clubs) and medical institutions or local governments, preventive healthcare measures advocated by health insurance unions, regional comprehensive care system designed for supporting independence of local residents. As nowadays lifestyle-related chronic diseases are more common than infectious diseases, it is imperative to promote healthy lifestyles in order to extend healthy life expectancy. Actively improving physical strength is widely acknowledged as a very important aspect of healthy lifestyles.

Under such background, special attention has been given to body trunk for the purpose of prevention injuries and fall, and many core training methods [2–5] have been introduced to increase trunk muscle mass. In dance sports, however, it is widely considered that the strength of body trunk is not characterized by the amount of muscle but by the cooperative use of body trunk and limb. Therefore, in order to support more integrative evaluation on trunk strength, we developed a mobile application named Axis Visualizer based on our proposed trunk torsion model for evaluating the smoothness of truck torsion movements. A user can obtain high score if he or she coordinately rotates shoulders and hips smoothly, with low vibration and high frequency.

The rest of the paper is organized as follows. The related work on trunk strength and movements is discussed in the next section. In Sect. 3, we present our proposed trunk torsion spring model and the evaluation measures of body trunk strength. In Sect. 4, we describe the implementation of the mobile application Axis Visualizer and a demo of the evaluation on users' torsion. We then give an overall picture of the health promotion community support that we are working on. The paper is concluded in Sect. 6.

2   Related Work

2.1   Definition of Trunk Strength

In order to discuss the body trunk strength, we first describe the definition of posture, movement, motion, action in kinematics.

- *Posture*: a posture consists of two elements: attitude and position. Attitude represents the relative positional relationship among each part of the body such as head, trunk, limb, and it can be measured through joint angle. On the other hand, position is used to represent the relationship between the body axis and gravity, and it can be indicated by standing, supine (face up), and so on.
- *Movement*: a movement refers to temporal change of posture. In other words, it is described as a change of attitude and position.
- *Motion*: a unit that analyzes the behavior as a task that is specifically carried out by a movement.
- *Action*: a unit when taking into consideration the context of the meaning and intention shown by a movement.

Body trunk is the torso which has the following three roles: (1) supporting and maintaining postures, (2) the foundation for producing movement, (3) serving as an axis. Several methods were proposed to increase the mass of surface muscle group (e.g., rectus abdominis muscle) and deep muscle groups (e.g., transverse abdominal muscle) [6–8], such as plank, elbow-to, and breathing techniques.

It is worth mentioning that the quality of movement is more important than the amount of movement, which is a key point in improving people's healthy life expectancy in the super-aged society in the future. Bad motion patterns caused by bad postures may lead to musculoskeletal pain syndrome. The prevention and treatment of pain is directly related to the activity in everyday life, therefore it is a very effective and efficient means for health promotion and preventive care. Based on this rationality, the MSI (Movement System Impairment) approach was proposed, which reduces mechanical stress by correcting the movements and motions and thereby enables the prevention and treatment of pain [9]. In addition, Shumway-Cook and Woollacott proposed a system theory which advocates that movement is not simply the result of muscle-specific exercise program or uniform reflection, but rather the result of the dynamic interaction among perception system, cognition system, and musculoskeletal system [10]. This theory has been applied in rehabilitation and has been proved effective in practice. For instance, the capability of independent walking in the elderly was improved after motion control exercise with repeated movement such as walking, even though muscle strength was not really improved, the capability of independent walking was increased. In physically expressive sports such as dance sports, it is widely known that smooth usage from deep muscles to the surface muscles is more important than muscle mass. And the core stability is the result of motion control and the muscle function of the Lumbar spine, pelvis, and hip joint complex.

Therefore, it is considered that system theory as well as MSI approach should be applied to health promotion and preventive medicine. In other words, rather than evaluating single function, such as muscle strength and range of motion, it is important to establish an easy and proper approach to evaluate and visualize the quality of movement pattern in a comprehensive manner by considering neuromuscular coordination. In this way, it will become possible to learn and acquire the optimal movement pattern without injury or secondary dysfunction. However, many services of health promotion and prevention activities still solely put emphasis on strength training.

2.2   Typical Trunk Movement

According to the WDSF technique book "Rumba" [11], there are four types of trunk movement.

1. *Left and right horizontal movement of pelvis* (Fig. 1 left). While keeping the pelvis and shoulder line horizontal, move pelvis left and right horizontally.
2. *Left and right tilt of pelvis* (Fig. 1 center). The left side of the body is compressed vertically while the right side of the body is stretched. Keep the left shoulder close to the left hip and the right shoulder away from the right hip. The right side is the same.

3. *Back and forward tilt of pelvis* (Fig. 1 right). For forward tilt, tilt the pelvis forward by moving the upper part of the pelvis forward and the bottom part backward, and vice versa for back tilt.
4. *Trunk torsion.* While keeping the pelvis and shoulder line horizontal, rotate around the vertical axis of the trunk.

The trunk can also make various movements by opening and closing the chest. In the case of standard dance, many movements involve the conjunction move of limbs and head. In the case of Latin dance, many movements only move the lower part of the body smoothly while keeping the upper part instable. In this paper, we focus on trunk torsion that may occur in walking and rotational motion, which in characterized by the angle change in the vertical axis of the shoulder line and the hip line.

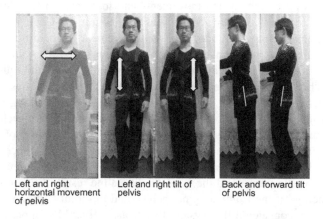

| Left and right horizontal movement of pelvis | Left and right tilt of pelvis | Back and forward tilt of pelvis |

Fig. 1. Examples of trunk movements in dance sports.

2.3   Existing Trunk Models

The most detailed trunk model is the musculoskeletal model [12]. As it models trunk components in great details, it can be used to describe complex movements. However, it is difficult to apply this on torsion movements due to large number of parameters involved. In addition, the trunk model for walking focuses on the waist and the lower limbs, which is not suitable for the purpose of our study. Even in the case of whole body models, the trunk is usually modeled as mass-point or cylinder, and there is no model of trunk torsion movements. Although there are models for body torsion while walking, they cannot be applied to the cases of repeated trunk torsions.

3   Proposal of Trunk Torsion Spring Model and Evaluation Method

3.1   Overview of the Proposal

In this paper, we propose a method for evaluating the smoothness of trunk movement. First, we propose the trunk torsion spring model. We selected the standard movements of trunk torsion as shown in Fig. 2 for easy evaluation on trunk movements. Second, we propose a method to use accelerometer on mobile phone for evaluating trunk movement. This method could be used more widely in comparison with motion capture systems or floor reaction force systems that are only available in laboratories.

3.2   Trunk Torsion Basic Movements

We selected two beginning and one intermediate movement for easy evaluation of trunk torsion. Since advanced movement such as Kuka Racha can only be performed smoothly by advanced dancers, we will not cover it in this paper. All the selected movements require stretching the body up and down by using abdominal muscle and abdominal oblique muscle as well as rotating trunk around the vertical axis naturally.

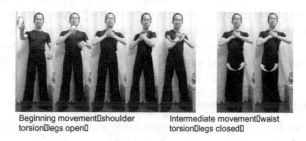

Beginning movement⬜shoulder   Intermediate movement⬜waist
torsion⬜legs open⬜   torsion⬜legs closed⬜

Fig. 2. Basic body torsion movements.

- Slow shoulder torsion(legs open)

Separate the legs at shoulder width while standing, as is shown in Fig. 2 (left). Slowly rotate the shoulder while keeping the head still (the waist is also rotated naturally). The shoulders and waist are almost in the same phase.

- Quick shoulder torsion(legs open)

Separate the legs at shoulder width while standing, as is shown in Fig. 2 (left). Quickly rotate the shoulder while keeping the head still (the waist is also rotated naturally). The shoulders and waist are almost in the opposite phase.

- Quick waist torsion(legs closed)

Close the legs while standing, as is shown in Fig. 3 (right). Rotate the waist so as not to move the upper chest. In practice the chest is also rotating slightly and is almost in the opposite phase as the waist.

3.3   Proposed Trunk Torsion Spring Model

Our proposed trunk torsion spring model is described by Eq. (1).

$$F = -k\theta \tag{1}$$

where,

F: the force in the vertical axis direction.

θ: torsion angel(rotating angle of the shoulder line to the pelvis.

k: spring constant (k_p + k_a).

k_p: the constant that characterizes the passive return of the trunk torsion to its original posture.

k_a: the constant that characterizes the force around the trunk axis generated by deep muscles, which is in the reverse direction of the rotation force.

The rationality of this model is that smooth body torsion movement is generated by the deep inner muscles along the body axis rather than the active linear force of outer muscles. The movement is supported by the passive restoring force caused by the torso, which is squeezed vertically by inner muscles. It is considered that k_p increases with the activities of the deep muscles, and we plan to measure it in the future. We will modify the model if the relationship was non-linear. Though k_a also increases with torsion force that accelerates the rotation of the deep muscles, it may also be affected by muscle activity while the frequency of rotation gradually changes. We plan to improve the accuracy of the model based on measurement using motion capture systems and floor reaction force meter.

In this model, oscillation frequency can be calculated using Eq. (2).

$$f = 1 \Big/ 2\pi\sqrt{(k/M)} \tag{2}$$

where M is the rotation moment. The Axis Index in the proposed model is defined as follows:

$$Axis\,Index : f(Naturalness, \ Elasticity, \ Position) \tag{3}$$

- *Naturalness:* if only deep muscles were used and surface muscles were not used, the movement satisfies Eq. (1) and is close to sine wave. It becomes coordinated motion and from chest to foot the body can move in harmony. In the implemented mobile app Axis Visualizer which will be described in the next section, peak ratio (the power of peak divided by the total power) is used to approximate *Naturalness*.
- *Elasticity:* refers to the oscillation frequency, or the square root of the restoring force (spring constant). The unit is [Hz] or [s^{-1}]. High frequency of torsion movement indicates stronger force to restore. Since it is in proportion to the square root of the value obtained by dividing the spring constant against the rotational moment of the trunk, stronger force is required if the body is large.
- *Position:* depending on the posture, the torsion center could shift forward or backward. This can be understood by plotting the trajectory of the sensor.

4   Implementation of Axis Visualizer

4.1   Overview

Axis Visualizer is a iOS app that evaluates the smoothness of trunk movements based on the proposed trunk torsion spring model described in Sect. 3. This app uses the imbedded accelerometer of mobile terminals and it performs simple analysis function with two types of visualization.

This app has the following three main characteristics: (1) adopting the evaluation method based on trunk torsion spring model; (2) offering easy measurement without the need of special devices; (3) providing straightforward visualization of the measurement results. As is shown in Fig. 3, the measurement procedure is as follows: physical condition check → practice of movement → practice of measuring method → measurement (12 s) → visualization of results → data export. In particular, the measurement method in step 4 can use two of the methods described in Sect. 3.3. If one becomes familiar with those methods, step 2 and 3 can be omitted. Similarly, step 6 is optional. In the following subsections, we will describe in detail the design of the application in step 4 and the data visualization in step 5.

4.2   Measurement: Sound Feedback

We implemented sound feedback during measurement to enhance the naturalness of movements. When the acceleration of the movement is greater than a fixed threshold value, the sound of "wheel" is played. If the timing deviates, the sound will not play. In the next step, we plan to refine the system to dynamically set the threshold value according to the motion of the user. One of the methods is to use the $th\%$ of the maximum value of the past N seconds. We will also conduct experiments to clarify the conditions for users to feel that the sound is played at good timing depending on their movement. Figure 4 presents two screenshots of the Axis Visualizer. Users simply need to input measurement duration (12 s by default) and nickname. The measurement starts when users tap the start button and stops when timer ends.

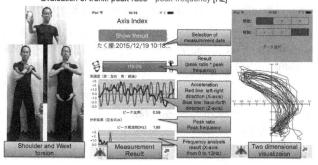

Fig. 3. Overview of Axis Visualizer.

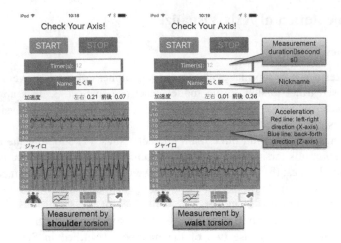

Fig. 4. The use of Axis Visualizer.

4.3   Result: Peak Ratio * Peak Frequency [Hz]

During a measurement, the sampling rate, FFT and sampling time are set to 50 Hz, 512 taps, and 10.24 s respectively. As is shown in Fig. 5, the final result that is given to the end user is the the value obtained by multiplying the peak frequency to the peak ratio of the movements. Figure 5 shows screenshots of measurement results. The percentage value shown on the top of the figure is a value obtained by multiplying the peak frequency to the peak ratio, which makes it easy to understand the measurement results. The graph in the center in Fig. 5 shows the acceleration. The red line indicates the acceleration in the left-right direction (X-axis), and the blue line indicates the acceleration in the back-forth direction (Z-axis). The value of the peak ratio and the peak frequency is presented below it. The graph at the bottom shows the frequency analysis results, illustrating which frequency components are often obtained during measurement. The fewer the peaks are, the more stable the torsion movement is. Peak ratios are obtained by dividing the peak power over full power. For this application, the peak power is calculated by summation from -2 to 2 taps, this means about 0.5 Hz width, of the FFT power result. The two screenshots on the right shows the evaluation of bad movements. The body axis shakes during waist torsion, generating both low frequency and high frequency. Therefore, the result was as low as 13.2 %.

Visualization of Analysis. The simple visualization function allows users to select two axis out of the X-axis, Y-axis, and Z-axis, and plot a graph of either acceleration or gyros on a two dimensional plane. The visualization helps users understand their movements straightforwardly. Figure 6 illustrates the plots of acceleration and gyros respectively on a two-dimensional plan with X-axis and Z-axis. This function not only helps users understand their own movements but also makes it possible to compare to previous measurement or the measurement results of others.

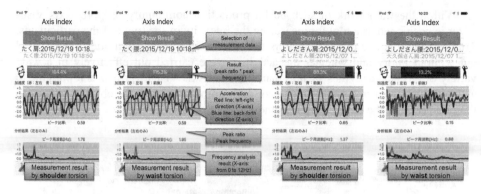

Fig. 5. Screenshots of measurement results.

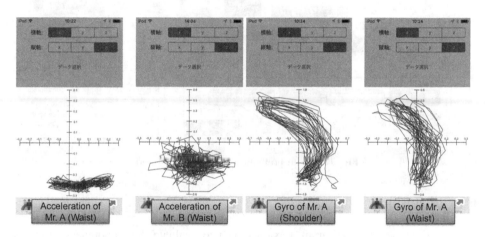

Fig. 6. Two dimensional trajectory of accelerometer.

5 Health Promotion Community Support

In this section, we describe our on-going health promotion community support, and shows the positioning of the implemented Axis Visualizer. As is shown in Fig. 7, health promotion community support refers to the repetitive cycle of performing physical activities within the organization, measuring, analyzing, visualizing, and re-designing (making strategic decision on tailored behavior change for better activity and better health state) the activity of community members. Health promotion communities can stay active by repeating this cycle. Furthermore, the measurement data and the insight of redesign can be aggregated in a database. After necessary processing such as anonymization, it is possible to share health community information /knowledge with other organizations. As a result, the useful information and knowledge obtained in one of the community can be utilized in other communities, and therefore the overall quality of health promotion community can be improved nationwide.

Within the framework of such health promotion community support, Axis Visualizer is positioned as a tool for measuring the intensity of the trunk of the participants. Trunk strength is one of the indicators to measure whether the activities were carried out without injury and whether the activities were carried out effectively in a wide variety of physical activities such as dance sports. Axis Visualizer makes it possible to autonomously measure trunk strength in each community and thereby contributes to the prosperity of the entire health promotion community.

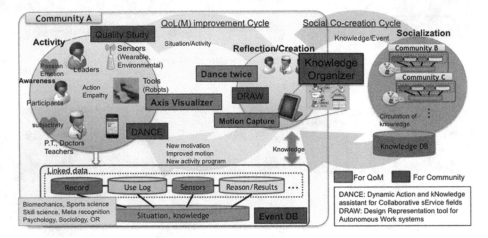

Fig. 7. Health promotion community support

6   Conclusions

In this paper, we proposed trunk torsion model to evaluate the smoothness of trunk movement. Based on the proposed model, we implemented and preliminarily evaluated a trunk movement evaluation application called Axis Visualizer. In the next step, we will refine the trunk torsion model based on measurement using motion capture systems or floor force plate systems, as well as assessing the model against users' subjective evaluation. We also plan to improve the real-time biofeedback in Axis Visualizer and to calibrate the constants in the proposed model. We will continue improve the trunk torsion model, the visualization of the analysis results, and the way to save and share the results after applying our system in practical use. In addition, we will build the modeling and evaluation techniques for other trunk movements and by doing so we will eventually promote the health promotion community support.

Acknowledgment.   This study was partly supported by Japanese METI's "Robotic Care Equipment Development and Introduction Project",NEDO's Artificial Intelligence Research Project and JSPS KAKENHI Grant Numbers 24500676 and 25730190. We would also like to thank the member of the health promotion project in Odaiba and Tsukuba for their kind support.

References

1. White Paper in 2015, Cabinet Office, Government Of Japan. http://www8.cao.go.jp/kourei/whitepaper/w-2015/html/zenbun/index.html [in Japanese]
2. Cowley, P.M., Fitzgerald, S., Sottung, K., Swensen, T.: Age, weight, and the front abdominal power test as predictors of isokinetic trunk strength and work in young men and women. J. Strength Cond. Res. **23**(3), 915–925 (2009)
3. Biering-Sørensen, F.: Physical measurements as risk indicators for low-back trouble over a one-year period. Spine **9**(2), 106–119 (1984)
4. McGill, S.M.: Low back stability: from formal description to issues for performance and rehabilitation. Exerc. Sport Sci. Rev. **29**(1), 26–31 (2001)
5. Baechle, T.R.: Essentials of strength training and conditioning, 3rd edition. National Strength and Conditioning Association (NSCA) (2008)
6. Bohm, D.G., Drinkwater, E.J., Willardson, J.M., et al.: The use of instability to train the core musculature. Appl. Physiol. Nutr. Metab. **35**(1), 91–108 (2010)
7. Panjabi, M.M.: The stabilizing system of the spine. J. Spinal Disord. 5(4), 390–397
8. Majewski-Schrage, T., Evans, T.A., Ragan, B.: Development of a core-stability model: a delphi approach. J. Sport Rehabil. **23**(2), 95–106 (2013)
9. Sahrmann, S.A.: Diagnosis and Treatment of Movement Impairment Syndromes, Mosby (2002)
10. Shumway-Cook, A., Woollacott, M.: Motor Control: Translating Research into Clinical Practice, 2nd Edition (1999)
11. WDSF Latin Technique Books and DVD, The World DanceSport Federation. https://www.worlddancesport.org/WDSF/Academy/Technique_Books
12. Nakamura, Y., Yamane, K., Suzuki, I., Fujita, Y.: Somatosensory computation for man machine interface from motion capture data and musculoskeletal human model. IEEE Trans. Rob. **21**(1), 58–66 (2004)

Design of Face Tracking System Using Environmental Cameras and Flying Robot for Evaluation of Health Care

Veerachart Srisamosorn[1(✉)], Noriaki Kuwahara[2], Atsushi Yamashita[1],
Taiki Ogata[3], and Jun Ota[3]

[1] Department of Precision Engineering, Graduate School of Engineering,
The University of Tokyo, 7-3-1 Hongo, Bunkyo-ku 113-8656, Tokyo, Japan
veera.sr@race.u-tokyo.ac.jp, yamashita@robot.t.u-tokyo.ac.jp
[2] Department of Advanced Fibro-Science, Kyoto Institute of Technology,
Kyoto-shi 606-8585, Japan
nkuwahar@kit.ac.jp
[3] Research into Artifacts, Center for Engineering (RACE), The University of Tokyo,
5-1-5 Kashiwanoha, Kashiwa-shi 277-8568, Chiba, Japan
{ogata,ota}@race.u-tokyo.ac.jp

Abstract. This paper presents a face tracking system for evaluation of health care service for elderly people in a care house. As face can show patient's smile and emotional response, it can be used for evaluation of the quality of health care and treatment provided to each patient, and therefore can be used to improve the quality of care. The conceptual system consists of cameras fixed in the environment to provide information about each person's location and face direction, and moving cameras for tracking the faces. To prove the concept, a system with 5 fixed Kinects and a quadrotor was set up to cover the area and track one person The experiment shows that the system can control the quadrotor to follow the movements by the person. By attaching a wireless camera to the quadrotor, facial images can be obtained from the system, proving the validity of tracking.

Keywords: Health care evaluation · Face tracking · UAV · Quadrotor

1 Introduction

In health care practice, the quality of the health care should be regularly assessed in order to maintain the quality of the care as well as adjusting measures to improve the performance. According to Donabedian Model [1], care can be evaluated according to their structure (organization, facility, and staff), processes (activities), and outcomes (symptoms, rate of reoccurence, etc.) Therefore, by observing the activities during health care and treatment as well as the outcome on the patient's expression, quality of the care can be evaluated. An example of health care provided to elderly people in care house is taken into consideration.

© Springer International Publishing Switzerland 2016
V.G. Duffy (Ed.): DHM 2016, LNCS 9745, pp. 264–273, 2016.
DOI: 10.1007/978-3-319-40247-5_27

Traditional method for evaluating the cares quality involves caretakers observing the patient's face for the smile and emotional responses. As the number of patients per staff is high, staff have difficulty in continuously observing patients while providing care. It is also necessary to record the activities and interactions between patients and caregivers as well as among patients to understand their social relationships. An example of Media Therapy is practiced with dementia patients, in which patient, family members, care managers and caregivers sit together around the table and pictures of important events in the past (for example wedding ceremony) are shown on the screen and they have discussion on the topic. Facial expression on the patient's face is recorded and evaluated by a camera placed on the table. Without movements, placing camera on the table is enough for recording the patient's face, but not interaction with others. There are also other therapies which include movements of patients and placing camera on the table cannot guarantee that face will always be recorded. Therefore, a system for tracking and recording person's position and face, both for the patients and the caregivers, in an area is important. The recorded video and images can be used for further analysis and as a part of the report by caregivers to transfer their observation on the patients to other caregivers in different shifts, giving them a hint on what needs to be carefully observed from the patients in the next shift. Care managers can also use the video to judge each caregiver if they did the right practice or not.

In order to achieve the record of people's faces and positions, a tracking system is required. There are a number of publications about systems for tracking people's positions, such as W^4 [2], and a system of multiple stereo cameras [3], without the effort on tracking people's faces. Face tracking at a distance sometimes uses the technique of multi-camera active vision system, in which wide field-of-view (WFOV) cameras detect and locate people while narrow field-of-view (NFOV) cameras are actively controlled to capture high-resolution faces by using pan-tilt-zoom (PTZ) commands. Examples of systems utilizing this method for face tracking are described in [4,5]. Face tracking can be achieved, but with the NFOV camera set in one direction, tracking is limited to the case of person walking in one direction, i.e. towards the camera. There are also robots tracking human beings and their faces [6–8], but the person to be tracked must be in front of the robot before tracking can begin. We also proposed a system of one depth-sensor and a flying quadrotor for tracking a person's face in [9]. This work expands the system to utilize multiple depth-sensors to enable tracking of the person in wider area and more various movements.

2   Problem Statement

Considering the application of recording the patient's face while receiving health care, a camera is required to be in front of each patient. The camera should be at appropriate angle and distance to ensure that the obtained face can be used in evaluation. The following assumptions are applied to the system:

- The environment (room and cameras' positions) is not changing during the tracking process.
- There is only one person in the area.
- The movement of the person being tracked is smooth and not too fast at standard speed (approximately around 1 m/s).
- The behavior of the person's face looking up and down is not considered.
- The person being tracked turns with the whole body, not by turning only his/her head.

3 System Design

3.1 Utilization of Cameras and Camera Configuration

Tracking position in indoor environment by using cameras was chosen as no device needs to be carried by the person or object to be tracked. The price is also relatively cheap. Accuracy is not so high but enough for the application. Depth camera was selected as it can provide 3D information of the positions.

Cameras can be configured for tracking in various methods. Utilizing only environmental cameras fixed in the environment is simple to implement, but requires large number of cameras in order to completely cover the whole area. Utilizing only moving cameras that follow the movement of people can ideally reduce the number of cameras down to one camera per person. However, searching for the person is required before tracking can begin, and it is necessary to search every time tracking is lost. Therefore, we propose to use the combination of both environmental cameras and moving cameras. Environmental cameras provide the information about the location and direction of each person as well as the position of each moving camera, while moving cameras use the information to move to the position where they can capture facial images at better quality. This method reduces the number of required cameras, as the environmental cameras do not need to see the face. Searching is also replaced by the use of position information from the environmental cameras. Moving cameras can also get closer to the faces and therefore give images with higher resolution.

3.2 System Overview

The system uses the combination of environmental cameras, depth cameras placed at fixed locations and orientations, and moving cameras, small cameras attached on moving robots. Environmental cameras provide information about each person's position and direction, as well as each moving camera's position (Fig. 1a). This information is used to set up the goal for each moving camera where the face of each person can be captured, i.e. in front of the person at an appropriate distance (Fig. 1b), and control the moving cameras so that they move to the goal position (Fig. 1c).

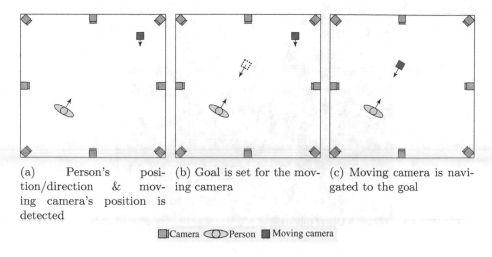

(a) Person's position/direction & moving camera's position is detected

(b) Goal is set for the moving camera

(c) Moving camera is navigated to the goal

□ Camera ⬭ Person ■ Moving camera

Fig. 1. Concept and steps of the system

4 Experiments and Results

4.1 System Implementation

The system was constructed in our laboratory as a test for the validity of the design. Xbox Kinect sensors were chosen as the sensor for acquiring depth information in the role the environmental cameras. Aerial robot was picked up for the choice of the robot carrying moving camera as its workspace does not overlap with human's moving space so it is more agile. Bitcraze's Crazyflie 2.0 quadrotor [10], shown in Fig. 2, was selected from among other flying robots for the task of moving camera in this experiment due to its small size and programmability.

Kinects were set up in the selected environment to cover the desired area of 3.0 m by 3.5 m, from the height of 0.7–2.5 m from the floor for both detection of the person and the quadrotor. Position and orientation of each Kinect was determined by optimization using the experimental space's dimension, possible location of cameras, and model of camera's field of view (FOV). Simulation was done to minimize the number of cameras and maximize the coverage of the whole area by adding one camera at a time. The best result uses 5 Kinects according to Fig. 3.

The system runs on Robot Operating System (ROS) [11]. The program is based on the package for Crazyflie control by Oliver Dunkley [12], which provides the control of the quadrotor by using joystick controller or inputting goal position via graphical user interface (GUI), obtaining the position of the quadrotor by background subtraction on the depth image from a single Kinect. Our modifications include multiple-Kinect integration, data fusion, human tracking and controlling based on human's position and direction.

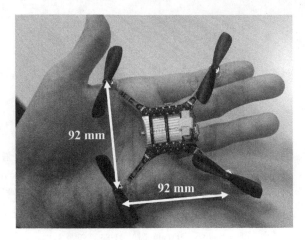

Fig. 2. Crazyflie 2.0

Human detection and tracking are done by OpenNI library, using ROS package `openni_tracker` [13]. The package provides approximation of position and orientation of each joint of the body, and the head's position and orientation are used. Data from multiple Kinects are fused together as the head of the same person if they are close together. The position and orientation of the fused head are used for setting up the goal for the moving camera to track each person, 1.5 m in front and 0.6 m above for safety and avoiding too direct observation of a person.

Positions of the quadrotor from different Kinects are also fused together when they are close together. Due to the size of the quadrotor, it is prone to false detection. To prevent the system from this false detection, the information about the number of Kinects observing the same object is used. There is higher chance that the detected object is real quadrotor and not the noise if there is more than one Kinect observing this object. Therefore, at the first time an object is detected, the number of sensors seeing that object is also obtained. If the number is more than one, it is considered as a real quadrotor, and tracking starts. If the number is one, it may be a noise. In the next observation, if there is no observation close to this object, there is high chance that it is a noise and it is removed from tracking. However, if there is more than one Kinect seeing it in the next observation, it is a real quadrotor and tracking starts. The number of quadrotors being tracked is limited to the number of quadrotors being used, which is known by the user beforehand.

As Kinect sensor utilizes unmodulated infrared light pattern for calculations of the depth [14], when multiple Kinects are used together in the same area, patterns overlap each other and pattern from one Kinect interferes with the patterns of other Kinects, resulting in confusion and loss of depth data in the intersected area. A vibration unit consisting of a DC motor and an unbalanced weight, as proposed in [15,16], is added to each Kinect in order to blur the patterns from other Kinects and keep its own pattern clear, as the pattern projector and receiver synchronously move together. The unit can solve the interference problem, as shown in Fig. 4 but also creates some disturbing noise. However, this will be ignored at this moment.

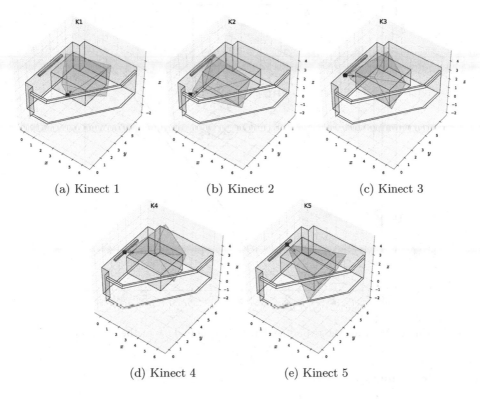

Fig. 3. 3D FOV of each Kinect and the region of interest

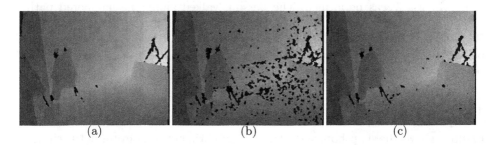

Fig. 4. Result of interference removal by vibration: (a) without interference, (b) with interference from other Kinects, (c) using vibration with interference from other Kinects

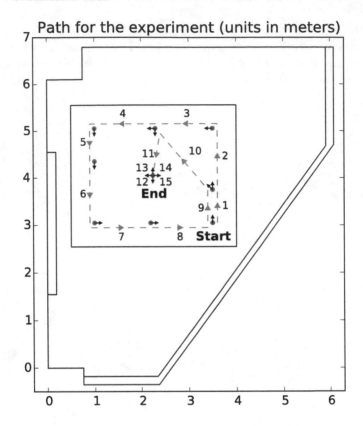

Fig. 5. Path for the experiment with the boundary of the setup area

4.2 Experimental Setup

To evaluate the tracking ability of the system, an experiment with a person, assuming the role of a patient, moving inside the area according to the path shown in Fig 5 was performed. The person walked along the numbered path, stopped at the markers on the floor (denoted by dots in the figure), facing in the direction of the arrows. The path ends in the center of the area, with the person turning around the point, stopping at around $-\frac{\pi}{2}$, $-\pi$, $\frac{\pi}{2}$, and 0 radian respectively, before finishing at $-\frac{\pi}{2}$ radian.

4.3 Results

Figure 6 shows the snapshots of the tracking experiment (quadrotor in the circle). The video can be found at http://youtu.be/OdvLoFQu5gk. From the video, we can confirm that the system can control the quadrotor to move and follow the motion of the person inside the designed area.

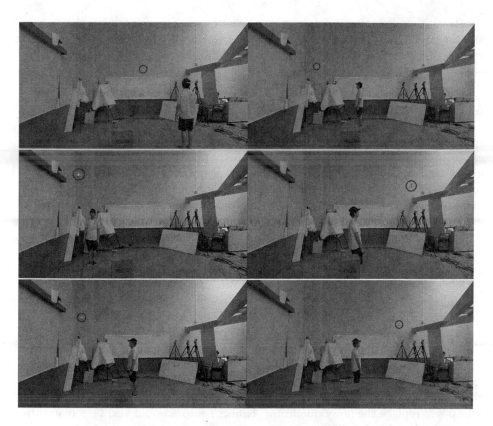

Fig. 6. Snapshots of quadrotor following the movement of a person

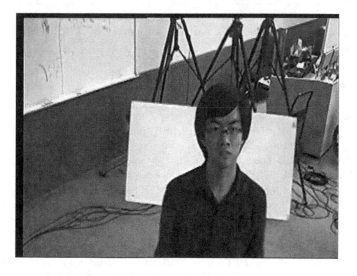

Fig. 7. A snapshot of the video taken by the camera on the quadrotor

By adding a small wireless camera to the quadrotor and testing the system again with random path, real facial images could be obtained from the on-board camera as shown in Fig. 7. Vibration and transmission noises were present so the quality of the video was not so high.

5   Conclusion and Future Works

In order to record elderly person's position and facial images for his/her facial expression in response to care and treatment provided in health care facility, a face tracking system utilizing environmental cameras and moving cameras is presented. The system is implemented by using multiple Kinect sensors, placed in positions and orientations obtained by optimization, and a small quadrotor. The experiment showed that with the system, the moving camera could move to follow the movement of the person inside the designed area. With a wireless camera attached to the quadrotor, facial images could be obtained by the proposed tracking system. The concept was proven to be effective for tracking of people's position and face in indoor environment.

Using quadrotors to move cameras has some drawbacks. Small quadrotors have quite short battery life (7 min without any loads for Crazyflie 2.0) and even larger quadrotors cannot fly longer than half an hour. Moreover, noise from the continuously rotating propellors are quite disturbing and can create the fear of falling and hitting the elderly people. This may have effects on the facial expression obtained and therefore alter the result of health care evaluation. In the next development, quieter, less power consuming, and safer helium-filled blimp will replace the noisy quadrotor. Kinect sensors would also be replaced by the new technology of 360-degree cameras so that activities and interaction of elderly people and caregivers can also be recorded.

Acknowledgments. This work was partially supported by JSPS KAKENHI Grant Number 15H01698.

References

1. Donabedian, A.: The quality of care: how can it be assessed? JAMA **260**(12), 1743–1748 (1988). http://dx.doi.org/10.1001/jama.1988.03410120089033
2. Haritaoglu, I., Harwood, D., Davis, L.: W^4: real-time surveillance of people and their activities. IEEE Trans. Pattern Anal. Mach. Intell. **22**(8), 809–830 (2000)
3. Zhao, T., Aggarwal, M., Kumar, R., Sawhney, H.: Real-time wide area multi-camera stereo tracking. In: IEEE Computer Society Conference on Computer Vision and Pattern Recognition, CVPR 2005, vol. 1, pp. 976–983, June 2005
4. Stillman, S., Tanawongsuwan, R., Essa, I.: A system for tracking and recognizing multiple people with multiple cameras. In: Proceedings of Second International Conference on Audio-Visionbased Person Authentication, pp. 96–101 (1998)
5. Wheeler, F., Weiss, R., Tu, P.: Face recognition at a distance system for surveillance applications. In: 2010 Fourth IEEE International Conference on Biometrics: Theory Applications and Systems (BTAS), pp. 1–8, September 2010

6. Ali, B., Qureshi, A., Iqbal, K., Ayaz, Y., Gilani, S., Jamil, M., Muhammad, N., Ahmed, F., Muhammad, M., Kim, W.Y., Ra, M.: Human tracking by a mobile robot using 3d features. In: 2013 IEEE International Conference on Robotics and Biomimetics (ROBIO), pp. 2464–2469, December 2013
7. Bellotto, N., Hu, H.: Multisensor-based human detection and tracking for mobile service robots. IEEE Trans. Syst. Man Cybern. Part B: Cybern. **39**(1), 167–181 (2009)
8. Vadakkepat, P., Lim, P., De Silva, L., Jing, L., Ling, L.L.: Multimodal approach to human-face detection and tracking. IEEE Trans. Ind. Electron. **55**(3), 1385–1393 (2008)
9. Srisamosorn, V., Kuwahara, N., Yamashita, A., Ogata, T., Ota, J.: Automatic face tracking system using quadrotors: Control by goal position thresholding. In: 2014 IEEE International Conference on Robotics and Biomimetics (ROBIO), pp. 1314–1319, December 2014
10. Bitcraze AB Company: Bitcraze. http://www.bitcraze.io/. Accessed 25 Aug 2015
11. ROS.org — Powering the world's robots. http://www.ros.org/. Accessed 25 Aug 2015
12. Dunkley, O.: GitHub omwdunkley/crazyflieROS, downloaded branch joyManager. http://github.com/omwdunkley/crazyflieROS. Accessed 15 April 2014
13. Field, T.: openni_tracker - ROS Wiki. http://wiki.ros.org/openni_tracker. Accessed 07 July 2015
14. Khoshelham, K., Elberink, S.O.: Accuracy and resolution of kinect depth data for indoor mapping applications. Sensors **12**(2), 1437 (2012). http://www.mdpi.com/1424-8220/12/2/1437
15. Maimone, A., Fuchs, H.: Reducing interference between multiple structured light depth sensors using motion. In: Virtual Reality Short Papers and Posters (VRW), pp. 51–54. IEEE, March 2012
16. Butler, A., Izadi, S., Hilliges, O., Molyneaux, D., Hodges, S., Kim, D.: Shake'n'sense: reducing interference for overlapping structured light depth cameras. In: Proceedings of the 2012 ACM Annual Conference on Human Factors in Computing Systems, pp. 1933–1936. ACM (2012). http://research.microsoft.com/apps/pubs/default.aspx?id=171706

Towards Person-Centered Anomaly Detection and Support System for Home Dementia Care

Kazunari Tamamizu[1(✉)], Seiki Tokunaga[1], Sachio Saiki[1],
Shinsuke Matsumoto[1], Masahide Nakamura[1], and Kiyoshi Yasuda[2]

[1] Graduate School of System Informatics, Kobe University,
1-1 Rokkodai, Nada, Kobe, Japan
tamamizu@ws.cs.kobe-u.ac.jp, masa-n@cs.kobe-u.ac.jp
[2] Chiba Rosai Hospital, 2-16 Tatsumidai-higashi, Ichihara, Japan
fwkk5911@mb.infoweb.ne.jp

Abstract. Anomaly detection is a crucial issue for people with dementia and their families to live a safe and comfortable life at home. The elderly monitoring system is a promising solution. However, the conventional systems have limitations in detectable anomalies and support actions, which cannot fully cover individual needs. To achieve more person-centered home care for people with dementia, our research group has been studying environmental sensing with IoT. In this paper, using the environmental sensing, we propose a new service that allows individual users to customize definition of anomaly and corresponding actions. Specifically, borrowing a mechanism of context-aware services, we regard every anomaly observed within the house as a context. We then define every care as an action bound to an anomaly context. This achieves the personalized anomaly detection and care. To demonstrate the feasibility, we implement a prototype system and conduct a practical case study.

1 Introduction

Japan is facing a hyper-aging society. In 2025, the total population will decrease to 120 million, while people over the age of 65 will increase to 37 million. Thus, approximately 30 % of the population will become the elderly [2]. Also, *people with dementia* increase to 7 million [7]. Many facilities of welfare and nursing care suffer from chronic shortage of workers. The job opening ratio is as high as 2.68 (as of Dec. 2014). The number of nursing home is not sufficient against the number of applicants, who are over 524,000 elderly people. The Japanese government starts to encourage *home care* rather than building new facilities [3]. Needless to say, the dementia care will rely more on home, which poses a burden to the family as care givers. Under these circumstances, *assistive technologies*, which support people with dementia using technologies, attract great attention.

Among many assistive technologies studied so far, this paper especially focuses on *anomaly detection and support for home dementia care*. An anomaly in this context is defined as any state or situation in home that can disturb safe and healthy life of the person with dementia and/or surrounding people. The

V.G. Duffy (Ed.): DHM 2016, LNCS 9745, pp. 274–285, 2016.
DOI: 10.1007/978-3-319-40247-5_28

elderly monitoring system is a well-known system that can detect such anomalies in home care. More specifically, a monitoring system observes a state of a patient using sensors or smart devices. If something wrong is observed, the system notifies it of the family or the caregivers. The existing systems include the wandering detection system [4], the dementia monitoring robot [10], and so on.

However, the conventional system covers only specific anomalies statically defined in the system. Also, the action for the anomalies is often limited to the alert to human caregivers. In fact, symptoms of dementia vary from one patient to another. The type and level of the anomaly are diverse among individual household. Thus, the static nature of the conventional systems cannot fully cover individual cases and needs. To achieve more *person-centered* home dementia care, our group is studying *IoT environmental sensing*, which measures multiple environmental values in a house (e.g., temperature, humidity, illumination, air pressure, sound volume, motion, vibration, etc.) with IoT sensors.

In this paper, we propose a new service that allows individual users to customize definition of anomaly and corresponding actions, based on the environmental sensing. More specifically, borrowing the concept of context-aware services [1], we consider every anomaly as a context (we call it *anomaly context*). An anomaly context is defined with the current and/or historical sensor values, obtained by the environmental sensing. Permitting individual users (i.e., family or caregiver) to define own anomaly contexts, the proposed service can cover a wide range of anomalies that vary one patient to another.

As for the cares for an anomaly detected, the proposed service provides three types of cares: *(a) Greeting, (b) Attract Attention, and (c) Invite to Activity*, in addition to the conventional alert to human caregivers. Greeting is a care that the service calls the name of a patient and speaks gently. Attract Attention is a care that a service attracts patient's attention to another interesting topic to distract the patient from being in a bad mode. Invite to Activity is a care that a service encourages the patient to an activity to be in a good mode. Using the virtual agent technology [5], we make the virtual agent (i.e., animated chat-bot) to provide these cares, instead of human caregivers. In the proposed service, a user freely binds any care to every anomaly context defined. The service continuously monitors the anomaly context via the environmental sensing, and automatically executes the corresponding care when the context is satisfied.

We have implemented a prototype of the proposed service as RESTful Web service, so that a client can easily consume anomaly contexts via Web. We also implemented GUI for defining anomaly contexts and registering cares. To evaluate the contexts and execute the cares, we have reused RuCAS [9], which is a context-aware service platform developed in our previous work. Using the prototype service, we conduct a practical case study, where a virtual agent conducts the "Greeting" care for the anomaly of "sudden screaming".

The proposed service can achieve flexible anomaly detection and anomaly care, which can meet individual circumstances of caregivers and people with dementia. Thus, the service can contribute to decreasing caregiver's burden, as well as sustainable and high-quality home dementia care.

2   Preliminaries

2.1   Dementia and Care

Dementia refers to syndromes composed of higher brain disorders developed by chronic or progressive brain diseases [6]. The symptoms of dementia include the *core symptom* and the *BPSD* (Behavioral and Psychological Symptoms of Dementia). The core symptom is developed directly by the brain impairment, including dysmnesia, disorientation, language disorder. All people with dementia have the core symptoms. On the other hand, the BPSD is developed by *personal factors* combined with the brain impairment, such as personality, physical condition, human relation, and living environment. Examples include screaming, wandering and depression. Since the BPSD is developed by personal factors, the type and intensity of the BPSD vary greatly among individuals.

Ideally, therefore, cares for the dementia should be *personalized*, considering individual situations. Typical dementia cares are as follows:

Greeting: A caregiver calls the name of the person with dementia, and speaks shortly and gently. This allows the caregiver to know what the patient is feeling, and to check the physical condition. The greeting also helps to easing anxiety and loneliness of the patient.

Attract Attention: A caregiver attracts attention of the person with dementia, and distracts the patient from any difficult circumstances. For example, a caregiver may attract attention by showing reminiscence pictures and videos, or by playing favorite music.

Invite to Activity: A caregiver encourages the person with dementia to do a certain activity. This care can help the patient to perform healthy thinking and actions. It can also prevents the day-night reversal. Doing an activity makes the patient feel confidence that there are many things the patient can do. Also, interacting with many people can resolve anxiety and loneliness. Concrete examples include singing songs, playing games, painting, folding origami paper, knitting, and joining a tea party.

2.2   Anomaly in Home Dementia Care

In the home of people with dementia, unusual circumstances (i.e., *anomaly*) are often caused by the dementia. An anomaly in this context is defined as any state (or situation) in home that can disturb a safe and healthy life of the person with dementia and/or surrounding people. Since the anomaly often occurs by BPSD, its type and severity are different from one home to another. Thus, it is essential to provide an appropriate care for each person. Concrete examples of the anomaly are as follows:

No air-conditioning in hot day: A person with dementia does not use air-conditioner even in an extremely hot day. This anomaly is often caused by a thrifty nature of a person with dementia, or a decline of sensitivity to temperature. This anomaly is characterized by a situation where high temperature, humidity and discomfort index are being kept in a room. If no action is taken, the person may get heat stroke or even die in the worst case.

Scream suddenly: A person with dementia suddenly screams with anger. It is often caused by anxiety, loneliness, confusion or delusion due to the dementia. In the home environment, the screaming can be observed by a situation where the sound volume in a room is raised suddenly. This anomaly leads to a problem that the family cannot sleep well or get stressed out. Therefore, it can be a burden to caregivers living with the patient.

Wandering: A person with dementia keeps walking without staying in the home, and sometimes goes out. In the home, the person repeats coming and going to same room many times in a short period of time. In case of outdoor, the person often gets lost, and may have an accident. Also, the person may strain legs because of long walking. The wandering can be a heavy burden for caregivers, since it must be always monitored.

2.3   Environmental Sensing and Context-Aware Service

In our research group, we are developing a *sensor box* [8] that autonomously measures the surrounding environment. It is a small box containing a single board computer connected with multiple sensor devices. The current version includes 7 sensor devices (temperature, humidity, light, air pressure, sound volume, motion and vibration) exposed as Web services. External applications access to the sensor box by platform-independent protocols (i.e., REST or SOAP) to retrieve the sensor data. That is, the sensor box is an IoT which can exchange data via the Internet. Multiple sensor boxes are deployed in some places in a home to conduct environmental sensing. The measured sensor values are uploaded to a cloud database, and are consumed by various applications.

The collected sensor data can be used for *context-aware service* [1]. A context is any information representing a state or situation of human, objects, environment and so on. A context-aware service is a service that automatically detects change of the context and provides actions appropriate to those changes. Generally, a context is defined or estimated by using the current and/or historical sensor values. In our study group, we have developed a service platform, called RuCAS, which facilitates creation and management of context-aware services using Web services [9]. Although the context-aware service has been widely studied so far, there are few examples used actively for home dementia care.

3   Anomaly Detection and Support Service for Home Dementia Care

3.1   System Achitecture

Figure 1 shows the system architecture of the proposed anomaly detection and care service. To achieve scalable services, the architecture exploits a cloud-based database and computing servers to be provided for a number of households. The architecture consists of *infrastructure layer*, *service layer* and *interface layer*.

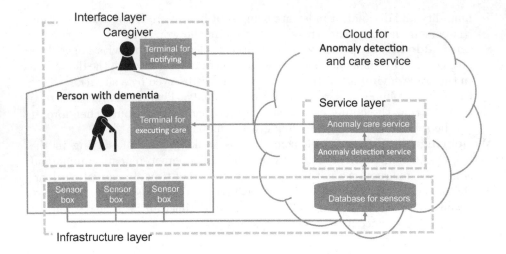

Fig. 1. Total architecture of proposed service

Infrastructure Layer: This layer includes sensor boxes that conduct environmental sensing of every house of a person with dementia, as well as a cloud database storing sensor data. The sensor boxes are deployed in some points at the home (e.g., living, entrance and bathroom). Each box periodically uploads sensor values to the database via a secure channel.

Service Layer: This layer detects the anomaly in a house and emits appropriate care actions. It consists of the *anomaly detection service* and the *anomaly care service*. The detection service detects the anomaly with sensor data provided by the infrastructure layer. The care service issues commands of cares to the home equipment based on the detected anomaly.

Interface Layer: This layer actually executes anomaly care, on receiving commands from the service layer. Examples of executed cares include the interaction with a virtual agent, status report, and alert to human caregiver.

Among the three layers, we especially focus on how to implement the service layer in this paper. For the anomaly detection service, we investigate *what kind of anomaly* should be detected *how*? For the anomaly care service, we study *what kinds of care* we should provide for the detected anomaly.

3.2   Key Idea

To implement primary features in the service layer, we borrow the concept of the context-aware service (described in Sect. 2.3). We consider every anomaly in the home as a *context* characterized by sensor data (we call it *anomaly context*). Note that the definition of anomaly should be adapted for individual cases, since the type and intensity of anomaly vary from one person to another (see Sect. 2.2). In the anomaly detection service, we therefore make it possible for individual users (i.e., caregivers or families) to customize definition of anomaly contexts and evaluation method. The anomaly detection service continuously evaluates every anomaly context and manages the state.

We then regard every care for the detected anomaly as an *action* of context-aware service. In the anomaly care service, we allow individual users to customize each care in Sect. 2.1, and to bind the care to an anomaly context. The anomaly care service monitors all the anomaly contexts. If a context is detected, the service automatically executes the actions bound to the context.

3.3   Anomaly Detection Service

The anomaly detection service allows a user to define and manage various anomaly in the home, by means of anomaly contexts characterized by sensor data. Let D be a set of all sensor data obtained by the environmental sensing. Then, an anomaly context c is defined by

$$c = [id, f : \mathcal{P}(D) \rightarrow \{true, false\}]$$

where *id* is an *identifier*, and f is an *evaluation function* that returns a boolean value for a given subset of D. That is, every anomaly contexts is evaluated as true (= anomaly) or false (= normal) based on a given set of sensor values. If c_1 and c_2 are both anomaly contexts here, $c_1\&\&c_2$ (AND), $c_1||c_2$ (OR) and $!c_1, !c_2$ (NOT) are also defined as anomaly contexts.

There are many possible ways to implement the evaluation function f. For example, an anomaly can be characterized only by the current sensor value. Another anomaly may require historical values. More sophisticated anomaly is derived by a learning algorithm with the sensor data. Therefore, in the anomaly detection service, we deploy a database to store various algorithms that implement f. The algorithms can be used as plug-in's based on user's demand. When defining an anomaly context, a user chooses an appropriate plug-in, and specifies parameters for the custom anomaly context.

The anomaly detection service periodically evaluates every anomaly context registered based on the given definition. For a given id of a context, the service returns the current value (true or false) of the context to the client.

For example, let us define the anomaly in Sect. 2.2 as anomaly contexts.

No air-conditioning in hot day: Using the observation that the high temperature lasts for long time, this anomaly can be defined as follows:

$$[hotWithoutAC, Continue(room1.temperature, >, 30C, 1\,h)]$$

Continue(sensor attribute, comparative operator, threshold, time) is an evaluation function that returns true if the value of the sensor attribute satisfies the condition for a given period of time until present. The context *hotWithoutAC* is defined by a condition that the temperature of room1 is kept greater than 30 degrees for an hour.

Scream suddenly: Using the observation that the sound volume in the room is raised suddenly, this anomaly can be defined as follows:

$$[loudVoice, Event(room1.sound, >, 75\,db)]$$

Event(sensor attribute, comparative operator, threshold) is an evaluation function that returns true as soon as the value of the sensor attribute satisfies the condition with the threshold. The context *loudVoice* is defined by a condition that the sound volume of room1 becomes larger than 75 dB.

Wandering: Using the observation that the person repeats coming and going to the same room many times, this anomaly can be defined as follows:

$$[wandering, Count(bath.presence == true, >=, 20, 10\,min)]$$

Count(condition, comparative operator, threshold, time) is evaluation function that returns true if the number of times where the given condition holds satisfies the condition with the threshold within a given moment. The context *wandering* is defined by a condition that the person comes to the bathroom more than 20 times within 10 min.

In addition to the above evaluation functions, more sophisticated algorithms can be added to the service, such as pattern mining and learning algorithms with the time-series analysis.

3.4   Anomaly Care Service

The anomaly care service allows a user to define cares for the anomaly, by means of as actions of context-aware services. The actions considered here are the ones in Sect. 2.1, including Notification to a caregiver (`notify()`), Greeting (`greet()`), Attract Attention (`attract()`), and Invite to Activity (`invite()`). We assume that the anomaly care service sends these actions as commands to the interface layer, and that the actions are actually executed in the interface layer (Fig. 1) with the virtual agent and other smart devices. Since there are many other possible actions considered (e.g., appliance control via smart home, Web services), we design the service so that more actions can be added later.

Furthermore, the anomaly care service associates each anomaly context with the corresponding care actions, by means of *ECA rule* [9]. Let c_1, c_2,... be contexts, and let a_1, a_2,... be actions. Then, an ECA rule r is defined by

$$r = [E : c_i, C : \{c_{j_1}, c_{j_2}, ..., c_{j_m}\}, A : \{a_{k_1}, a_{k_2}, ..., a_{k_n}\}]$$

where E is a *event*, C is a *condition* and A is an *action*. We say that the event E *occurs* when c_i changes from false to true. When E occurs, if all $c_{j_1}, c_{j_2}, ..., c_{j_m}$ are true, r is *executed*. When r is executed, all $a_{k_1}, ..., a_{k_m}$ are sequentially executed. To achieve personalized anomaly care, we assume that individual users define ECA rules, according to the individual status of patients. The user-defined anomaly contexts in the anomaly detection service are used to specify E and C. Also, the user chooses appropriate actions for A with parameters.

Let us define ECA rules of cares for the three contexts in Sect. 3.3.

No air-conditioning in hot day: We consider a care that lets the person know that the room is unusually hot, using Greeting.

```
r1 = [E:hotWithoutAC, C:isPresent, A: greet(''Mr.Tamamizu, this room is very hot.
Please turn on an air-conditioner.'')]
```

In the rule, we specify the context hotWithoutAC in Sect. 3.3 as an event, specify the context that the person is present in the room as a condition, and specify Greeting as an action. In case that greeting does not work well for the person, we should consider to add extra rules that notifies to human caregivers, or turns on an air conditioner via smart home.

Scream suddenly: We consider a care that asks the person what happened and attracts attention by showing memorable pictures.

```
r2 = [E:loudVoice, C:isPresent, A: greet(''Mr.Tamamizu, what happened? I get the pictures
with a memory. Let's have a look.''), attract(''Memorable_picture.jpg'')]
```

Inviting to an activity such as origami papers can be another care.

Wandering: We consider a care that asks the person what happened with greeting. If the service finds the reason of wandering, it provides cares to get rid of the reason (e.g., lead to the toilets). If no reason is found, it invites games to distract the patient from wandering.

```
r3 = [E:wandering, C:true, A:greet(''Mr.Tamamizu, where do you want to go?'')]
r4 = [E:reasonToilet, C:wandering, A:greet(''A toilet is this way, please.'')]
r5 = [E:reasonUnknown, C:wandering, A:invite(''game'')]
```

4   Implementation

4.1   Prototype Service

We have developed a prototype of the proposed anomaly detection and care services. Technologies used for the implementation are summarized as follows:

- Development language: Java 1.7.0_75
- Database: MongoDB
- Web server: Apache Tomcat 7.0.59
- Web service framework: Jersey 1.19

The anomaly detection service and the anomaly care service are deployed as Web services. Therefore, both services can be consumed with the platform-indepent REST protocol. Regarding the plug-in mechanism of the evaluation functions, we used Java reflection to dynamically add new plug-ins only by putting jar files. In the current version, we have implemented basic plugin that evaluates the current sensor value with a threshold. As for the action, we have implemented greet() in the anomaly care service. We have reused RuCAS [9] as the engine to execute ECA rules.

Moreover, we have implemented GUI Web application with which a user registers anomaly contexts and actions. Technologies used for the GUI are summarized as follows:

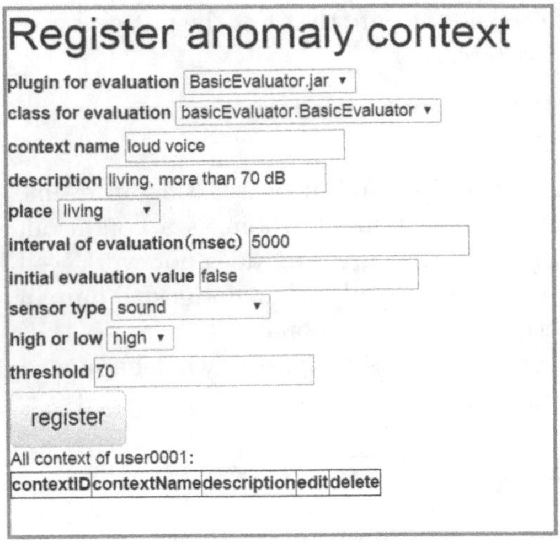

(a) Registration of anomaly context 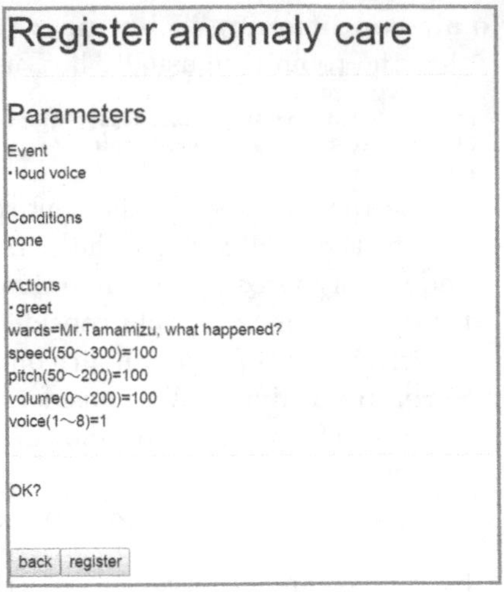   (b) Registration of anormaly care

Fig. 2. Screenshot of GUI

- Development language: HTML, Javascript
- Javascript library: jQuery 2.1.4
- CSS framework: Twitter Bootstrap 3.1.1

Figure 2(a) shows a screenshot of the registration screen of anomaly context. In the screen, a user inputs parameters for plugin and class for the evaluation function, context name, place, interval of evaluation, comparative operator, threshold value, and so on.

Figure 2(b) shows a screenshot of the registration screen of ECA rule for the anomaly care service. A user chooses contexts for the event and the condition. Then, the user specifies parameters of greet(), designated as an action for this rule. The parameters for greet() include speech text, speed, pitch, volume and voice type.

4.2 Case Study

As a practical case study, we have conducted the anomaly detection and care for "Scream suddenly" described in Sect. 3.4. In this case study, we registered greet() only for the action using the developed prototype. We used an actual smart home installed in our experimental room S101. We assume that the room S101 is the home of the patient, set a threshold of sound volume to 70 dB. More specifically, we have specified parameters shown in Table 1 to define the anomaly context. Next, we configured parameters shown in Table 2, to register greet() as the anomaly care when "Screaming suddenly" is detected.

Table 1. Parameters for registering scream suddenly

Parameter	Value
Plugin for evaluation	BasicEvaluator.jar
Class for evaluation	basicEvaluator.BasicEvaluator
Context name	loud voice
Description	livingCmore than70 dB
Place	living
Interval of evaluation(msec)	5000
Initial evaluation value	false
Sensor type	sound
High or low	high
Threshold	70

Table 2. Parameters for registering care for scream suddenly

Parameter	Value
Event	loud voice
Conditions	none
Actions	greet
Speech text	Mr. Tamamizu, what happened?
Speed	100
Pitch	100
Volume	100
Voice type	1

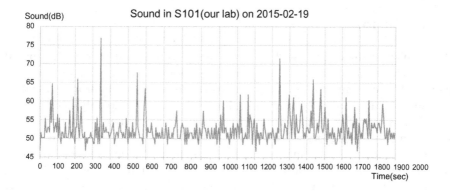

Fig. 3. Ambient sound volume in S101

Figure 3 shows a graph of the sound volume observed in S101 (19 Feb. 2015). The horizontal axis represents the time, while the vertical axis represents the sound volume. In the graph, it can be seen that the sound volume exceeds the threshold of 70 dB at approximately 345 seconds. Hence, the execution of greet() is expected approximately 345 seconds after the registration is complete.

Indeed in the experiment, the greet() was executed after 350 seconds since we registered the anomaly context and an ECA rule for the care. Therefore, we have confirmed that the prototype system worked as expected.

4.3   Discussion

From the result of the case study, we have confirmed that the proposed service as expected for the used sensor data. As for the anomaly detection, there may exist a certain latency between the actual anomaly event and its detection by the service. However, we consider it to be a trivial problem since the interval of the context evaluation can be optimized freely by the user.

In the case study, we were unable to check if someone actually screamed in the room, since we used historical sensor data for the evaluation. Preferably, we should conduct online validation in the real home of a person with dementia.

The prototype can cover only simple anomaly contexts. Therefore, it cannot distinguish actual screaming from other environmental noise, which may result in mis-detection of anomaly context. Also the prototype cannot cover complex contexts that require time-series data analysis for the evaluation (e.g., wandering). Implementation of plug-ins for more sophisticated evaluation functions will be left for our future work.

The definition of anomaly contexts and cares requires certain technical knowledge (e.g., threshold, plugin for evaluation, class for evaluation) within the current version of GUI Web application. This becomes a burden for non-expert users to define them. To cope with the problem, we plan to add intuitive interface for the registration. For example, we would use an slider bar [sensitive - general - insensitive] for specifying a threshold value, instead of using absolute value.

5   Conclusion

In this paper, we have proposed an anomaly detection and care service based on the environmental sensing, in order to support home care of people with dementia. Borrowing the concept of context-aware services, the proposed service allows individual users to customize flexibly definition of anomaly and the corresponding cares. This promotes person-centered home dementia care. We have also implemented a prototype service and evaluated the practical feasibility.

In our future work, we implement plug-ins that can be used for advanced anomaly contexts. Integration with smart home and virtual agent for advanced care actions is also interesting topic. Finally, it is also essential to conduct experiment in actual patient's home, by elaborating the GUI for non-experts.

Acknowledgments. This research was partially supported by the Japan Ministry of Education, Science, Sports, and Culture [Grant-in-Aid for Scientific Research (B) (No. 26280115, No. 15H02701), Young Scientists (B) (No. 26730155), and Challenging Exploratory Research (15K12020)].

References

1. Baldauf, M., Dustdar, S., Rosenberg, F.: A survey on context-aware systems. Int. J. Ad Hoc Ubiquit. Comput. **2**(4), 263–277 (2007)
2. Cabinet Office: Heisei 27nendoban koreishakai hakusho (white book on aged society published in 2015). http://www8.cao.go.jp/kourei/whitepaper/w-2015/zenbun/27pdf_index.html
3. Daiwa Institute of Research Ltd: Chokoureikashakai ni okeru kaigo mondai (nursing care problem in super-aging society). http://www.dir.co.jp/research/report/japan/mlothers/20140509_008508.pdf
4. Francebed, C.O., LTD.: Ninchisho gaishutsu tsuho sisutemu: OdekakekyattiWS-01 (system notifying of outgo of peoplo with demetia: Odekake catch ws-01). http://www.francebed.co.jp/medical/news/detail.php?id=295
5. Horiuchi, H., Saiki, S., Matsumoto, S., Nakamura, M.: Designing and implementing service framework for virtual agents in home network system. In: 2014 15th IEEE/ACIS International Conference on Software Engineering, Artificial Intelligence, Networking and Parallel/Distributed Computing (SNPD 2014), pp. 343–348, Las Vegas, USA, June 2014
6. Japanese Society of Neurology: Ninchisho shikkan chiryo gaidorain2010 konpakutoban2012 (guideline version2010 for therapying dementia compact edition in 2012). http://www.neurology-jp.org/guidelinem/nintisyo_compact.html
7. Ministry of Health, Labour, Welfare: Ninchishoshisaku suishin sougou senryakushin orenji puran (comprehensive strategy for the promotion of measures for dementia (Shin Orenji Puran)). http://www.mhlw.go.jp/file/04-Houdouhappyou-12304500-Roukenkyoku-Ninchishougyakutaiboushitaisakusuishinshitsu/01_1.pdf
8. Okushi, A., Matsumoto, S., Saiki, S., Nakamura, M.: A framework for personal sensor box in mobile environmental sensing. In: IEICE Technical report, vol. 113, pp. 51–56, November 2013
9. Takatsuka, H., Saiki, S., Matsumoto, S., Nakamura, M.: Rucas: rule-based framework for managing context-aware services with distributed web services. Int. J. Softw. Innov. **3**(3), 57–68 (2015)
10. Technos Japan Corp: Zaitakukea: mimamori kaigo robotto "Kea robo" (in-home care: monitoring nursing-care robot "Care robo"). http://www.technosjapan.jp/product/tascal/index.html

Physicians' Code of Conduct and Further Requirements for a Productive Patient Physician Relationship Exemplified in the Area of Orthognathic Surgery

Luisa Vervier[✉] and Martina Ziefle

Human-Computer Interaction Center,
RWTH Aachen University, Aachen, Germany
{vervier, ziefle}@comm.rwth-aachen.de

Abstract. Ever since healthcare has been of enormous importance for individuals and societies. However, healthcare represents still a fragile system which needs to be strengthened and improved especially regarding communication and psychological support. The better the healthcare process is balanced with the information and communication needs, the more patients feel understood. As an exemplary field, orthognathic surgery was selected as one kind of a very intensive treatment. The overall purpose of the current study is to understand the patients' emotional experience during treatment, their way of information seeking and their advice to physicians. The aim is the development of an information and communication concept. In the current longitudinal study approach, 22 patients were accompanied over 6 months during treatment, starting from surgery to half a year follow-up. Results portray a code of conduct for physicians as well as a first approach of possible app content guideline as an electronic support service.

Keywords: Orthognathic surgery · Medical treatment · Information and communication concept · Physician-patient-relationship · Electronic support service in medicine

1 Introduction

The precise amount of information and appropriate kind of communication is known to be one of the most important factors for patients in treatment in order to maintain a positive outcome [1]. Characteristically, only patients can determine the adequateness of information and communication. Physicians need to tell them "everything" in order to prevent unexpected encounters. On the other hand, physicians should not go into unnecessary detail in order to prevent them to panic. Finally, physicians should have the ability to take patients' positions and find the right word and tone (sensible, warm, but not schoolmasterly or patronizing). Physicians find it often challenging to do justice to the individual patients need due to time restrictions and the time requirement in hospitals. Especially patients who are confronted with a drastic surgery are reliant on a sensitive and well-elaborated treatment. Orthognathic surgery is e.g. one kind of a very

© Springer International Publishing Switzerland 2016
V.G. Duffy (Ed.): DHM 2016, LNCS 9745, pp. 286–297, 2016.
DOI: 10.1007/978-3-319-40247-5_29

intensive and radically treatment. Patients with jaw modulation often suffer from functional problems such as chewing or swallowing. Additionally, psychological side effects such as emotional instability or low-self esteem because of "abnormal" appearance are very common and portray just a few of associated psychological difficulties [2, 3]. The main purpose of orthognathic surgery is finally to correct these functional and aesthetic problems due to underlying jaw deformities. However, psychological consequences of such a surgery and its treatment tend to be neglected. The result of an aesthetic improvement does not always correspond with the patients' self-concept [4]. To integrate one's facial appearance into the individual self-concept requires a well elaborated support. Therefore, the main research purpose and question is with what kind of expectation patients enter the treatment, how far they deal with such a decisive medical treatment, how they inform themselves and experience the process. Besides, in order to improve the common physician-patient relationship and way of communication, the question occurs in which way physician should act with their patient. The study will represent a potentially code of conduct for physicians. Furthermore, a first approach of possible app content guidelines as a further electronic support service for improving the physician patient communication will be described.

1.1 Clinical Picture

A malocclusion (jaw modulation) is an incorrect relation between the teeth of the two dental arches when they approach to each other. The term "bad bite" is also in common use. People with this deformity are often not able to close their mouth properly due to the misalignment of teeth. The misalignment may be due to the misplacement of some teeth or to an abnormality of the position of the jaws. This physical appearance may imply functional and social consequences [5]. Ability to eat or to speak may be affected as well as comorbid disorders such as headache may appear. Furthermore, social side effects such as dissatisfaction with the facial appearance lead to a lower self-esteem and may affect people's life from childhood to adulthood.

1.2 Medical Treatment

Orthognathic surgery is recommended for people who suffer from severe functional problems such as not being able to chew properly among others. The malocclusion is restructured by cutting the specific bone and repositioning the bone segments thus the upper and the lower jaw match with each other again. This intervention requires a long recovery period of at least 6 months. Common problems after surgery which might appear are numbness of the upper or lower lip or other risks such as infection, swelling or muscle spasm among others. Besides, psychological consequences also belong to problems after surgery. The change of the familiar facial appearance often causes adaption disorders or a general negative psychological well-being [6–8]. In a first consultation with the physician possible treatment procedures are discussed. Once the patient has agreed on a surgery, X-ray images and plaster models are manufactured. With the help of plaster models, the patient receives medical education by the physician.

The physician explains the exact procedure, describes all possible risks and answers all questions which remain on the patient side. The patient will stay at hospital at least 7 days. After 10 days, 1 month, 3 months and 6 months follow-up cares are offered. After 6 months a second surgery is done to remove the metal brace.

1.3   Psychological Requirements and Communication

The communication and relationship between patient and physician can be seen as the main component in medical care. This topic has been popular over decades in research. The phenomenon has been divided into distinct aspects by different authors, such as the (1) different purposes of medical communication, (2) the analysis of physician-patient communication, (3) the specific communicative behaviors displayed during consultations and (4) the influence of communicative behaviors on certain patient outcomes [9, 10]. It has also been reported that the specific phyiscians behavior has an influence on certain patient outcomes, namely: satisfaction, compliance/adherence to treatment, recall and understanding of information and health status/psychiatric morbidity. Moreover, the physician-patient relationship has been shifted from a predominantly physician-dominant, one-sided relationship to a proactive one from both sides. This is mainly attributed to the amount of information available to patients via the Internet. Nowadays, a patient-centered approach is practised and describes a new alliance between physician and patient, based on a co-operation rather than a confrontation [11]. Taking this theoretical research findings into account the physician´s challenge in this patient-centered model is "(...) to bridge the gap between the world of medicine and the personal experiences and needs of his patients" [11]. Even though, theoretically this model is comprehensible, the reality often lacks of the implementation of these findings in the daily practical work. Correcting a jaw modulation involves further changes in the face, such as the position of the nose, cheeks, etc. which might imply a kind of identity change. The face, as being one of the most complex part of the body, reflects the individuality and social identity [12]. Therefore, this intervention has to be handled with sensitivity and with a good psychological support in order to support patients in an optimal way. Physicians challenge is to find the right balance between explaining risks and in the same way not to scare patients but still deliver the adequate dose of necessary information. Further more, explanation with the help of the plaster model are hard to understand which also cause uncertainty of comprehension among patients.

1.4   Requirements for Electronic Support

The usage of smartphone applications –so called apps- is nowadays very common. Among the huge range of app purposes, the number of healthcare apps is growing [13]. The area of use is diverse. Mosa et al. [14] stated in their review of healthcare applications areas, such as e.g. disease diagnosis, drug reference, medical calculators, clinical communication. Communication between patient and physician via an application is still rarely common in daily medical work. However, the benefits of integrating smartphones into the practice of medicine and one's personal life are numerous [15]. Since the main focus of this study is placed on patient and physician communication and how it can be improved, the application approach also considers this fact. Therefore, a possible app solution in the area of patient-physician communication should support and not hinder aspects of the face-to-face dialogue between patient and physician. It could support the information process on both sides. For physicians, information about patients such as character traits could be provided. Patients would answer specific questions prior the medical education. On the other hand, patients could e.g. use the app to keep a pain diary. Physicians would be able to intervene directly in case of emergency. More over, the app could easily be used when the patient is already at home. Occurring questions dealing with the recovery e.g. could be directly leaded to the physician. Besides, the app could offer a patient network that provides the possibility for patients to exchange experience, support, encourage and advise other affected patients. Finally, general information material as well as FAQ's could be included.

1.5   Question Addressed and Logic of Procedure

The study aims to explore the individually experienced process of treatment of each patient as well as to sense the patient's needs. Since every patient has its own way of handling such a decisive experience, first insights into the patients'way of dealing with it are collected. Thus, four main research questions are guiding the study: (1) What are the expectations (cognitive and affective) regarding consequences of surgery? (2) How far and in what ways do patient inform themselves and which attitudes do they recommend a physician to be?, (3) What kind of impact has the surgery on quality of life?, (4) How far does the patient's mood change due to the surgery?

2   Method

In order to understand the individual experience of such a decisive intervention, a longitudinal study design over a time period of 6 months was chosen. The study accompanied patients while they were going through treatment. Thus, it was possible to collect data at each important state of treatment. In order to conduct the study as economically as possible for patients as well as physicians, the questionnaire method was selected. Patients who were going to receive surgery participated and assessed on five different periods of time the treatment; one day before surgery, 10 days after, 1 month after, 3 and 6 months after surgery. Therefore, five different questionnaires were designed, collecting qualitative and quantitative data (Fig. 1).

2.1   Survey Structure

The survey contains five questionnaires, one for each period of time. In order to compare questionnaires individually for each patient and still provide anonymity, patients had to create an individual code which they had to provide for each investigation.

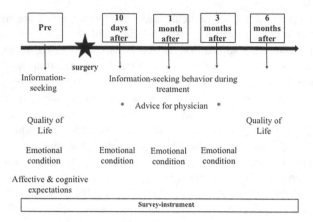

Fig. 1. Structural figure of current longitudinal study design

Demographic data. The questionnaire before surgery measured demographical data such as gender, age, educational level as well as the reason for undergoing surgery.

Information type. Participants were asked to state their source of information seeking for the upcoming surgery. Multiple replies were possible (Internet, research literature, etc.). During the treatment patients were again asked where they inform themselves with three items which had to be answered on a 6-point-likert scale.

Advice to physician. Participants were asked to give advice to physician by finishing following sentences: (1) "The physician should be…" (2) "It would be helpful for treatment, if…." (3) "For future patient it would be helpful,…" (4) "The physician should avoid…" Multiple replies were possible.

Affective and cognitive expectations. Before surgery, patients were requested to describe their positive and negative expectations of the intervention. The question was stated in an open way. Multiple answers were permitted.

Quality of life. To assess the level of life satisfaction, the standardized questionnaire by Fahrenberg et al. [16] was included in the questionnaire at two times of the investigation: before surgery and 6 months after surgery. This instrument measures the following areas of life satisfaction: health, job and profession, finances, leisure, spouse/partner, friends and relatives, and home. All of the items were formulated as followed: "How satisfied are you with your (health, etc.)?" and had to be rated from 1 (very dissatisfied) to 5 (very satisfied). High scores indicate high satisfaction with the areas of life.

Emotional condition. The adjective mood scale, developed by Zerssen [17], represents 24 bipolar item meanings such as e.g. happy versus unhappy, irritated versus calm, etc.. Patients are requested to select the most appropriate alternative or if they can not decide the "neither nor" alternative. The emotional condition was assessed before, 10 days after, 1 month and 3 months after surgery.

2.2   Procedure

In the beginning of each treatment, the patient was informed about the study and its purpose. The participation of the study was optional. Most of the patient undergoing surgery, decided to take part into the study. To each period of time (one day before surgery, 10 days after, 1 month after, 3 months and 6 months after) patients were asked to fill out the questionnaire via a tablet or computer.

2.3   Sample

Data was collected from patients undergoing orthognathic surgery at the RWTH clinic, Aachen University. Participants were invited to participate in the study via the attending physician. Completion of the questionnaire took approximately 30–40 min. 22 patients fulfilled the study from its beginning to its end. The mean age of the participants was M = 24.95 years (SD = 9.89, 17–48 range years). 19 participants were female and 3 were male. The profession of patients compasses a wide range of activities (student, employees, free-lancer, etc.). Asked for the reason of surgery, the most mentioned was the functional one (58 %; problems when chewing), followed by reasons of pain (25 %; jaw pain, headache) and recommendation by ambulant physician (17 %).

3   Results

Results were analysed by frequencies, qualitative data analysis by Mayring [18] and with non-parametric tests due to the small sample size. Friedman test was calculated.

Cognitive and affective expectations. Patients stated various hopes and worries. Multiple responses were possible by each patient with an open stated question. Answers were differentiated by cognitive (beliefs and thoughts towards surgery) and affective (feelings and emotional reaction towards surgery) meanings following the guidelines of the qualitative data analysis by Mayring. Cognitive hopes were described as *"general improvement of appearance*, such as the improvement of the face and

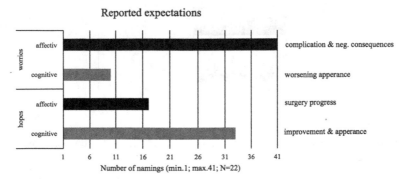

Fig. 2. Reported expectations (affectiv worries and hopes; cognitive worries and hopes). Multiple responses possible ($\sum$ = 101 responses; N = 22).

smile (11 namings) and *"general functional improvement"* such as jaw position, speech and less pain (22 namings). Affective hopes were described with the category *"process of treatment"* (17 namings).

Patients stated hopes such as to recover totally, to have no complication and pain during treatment, receiving a socially accepted appearance as well as hoping to have a lifelong solution. Worries were divided into *"worsening of appearance"* as the cognitive component with 10 namings (e.g. worry about functional decline). As affective worries, two categories were developed: *"complication in recovery process"* (19 namings e.g. pain during recovery, restriction in life, inflammation during recovery, etc.) and *"negative consequences of surgery"* (22 namings; e.g. neural damage, numbness, other remaining pain, weightloss, death, no recognition because of facial change) (see Fig. 2).

Information. Asked about where patients inform themselves about surgery and treatment over 55 % stated to receive their information from the Internet, followed with 36 % by questioning the attending physician. 32 % also stated to ask other experienced patients (multiple replies were possible). During the process of treatment patients were asked where they inform themselves when having questions. On a 6-point rating scale from 1 = I do not agree at all to 6 = I agree at all, patients rated to ask the attending physician over the whole period of time rather the nurse staff, other patients or even the Internet (see Fig. 3 left).

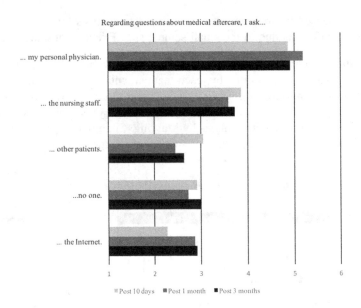

Fig. 3. Information source during treatment (response scale from 1 = do not agree at all – 6 = do agree at all).

Advice to physician. Since the physicians' behaviour has a main influence on certain patient outcomes such as satisfaction among others, patients were asked to give advice to physician regarding four different aspects: physicians' character, helpful information for treatment, advice for future patients, information which should not be mentioned. Multiple replies were possible on the open question. Figure 4 (left) protrays the results on the physicians' character. Being "friendly" (12 namings), followed by "being open-minded" (8 namings) and being "honest" (6 namings) seem to be the most important character traits, a physician should have. The outstanding advice regarding behaviour a physician should avoid, were the "usage of medical language" (10 namings) as well as fearing the patient (4 namings) among others (see Fig. 4 right).

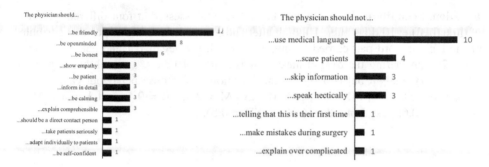

Fig. 4. Reported advice; left multiple responses possible ($\Sigma = 44$ responses; N = 22); right multiple responses possible ($\Sigma = 23$ responses; N = 22).

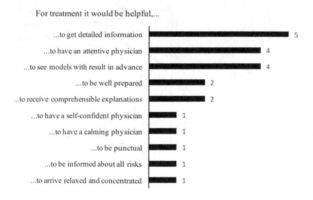

Fig. 5. Reported advice; multiple responses possible ($\Sigma = 44$ responses; N = 22)

Regarding the question what would be helpful for treatment, the most important advice were (Fig. 5): *"receive detailed information"* (5 namings), *"have attention"* (4 namings) and *"to show models which portray the future face"* (4 namings).

Asked about what current patients would wish for future patients, the following aspects were mentioned (multiple answers were possible): *"Future patients should have their questions and concerns discussed in detail"* (7 namings), *"(...) should be patient*" (3 namings), "*(...) should meet a competent physician*" (2 namings), and as one time mentions "*(...) should see a better visualisation model of future face*", "*(...) should have courage*" and "*(...) should meet a physician who explains comprehensible*".

Quality of life. An overall mean score was computed with all the items before surgery and a second one 6 months after surgery. The overall mean value before surgery was M = 3.4 and SD = 0.7 on an answering scale of 5 points max. A similiar responsiveness was found 6 months after surgery with M = 3.65 and SD = 0.6. No statistically significant difference could be found from the first assessment before surgery and the last after 6 months.

Emotional condition. The emotional condition was assessed at four different periods of time (before, 10 days after, 1 month after and 3 months after). The positive attribute of the bipolar word pair carried the higher value 3, the negative 1 and neither nor the value 2. Considering the overall mean values before, 10 days, 1 month and 3 month after surgery a slight but non significant deviation of response behaviour can be registered (pre M = 2.3, SD = 0.3; post 10 days M = 2.4, SD = 0.4; post 1 month M = 2.3, SD = 0.6; post 3 months M = 2.3, SD = 0.5).

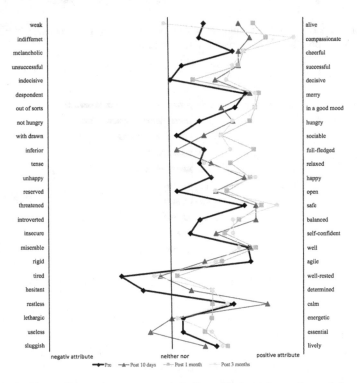

Fig. 6. Emotional condition; response pattern before, 10 days, 1 months and 3 months after surgery (1 = negative attribute; 2 = neither nor; 3 = positive attribute; N = 22).

Figure 6 shows the assessment of each word pair to each time of investigation. Taking a general look at the figure, the assessment of attributes is rated throughout positively. However, a few deviations are noticeable during the course of time. Before surgery patients feel rather "tired" and "hesitant" in comparison with further times of treatment. 10 days after surgery patients feel outstanding useless. 1 month after surgery a very homogenous picture appears. 3 months after surgery two emotional conditions are more outstanding. The feeling of "safety" is rated as being very strong. The emotional condition of feeling "weak" is remarkably negatively attributed in comparison with the other times of investigation.

4 Discussion and Outlook

In this paper a longitudinal study is represented as an empirical approach to an improvement of the patient and physician relationship of patients undergoing orthognathic surgery. The overall purpose of the current study is the development of a data base for an information and communication concept. Thus, 22 patients were accompanied over six months during treatment. Patients who were going to receive surgery participated and assessed on five different periods of time the treatment. The main research aims were to identify expectations of patients entering the treatment, coping strategies, information behaviour and recommended physician behaviour stated by patients. The data portrays that patients with jaw malposition suffer from psychological and physical difficulties. Patients mainly decided to undergo surgery in order to improve the function of chewing, as being a basic necessity. The expectation to receive an improvement of general functions such as chewing and biting is obvious and can also be seen in the data of patient´s reported expectations. Having divided the stated expectations into cognitive and affective hopes and worries, it turns out that the reported affective worries outnumber the hopes and seem to be of special importance. Main topics are *complication in recovery process* and *negative consequences of surgery*. Information about treatment before surgery was mainly collected in the medical education by the attending physician as well as in the Internet. A similar behaviour pattern occurs in information seeking during treatment. The attending physician is the most contacted person followed by other experienced patients and the Web. Therefore, medical education and especially the physician as a person is among the whole treatment the essential source for patients receiving answers on their questions and needs special focus regarding an information communication concept. Even though essential necessities as e.g. being able to chew properly were reported as a main reason for surgery with the intention to improve it, no effects on the patient´s quality of life especially before and after surgery could be detected. It seems that generally the group of patients has a well rated quality of life and does not show any remarkable losses due to their jaw deformity, at least not in the experimental time frame of 6 months. However, the opposite has been discovered in studies [19] and still needs to be focused on in further studies. The course of emotional conditions was also throughout positive which leads to the assumption that patients who have decided on such a severe treatment are likely to be highly motivated to make changes to their facial appearance and quality of life.

As a code of conduct patients of this underlying study recommended the physician to be friendly, to be open-minded, and honest. The physician should use comprehensible words in his explanations, calm patients and inform in detail. Furthermore, a model with the facial result in advance would be appreciated as well as to have an attentive physician who takes patients' concerns serious. Now, the question occurs during what time of treatment the patient needs special support. The scale of emotional conditions provides first insights into the patient´s well-being and delivers hints at which point an intervention could take place in order to maintain a positive emotional condition. It is known that the better the emotional well-being the better the treatment outcome [20]. Before treatment the emotional condition of patients is described as being tired and hesitant. Psychological support and motivation for doing this decisive step needs to be offered to the patient thus the patient does not need to be hesitant. Also 10 days after surgery the emotional condition, described as feeling rather useless, needs special focus. The feeling may originate from medication and physical limitations due to the recent surgery but still encouraging attention is necessary. Taking all this results into account, a first approach to app content guidelines is to offer more information about complication in recovery process and negative consequences of surgery in detail. It is important to describe possible consequences in comprehensible language. An included medical dictionary needs to be integrated at this point. Experience reports of patients who have already undergone surgery should be provided. As results show, many patients inform themselves via Internet besides the dialogue with physician. However, to receive emotional support, get encouraged especially in severe times right before and after surgery a patient-network needs to be generated. Generally, risks need to be mentioned however in a calming way. Regarding information about surgery, information about the different treatment steps and possible psychologically and physically recovery stages should be offered as well as recommendation what to do for well-being. Thus, a patient could wonder at which time the swelling declines. The app would offer the information of recovery at four times of assessment as executed in this study (before, 10 days, 1 month, 3 months and 6 months after surgery). Since the app is supposed to be a communication tool between patient and physician, the physician could easily intervene and encourage or calm the patient. Additionally, motivational support before and directly after surgery needs to be offered.

So far the study only describes possible contents for an app guideline. The assessment of such an idea, specific contents and its structure necessarily has to be investigated in a first step. In a further study, a real prototype should be developed and tested regarding the (TAM Model by Davis [21]) attitude towards using it, the perceived usefulness, the perceived ease of use and intention to use it. A further aspect is the size of our sample. In order to report representative data, the sample has to be enlarged. On a long term, the question appears how far an information and communication strategy in the field of jaw malposition under regard of technical devices for patient information is transferable to other medical fields. An interesting research question could be how far this kind of electronic support has an impact on the patient´s well-being and a positive outcome of treatment. Finally, the question appears, if this kind of information and communication concept is transferable to other medical fields.

Acknowledgements. Authors would like to thank Dr. Ali Modabber, Dr. Evgeny Goloborodko, Florian Peters and Sarah Völkel for their research support. A special thank goes to all the participants who took part. The Excellence Initiative of the German Research Foundation DFG funded this work.

References

1. Stewart, Moira A.: Effective physician-patient communication and health outcomes: a review. CMAJ: Can. Med. Assoc. J. **152**(9), 1423 (1995)
2. Philipps, C., Asuman Kiyak, H., Bloomquist, D., Turvey, T.: Perceptions of recorvery and satisfaction in the short term after orthognathic surgery. J. Oral Maxillofac. Surg. **62**(5), 535–534 (2004)
3. Modig, M., Andersson, L., Wårdh, I.: Patients' perception of improvement after orthognathic surgery: pilot study. Br. J. Oral Maxillofac. Surg. **44**(1), 24–27 (2006)
4. Cunningham, S.J., Crean, S.J., Hunt, N.P., Harris, M.: Preparation, perceptions, and problems: a long-term follow-up study of orthognathic surgery. Int. J. Adult Orthod. Orthognathic Surg. **11**(1), 41–47 (1996)
5. Rateitschak, K.H., Rateitschak, E.M., Wolf, H.F.: Parodontologie. Farbatlanten der Zahnmedizin, Bd 1. Thieme. (1984)
6. Frost, V., Peterson, G.: Psychological aspects of orthognathic surgery: how people respond to facial change. Oral. Surg. Oral. Med. Oral. Pathol. **71**(5), 538–42 (1991)
7. Sykes, J.M.: Managing the psychological aspects of plastic surgery patients. Curr. Opin. Otolaryngol. Head. Neck. Surg. **17**(4), 321–5 (2009)
8. Vuyk, H.D., Zijlker, T.D.: Psychosocial aspects of patient counseling and selection: a surgeon's perspective. Facial Plast. Surg. **11**(2), 55–60 (1995)
9. Ong, L.M., De Haes, J.C., Hoos, A.M., Lammes, F.B.: Doctor-patient communication: a review of the literature. Soc. Sci. Med. **40**(7), 903–918 (1995)
10. Wilkins, S.: Physician-Patient Communication. Mind the Gap Academy Publishing (2014)
11. Kaba, R., Sooriakumaran, P.: The evolution of the doctor-patient relationship. Int. J. Surg. **5**(1), 57–65 (2007)
12. Ekman, P., Friesen, W.V.: Constants across cultures in the face and emotion. J. Pers. Soc. Psychol. **17**(2), 124 (1971)
13. Boulos, M.N.K, et al.: Mobile medical and health apps: state of the art, concerns, regulatory control and certification. Online J. Public Health Inform. **5**(3) (2014)
14. Mosa, A.S.M., Yoo, I., Sheets, L.: A systematic review of healthcare applications for smartphones. BMC Med. Inform. Decis. Mak. **12**(1), 67 (2012)
15. Ozdalga, E., Ozdalga, A., Ahuja, N.: The smartphone in medicine: a review of current and potential use among physicians and students. J. Med. Internet Res. **14**(5), e128 (2012)
16. FLZ: Fragebogen zur Lebenszufriedenheit. Hogrefe Verlag für Psychologie (2000)
17. Zerssen, D., Petermann, F.: Bf-SR - Die Befindlichkeits-Skala - Revidierte Fassung. Hogrefe, Göttingen (2011)
18. Mayring, P.: Qualitative inhaltsanalyse. VS Verlag für Sozialwissenschaften (2010)
19. De Sousa, Avinash.: Psychological issues in oral and maxillofacial reconstructive surgery. Br. J. Oral Maxillofac. Surg. **46**(8), 661–664 (2008)
20. Meade, E.A., Inglehart, M.R.: Young patients' treatment motivation and satisfaction with orthognathic surgery outcomes: the role of "possible selves". Am. J. Orthod. Dentofacial Orthop. **137**(1), 26–34 (2010)
21. Davis, F.D.: Perceived usefulness, perceived ease of use and user acceptance of information technology. MIS Q. **13**(3), 319–339 (1989)

AtHoCare: An Intelligent Elder Care at Home System

Tao Xu[1,2(✉)], Yun Zhou[3], and Zhe Ma[1]

[1] School of Software and Microelectronics,
Northwestern Polytechnical University, 127 West Youyi Road,
Xi'an 710072, Shaanxi, People's Republic of China
xutao@nwpu.edu.cn, mazhe1994@126.com
[2] State Key Laboratory for Manufacturing Systems Engineering,
Xi'an Jiaotong University, No. 99 Yan Cheung Road, Xi'an 710072, Shaanxi,
People's Republic of China
[3] School of Education, Shaanxi Normal University, 199 South Chang'an Road,
Xi'an 710062, Shaanxi, People's Republic of China
zhouyun@snnu.edu.cn

Abstract. In recent years, the shortage of nursing home and the demand from elders have made the balance inclined. Additionally, the increased numbers of elders per year have not deemed fit to wait for growth rate of nursing home. Therefore, more and more elders have to stay at home and live alone, which easily leads them to be in danger, especially when unexpected emergency occurring like falling. To investigate this issue, we have designed AtHoCare, an intelligent elder care at home system, which employs Microsoft depth camera sensor Kinect to detect fall and an intelligent sever to send alarms to nurses' smart phones. In this way, medical staffs could easily monitor several elders at the same time, which greatly increases work efficiency. It is worth stressing that AtHoCare also proposes an algorithm of fall detection based on skeleton data of elders only. It protects elders' privacy much more than other vision based algorithm of fall detection. Results from our preliminary lab-environment test showed that AtHoCare has a well-done performance on detection.

Keywords: Healthcare · Fall detection · Intelligent system

1 Introduction

Nowadays, population ageing has become a worldwide serious problem and drawn public attention. Limited resources and labor force of nursing home and a huge requirement from elders made this issue acute that all countries have to face. The data from Ministry of Civil Affairs of P. R. China indicates that every one thousand elders in China have only 25 beds in nursing house. With no choice, many elders have to stay at home. However, these elders may not get an in-time treatment when some health emergencies happen, such as stroke, heartache, and especially fall. Falls of elderly people are the main cause of admission and extended period of stay in a hospital.

V.G. Duffy (Ed.): DHM 2016, LNCS 9745, pp. 298–305, 2016.
DOI: 10.1007/978-3-319-40247-5_30

It is also the sixth cause of death for people over the age of 65, the second for people between 65 and 75, and the first for people over 75 [1]. A number of studies have been carried out to detect falls. These investigations can be classified into three main types: wearable device based approaches, ambience sensor based approaches, and camera based approach. Camera based approaches have been increasingly adopted in home assistive/care system recently, since these approaches can be used to detect multiple events simultaneously with less intrusion [2]. Bevilacqua et al. [3] proposed a fall-detection tool based on commercial RGB-D camera that was capable of accurately detecting several types of falls. Stone et al. [4] presented a two-stage fall detection system detecting falls in the houses of old adults using the Microsoft Kinect. Miaou and his colleagues [5] designed a fall detection system that used a MapCam (omni-camera) to capture images and performed image processing over the images. The personal information of each individual has been also considered in the processing tasks. Wu [6] used the velocity profile for detection of normal and abnormal (i.e., fall) activities, which made the automatic detection of falls during the descending phase of a fall. Williams et al. [7] designed a system based on distributed network of smart cameras, whose function was to detect and localize falls. In this work, they designed and implemented an important application in elderly living environment. However, these studies usually lacked strategies to protect data privacy [8].

To crack this hard nut, we design an intelligent elder care system, which can help medical staffs to monitor elders' falls and other activities in door at home and protect their sensitive data. The model of system consists of three main components: sensors (Kinect), intelligent server and clients. This system only employs Kinect to get elders' skeleton data for monitoring elders' activities, without gathering other biometrics data like facial expression. Through computing body's centroid changing and the recovery time, we can detect the status of elder, that is, falling or not. When falls happen, the medical staffs will be informed at different urgent levels. This paper is organized as follows. It starts with describing the intelligent elder care at home system structure at first. Then a fall detection algorithm based on center of mass (COM) is proposed. Finally, results and discussion are stated based on a preliminary lab study.

2   AtHoCare: The Intelligent Elder Care at Home System

2.1   System Structure

AtHoCare is designed to help elders take care themselves in their homes. It consists of three main parts: intelligent server, clients and sensors (Kinect). The system structure is shown in Fig. 1.

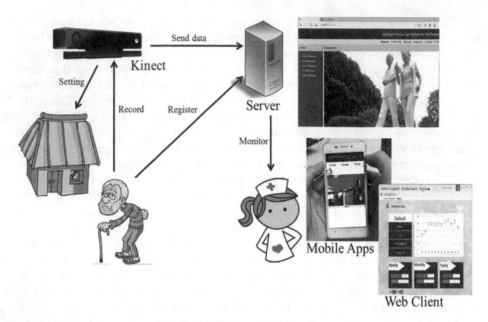

Fig. 1. Intelligent elder care system

Intelligent server has two main functions. One is responsible for storage personal information for elders, including: name, gender, age, telephone number and medical record. Elders can easy to sign it up via internet. Another one is to collect elders' activity information, which can be used to analyze elders' body movements, habit and health status. When a fall or other abnormal activities occur, the data relating to these activities will be sent to the server. Also, it employs web service to provide access to PC and mobile.

The client is designed to help medical staffs to easily find elders in emergency situation anywhere at any time. It has two methods to access to intelligent server: web client and mobile application (with regard to testing version, we develop an app running on Android OS). When elders falling in their homes, client will receive an alarm from intelligent sever.

The core part of AtHoCare is to monitor elders' daily activity and to detect elders' abnormal activity: fall when it taking place. We employ Kinect to trace elders' daily activities; it is a line of motion sensing input devices by Microsoft for Xbox 360 and Xbox One video game consoles, as well as Windows PCs. Based on an IR depth-finding camera and a RGB camera, Kinect enables advanced gesture recognition, facial recognition and voice recognition [9]. Besides this, Kinect is capable of simultaneously tracking up to six people, including two active players for motion analysis with a feature extraction of 20 joints per person. We set Kinect in the high corner of room to monitor elders' daily activities. With regard to privacy concerns, we block the RGB data and leverage skeleton joint data to detect elders' accidental fall and other abnormal activity. It can not only get elders' precise behavior information in a small data quantity but also protect their privacy to maximum extent.

2.2   Fall Detection Algorithm

Based on AtHoCare as described above, we propose an algorithm of fall detection based on COM. We use the acceleration of COM, the distance changed of COM, and the recovery time as three key features to detect a fall. Then we combine the fall type and contextual information to evaluate the danger level.

De la Leva's work [10] segments human (female and male) into eight parts: head, trunk, upper arm, forearm, hand, thigh, shank, and foot. The Kinect can get 3D position data of 20 joints' of human body, which cannot match Leva's work directly. Thus, we consider dividing the human body into six parts anew: head, trunk, two arms, and two legs to match the motion of people with the segment of body mass. The segment mass is the weight ratio of body part to the whole body. As shown in Table 1, we listed these common ratios or percentages from Leva's work. Since Kinect cannot identify the gender from skeleton data, we compute the average percentage based on female's and male's percentage. The last column in Table 1 shows the calculated average. Finally, we also use the average body mass as 67.45 kg, based on Leva's work (male, 73.0 kg; female, 61.9 kg).

Table 1. Human's Segment Weight data

Segment	Quantity	Female's percentage (%)	Male's percentage (%)	Average percentage (%)
Head	1	6.68	6.94	6.810
Trunk	1	42.57	43.46	43.015
Total arm	2	4.49	4.92	4.715
Total leg	2	20.88	19.86	20.370

Based on the position information and the average body mass, we convert 20 joints into six parts to represent human body, as shown in Fig. 2. The whole body's COM data can be computed as the weighted sum of the whole body [11].

We get the real-time vertical acceleration of COM from each interval two frames based on function (1):

$$a_{COM} = P_{frame\ n} - P_{frame\ n-1} / \Delta t \tag{1}$$

Based on Li's work [12], we define threshold value as: 2.5 g ($g = 9.8m/s^2$). When a_{COM} is bigger than the threshold value, we consider it as a fall-prone action.

In order to obtain the distance changed of COM, we measure the angle between the Kinect and the vertical wall, as shown in Fig. 3. Through the calculation of the coordinate system of Kinect, we then infer and obtain the actual distance changed of COM.

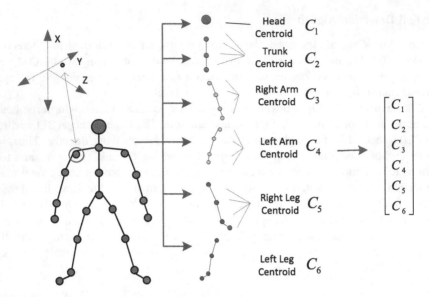

Fig. 2. The model of activities based on skeleton joints' centroid

With respect to the recovery time, we define it as the interval lasting from a fall-prone action occurring to the COM that is higher than that of the sitting posture on the ground. We detect the fall-prone action by using the rule set method, which is based on the acceleration of COM and distance changed of COM. The fall type is determined by the recovery time. We classify the falls into three main categories: non-risk falls, low-risk falls and high-risk falls.

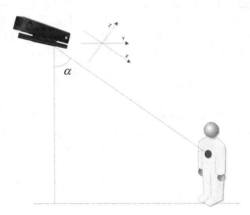

Fig. 3. The framework to obtain the distance changed of COM

Finally, we get the danger level of the fall based on fall type and elder's context at that time, as shown in Fig. 4. This level helps the system to distinguish the fall is danger or not. For instance, some elders in Asian countries are accustomed to take a nap after lunch, sleeping directly on the ground.

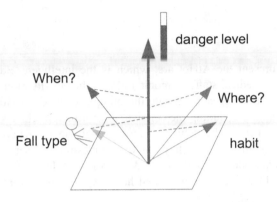

Fig. 4. The danger level (Color figure online)

3 Results and Discussion

We test AtHoCare in a lab environment. The AtHoCare is built based on a PC, withIntel(R) Core(TM)i7-3520 @2.9 GHz, 12.0 GB RAM, Windows 8.1 Operation System, a Kinect, a smart phone on Andoid, and five volunteer participants. The kinect is fixed at the high corner in the test room to record users' activities. The intelligent sever is developed in Java, which provides web service based on AXIS2.

We select and define three common activities in daily life: walking, siting and jumping, to make a comparison with falling.

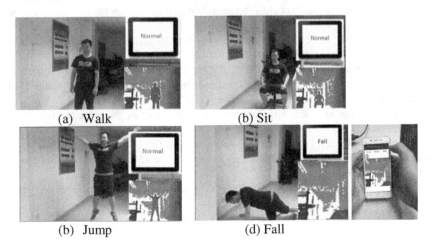

Fig. 5. The test in a lab-environment

The results are shown in Fig. 5. From results, the system can easily detect falls from other normal activities. Due to the use of the skeleton data as source data, we could ensure the protection of users' privacy and make the data small enough to be easily and quickly transferred. The client end can be alarmed immiditely while the volenteer falling, even in cellular networks.

4 Conclusion

In this paper, we present the AtHoCare, which is the intelligent elder care at home system and can help medical staffs to moniter elders' health situation distantly. In this system, the intelligent server can estimate the danger level of activities based on fall type and users' situation, including the contextual information, elder's behavior habits, etc. Medical staffs can check the status of elders through the mobile app and web client. Based on the in-time information, they could provide medical services immediately. Finally, the system is evaluated in a lab-based environment. In our future work, we will set our intelligent elder care system on real house to test its performance in the real environment.

References

1. Abbate, S., Avvenuti, M., Corsini, P., Light, J., Vecchio, A.: Monitoring of human movements for fall detection and activities recognition in elderly care using wireless sensor network: a survey. In: Tan, Y.K. (ed.) Wireless Sensor Networks: Application-Centric Design. InTech, Rijeka (2010)
2. Mubashir, M., Shao, L., Seed, L.: A survey on fall detection: principles and approaches. Neurocomput. **100**, 144–152 (2013)
3. Bevilacqua, V., Nuzzolese, N., Barone, D., Pantaleo, M., Suma, M., D'Ambruoso, D., Volpe, A., Loconsole, C., Stroppa, F.: Fall detection in indoor environment with kinect sensor. In: Proceedings of 2014 IEEE International Symposium on Innovations in Intelligent Systems and Applications (INISTA), pp. 319–324 (2014)
4. Stone, E.E., Skubic, M.: Fall detection in homes of older adults using the Microsoft Kinect. IEEE J. Biomed. Health Inform. **19**, 290–301 (2015)
5. Miaou, S.-G., Sung, P.-H., Huang, C.-Y.: A Customized human fall detection system using omni-camera images and personal information. In: 1st Transdisciplinary Conference on Distributed Diagnosis and Home Healthcare, D2H2, pp. 39–42 (2006)
6. Wu, G.: Distinguishing fall activities from normal activities by velocity characteristics. J. Biomech. **33**, 1497–1500 (2000)
7. Williams, A., Ganesan, D., Hanson, A.: Aging in place: fall detection and localization in a distributed smart camera network. In: Proceedings of the 15th International Conference on Multimedia (2007)
8. Igual, R., Medrano, C., Plaza, I.: Challenges, issues and trends in fall detection systems. Biomed. Eng. OnLine. **12**, 1–24 (2013)
9. Kinect (2016). https://en.wikipedia.org/w/index.php?title=Kinect&oldid=702574374

10. de Leva, P.: Adjustments to Zatsiorsky-Seluyanov's segment inertia parameters. J. Biomech. **29**, 1223–1230 (1996)
11. Winter, D.A.: Biomechanics and Motor Control of Human Movement. Wiley, Hoboken (2009)
12. Li, N., Hou, Y., Huang, Z.: Implementation of a real-time fall detection algorithm based on body's acceleration. J. Chin. Comput. Syst. **33**(11), 2410–2413 (2012)

The Transfer of Expertise in Conducting a Participatory Music Therapy During a Combined Rehabilitation-Recreational Program in an Elderly Care Facility

Akiyoshi Yamamoto[1], Henry Cereno Barrameda Jr.[1(✉)],
Tatsunori Azuma[1], Hideaki Kasasaku[1], Kayoko Hirota[1],
Momo Jinno[1], Maki Sumiyama[1], Tomoko Ota[2], Akihiko Goto[3],
Noriyuki Kida[4], Noriaki Kuwahara[4], and Hiroyuki Hamada[4]

[1] Super Court Co., Ltd., Osaka, Japan
{yamamoto,henrybarramedajr,
azuma,kyo-shijyuoomiya}@supercourt.co.jp,
organ0412@gmail.com, zimal031@gmail.com
jiayuzi-5963@ezweb.ne.jp
[2] Chuo Business Group, Osaka, Japan
tomoko.ota@k.vodafone.ne.jp
[3] Osaka Sangyo University, Osaka, Japan
gotoh@ise.osaka-sandai.ac.jp
[4] Kyoto Institute of Technology, Kyoto, Japan
{kida,nkuwahar,hhamada}@kit.ac.jp

Abstract. As the population ages, the number of elderly people who require nursing care continuously increases. In Japan, as of October 2012, a total of 5.49 million qualification certificates were issued to those elderly requiring support, as well as those requiring long-term care in their daily life. Japan's long-term care system is being promoted based on the philosophy of a society supporting individuals to preserve a dignified lifestyle. However, along with Japan's rapid aging society, experts in nursing care among experts on different fields are also growing old, remarkably low birth rate poses another challenge in transfer of these expertise to young generations later. In this study we present an experiment that will analyze the attributes of every core skill we identified during our previous study which mapped the core skills of the expert that is needed in conducting an effective participatory music therapy in a nursing home facility. By identifying attributes, much deeper understanding of every core skill was gained, and a better and smoother skill transfer from an expert to a successor performer was attained.

Keywords: Caregiver · Paid elderly facility · Recreation · Participatory music therapy

© Springer International Publishing Switzerland 2016
V.G. Duffy (Ed.): DHM 2016, LNCS 9745, pp. 306–316, 2016.
DOI: 10.1007/978-3-319-40247-5_31

1 Research Background

1.1 Introduction

The number of elderly people who require nursing care is increasing as the population ages. As of October 2012, there were 5.49 million people in Japan with Certificates of Required Support or Certificates of Required Long-Term Care, who require some kind of care in their daily lives. Therefore, high quality caretaking services are being promoted based on the idea of a society supporting "individual, dignified lifestyles.

However, along with Japan's rapid aging society, experts in nursing care among experts on different fields are also growing old, remarkably low birth rate poses another challenge in transfer of these expertise to young generations later. (The Transfer of Expertise in Conducting a Participatory Music Therapy during a Combined Rehabilitation-Recreational Program in an Elderly Care Facility, Yamamoto 2015).

In Japan, music therapy has been introduced not so long ago as a new recreational and rehabilitation therapy. Activation of the brain, strengthening of the muscles for swallowing, and emotional and mental stability are just few of the most common beneficial effects improving the mind and body functions. It as well aim to improve of daily quality of life among the recipients. It has since been a standard for the elderly welfare care facilities of to provide recreational events, and recreation has also been the main in the life support provided by Day Service Institutions (Yamamoto 2015).

The setting of our study is a paid nursing home facility in Japan. Providing music therapy in the said facility has yield positive results, and we have felt the need for the expansion of the program to our other facility so that other residents could have access to music therapy.

However, offering sustainable service has always been a challenge to the currently short-staffed and notoriously high turn-over rate caregiver work in Japan (Yamamoto 2015).

Another condition that poses challenge to skill transfer is that studies found that as the expert's expertise increases, mental representations become more abstract, making it hard for them to give educational instructions to successor. For example in an electronics trouble-shooting task, Gitomer 1988 found that more skilled technicians viewed an electronic device as a system of components, and conducted trouble shooting by following a conceptual model of the circuit. Less skilled technicians assumed that "there must be a short somewhere" and spent more time switching, using a trial-and-error procedure (Hinds et al. 2001).

Trial and error skill transfer procedure in the already time constraint working environment in nursing home would cause great burden to the expert staff. So, in order to cope up and meet the increasing demand for the provision of higher quality nursing service to the residents in the elderly facilities, we believe that researches on transfer of certain nursing skills is indispensable (Yamamoto 2015).

Many research works are being carried out to improve nursing services, however, studies related to sustainability of operation like research on skills transfer are not given much emphasis. In fact, our query on any research pertaining to transfer of expertise and skills in the nursing field in Japan yield us very limited result. (Yamamoto 2015).

In our previous study, we studied how to be able to transfer skills effectively by careful analysis of the technique used while performing. It was aimed to identify the set of skills needed for the rendition of an effective music therapy. We begin by analyzing the common techniques employed by expert performer, as characterized by her use of time, decisions and actions while performing a participatory music therapy in a paid nursing facility.

However, in this particular study, our aim was to define the attributes of every skill identified in the previous research.

1.2   Research Trends and Significance of the Study

In Japan, in the paper, Effects of Music Therapy for Dementia: A systematic review (Watanabe 2005) suggested that after reviewing researches published within the past 20 years, they have found out that along with the findings of Koger, music therapy is an effective intervention for dementia.

In a separate study, that was conducted in a long term-care health facility, Kuwahara (2001) stated that music has physiological and mental effects on human being. Their work found significance on the activities, whether it is a music therapy or music recreational activity.

However, along with Japan's rapid aging society, experts on different fields are also growing old, remarkably low birth rate poses another challenge in transfer of these expertise to young generations later. Problems in skills transfer is not just being a business entity issue but becoming a Japan national issue as well (Gijutsu•Ginou Denshou no tame no Ginou Bunseki to Manyuaru Kousei no Houhou, Mori 2001).

Having the same commitment with our previous study, this study will be a significant endeavor in the transfer of expertise in music therapy. Not only the expert and successor performers would benefit when they employ the learning from the training tool for transfer of expertise that will be created, but if we are able to create more successor performers, it is the end-user of music therapy, who are residents in the paid nursing facility suffering from dementia would greatly benefit from this study. By understanding the specific skills to consider in order to render an effective music therapy, smooth transfer of skills from expert and successor will be assured.

2   Design

2.1   Grounded Theory Methodology

As with the previous experiment, we have employed grounded theory method, it is a systematic generation of theory from data that contains both inductive and deductive thinking. One goal is to formulate hypotheses based on conceptual ideas. Generally speaking, grounded theory is an approach for looking systematically at (mostly) qualitative data (like transcripts of interviews or protocols of observations) aiming at the generation of theory. Sometimes, grounded theory is seen as a qualitative method, but grounded theory reaches farther: it combines a specific style of research (or a paradigm) with pragmatic theory of action and with some methodological guidelines.

Grounded theory method does not aim for the "truth" but to conceptualize what is going on by using empirical research. In a way, grounded theory method resembles what many researchers do when retrospectively formulating new hypotheses to fit data. However, when applying the grounded theory method, the researcher does not formulate the hypotheses in advance since preconceived hypotheses result in a theory that is ungrounded from the data (Glaser and Strauss 1967).

2.2 Subjects and Location of Study

The same two subjects from our previous study were considered in this experiment: An expert music performer, (Female, 54 years old, with a total of 49 years of piano recital experience, 6 years of which is music therapy related, with averaging 2 performances a month) and a successor, (Female, 25 years old, with 19 years piano recital experience. Both subjects were working in the elderly nursing facility. The expert is a care manager with a total of 13 and half years of experience in the field of caregiving, and the successor is a caregiver with 1 year and 10 months experience in caregiving field. See Table 1.

Table 1. Data of the subjects

Subject	Age	No. of times performed music therapy	No. of years performing piano recital	No. of years of experience in caring for elderly suffering with dementia
Expert	54	72	49	13.5
Successor	24	2	20	1.8

The setting of our study is a paid nursing home facility in Japan. The facility houses 73 residents, with about 80 % of them affected by dementia or having dementia symptoms. We have created the music therapy program to address dementia as well as to prevent it's onset on the residents.

The facility is within a network of 40 paid nursing care branches which caters different kinds of recreation to their residents. The mean participation rate for every event is shown below. See Table 2.

Table 2. Recreation participation rate

Participation Rate		
	No. of times	Participation rate for every event
Recreation within 40 facilities	7680	48.8%
Recreation in the facility where the expert is deployed	216	54.4%
Music recreation within 40 facilities	1923	63.2%
Music recreation by the Expert	24	88.2%

2.3   Objective of Analysis

Our objective is to formulate hypotheses based on conceptual ideas presented by the expert performer. This study is sought to define the attributes of the skill set identified in the previous research. We then validated the effectiveness of the skill transfer process by looking into the data on the resident's mean participation rate for music therapy performed by the expert and successor.

2.3.1   Video Recorded Participatory Music Therapy

Video footage of the actual performance served as an important medium that was used in analyzing the performance process, and profiling the core skill requirements. After which when the core skills were identified in the previous study, every core skill attributes were defined in this study.

Camera Position. Figure 1 shows that, three video cameras were used, all were set on a tripod. One camera is positioned at the back of the Audience, capturing the entire general setting. This camera also is used for observing the performer in the direct view. The other two video cameras were position to the front left and to the right of the performer, aimed to capture the general movement of the performer, as well as some part of the audience. All of the video cameras were set to wide angle or zoomed-out to be able to capture wide area. The same camera set-up was used for both the expert and the successor performance analysis.

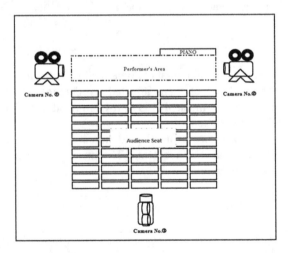

Fig. 1. Camera position

2.3.2   Video Recorded Interview

While watching the video footage of their own performances, the expert and successor were ask questions focusing on analyzing the performance protocol. Data gathered from these recorded interviews were used in mapping the core skills in the previous study and then later on, was also used in this study to define the attribute of every skill (Fig. 2).

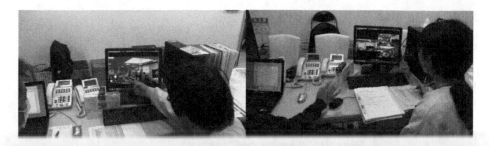

Fig. 2. Interview

2.3.2.1 Core Skill Mapping Based on Interview Data. Interview data which consisted 30 pages has been compiled for process analysis and core skill mapping in the previous study and then used here in order to be able to define the attributes of the skills (Fig. 3).

広田：・・・というのをやるというので分けているんです。それと、もう一つは、"京都を入れる"、お座敷小唄という曲は、"京都"が入っているでしょ。それともう一つは、"季節を入れる。"だからこのあたりの曲は秋の曲が並んでいます。また、楽しい雰囲気というので、最初はみんなの知っている歌 "ドレミの歌"、みんなを一つにしないといけないので、注目を集める。みんなが集まってきた状態だったら、固まった状態です。まだ、準備ができていない、気分的に楽しい雰囲気というので、最初が "ドレミの歌"、みんな知っている歌を入れる。また、声がまだ出ていないから、発声練習を、発声練習も難しい発声練習をしない。だから、"ア""イ""ウ""ベ"と言って、本当に単純で、表情を知らげる意味もあるのをや

る。わざと「旗が立つ人が昔ました！はい。その人に向かって "イ～ッ！"ダメ、もっと"イ～ッ！"としましょうか！？」というように、わざとオーバーにやることで、リラックスするのが意図なんです。"ベ～"と言うのもただ、「出してください！」と言うより、「はい、横の人に "あっかんべ～" としてください。」と言う方が、親近感、ぐっと距離が縮まる、一体感があるようになってくると思います。かと言って、大きな声を出すのが発声練習かというと違って。"ウ～"というのだけが、「大きい声を出さないで、長く細く息を出しましょうか。」としている。私は声楽を学んでいたので、先生から「頭蓋の炎をふぅ～と吹き消すように、息長くふぅ～とやりなさい。」と言われていた。その意図もあり、大きな声で"ア～ッ！"

Fig. 3. Interview data

2.3.2.2 Analysis on the Usage of Time During Performance. Attention is a high-priced commodity especially in performances (Yamamoto 2015). In this experiment, we tried to analyze the difference in usage of time between the expert and successor. Rendition time of song and exercise as well as time used in between songs were analyzed. A much easier to understand graphical representation was employed in this study than in the previous one.

2.3.2.3 Validation of Result. To measure the effectiveness of the skill transfer, we have gathered the data on the participation of the residents in all recreational activities for the period of one year in all our 40 paid nursing care facilities and compared it to the data gathered after the skills transfer.

3 Results and Consideration

3.1 Video Recorded Participatory Music Therapy

Figure 4 shows the flowchart we followed starting from video shoot of the actual music therapy until the performance process analysis.

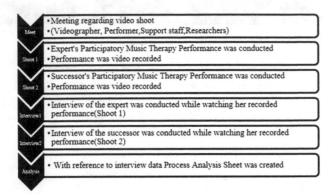

Fig. 4. Performance process analysis flowchart

Core Skill Mapping Result. As shown in Fig. 5, upon careful consideration of the collected data, it is suggested that in order to perform an effective music therapy performance, core skills such as, (1) Ability to identify suitable song rendition and exercises, (2) Knowledge on songs of the same era as the audience, (3) Knowledge on the varied effect of songs, (4) Knowledge on the use of props related to music therapy, (5) Ability to assess the audience response to performance and adjust for it, (6) Ability to continuously communicate with the audience, (7) Ability to create variation for an emotionally enjoyable music experience, (8) Ability to assess for audience exhaustion, (9) Ability to observe the standard performance sequence while making minute modifications midway, are required. Interview yield results that cooling down of the audience is proportionally important as preparation of the audience for the activity. It was known that the performer's knowledge of songs familiar to most of the audiences, like songs related to hometown were essential components of the performance. Moreover, performer's ability to observe and make changes in tempo, rhythm, tone of the song is indispensable to be able to maintain the audience attention.

Analysis on the Usage of Time During Performance. We have found that the skill (1) Ability to identify suitable song rendition and exercises, is attributed to communication with audience before the rendition; (2) Knowledge on songs of the same era as the audience, is attributed to learning the history of songs, and singers; (3) Knowledge on the varied effect of songs, is attributed to identifying songs that has cool down and excite effect, and identifying the effects of adjusting the song tempo and pitch; (4) Knowledge on the use of props related to music therapy, is attributed to learning the

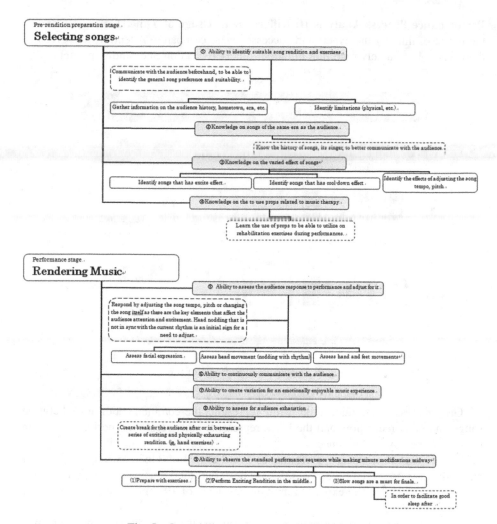

Fig. 5. Core skill mapping result (skill attributes)

utilization of props for rehabilitation; (5) Ability to assess the audience response to performance and adjust for it, is attributed to assessing the facial expression of the audience, hand and feet movement, and rhythmic nodding; (6) Ability to continuously communicate with the audience, is attributed to the vigilant observation; (7) Ability to create variation for an emotionally enjoyable music experience, is attributed to the use varied songs; (8) Ability to assess the audience exhaustion, is attributed by creating breaks after or in between a series of physically demanding activities; (9) Ability to observe the standard performance sequence while making minute modifications mid-way, is attributed by preparing for a music performance with an exercise from the start, exciting renditions in the middle, and lastly, slow song for the finale.

Performance Process Analysis II: Difference in Usage of Time. On Figs. 6 and 7, the usage of time by the expert and successor were compared. Attention was given to three variables, namely rendition duration, others recreation and rendition interval.

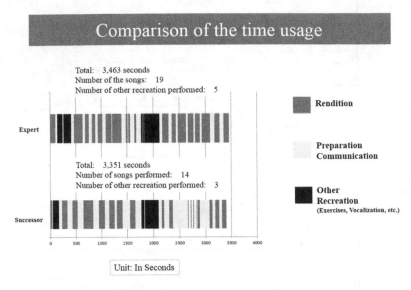

Fig. 6. Comparison in usage of time

Gray represents rendition time, white represents the communication took between songs and other recreation, and the black represents other recreation performed within the music therapy performance.

The expert music therapy performance timed a total of 3463 s, while on the other hand, the successor total time was 3351 s. The expert total music therapy performance time is 112 s longer. The expert's rendition consisted of 19 songs while the successor consisted of 14 songs.

The time spent on preparation communication by the expert was short and was proportionately used. On other recreation, longer time was used by the expert, it consisted of 5 performances while on the other hand, the time spent by the successor was shorter and it only consisted of 3 performances.

Validation of Result. Based on the result below, after the transfer of skill was carried out, the mean participation rate for the successor's performance was 80.9 %. Although the mean participation rate of 88.2 % during music therapy performances of the expert has not been surpassed by the successor, high participation rate is maintained, thus effectiveness of the transfer of skill is validated. See Table 3.

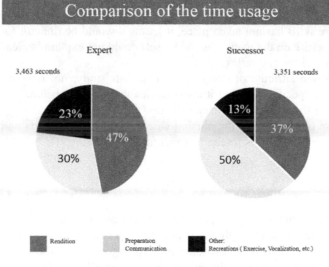

Fig. 7. Comparison in usage of time

Table 3. Participation rate after the transfer

Participation Rate

	No. of times	Participation rate for every event
Recreation within 40 facilities	7680	48.8%
Recreation in the facility where the expert is deployed	216	54.4%
Music recreation within 40 facilities	1923	63.2%
Music recreation by the Expert	24	88.2%
Music recreation by the Non Expert	9	80.9%

4 Discussion

Transfer of expertise. Explicit knowledge like improving performance through optimization in the usage of time is comparably easier to attain because there are exact representation for every unit of time. However, tacit knowledge which is learned through experience is comparable to a very complicated formula, whereas sometimes the expert himself experiencing difficulty in articulating the knowledge in words, thus difficult to share with others.

As there were visual reference, devising a technique on the effective use of time seemed it will not require enormous effort to get solved, however, we feel that, if mapping of core skills has not taken place, it seems it would be difficult for the expert to share her expertise on the matter, as she herself could not explain in clear details the specifics of her actions and reflex.

By defining the attribute of every skill, as in this study, not only it reveals the foundation of the specific skill, but it also clarifies the rationale behind the need for a particular skill in the whole performance process.

As there are other fields in the nursing care needing more experts and specialist, more of the same kind of this research is recommended.

5   Conclusion

This study also implies that good performance depends on the preparation and utilization of the core skills. Through the mapping of the core skill, as well as being able to define the attribute of each skill, requirements for a good music therapy performance had been made clear not only to the successor, but as well as to the expert herself.

References

Yamamoto, A., et al.: The transfer of expertise in conducting a participatory music therapy during a combined rehabilitation-recreational program in an elderly facility. In: Duffy, V.G. (ed.) DHM 2015, Part II. LNCS, vol. 9185, pp. 500–511. Springer, Switzerland (2015)

Yamamoto, A., et al.: Research of work climate at nursing home - from job separation and management capability point. In: Duffy, V.G. (ed.) DHM 2015, Part II. LNCS, vol. 9185, pp. 512–523. Springer, Switzerland (2015)

Gitomer, D.H.: Individual differences in technical troubleshooting. Hum. Perform. **1**(2), 111–131 (1988)

Kuwahara, K.: Kaigo Roujin Hoken Shisetsu ni okeru Ongaku Ryouhou to Ongaku wo Riyou Shita Rikuriesyon (2001). (in Japanese)

Mori, K.: Gijutsu•Ginou denshou no tame no ginou bunseki to manyuaru kousei no Houhou (2001)

Watanabe, T.: Chihousei koureisha ni tai suru ongaku ryouhou ni kansuru systematic review. Aichi Kyouiku Daigaku Kenkyuu Houkoku 54, pp. 57–61 (2005). (in Japanese)

Hinds, P.J.: Bothered by abstraction: the effect of expertise in knowledge transfer and subsequent novice performance. J. Appl. Psychol. **86**, 1232–1243 (2001)

Glaser, B., Strauss A.: The discovery of grounded theory: strategies for qualitative research. Aldine Transaction (1967)

Videophone Conversation of Two Individuals with Dementia Using an Anime Agent System

Kiyoshi Yasuda[1,2(✉)], Masao Fuketa[3], Kazuhiro Morita[3],
Jyun-ich Aoe[3], and Noriaki Kuwahara[4]

[1] Department of Rehabilitation, Chiba Rosai Hospital Tatsumidai-Higashi 2-16,
Ichiharasi 290-0003, Japan
fwkk5911@mb.infoweb.ne.jp
[2] Augumented Community AID Research Center,
Kyoto Institute of Technology, Kyoto, Japan
[3] Faculty of Engineering, University of Tokushima, Tokushima, Japan
{fuketa,kam,aoe}@is.tokushima-u.ac.jp
[4] Graduate School of Engineering and Science,
Kyoto Institute of Technology, Kyoto, Japan
nkuwahar@kit.ac.jp

Abstract. We reported that videophone conversation was effective in increasing psychological stability of individuals with dementia. We als developed an anime agent system to serve as a conversation partner for individuals with dementia. The computer screen showed an animated face resembling "a 5-year-old grandchild". The agent was programmed to ask any of 120 pre-set reminiscence questions, automatically detect the ends of replies, and follow with new questions. In the third experiment, the remote multi-party conversation system Skype™ was integrated with the agent system. The agent participated as a presenter of conversation topics for the multi-party interaction. Three pairs conversed under two conditions: conversation of two subjects and a chairperson (human condition) and conversation in which the agent participated as a topic presenter to the above groups (agent condition). The quality of the conversation was scored by three evaluators. The average score of the evaluation was 3.9 (78 %) in the agent condition and 4.9 (100 %) in the human condition. With further improvement of this agent system, it will become practical as a topic presenter for multi-party conversation of individuals with dementia.

Keywords: Agent · Dementia · Conversation · Videophone · Intervention

1 Introduction

The progression of dementia often begins with amnesia and involves behavioral disturbances such as agitation and incontinence [1]. To reduce the stress of individuals with dementia and the burden on their caregivers, various therapeutic approaches have been proposed, such as validation and music therapy [2]. Reminiscence intervention aims to increase self-esteem and psychosocial well-being [3] and to decrease behavioral disturbances [4]. A conversation is a common and enjoyable activity for most individuals [5]. Individuals with dementia, however, tend to be isolated, with few

© Springer International Publishing Switzerland 2016
V.G. Duffy (Ed.): DHM 2016, LNCS 9745, pp. 317–326, 2016.
DOI: 10.1007/978-3-319-40247-5_32

opportunities to converse [5]. Therefore, providing them with opportunities to converse with people is an important intervention. As the number of individuals with dementia is rapidly increasing, it is becoming difficult to find sufficient numbers of talking partners. In the last decades, many talking dolls and toys for the elderly have become available in the market. Recently, several talking robots have been developed.

One such alternative intervention is conversation with animated agents on a computer screen. Previous studies have investigated the acceptance of such agents by the elderly. They suggested that it was important for the agents to display social signals such as smiling and head nods [6–8]. Sakai et al. [9] developed a computer agent system that could serve as a talking partner for individuals with dementia in clinical settings such as hospitals and clinics. The results revealed that all the individuals with dementia replied and were satisfied with the conversation with the agent. However, the above agent systems could not conduct long conversations such as a 30-min reminiscence or review of life [10]. Short conversations may not be enough to satisfy and stabilize individuals with dementia. To conduct long conversations, we have developed another computer agent system for individuals with dementia [11, 12]. We evaluated the efficacy of this agent system in the three experiments discussed below.

2   An Anime Agent System for Conversation of Individuals with Dementia (Yasuda et al. 2013)

In our agent system [11, 12], the computer screen shows an animated face of a child agent resembling "a 5-year-old grandchild". When the subject speaks, the agent reacts to them, automatically showing nods, mouth movements, and acknowledgement.

2.1   Methods

We prepared eight categorical sets of approximately 15 (total 120) reminiscence questions, such as those about parents, hometowns, and school life. These were spoken

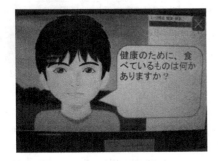 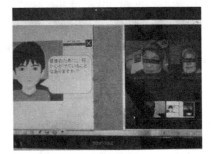

Fig. 1. Face of the anime agent. Note. The agent is asking: What are you eating for your health?

Fig. 2. Multi-party conversation in the agent condition. Note. Agent is on the left. The upper right shows two subjects. The lower right is the chairperson.

aloud through the synthesized voice of the agent. In the preliminary trial, the continual questioning of the agent yielded an atmosphere like "a police interrogation". To improve this atmosphere, each question was composed of two parts. The first was composed of introductory comments by the agent. The agent introduced his own reminiscences, e.g., "I used to eat watermelon in the summer". The second part was a question for the subjects, e.g., "what kind of fruits do you like?" Introductory comments and questions were also shown in the written form on the screen for the visual confirmation of questions and compensation for hearing difficulty (Fig. 1).

According to the results of Sakai et al. [9], the waiting time was very important for smooth conversation with this type of agent system. Because of the analysis of Sakai et al. [9], the wait time was set to 3.5 s for this experiment. If speech sounds were not detected during the 3.5 s waiting time, the agent moved to the next question.

Eight subjects with mild Alzheimer's disease participated in the first experiment. The average age was 78.5 years, and the mean Mini-Mental State Examination (MMSE) [13] score was 22.2. To evaluate the effectiveness of this system, subjects replied to questions by the agent (agent condition) and by a chairperson (human condition). In both conditions, almost the same 15 questions were asked. Each conversation took approximately 20 min.

2.2 Results and Discussion

Recently, several robots and smart phones have speech recognition systems installed to enable them to converse with people. However, the robustness of such systems for speech recognition remains unstable. Furthermore, elderly individuals do not always speak clearly. Because robustness is quite important for the practical use of this system, we employed a sound-detection system.

In this experiment, the syllable number in the subjects' replies was calculated for the two conditions. The subjects uttered a total of 5494 (74 %) syllables in the agent condition compared with 7406 (100 %) syllables in the human condition. Although the number of syllables was lesser in the agent condition, the system could elicit 74 % syllables from subjects with dementia. This percentage means that this system may become a valuable alternative method to elicit conversation when no human conversation partner exists.

The interview after the experiment was very impressive. A female subject was moved to tears while conversing with the agent because it was "so enjoyable for" her. This suggests that she may have felt the agent was a real boy. Another male subject said "With this system, I can speak freely without any hesitation or anxiety." Conversations with normal people were stressful to him because of their difficult questions, to which he could not reply. Therefore, we consider that this type of artificial conversation system is required to provide enough chances to speak without hesitation and worry for subjects like him.

3   Multi-party Conversation Between the Agent and Two Subjects (Yasuda et al. 2014)

The number of individuals with dementia is increasing. Because of the shortage of talking partners, even one-(agent)-to-one-(individual with dementia) conversations such as those in experiment 1 are becoming difficult. Therefore, a one-(agent)-to-multi-party conversation will be required. In our second experiment, we performed a multi-party conversation between the agent and two subjects with mild dementia [14].

3.1   Methods

Five pairs (10 subjects in total) conversed with the agent (agent condition) or without it (human condition). Their average age was 75.9 years, and their mean MMSE score was 24. In the human condition, they spoke freely with each other for 10 min. In the agent condition, the agent participated with each pair as a topic presenter. One categorical set, namely *health and disease*, was selected from among eight categorical sets of reminiscence questions. This category includes 12 questions (see the Appendix). This waiting time was fixed to 3.5 s, as in experiment 1. If the conversation in each pair stopped or speech sounds were not detected during the waiting time, the agent uttered the next question. After the question, they talked freely. The 10 conversations (five pairs × two conditions) were videotaped. We evaluated the influence of the agent participation on the quality of their conversation using original five-scale ratings in five categories (Table 3). In this evaluation, higher scores mean better-quality conversation.

3.2   Results and Discussion

The three evaluators scored the quality of the 10 conversations independently. The total average score was 2.7 (77 %) for the agent conditions and 3.54 (100 %) for the human conditions. Among the five categories, the average score for the category *Flow of conversation* was the worst in the agent condition. The 3.5 s waiting time was too short: the agent often interrupted the speech flow of subjects. On the other hand, this agent system succeeded in raising the interactivity of conversation; in other words, it prevented monopolization by one subject. One participant said "This agent was good at providing topics for the conversation". Although further improvements are required, this system will be practical as a presenter of topics.

4   Videophone Conversation of Two Subjects with the Participation of an Anime Agent System

Over the last decade, videophone conversations have been proposed for the assistance of individuals with dementia [15]. Kuwahara et al. [16] and Yasuda et al. [17] demonstrated that a combination of videophones and reminiscence interventions was more effective for psychological stability. Some subjects remained psychologically stable for more than 3 h after the conversation session ended [16, 17]. The number of people with dementia is increasing. Because of the deficit of talking partners, even agent-to-multi party conversations [14] such as those in experiment 2 will become difficult in the future. Therefore, an agent-to-multi-party conversation via a videophone will be required. To determine the effectiveness of anime agent participation in remote conversation, we created two types of multi-party conversation for our third experiment.

One is conversation between the two subjects and a chairperson (human condition). In the other conversation, the agent participated as a topic presenter for the above groups (agent condition). By evaluating the quality of these conversations, we discussed the effectiveness of agent participation in multi-party conversations via a videophone and necessary revisions for further improvement.

4.1   Methods

Subjects. The participants were six subjects with mild and moderate dementia. Their average age was 75.0 years, and their mean MMSE score was 19.4. They were classified into three pairs (Table 1).

Table 1. The Participants

Pairs	Subjects	Sex	Age	MMSE	Etiology
A	Ik	f	78	21	Alz
	Mu	f	78	19	Alz
B	Ok	m	82	24	Alz
	Mu	m	77	20	VD
C	Sh	f	61	14	Alz
	Fu	f	74	20	Alz
	Mean		*75.0*	*19.4*	

Note. Alz, Alzheimer's dementia VD, Vascular
Dementia MMSE, Mini-Mental State
Examination

Procedure. A volunteer engineer set up hardware such as a PC and a webcam in the home of each subject. The engineer connected the PCs to the Internet via fiber optic cables. Skype™ was set up so that it automatically launched when a chairperson (a speech-language pathologist, one of authors of this study) clicked the subject's Skype™ name. The caregivers were asked not to turn off or unplug the PC. Recently, Skype™ has acquired the capability to conduct a multi-party videophone conversation with up to 10 persons simultaneously without charge (Fig. 2).

Each pair conversed in the following two conditions: conversation between two subjects and a chairperson with the participation of an agent on the PC monitor (agent condition) and conversation without the agent (human condition). The order of the two conditions was randomized. In both conditions, one categorical set, namely *health and diseases*, was used. The 12 questions used were the same as those in experiment 2 (see the Appendix). The supposed age of the agent was 5 years. The chairperson's age was 62 years. Therefore, the introductory comments were slightly modified to suit the age of the speaker (see the Appendix).

In experiment 2, the main waiting times were set to 3.5 s, which interrupted the flow of the conversations. Because two subjects and a chairperson talked in this experiment, the main waiting time was extended to 10 s. These six conversations (three pairs × two conditions) were videotaped for the following evaluation.

In both conditions, the chairperson encouraged the subjects when another subject did not reply or when their replies were short, with the following prompts: "Mr./Ms. _, let's talk now," or "Mr./Ms. _, let's talk about it in detail".

We evaluated the effectiveness of these conversations using a psychological five-point scale rating (Table 3) with three evaluators. They independently evaluated the quality of these six conversation videos in random order. Three evaluators, with an average age of 70 years, were talking volunteers for elderly patients at a hospital.

4.2 Results

The average conversation time was 13.72 min for the agent condition and 12.28 min for the human condition. Table 2 shows the average quality scores for the six conversations by the three evaluators. A higher score means better conversation quality. The total average score was 3.9 (72 %) for the agent condition and 4.9 (100 %) for the human condition.

Table 2. Average scores by three evaluators

Pair	Human	Agent
Pair A		
Naturalness of conversation	4.3	3.3
Liveliness of conversation	4.3	3.7
Flow of conversation	4.3	3.3
Interactivity of conversation	4.7	3.6
Mean	*5.9*	*4.6*
Pair B		
Naturalness of conversation	4	3.7
Liveliness of conversation	4	3.3
Flow of conversation	4	3.3
Interactivity of conversation	4	4
Mean	*4*	*3.6*
Pair C		
Naturalness of conversation	5	3.3
Liveliness of conversation	5	3.7
Flow of conversation	4.7	3.7
Interactivity of conversation	4.3	3.7
Mean	*4.8*	*3.6*
Total average	*4.9*	*3.9*

Note. Another: encourage another subject to talk; more: encourage subject to explain more.

The number of times the chairperson encouraged another subject to talk or to explain more was calculated. The total number of encouragements was 47 for the agent condition and 38 for the human condition. The number of encouragements by the chairperson, particularly encouragements for another subject to talk, was greater in the agent condition than in the human condition (Table 3).

Table 3. Number of encouragements for subjects

		Human		Agent	
		another	more	another	more
Pair	A	5	8	16	6
	B	10	3	6	6
	C	4	8	12	1
Subtotal		19	19	34	13
Total		38		47	

Observations by evaluators. In the agent conditions, some subjects unconsciously made noises such as table tapping. The computer of one subject emitted an electronic whine. These events prevented the agent system from uttering the next question. Direct conversation between subjects did not occur, except in the human condition of pair C. In pair C, the two subjects asked questions to each other and cracked jokes. In most cases, the turns to reply was naturally fixed. Some subjects did not start replying until the chairperson urged them, in both conditions.

4.3   Discussion

The videophone is an appropriate communication tool for individuals with dementia to understand what is said in a conversation with gestures and body language. Some individuals were even stable for more than 3 h after the end of a videophone conversation session [16, 17]. Insufficient communication was considered to be a cause of stress, worry, or instability, which may have been reduced by the videophone conversation. These studies suggest that conversation itself has the potential to prevent individuals with dementia from showing anticipated behavioral disturbances such as "evening syndrome" [16, 17].

However, the number of individuals with dementia is rapidly increasing; it is very difficult for them to engage in conversation at all times. Frequent and regular videophone conversation is becoming difficult to perform. As a possible resolution of these situations, we incorporated an agent as topic presenter in the videophone conversation. Although a prototype has been proposed [8], this is the first clinical trial of the participation of an agent in a videophone conversation.

We observed a multi-party conversation with an agent (agent condition) and without an agent (human condition). The time required to conduct these conversations was almost the same. However, conversations in this experiment were, strictly speaking, not normal conversations. The topics of the conversations were preset. Flexible reactive comments to the replies of subjects were impossible in the agent conditions (system) and were restrained by the chairperson in the human conditions to balance the conversation style in the two conditions. Although these operational procedures prevent intrinsic comparison on the quality of conversations between two conditions, all average scores of the quality of conversations were better in the human conditions. However, the percentage of the scores was 72 % for the agent condition compared with 100 % for the human condition. We consider that this percentage means it is worth applying this system in supporting group conversations via a videophone.

From the number of encouragements, conversations in the agent conditions seemed to need more prompts, particularly encouragements for another subject to talk, than those in the human conditions. In the agent conditions, some subjects may have felt hesitation from speaking at will. In future revisions, encouraging words should be used to prompt more reserved participants to talk, such as "how about another person?" as well as "please explain in detail".

Direct conversation between subjects occurred naturally in the human condition of pair C. To compensate the technical insufficiency of the agent system, direct talking between participating subjects should be augmented by prompts such as "Let's talk to each other". Furthermore, to increase the benefit of the agent system or of ICT interventions, use of various internet resources such as pictures, music, and short movies will be greatly beneficial.

Smooth transfer to the next question was sometimes disturbed by the subject's unconscious noises and electronic whines. Although this system may work well under quiet circumstances, some methods of coping are required in these cases, such as a forced transfer function to next question. Future revision will incorporate the above prompts and functions in the agent system to increase the usability of this system.

Most individuals with mild or moderate dementia still have the ability to talk to each other. They also say that "I would like to make a social contribution, even though I have dementia". Talking volunteers are one of the few remaining employments for them. Indeed, they are even more suited to be talking volunteers for other individuals with dementia. They easily forget what has been already said; therefore, they are not annoyed by repetition by other individuals with dementia. However, it is often difficult to recollect topics because of their degraded recall abilities. This agent system can work as a topic-providing system for them. Most families in advanced nations have computers and access to the internet. Younger seniors with dementia who are accustomed with the operation of PCs and smart phone are increasing. The operation of SkypeTM will not be difficult for such individuals.

In this field study, the quality of conversation was based on the evaluator's impressions. In the future, the use of artificial intelligence tools such as facial expression analysis and laughing voices analysis is desirable for the objective proof of efficient and enjoyable conversation. Procedural limitations and the small number of subjects require caution in the interpretation of the results in this experiment. However, agent participation in multi-party videophone conversations showed the possibility of supporting individuals with dementia.

4.4 Conclusion

An anime agent participated in multi-party videophone conversations as a conversation topic presenter. Although further improvements are required, this agent system may become a promising intervention for assisted conversation of individuals with dementia.

Acknowledgments. The authors wish to thank the cooperation of the six subjects and their caregivers, the three evaluators, Hachiro Kiyoto, and Shingo Aoe.

A Appendix: List of Questions

The underlined are introductory comments. In the human condition, the words before the parentheses were changed with the words within them.

My father (I) has (have) back pain. Do you have any chronic pain?

My older sister (I) eats (eat) fruit (yogurt) every morning for maintaining health. What are you eating for health?

Last night, I had a dream in which I was flying in the sky. Do you have dreams while you are sleeping?

I am going to bed as early as possible for my health. Are you doing anything to maintain your health?

My father (I) is (am) wearing eyeglasses. How is the condition of your eyes?

I am enjoying vigorous health (I go to swimming once a week). My mother says not to run indoors. How is your health recently?

My grandmamma (I) is (am) taking medicine to reduce high blood pressure. Is your blood pressure high?

Usually, I go to bed at nine o'clock. What time do you go to bed?

My father (I) smokes (smoke) a cigarette after supper. Do you smoke?

I was hospitalized due to bone fracture. Have you been hospitalized?

Recently, I fell and cut my knee. Have you have experienced serious disease or injuries?

If I had a lot of money, I would like to go traveling. What would you want to do if you were 30 years younger?

References

1. Davis, R.N., Massman, P.J., Doody, R.S.: Cognitive intervention in Alzheimer disease: A randomised placebo-controlled study. Alzheimer Dis. Assoc. Disord. **15**, 1–9 (2001)
2. De Vreese, L.P., Neri, M., Fioravanti, M., Belloi, L., Zanetti, O.: Memory rehabilitation in Alzheimer's disease: A review of progress. Int. J. Geriatr. Psychiatry **16**, 794–809 (2001)
3. Lai, C.K., Chi, I., Kayser-Jones, J.: A randomised controlled trial of a specific reminiscence approach to promote the well-being of nursing home residents with dementia. Int. Psychogeriatr. **16**, 33–49 (2004)
4. Finnema, E., Droes, R.M., Ribbe, M., Van, W.: The effects of emotion-oriented approaches in the care for persons suffering from dementia: A review of the literature. Int. J. Geriatr. Psychiatry **15**, 141–161 (2000)
5. Yasuda, K., Kuwabara, K., Kuwahara, N., Abe, S., Tetsutani, N.: Effectiveness of personalised reminiscence photo videos for individuals with dementia. Neuropsychological Rehabil. **19**, 603–619 (2009)
6. Cassll, J.: Embodied conversational agents. In: Cassell, J., Sullivan, J., Prevost, S., Churchill, E. (eds.) EC Agents, pp. 1–27. The MIT Press, Cambridge (2000)
7. Heerink, M., Krose, B., Evers, V., Wielinga, B.: Studying the acceptance of a robotic agent by elderly users. Int. J. ARM **7**, 33–43 (2006)
8. Smith, C., Crook, N., Boye, J., Charlton, D., Dobnik, S., Pizzi, D., Cavazza, M., Pulman, S., de la Camara, R.S., Turunen, M.: Interaction strategies for an affective conversational agent. In: Safonova, A. (ed.) IVA 2010. LNCS, vol. 6356, pp. 301–314. Springer, Heidelberg (2010)
9. Sakai, Y., Nonaka, Y., Yasuda, K., Nakano, Y.: Listener agent for elderly people with dementia. In: Proceedings of the Seventh annual ACM/IEEE International Conference on Human-Robot Interaction (HRI2012), pp. 199–200 (2012)
10. Butler, R., Butler, N.: Successful aging and the role of the life review. J. Am. Geriatr. Soc. **22**, 529–535 (1974)
11. Yasuda, K., Aoe, J., Fuketa, M.: Development of an agent system for conversing with individuals with dementia. In: The 27th Annual Conference of the Japanese Society for Artificial Intelligence (2013). https://kaigi.org/jsai/webprogram/2013/pdf/979.pdf
12. Fuketa, M., Morita, K., Aoe, J.: Agent-based communication system for elders using a reminiscence therapy. Int. J. Intell. Syst. Technol. Appl. **12**, 3–4 (2013). doi:10.1504/IJISTA.2013.056533
13. Folstein, M.F., Folstein, S.E., McHugh, P.R.: "mini-mental state": A practical method for grading the cognitive state of patients for the clinician. J. Psychiatr. Res. **12**, 189–198 (1975)
14. Yasuda, K., Fuketa, M., Aoe, J.: An anime agent system for reminiscence therapy. Gerontechnlogy **13**, 118–119 (2014)
15. Sävenstedt, S., Brulin, C., Sandman, P.O.: Family members' narrated experiences of communicating via video-phone with patients with dementia staying at a nursing home. J. Telemedicine Telecare **9**, 216–220 (2003)
16. Kuwahara, N., Yasuda, K., Tetsutani, N., Morimoto, K.: Remote assistance for people with dementia at home using reminiscence systems and a schedule prompter. Int. J. Comput. Healthc. **1**, 126–143 (2010)
17. Yasuda, K., Kuwahara, N., Kuwabara, K., Morimoto, K., Tetsutani, N.: Daily assistance for individuals with dementia via videophone. Am. J. Alzheimer's Dis. Other Dementias **28**, 508–516 (2013)

Design for Health

MEDEDUC:
An Educational Medical Serious Game

Vitor Manuel Fragoso Ferreira, Rosa Maria E. Moreira da Costa[✉],
and Vera M.B. Werneck

Universidade do Estado do Rio de Janeiro – UERJ,
Instituto de Matemática e Estatística –IME,
Mestrado em Ciências Computacionais,
Rua São Francisco Xavier 524-6° andar – Bl. B, Rio de Janeiro
RJ 20550-013, Brazil
vitor@fragoso.me,
{rcosta,vera}@ime.uerj.br

Abstract. In general, serious games motivate people from all ages and have been applied in many areas to stimulate the learning processes. However, the adoption of specific methodologies to construct these games is still rare. This paper aims at presenting an experiment that applied an agile methodology to develop the MEDEDUC. It is a multi-agent game to improve learning and clinical performance of students from the health care area. This game allows the student to learn pulmonology by answering questions, in five levels of difficulty and exploring multimedia presentations. MEDEDUC was developed using SCRUM agile methodology and the results stressed some difficulties associated to the adoption of this agile methodology.

Keywords: Multi-agents systems · Scrum methodology · Agile methodologies · Medical serious games

1 Introduction

Serious games provide a problem situation environment [5] and there is a potentially effective use of games for medicine students; however there are a limited number of studies [2].

Multi-agent systems (MAS) are composed of autonomous modules that perform activities and communicate with each other in order to achieve a common goal. The construction of multi-agent systems involves different characteristics from those employed in traditional software development. According to Jubilson [8], the conception, design and implementation of such systems that operate in distributed environments, must consider new development process perspectives.

Some agent-oriented methods have been proposed for building MAS but there is no consensus about the best one that must be applied in MAS development [12]. In general, these methodologies are complex to use, the time consuming is high and generate a great number of diagrams and documentation. In addition, these processes have not been able to reach the desired flexibility.

© Springer International Publishing Switzerland 2016
V.G. Duffy (Ed.): DHM 2016, LNCS 9745, pp. 329–337, 2016.
DOI: 10.1007/978-3-319-40247-5_33

To overcome these problems in the MEDEDUC development process we considered concepts of agile methodologies such SCRUM. This methodology improves software production focusing on customers' requirements, frequent deliveries, daily meetings, review meetings and retrospective meetings.

The Agile SCRUM [10] proved to be able to deliver a final product with better requirements; the modules were completed and presented to clients' review with a short iterations period. In addition, the development team is always ready to include all the desired requirements and improve the game.

The MEDEDUC game focuses on the pulmonology area by letting the student answer questions with different levels of difficulty. The questions present images, sounds and videos to enrich the communication and the learning process.

The game starts testing the students' previous knowledge to direct him to the respective game level. If the game identifies that the student is having a high number of errors a basic knowledge module will be active by the intelligent agents. The student is rewarded when each module ends with success. The awards are medical equipments which compose the student virtual office such as stethoscope, x-ray machine, computer or others. At the end of the game, the student will have his office set up. The intelligent interactive interface opens new possibilities to have fun in the learning process and to keep the student involved into the game activities.

The relevance of this study is based on the lack of experiments that integrate, in a practical way, issues such as multi-agent systems, medical educational games and agile methodologies.

2 Serious Games

According to Blackman [4], serious games compose a special category of games that complement a fun activity with specific content.

Serious games in Educational area promote a competitive universe with pre-established rules [7]. The playful and challenging approaches motivate users to accomplish tasks.

Specifically, in the health care area, the serious games offer a great potential to improve the clinical performance of medical students. In this case, they can transfer the game situations to real life. Several studies have suggested beneficial effects in the use of educational games in health and education [13]. In this context, we have some examples of success.

Abreu et al. [1] created a multi-agent 3-D serious game to stimulate cognitive functions of people with different disabilities due to trauma or brain accident. Scarle et al. [9] developed the Match-3 serious game that was designed to combat childhood obesity using the Wii-system. Atkinson and Narasimhan [3] created a medical gaming environment for diagnosis and management of Parkinson's disease using a haptic interface.

When these products are created we must consider some aspects related to costs, time and effort required for their development. The adoption of a software development methodology can aid to avoid some of problems related to those items.

Next we present the SCRUM methodology which considers a dynamic process to create software.

3 SCRUM Methodology

Scrum [11] is an agile development methodology with incremental and iterative processes that has good management practices set providing quick adjustments, monitoring, constant visibility and realistic plans.

The Scrum development process iterations are called sprints, which should last two to four weeks. This time aims at promoting greater visibility throughout the development process by the possibility to delivery small functionalities system with features being validated with the customer and, if necessary, modified promptly to avoid waste of work. The team, as far as possible, should be kept in the constant size, allowing the collected metric and estimates become efficiently [11].

Scrum is an open model and is not predictable [10]. In general, we can identify some important points: (i) self-organizing teams; (ii) development progress through sprints, sprint being a Scrum development cycle, characterized by a short period, where the team focus to achieve a specific goal; (iii) Requirements of products organized in a list of items called Product Backlog; (iv) Closed concept of time (Timeboxed) that are all tasks within the Scrum having maximum time set for its implementation and must not supplant these times [11].

The customer is close to the process and becomes almost part of the team, indicating how they want their product and how it should be output. Their stories are told and requirements appear spontaneously.

The sprint is divided into stages, the planning meeting (Sprint Planning) is the first stage, where the team (Scrum Team) together with the customer (represented by the product owner), define what will be developed and implemented in the iteration, creating the Product Backlog. The Product Backlog (Sprint Backlog) is a list containing the business features, technical requirements and the errors found in the system, that need to be developed or improved. This list is in constant evolution, because new business requirements can appear and also the software must be maintained or re-factored. Each increment of the Product Backlog must be implemented during the Sprint.

The Product Owner role has the responsibility of maintaining the list of priorities and shows the prospects of the project to the team. A Scrum challenge is to keep an organized Project Backlog, either with the priorities or with respect to the complexity necessary for the stories fulfillment.

After prioritizing the Project Backlog items, the details of the software are described by creating stories and tasks necessary for the Sprint development. The story is the element that describes a feature, an improvement or correction to be implemented, indicating what will be developed and how it will be done.

In Scrum there are tasks follow-up meetings of each Sprint [11]. For this, there must be a plan that should contain the goal, team members, the Sprint itself, the date and time of presentation of the Sprint.

During the Sprint the team performs Daily Meeting, that should not take more than 15 min, and they aims at investigating the development progress using for this the Burn-down Chart which is a graph used for tasks monitoring in progress and finished.

In the whiteboard, the goals and requirements are written on Post-it notes and are placed in order of their priority. They are then allocated to the phase in which its implementation is: not started, in progress or completed. Their team members change the status of each requirement in the frame. In this white board, too, is the Burn-down Chart, which is a graph showing the progress of work.

At the end of Sprint are held two other meetings, one for the delivery validation (Sprint Review) where the customer and others who are interested in the product can verify if the sprint goal was achieved. After, sprint retrospective meeting is performed only by the staff, evaluating the Sprint in the process perspective, team or product, noting the successes and mistakes in order to improve the work process for the next Sprints.

In addition to the Sprint planning meeting, the Scrum addresses other follow-up meetings of the processes, such as: (i) Sprint Review that is the presentation of the increases made at the end of each Sprint Backlog; (ii) Daily Scrum which is tracking and monitoring processes; (iii) Retrospective Meetings which is the reflection of what has passed and planning of actions to be taken to achieve the objectives; (iv) FUP Meeting which is the detailing and elucidations concerning requirements; (v) Re-Estimate Meetings which is an application of techniques such as Poker Planning for estimating requirements; (vi) Sprint Planning 2 which is the discussion of technical aspects, such as product architecture, component reuse, etc.

There are different roles in Scrum: Scrum Master, Product Owner and Team (team working on processes). The Scrum Master is responsible for facilitating the work, by helping the team to solve problems and difficulties during the sprints and by disseminating and applying the process in the organization. The Product Owner has the function of representing the interests of all involved in the process (stakeholders), defining the product features and prioritizing items in the Product Backlog. The Product Owner is responsible for creating a guideline for the Sprint Planning.

The Scrum team should be multidisciplinary, self-organized and small with a maximum of 10 to 15 participants. The team should be also independent and have control over the development process, and the responsibility, at the end of each sprint, to present the results of the work for the customer.

Scrum features are: (i) Customers become part of the development team; (ii) transparency in the planning and development; (iii) frequent meetings with stakeholders (all involved in the process) to monitor progress; (iv) problems are not "left out" and no one is penalized for recognize or describe any unseen problem; (v) working hours should be optimized in the sense that "overtime" does not necessarily mean "produce more"; (vi) Teamwork is critical to the success of the process.

4   MEDEDUC: A Medical Serious Game

MEDEDUC is a medical educational game developed to support Medical students by teaching concepts of Pulmonology, combining fun and learning.

The students must answer questions organized in difficulty levels and are rewarded at end of each module. This award is medical equipment such as stethoscope, x-ray machine, computer or others, and this award will compose his/her virtual office. By the end of the game (fifth level), the student will have his/her office set up.

A test is performed to verify the student previous knowledge, thus the game can directed the student to the respective level of knowledge. During the game if the student is having a high number of errors, he/she will have to learn basic subjects related to the active module. The interactive, fun and intelligent environment are fundamental to keep the student involved into the game activities.

The MEDEDUC has 110 questions with three answer options for each, divided into 5 knowledge levels (Fig. 1) and the Reinforcement Level.

The basic requirements for the game are: (i) each module will be available to the user gradually, according to his/her progress in the game; (ii) the user should be informed when the result of a module is positive or negative; (iii) the higher the level, the greater the complexity assigned to each question [6].

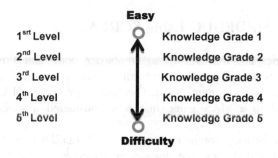

Fig. 1. Knowledge grade by level

The game behavior requirements for Level and Reinforcement modules are: "(i) the questions explore audio, video, images and text items; (ii) Each question has three response options (A, B and C); (iii) When selecting an incorrect option, the user must be informed of the correct option; (iv) When selecting an incorrect option, the user must receive a return with a justification reporting why the chosen option is incorrect. (v) Upon entering the game for the first time, you must perform the Leveling and other features will be unavailable; (vi) During the Leveling, the user must answer 10 questions related to five levels. For each level, there are two questions distributed randomly; (vii) When the user hit a question, a green indicator in the status bar should be shown. For errors, the user sees a red indicator. (viii) By clicking on the indicative position of each question on the status bar, the user should be able to review the question, answer and return. However, the user cannot change the selected option; (ix) The user should perform the Level 5, even if it hits all the questions. When the user finish answering the questions of the Leveling, the user should receive a return stating the level reached." [6]. Figure 2 presents a Leveling Module interface.

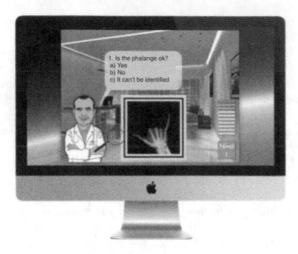

Fig. 2. MEDEDUC level model prototype [6]

5 Developing MEDEDUC Using SCRUM

Agile methodologies are well known to emphasize communication and customer engagement. However, for complex problems, modeling methodologies helps the solution design and team communication. This section presents SCRUM development experience applied to a MAS game that was considered a successful operation prototype.

We needed almost four months to construct the MEDEDUC prototype. The team was composed of five undergraduate students in computer science, a master's student and two research professors. The master student is an expert of agile methodologies and performs the Product Owner role with the support professors that are expert in Multi-agent System development and Virtual Reality games in the health care area. At first a Medicine professor supported the definition of the MEDEDUC requirements as defined in Sect. 3 but this professor did not have the contact with the whole team.

The team has experience in software development processes but never developed MAS. Some of them had already worked constructing games and had theoretical knowledge about Scrum. However, they have a few experiences in real projects. So the first two weeks they attend lectures about agents, MAS and Scrum methodology. After that they present a Sprint Planning of the first sprint. Table 1 shows the Sprint Planning of this step.

For each Sprint, the group and the Product Owner held a meeting, where members of the group summed up the work evolution. This meeting was performed in about two weeks. The team members thought that sometimes the Sprint duration was short of time, especially when they had to developed complex algorithms to represent the agents' behaviors. Another point considered was that the several changes resulted of these review meetings required them to understand and integrate these new functionalities in the system in a short time, to be ready for the next meeting. Figures 3 and 4 show the user interface of MEDEDUC.

Table 1. Sprint planning report

	Artefact	Preview date	Real data	# Days late
1	Report of Product Delivers Sprint 1	22/10/2014	22/10/2014	0
2	Sprint 1 Revision Meeting	04/11/2014	04/11/2014	0
3	Report of Product Delivers Sprint 2	05/11/2014	06/11/2014	1
4	Sprint 2 Revision Meeting	18/11/2014	18/11/2014	0
5	Report of Product Delivers Sprint 3	19/11/2014	19/11/2014	0
6	Sprint 3Revision Meeting	02/12/2014	02/12/2014	0
7	Report of Product Delivers Sprint 4	03/12/2014	03/12/2014	0
8	Sprint 4 Revision Meeting	16/12/2014	16/12/2014	0
9	Report of Product Delivers Sprint 5	17/12/2014	17/12/2014	0
10	Sprint 5 Revision Meeting	13/01/2015	13/01/2015	0
11	Game deliver	19/01/2015	19/01/2015	0
12	Game presentation	22/01/2015	22/01/2015	0

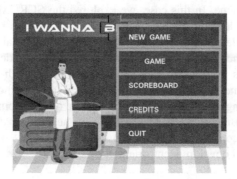

Fig. 3. Main screen

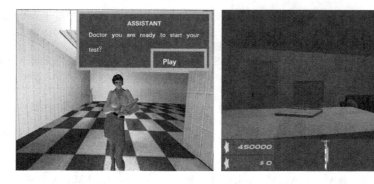

Fig. 4. Game final screens with a character and the office

At the end of the development process, the owner considered that the final product met the proposed requirements.

In Scrum, the client must be all the time available to the team. However, despite this, as this methodology is not specific to work with intelligent agents, we observed some problems to identify and implement agents' features. The lack of models created difficulties for developing the agent architecture. In general, agile methodologies do not consider a high quantity of documentation. Then, to alleviate these problems, the team documented some agents' features to improve the understanding of its functionalities.

Another point observed was that the excess of meetings during the development process can increase the number of client requirements because the client sees the system working and proposes new features to be incorporated in the system. In this case, the system is never considered finished.

6 Conclusions

This paper described the adoption of an agile methodology to develop an agent oriented medical educational game. In this case, we explored the SCRUM agile methodology that is not specific to develop MAS.

By one side, the related experiment tried to verify the potential of this methodology to develop MAS. At the other side, our current researches try to develop serious games to be used by students from health care areas as a learning method.

We identified some fragility in the adoption of this methodology, which can overcome by integrating usual practices imported from other specific methodologies for MAS' development. But, as we had a decrease in the time of development of such complex system, we considered that we can use the SCRUM, which is non specific MAS methodology, to develop agent oriented systems.

References

1. Abreu, P.F., Carvalho, L.A.V., Werneck, V.M.B., Costa, R.M.E.M.: Employing multi-agents in 3D game for cognitive stimulation. In: Proceedings of the XIII Symposium on Virtual and Augmented Reality, Uberlândia, vol. 1 (2011)
2. Akl, E.A., Sackett, K., Pretorius, R., Erdley, S., Bhoopathi, P.S., Mustafa, R., Schunemann, H.J.: Educational games for health professionals. Cochrane Database Syst. Rev. (1), CD006411 (2008)
3. Atkinson, S.D., Narasimhan, V.L.: Design of an introductory medical gaming environment for diagnosis and management of Parkinson's disease. In: Proceedings of the 2nd International Conference on Trendz in Information Sciences and Computing (TISC 2010), pp. 94–102, December 2010
4. Blackman, S.: Serious Games... and Less! Comput. Graph. 39(1), 12–16 (2005). ACM
5. Connolly, T.M., Boyle, E.A., MacArthur, E., Hainey, T., Boyle, J.M.: A systematic literature review of empirical evidence on computer games and serious games. Comput. Educ. 59(2), 661–686 (2012)

6. Ferreira, V.M.F., Carvalho, J.C.C., Werneck, V.M.B., Costa, R.M.E.M.: Developing an educational medical game using AgilePASSI multi-agent methodology. In: IEEE 28th International Symposium on Computer-Based Medical Systems, pp. 298–303 (2015)
7. Janarthanan, V.: Serious video games: games for education and health. In: Proceedings of the 9th International Conference on Information Technology (ITNG 2012), pp. 875–878, April 2012
8. Jubilson, E.A., Joe Prathap, P.M., Vimal Khanna, V., Dhanavanthini, P., Vinil Dani, W., Gunasekaran, A.: An empirical analysis of agent oriented methodologies by exploiting the lifecycle phases of each methodology. In: Satapathy, S.C., Govardhan, A., Srujan Raju, K., Mandal, J.K. (eds.) Emerging ICT for Bridging the Future - Proceedings of the 49th Annual Convention of the Computer Society of India (CSI) Volume 1. AISC, vol. 337, pp. 205–214. Springer, Heidelberg (2015)
9. Scarle, S. et al.: Complete motion control of a serious game against obesity in children. In: Proceedings of the 3rd International Conference on Games and Virtual Worlds for Serious Applications (VS-Games 2011), pp. 178–179, May 2011
10. Schwaber, K.: Agile Project Management with Scrum. Microsoft Press, Redmond (2004). ISBN: 978-0-7356-1993-7
11. Schwaber, K.: Scrum Guide (2009). http://www.trainning.com.br/download/GUIA_DO_SCRUM.pdf. visited in 2016 (in Portuguese)
12. Shehory, O., Sturm, A.: A brief introduction to agents. In: Shehory, O., Sturm, A. (eds.) Agent-Oriented Software Engineering, pp. 3–11. Springer, Heidelberg (2014)
13. Wattanasoontorn, V., Hernandez, R.J.G., Sbert, M.: Serious games for e-health care. In: Cai, Y., Goei, S.L. (eds.) Simulations, Serious Games and Their Applications. Gaming Media and Social Effects, pp. 127–146. Springer, Singapore (2014)

Analysis of CS Survey and NPS Numbers in Japanese Wedding Market

Shigeyuki Takami[1(✉)], Nobuyuki Kitada[2], and Tomoko Ota[3]

[1] Takami Bridal Co., Ltd., Kyoto, Japan
shigeyuki@takami-bridal.com
[2] Kyoto Institute of Technology, Kyoto, Japan
kida@kit.ac.jp
[3] Chuo Business Group Co., Ltd., Osaka, Japan
promotl@gold.ocn.ne.jp

Abstract. Wedding market in Japan is about 3 trillion yen conjunction with marriage costs and new life preparation costs, and the number of marriage couples is estimated to be approximately 650,000 pairs. Domestic population is in the medium- and middle-long term downwards due to the declining birth rate. It has been presumed that there is also decreasing number of marriages, compare to this number, the implementation rate of the wedding reception is about 50 %. It can be recognized as the wedding market still has a certain amount of potential market. Against a backdrop of this, it is essentially to be impressed the "customer", satisfied more than what they expected. Far beyond that, the most important thing is made them influencers to dig up potential customers. Wedding reception is not only goods itself, because it is the market that is selling the services too, and to survey on the CS (Customer Satisfaction) through survey after the enforcement wedding reception is estimated to be higher. Thus, the author focused on and decided to study on what products and services to either contribute to the overall CS improvement.

Index that becomes the axis in this study is the NPS (Net Promoter Score).

This is an indication of the investigation method for measuring customer's loyalty proposed by Frederick F. Reichheld. To classify into 3 groups by scores (the range of 0–10) through questions the possibility of recommendation the company (products, services or brands) to friends or colleagues along with the answer.

Among the Fortune 500 ranking of the US sales higher 500 companies in 2014, there are statistics that indeed 35 % of companies adopted with the NPS.

The wedding market as well as others, the important factor is the customer's reviews, word of mouth and word of mouse (through internet). We have given the NPS survey to the customers after wedding reception, with 400 couples at 5 different locations (Tokyo, Nagoya, Kobe, Kyoto and Fukuoka) and also provided the questionnaire in 40 questions about products and services In this paper, the author analyzes relationship between NPS numbers and other 40 questions of the questionnaire, the customer will be revealed by multiple regression analysis.

Keywords: NPS · CS · Marketing mix · Encounter marketing mix

© Springer International Publishing Switzerland 2016
V.G. Duffy (Ed.): DHM 2016, LNCS 9745, pp. 338–344, 2016.
DOI: 10.1007/978-3-319-40247-5_34

1 Introduction

Wedding market in Japan is about 3 trillion yen [1] conjunction with marriage costs and new life preparation costs, and the number of marriage couples is estimated to be approximately 650,000 pairs [2]. Domestic population is in the medium- and middle-long term downwards due to the declining birth rate. It has been presumed that there is also decreasing number of marriages, compare to this number, the implementation rate of the wedding reception is about 50 % [3]. It can be recognized as the wedding market still has a certain amount of potential market. Against a backdrop of this, it is essentially to be impressed the "customer", satisfied more than what they expected. Far beyond that, the most important fact is made them influencers to dig up more potential customers. The marketing researches market of interest has been changed in 2 decades from spending on the expenditure non-durable goods such as food in everyday of life to the services in providing. This means that consumer spends more on "buy goods" to "usage of the service" [4]. Wedding reception is not only goods itself, because it is the market that is selling the services too, and to survey on the CS (Customer Satisfaction) through survey after the enforcement wedding reception is estimated to be higher. Also, especially in the marketing mix, it is said to be important part that is post Encounter marketing mix (after customers received the service) [5, 6], what products and services to customers is to contribute to the overall CS improvement attention is focused, and decided to research.

Index that becomes the axis in this study is the NPS (Net Promoter Score). This is an indication of the investigation method for measuring customer's loyalty proposed by Frederick F. Reichheld. To classify into 3 groups by scores (the range of 0–10) through questions the possibility of recommendation the company (products, services or brands) to friends or colleagues along with the answer.

Among the Fortune 500 ranking of the US sales higher 500 companies in 2014, there are statistics that indeed 35 % of companies adopted with the NPS [7].

The wedding market as well as others, the important factor is the customer's reviews, word of mouth and word of mouse (through internet). We have given the NPS survey to the customers after wedding reception, with 235 couples at 5 different locations (Tokyo, Nagoya, Kobe, Kyoto and Fukuoka) and also provided the questionnaire in 40 questions about products and services to contribute more developing in hospitality industry [8].

In this paper, the author analyzes relationship between NPS numbers and other 40 questions of the questionnaire, the customer will be revealed by multiple regression analysis.

2 Methodology

2.1 Overview of the Experiment

NPS numbers and other 40 questions of NPS numerical value to analyze the relationship with the impact of the post-wedding reception enforcement in order to determine the relevant with categories of 40 questions to evaluate high and low scores at the locations (Tokyo, Nagoya, Kyoto, Fukuoka). Couples of 235 pairs were examined for NPB numbers as the customer's questionnaires, and also another survey for the customers more likely purchased which goods and services related to the 40 questions to examine multiple regression analysis.

2.2   Experiment Method

Using the A3 size of the questionnaire that NPS and 40 questions of Fig. 1 is described, for survey the bride and the groom after the wedding reception in the products and services provided during the reception. The categories will be described in detail in Sect. 2.3.

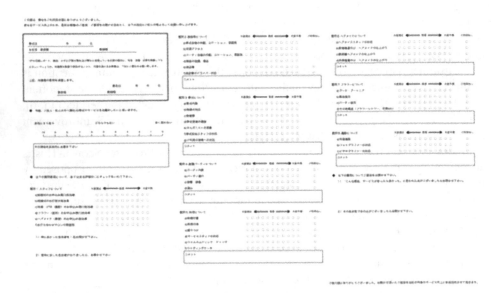

Fig. 1.   NPS and 40 questions of survey

2.3   The Details of the Questionnaire

Question details of the questionnaire data, as a NPS question is "would you recommend your friends and acquaintances to our wedding and services?" And for 40 categories of questionnaires are;

(1) About staff- (1-a) Application contact person in charge of the ceremony and reception, (1-b) meeting contact the person in charge of the ceremony and reception, (1-c) the contact person in charge of tuxedo and wedding dress, (1-d) application contact the person in charge of the photo/VTR (shooting), (1-e) application contact the person in charge of the Flower (flower arranging), (1-f) hair and makeup (beauty) of your application personnel, (1-g) the atmosphere of meeting Salon.

(2) About facilities- (2-a) the wedding venue appearance, location, atmosphere, (2-b) transportation access, (2-c) the party venue introspection, location, atmosphere, (2-d) property amenities and fixtures, (2-e) courtesy car, (2-f) the courtesy car driver's attitude

(3) About the wedding, (3-a) wedding content, (3-b) pastor compatible, (3-c) choir, (3-d)the selection of wedding music, (3-e) organist playing, (3-f) the wedding correspondence of staff, (3-g) the guest attendance

(4) About wedding reception, (4-a) party content, (4-b) party progress, (4-c) audio-video, (4-d) production

(5) About cuisine, (5-a) the amount of dishes, (5-b) taste of dishes, (5-c) Serve, (5-d) the service staff support, (5-e) providing welcome drinks, drinks, (5-f) wedding cake

(6) About hair makeup and makeup, (6 a) correspondence of hair make up staff (6 b) dressing bride, hair and makeup finish, (6-c) groom dressing hair and makeup, (6-d) guests dressing, hair and makeup finish

(7) About Flower arrangement, (7-a) Bouquet and boutonniere, (7-b) church flower arranging, (7-c) party flower arranging, (7-d) Other items (flower shower, bouquet etc.)

(8) About shooting, (8-a) photography, (8-b) of the corresponding photographer, is (8-c) videographer corresponding more.

2.4   The Details of the Questionnaire

At the time of the counting of the questionnaire from the national 235 set (1) wedding reception invitation number of people (2) bride age (3) bride Hometown (4) bride profession (5) groom age (6) groom Hometown (7) groom profession (8) wedding reception final payment amount the has been added to the questionnaire, Table 1 is it.

Table 1. The results and data addition table

2.5 The Duration of Collection Questionnaire and Categorized by Area and Samples

Table 2 is the number of samples Questionnaire period and area.

Table 2. The number of samples of the survey area

	Data collection period		
	2014	2015	Total
Tokyo 1		14	14
Tokyo 2	8	56	64
Nagoya	21	39	60
Kyoto 1	5	19	24
Kyoto 2	1	12	13
Fukuoka		60	60
Total	35	200	235

3 Observation

3.1 Relevant to the NPS

Groom age to questions of NPS and 40 of 2.3, bride age, add a wedding reception last payment amount, a numeric indication of the correlation between the NPS number is a Table 3. Is referred to as a comprehensive evaluation of Table 3 what you have is in conjunction with the number of NPS, next to the comprehensive evaluation ✕ high number relation to the evaluation the greater of the mark, the more does not have a rating in the relationship at all if no. of comprehensive evaluation number is higher, it comes to a high NPS numerical value. blue and item that is highlighted is made to item high relationship with the NPS in, especially 1 high relationship item, wedding-reception of your meeting contact person 2, wedding staff of the corresponding 3, photography of the corresponding 4, your application contact person 5 of wedding-reception, was a sign up contact the person in charge of the dress tuxedo. Both five items the impact of people to provide services is considered to be large.

3.2 Unrelated Categories with NPS

Items that are not affected at all to the NPS figures become item no comprehensive evaluation beside ✕ mark in Table 3. They are, traffic access, courtesy car, choir, wedding music selection, wedding cake, the music, both in the service item no it was found that a product item.

Table 3 is a distribution with respect to sample 235 set of NPS (Fig. 2).

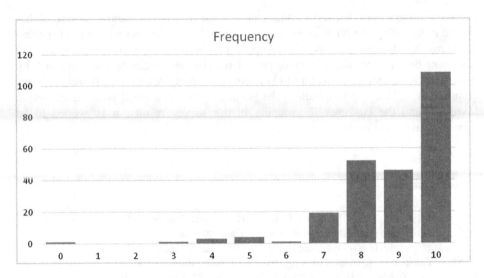

Fig. 2. NPS results

Table 3. Correlation between each variable and the NPS

◆Correlation between each variable and the NPS numerical value

If the number is large, a high relationship with the NPS
∗∗∗∗∗The number is higher, it affected the value of the NPS.
∗∗∗∗The number is higher, it affected somewhat to a number of NPS.
Blue area∗∗very high relevance to the NPS

	The age of bride		The age of groom		The final amount of price		Overall rating	
The age of bride			.583	∗∗	−.187	∗	.023	
The age of groom	.583	∗∗			−.171		−.051	
The final amount of price	−.187	∗	−.171				.032	
The person who is in charge of receiving wedding and itemization request	−.146		−.066		.129		.353	∗∗
The person who is in charge of meeting about wedding and itemization	−.106		−.131		.143		.456	∗∗
The person who is in charge of meeting down and itemize request	.019		.029		.180	∗	.352	∗∗
The person who is in charge of receiving photos and shooting a video request	−.163	∗	−.117		.166		.229	∗∗
The person who is in charge of receiving flower arrangement request	.004		−.101		.095		.210	∗∗
The person who is in charge of receiving hair make up request	−.013		−.002		.059		.325	∗∗
Atmosphere of the meeting Salon (concierge)	−.072		−.170	∗	.094		.274	∗∗
Appearance of the buildings, location and atmosphere	.028		.076		−.086		.366	∗∗
Accessibility	.169	∗	.080		−.314	∗∗	.095	
Interiors of the party room, location and atmosphere	.068		−.024		−.133		.233	∗∗
Facilities	−.071		−.100		−.050		.175	∗∗
Limousine	−.269		.081		−.147		.207	∗∗
Customer support of the limousine driver	−.241		.077		−.146		.266	∗
Content of the wedding	.027		.064		−.027		.232	∗∗
Customer support of pastor	−.097		−.125		.106		.151	∗
Choir	−.064		−.141		−.050		.101	
Selections of music	−.040		−.163	∗	−.060		.112	
Performance of organist	−.080		−.153		−.039		.230	∗∗
Customer support of the wedding staff	−.024		−.020		−.062		.441	∗∗
Customer support for the guests	−.055		−.140		.012		.429	∗∗
Content of solemnization	−.046		−.037		.074		.302	∗∗
Performance of MC	−.001		−.081		−.045		.263	∗∗
Sound and videos	−.085		−.060		−.071		.240	∗∗
Performance (Candle Service and Fairly Illusion etc)	−.059		−.157		−.014		.347	∗∗
The amount of the cuisine	−.076		−.044		.045		.204	∗∗
The taste of the cuisine	−.062		−.045		.064		.240	∗∗
Dish appearance	−.029		−.001		−.088		.223	∗∗
Customer support of the waitresses	.054		−.047		−.033		.155	∗
Welcome drinks and normal drinks	−.008		−.131		.073		.213	∗∗
The wedding cake	−.114		−.060		.108		.129	
Dress and hair make up of the bride	.075		.076		−.038		.344	∗∗
Dress and hair make up of the groom	.102		.110		−.180		.392	∗∗
Dress and hair make up of the guests	.015		−.064		.002		.159	∗
Bouquet and boutonniere	.007		−.009		−.068		.257	∗∗
Flower arrangement inside the church	−.051		−.047		−.044		.324	∗∗
Flower arrangement of the solemnization	−.037		−.086		.037		.300	∗∗
The other flowers (e.g. flower shower, flower gift and headpiece)	−.107		−.189	∗	.055		.378	∗∗
Photo	.007		−.021		−.085		.426	∗∗
The customer support of the photographer	.010		.066		−.105		.292	∗∗
The customer support of the videographer	−.022		.097		−.153		.294	∗∗
Comprehensive evaluation	.023		−.051		.032			

4 Conclusion

From the observation that factors that can be seen in service categories were highly related to the NPS. The NPS scores made lower in factor was also related to the person who provided the service, thus, to keep up earning high points from the groom and the bride satisfied needed quality service providers. The results can be grouping in 5 by using the factor extraction method; (1) cuisine, (2) party reception, (3) wedding ceremony, (4) service, (5) hospitality. The hospitality is categorized contents of people involved, and the customer is grouping in the survey results. It is needed to be deepened in the future further research.

References

1. Recruit: Investigation of Wedding Trend, p. 123. Bridal Souken (2014)
2. Report in 2015 by Ministry of Health, Labour and Welfare
3. Recruit: Investigation of Wedding Trend, p. 83. Bridal Souken (2015)
4. Shoji Yamamoto: Service Marketing, pp. 23–24. Nikkeibunko (2007)
5. Bowie, D., Buttle, F.: Hospitality Marketing, pp. 31–32. Elsevier (2004)
6. Kral, J.M.: Net Service design, pp. 35–36. BNN社 (2015)
7. Reichheld, F., Markey, R.: Net Promoter System, p. 60. President.co (2013)
8. Kotler, P.: Marketing Professional Service, p. 204. Pearson Education Japan Co (2002)

Integrating Human Factors in Information Systems Development: User Centred and Agile Development Approaches

Leonor Teixeira[1,3(✉)], Vasco Saavedra[1], Beatriz Sousa Santos[2,3], and Carlos Ferreira[1,3]

[1] Department of Economics, Management and Industrial Engineering,
University of Aveiro, Aveiro, Portugal
{lteixeira, vsaavedra, carlosf}@ua.pt
[2] Department of Electronics, Telecommunications and Informatics,
University of Aveiro, Aveiro, Portugal
bss@ua.pt
[3] Institute of Electronics and Informatics Engineering of Aveiro (IEETA),
Aveiro, Portugal

Abstract. This paper presents an overview and discussion based on the literature review of recent research of some practices that incorporate human factors, emphasizing the user-centred design (UCD) and agile software development (ASD) approaches. Additionally, this article presents an experience of the development of a web-based application that aims to manage the clinical information in haemophilia care, which benefited from these practices, making use of some methods to support the collaboration and communication between designers, users, and developers. The results of our experience show that the hybrid approach, that combines the principles of UCD with values of ASD can help to integrate human factors into the software development process in a highly complex environment, characterized by missing information, shifting goals and a great deal of uncertainty, such as the healthcare field.

Keywords: Human factors · Information system development · User-Centred design · Agile software development · Interactive software

1 Introduction

The dynamics that currently characterize the software market also require the same dynamic and some flexibility when managing the software requirements. On the other hand, the traditional models of software engineering (SE) and management practices for the development of this type of projects limit the flexibility for the adaptation of those requirements, often compromising the quality of the final product.

In SE, it has been intuitively accepted that user involvement during the Systems Development Life Cycle (SDLC), leads to a better management software requirements, and consequently can lead to system success [1]. User involvement in SDLC facilitates the understanding of their work environment and can improve the quality, accuracy and completeness of the requirements.

© Springer International Publishing Switzerland 2016
V.G. Duffy (Ed.): DHM 2016, LNCS 9745, pp. 345–356, 2016.
DOI: 10.1007/978-3-319-40247-5_35

Users typically have important tacit knowledge about the system domain and context of the system usage [1] that can be difficult to be articulated with traditional techniques from SE. For this reason, the development process of interactive software (IS), albeit with major contributions coming from the SE, recently has integrated methods from other knowledge areas to cover the social and human aspects associated with the interaction component.

On the other hand, aspects such accelerate of time to market, increase the final product quality, align the information and communication technologies (ICT) with business strategies, and promote flexibility [2, 3] are increasingly important values in the software development context. In order to consider this values, the software development industry has been adopting agile methods, because they are more flexible and can promote benefits such productivity gains and business alignment [2].

The user-centred design (UCD) and agile software development (ADS) emerge as appropriate counterproposals to traditional development methodologies, changing the values of project management, and centring the focus on people.

This paper presents an overview of these two approaches based on a literature review of recent research. Additionally it describes an experience of developing a Health Information System that benefited from these practices.

The remainder of this paper is organized as follows. Section 2 shows some concepts related to human factors in the software development process with focus on UCD and ASD approaches. Section 3 describes an experience of developing a Health Information System that benefited from a hybrid approach, combining traditional methods with UCD and ASD practices. Finally, Sect. 4 presents some conclusions.

2 Background: Human Factor in Software Development Process

Actually, the human factors play a very important role in the software development (SD) with a major impact on the process performance and product success. In this area of research, the growing importance of human factors are proved by the existence of specific tracks devoted to this topic in conferences related with SE, as well as the specific issues in some important journals in the field, such as Information and Software Technology [4].

SD has been characterized as a set of activities comprising a set of tasks grouped in system analysis, system design, coding, and testing. Moreover, the SD has been considered a socio-technical endeavour, and particularly in the case of SE, the effectively communication with users and team members is increasingly important.

Actually, in the development of interactive software (IS), it is important to consider, not only the functional and technical specifications, but also all the aspects related to the user interface and the interaction process. From the user's point of view, the system is usually used and evaluated as a whole, and the separation between technical/functional components and the user interface is not possible. Conceptually these components can be designed using concepts from different knowledge areas. While the former is defined from the user's specification, and is generally addressed by SE, the interface component, which deals with issues related to the interaction between the user and the IS, is associated with Human-Computer Interaction (HCI) and/or Usability Engineering (UE).

In order to facilitate the development process of IS, several methods and techniques have been proposed to provide solutions for the effective involvement of users and that take into account the human factors. Joint Application Development (JAD) [5], Agile Software Development (ASD) methods [6, 7], Lean Software Development (LSD) [8, 9], Effective Technical and Human Interaction with Computer based Systems (ETHICS) [1] are some examples of those techniques. Other contributions attempt to accommodate methods from SE and HCI areas in the same process. For example, Harmelen [10] suggests the Object Oriented and Human Computer Interaction (OO&HCI) method, which integrates object-oriented (OO) modelling techniques, and HCI concepts for developing IS. Other prominent proposals in this area are the Design for User-Centred Innovation (DUCI) presented by Zaina and Álvaro [11], which attempt to integrate HCI into the traditional OO development, combining the merits of both approaches in order to design software that is both usable and useful. The proposal by Mayhew [12], implemented through the Framework 'Usability Engineering Life-cycle', also resulted from an attempt to redesign the process of software development involving methods and activities of the UE.

In fact, the terms 'user-centred' and 'customer-focus' are the most used in the human factors' community.

Nowadays, the set of most well-known techniques used by software development industry to include human factors has been characterized by two major approaches: on the one hand the techniques that follow the principles of agile software development (ASD), which aims to achieve increased velocity and flexibility during the development process; on the other hand the techniques which put the goals and users' needs at the centre of software development, in order to deliver software with appropriate usability, known as user-centred design (UCD).

According to Brhel et al. [13], while the agile methods focus on the question of "how useful software can be developed, with customer value being understood as primarily driven by providing an appropriate functional scope"; the UCD ensures that the "goals and needs of the system's end-users is the focus of the product's development" [13].

Given that the UCD approach focuses on the *user* and produces *usable* software and ASD focuses on the *customer* and produces *useful* software, hybrid developments can contribute to the production of usable and useful software, trying to combine the merits of both approaches.

2.1 About User-Centred Development Approach

In recent years, the methodologies for the development of IS have placed great emphasis on iterative and incremental development practices, with evaluation processes throughout the entire development cycle. On the other hand, important advances in the SE area have emerged from adaptations of traditional development methods, based on iterative and incremental models supported by the principles of user-centred design (UCD).

The literature reports that the UCD methodologies, with a central focus on continuous evaluation, in iterative processes of a formative evaluation, have been the most sought for the development of IS. UCD is an approach to interactive system development that focuses specifically on making usable systems [14]. UCD is defined by Vredenburg *et al.* [15], as "an approach to designing ease of use into the total user experience with products and systems, involving two fundamental elements: multidisciplinary teamwork and a set of specialized methods of acquiring user input and converting it into design".

The development according to principles of UCD arises from the attempt to merge the best practices from SE and HCI and/or UE, and is defined as a philosophy that puts the user into the centre of the development process. In this approach, apart from the user, the tasks and the environment or usage-context emerge as important requirements, having as a main objective the creation of systems after a solid knowledge about the characteristics of users and the tasks they perform. Thus, the result of a good design is reflected in a usable system.

Considering the standard on human-centred design by ISO 13407 [14], there are five critical processes that should be performed in order to incorporate usability into the software development process: (i) plan the human-centred design process; (ii) understand and specify the context of use; (iii) specify the user and organizational requirements; (iv) produce designs and prototypes; and (v) perform user-based assessment.

There are several works which attempt to incorporate usability into the software development process, following a methodological approach based on the principles of UCD. However, these approaches are not governed by formal methods, but by a set of techniques and principles that put the user at the centre of development [16].

The International Usability Standard, ISO 13407 [14], specifies the principles and activities that underlie UCD:

- The process is iterative;
- Users are involved throughout design and development;
- The design addresses the whole user experience;
- The design is based on explicit understanding of users, their tasks and environment;
- The design is driven and refined by user-centred formative evaluation.

A good example is the Framework presented by Kushniruk [17] that depicts a structure relating the main techniques and assessment methods with the respective stages of the IS development cycle, combining a set of techniques from HCI and/or UE, with the traditional methods of SE (see Fig. 1).

Typically, as shown in the Framework of Fig. 1, the UCD approach is a philosophy that uses a set of techniques and methods already known in other knowledge areas, aiming to produce usable systems that meet the needs of those who use them.

Techniques coming from the Social and Cognitive Sciences, such as questionnaires, interviews, documentation analysis, and ethnographic techniques (direct observation) are the most used for the knowledge of the problem and system analysis.

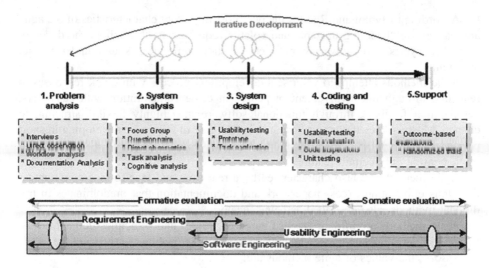

Fig. 1. Framework of IS development considering techniques and methods from different knowledge areas (adapted from [17])

For a better understanding of the mental model of the users, there are other techniques coming from HCI and/or UE, including task analysis and cognitive analysis, useful for validating the requirements previously found and for stabilizing the most volatile requirements. Prototypes accompanied by usability testing and task evaluation represent also excellent tools for requirements validation and evaluation of the solution acceptance by the users that can be used in system design, as well as in the remaining phases of the SDLC.

2.2 About Agile Software Development Approach

The term Agile Software Development (ASD) was created in 2001, by a group of people involved in defining new software development methods around a common name '*Agile Manifesto*' [18].

One of the main beliefs of the promoters of the '*Agile Manifesto*' is that the traditional methods of SE, strongly based on a strict specification and supported by formal contracts, cannot cope with the rapid change and uncertainty that the processes of a dynamic and competitive economy require.

The '*Agile Manifesto*' was developed in response to the emphasis placed by main stream software development research on planning, control, and efficiency [19], providing "a set of practices that allow for quick adaptations matching the needs of the software development" [20]. The ASD implements evolutionary and flexible software processes that answer to changes in customer requirements based on cooperation and communication, rather than on bureaucracy with models and written documents, to communicate the requirements and validate the solution [19].

According to Jyothi and Rao [3] the two most important characteristics of the agile approaches are "handling unstable and volatile requirements throughout the development life cycles and delivering products in short time frames and under budget constraints".

Agile methods attempt to valorise a development process with quick responses in real time through the involvement of people in close collaboration with customers, getting their feedback through functional software in a highly flexible structure to change. Most agile methods tries to minimize the risk of failure by developing in short periods, called iterations. Each iteration works as the development of a small project, implementing only certain features.

Agile methods are also characterized by a real time and face-to-face communication, thus eliminating excess paperwork and documentation that predominates in traditional methods, also described as being 'heavy'.

Agile methods are in their essence based on values and principles defined on the 'Agile Manifesto' and composed by agile practices [18]. Taking into account the 'Agile Manifesto', the values of agile methods are:

- Individuals and interactions rather than processes and tools;
- Functional software, rather than comprehensive documentation;
- Collaboration with the customer rather than contract negotiation;
- Response to changes, rather than follow a predefined planning.

With regard to the agile practices, Table 1 reports the 16 most used, taking into consideration the survey study in Version One State of Agile 2014 Research [21].

Table 1. The agile practices most adopted (%) according a survey study in [21]

Position	Practices	%	Position	Practices	%
1	Daily stand-up	80 %	9	Iteration reviews	53 %
2	Short iterations	79 %	10	Task board	53 %
3	Prioritized backlogs	79 %	11	Continuous integration	50 %
4	Iteration planning	71 %	12	Dedicated product owner	48 %
5	Retrospectives	69 %	13	Single team	46 %
6	Release planning	65 %	14	Coding standards	43 %
7	Unit testing	65 %	15	Open work area	38 %
8	Team-based estimation	56 %	16	Refactoring	36 %

According to Campanelli and Parreiras [2], the different agile practices can be grouped into (i) management practices, (ii) software process practices, and (iii) software development practices. While management practices are principles such as: on-site customer, daily stand-up meetings, release planning and open work area; the software process practices include simple design, coding standards and collective code ownership, and the software development practices correspond to, for example, pair programming and unit testing.

However, the various existing practices all share the same principles, following an iterative development process, based on strong communication between the development team members, applying minimal effort in documentation or in the creation of intermediate artefacts. Delivering working software in short time periods, with high quality and under budget and handling unstable requirements, are the main distinctive characteristics of agile methods when compared with traditional ones [2].

There are several agile methods, some of them hybrids, benefiting the best from several other methods, with slight differences in the practices they apply. eXtreme Programming (XP) [22], Scrum [23], Crystal Methods [24], Adaptive Software Development (AdapSD) [25], Feature-Driven Development (FDD) [26], Lean Software Development (LSD) [9], and Dynamic Systems Development Methodology (DSDM) [2] represent the most popular agile methods.

3 Experimental Study Using User-Centred Design and Agile Development Approaches

Although the literature often refers to the UCD and ASD approaches as methodologies, in fact they are philosophies that define a set of practices based on certain principles, using for this purpose a set of techniques and methods coming from other knowledge areas.

As these approaches have different focuses at different stages of system development, they can become useful as complementary approaches in some projects.

While the UCD approach requires more investment in the early stages of the lifecycle, reducing the risk of unexpected changes in requirements, the ASD can provide a great contribution in coding phases, reducing service costs and all associated bureaucracy.

Given the complementary nature of these approaches, there are already several projects that experienced hybrid approaches, trying to combine the merits of UCD and ASD approaches in order to design software that is both *usable* and *useful* [13, 27–32]. The experimental study briefly presented in this paper is one such example which adopts a hybrid approach, taking advantage of both the UCD and the ASD, and having been applied in the development of an application to manage the clinical information in the hemophilia care.

3.1 Overview of the Project and Brief Characterization

The project at issue aimed to develop a technological application to manage the clinical information in haemophilia care, as well as to support the process of registry and submission of the data generated in the home-treatments by patients [33]. In order to manage the data, this application integrates three actors: (i) Patient who has access to a restrict online area allowing the registry of all data generated from home treatments; (ii) Physician responsible for the management of all patient's clinical data; and (iii) Nurse responsible for managing the stocks of the drugs used, as well as the registry of the hospital-treatments (see more details of application in [34–36].

The problem emerged in the scope of a highly complex environment, characterized by missing information, shifting goals and a great deal of uncertainty. Given the type of the problem and the peculiarities of the project, the development of the technology involved a strong interaction with the domain experts in the early stages of the SDLC, once the users were the main holders of the tacit knowledge needed to define the system requirements. Actually, decisions in healthcare are complex processes strongly based on tacit knowledge, which contributes for a difficult process of requirement elicitation using traditional methodologies. For this reason, it was decided to incorporate the principles of the UCD approach in the early stages of the project, more specifically in the requirement engineering phase [37].

On the other hand, and since the developers team was physically displaced, there was the need to mediate the process between users and the team of developers through a figure of the analyst. The analyst was responsible for understanding the problem, collecting the requirements and validation with the users, ensuring also a proper communication of the requirements with development team.

3.2   Framework with the Overview of the Development Approach

The approach used in the development of the present technological solution was inspired by a hybrid approach, combining UCD and ASD techniques (see Fig. 2).

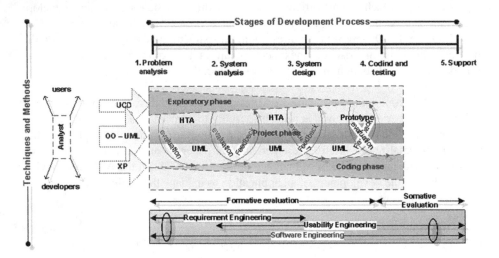

Fig. 2. Framework of development proposed based on experimental study

As shown in the framework presented in Fig. 2, the development approach adopted was based on an iterative and incremental model comprising three main phases: (i) exploratory phase, (ii) project phase and (iii) coding phase.

While the exploratory phase focused its work in the early stages of the development process, the coding phase was more prominent in the final stages, although it had begun at the same time as the requirement analysis.

The exploratory phase used some contextual techniques for understanding the problem, focusing on the document analysis, direct observation, and informal interviews with the domain experts.

As the knowledge of the domain problem was increasing, and the first requirements were collected, the first version of the conceptual model was created, using the UML notation (Use-Case diagram and Class diagram). The choice of this notation was due to UML being Object-Oriented (OO) and therefore suitable to the evolutionary characteristic of the project (incremental development). In order to validate the models with users, techniques derived from HCI were selected, specifically techniques for task analysis - hierarchical task analysis (HTA) [38], and prototypes [39].

The assessed requirements were implemented (coding phase) using the principles of the eXtreme Programming (XP) approach. As the programming team was geographically displaced from the users responsible for defining the requirements, the analyst had an important role in the process of mediation, using techniques for proper communication with each of the stakeholders.

3.3   Some Remarks About Proposed Framework

In the project development cycle (see the framework of Fig. 2 from left to right), it can be seen that the uncertainty in terms of requirements decreases, the importance of the activities of each phase changes, reversing the effort and the work required, particularly in the exploratory phase and coding phase. The project phase is the communication link between the front-end component of the project, where are the users and customers, and the back-end component, where are the developers. As such, and given the importance of the work on this level and its impact on the final result, the framework recommends a double approach to the work at this stage. First, one OO analysis using UML to build the conceptual solution in an iterative way so it can be understood by the programmers working on the back-end component of the project. On the other hand, in order to interface with users and customers on the validation component, verification and gathering new requirements, models less abstract and more easily interpretable by people without computer knowledge are recommended, such as HTA models and prototypes.

The UML has a great potential for documenting evolving projects and for communicating with developers; however, is not an easy language to interpret and, as such, is not ideal for interfacing with users without a computer background. For this reason, it is concluded that the interface with users in order to validate and complete the data previously obtained, should be made based on simple models coming from HCI and/or UE areas.

In this experiment, the HTA model and prototypes revealed having a great potential for communication with users, integrating the proposal as an essential component in the Requirements Engineering process. Regarding the type of prototype, the vertical one could be the best solution, being in line with evolutionary prototype that characterizes the XP approach.

This approach combining techniques coming from HCI with ASD, not only allowed more easily capture and validate the requirements with the end user, as also provided an excellent basis for obtaining new requirements, particularly for the most difficult requirements to capture (emerging requirements).

4 Conclusion

The present work discussed the development process of usable and useful software, focusing on human factors, based on some recent literature. The literature points to the existence of several methods that attempt to incorporate human factors in the development process, highlighting two categories: (i) the approaches that are governed by the principles of UCD; and (ii) the approaches that follow the values of ASD.

Although the UCD and the ASD have different approaches, they do have some similarities. Both philosophies are iterative, i.e., they progress in small steps providing opportunities for validation and refinement the results during the development process, and both are human-centred approaches, despite the UCD being focused in the user and the ASD focused in the customer.

Given their complementarity, there are already several proposals reported in the literature that attempt to combine the principles of the two approaches, taking advantage of the best each has to offer. However, the literature shows a clear need for more empirical and/or experimental studies regarding UCD and Agile Methods.

This paper presented an experimental study relating to the development of an Information System in healthcare, which used a hybrid approach, following the principles of UCD and ASD, aiming to reach a useful and usable final product.

The results of our experience show that a hybrid approach, that combines the principles of UCD with values of ASD can help to integrate human factors into the software development process in a highly complex environment, characterized by missing information, shifting goals and a great deal of uncertainty, such as the healthcare field.

Finally, it should be noted that despite the successful experience with this approach, this proposal has some limitations, having to be adjusted according to the type of project. It should be emphasized the high degree of demand in terms of availability from the analyst and the motivation and willingness of users who will participate in the process.

Acknowledgments. This work is funded by National Funds through FCT - Foundation for Science and Technology, in the context of the project PEst- OE/EEI/UI0127/2014.

References

1. Bano, M., Zowghi, D.: A systematic review on the relationship between user involvement and system success. Inf. Softw. Technol. **58**, 148–169 (2015)
2. Campanelli, A.S., Parreiras, F.S.: Agile methods tailoring – A systematic literature review. J. Syst. Softw. **110**, 85–100 (2015)

3. Jyothi, V.E., Rao, K.N.: Effective implementation of agile practices ingenious and organized theoretical framework. Int. J. Adv. Comput. Sci. Appl. **2**, 41–48 (2011)
4. Amrit, C., Daneva, M., Damian, D.: Human factors in software development: On its underlying theories and the value of learning from related disciplines. A guest editorial introduction to the special issue. Inf. Softw. Technol. **56**, 1537–1542 (2014)
5. Duggan, E.W., Thachenkary, C.S.: Integrating nominal group technique and joint application development for improved systems requirements determination. Inf. Manag. **41**, 399–411 (2004)
6. Inayat, I., Salim, S.S., Marczak, S., Daneva, M., Shamshirband, S.: A systematic literature review on agile requirements engineering practices and challenges. Comput. Human Behav. **51**, 915–929 (2014)
7. Losada, B., Urretavizcaya, M., Fernández-Castro, I.: A guide to agile development of interactive software with a "user objectives"-driven methodology. Sci. Comput. Program. **78**, 2268–2281 (2013)
8. Ebert, C., Abrahamsson, P., Oza, N.: Lean software development. IEEE Softw. **29**, 22–25 (2012)
9. Poppendieck, M., Cusumano, M.A.: Lean software development: A tutorial. IEEE Softw. **29**, 26–32 (2012)
10. van Harmelen, M.: Interactive system design using OO&HCI methods. In: Object Modelling and User Interface Design: Designing Interactive Systems, pp. 365–427. Addison Wesley (2001)
11. Zaina, L.A.M., Alvaro, A.: A design methodology for user-centered innovation in the software development area. J. Syst. Softw. **110**, 155–177 (2015)
12. Mayhew, D.J.: The usability engineering lifecycle. Morgan Kaufman, San Francisco (1999)
13. Brhel, M., Meth, H., Maedche, A., Werder, K.: Exploring principles of user-centered agile software development: A literature review. Inf. Softw. Technol. **61**, 163–181 (2015)
14. ISO: ISO 13407 - Human-centred design processes for interactive systems. Ergonomics (1999)
15. Vredenberg, K., Isensee, S., Righi, C.: User-Centered Design: An Integrated Approach with Cdrom. Prentice Hall PTR, Upper Saddle River (2001)
16. Norman, D.A., Draper, S.W.: User Centered System Design: New Perspectives on Human-Computer Interaction. L. Erlbaum Associates Inc., Hillsdale (1986)
17. Kushniruk, A.: Evaluation in the design of health information systems: application of approaches emerging from usability engineering. Comput. Biol. Med. **32**, 141–149 (2002)
18. Beck, K., Beedle, M., van Bennekum, A., Cockburn, A., Cunningham, W., Fowler, M., Grenning, J., Highsmith, J., Hunt, A., Jeffries, R., Kern, J., Marick, B., Martin, R.C., Mellor, S., Schwaber, K., Sutherland, J., Thomas, D.: Agile Manifesto. http://www.agilemanifesto.org
19. Hansson, C., Dittrich, Y., Gustafsson, B., Zarnak, S.: How agile are industrial software development practices? J. Syst. Softw. **79**, 1295–1311 (2006)
20. Papadopoulos, G.: Moving from traditional to agile software development methodologies also on large, distributed projects. Procedia - Soc. Behav. Sci. **175**, 455–463 (2015)
21. VersionOne: 9th Annual State of Agile Survey (2015)
22. Beck, K., Andres, C.: Extreme Programming Explained. Addison Wesley, Pearson Education, Reading, Upper Saddle River (2005)
23. Schwaber, K., Beedle, A.: Agile Software Development with SCRUM. Prentice- Hall, Upper Saddle River (2002)
24. Cockburn, A.: Crystal Clear: A Human-Powered Software Development Methodology for Small Teams. Addison-Wesley, Reading (2001)

25. Highsmith, J.: Agile Software Development Ecosystems. Addison-Wesley Longman Publishing Co., Boston (2002)
26. Coad, P., Palmer, S.: Feature-Driven Development. Prentice Hall, Englewood Cliffs (2002)
27. Sohaib, O., Khan, K.: Integrating usability engineering and agile software development: A literature review. In: 2010 International Conference on Computer Design and Applications (ICCDA), pp. V2-32–V2-38 (2010)
28. da Silva, T.S., Martin, A., Maurer, F., Silveira, M.: User-centered design and agile methods: a systematic review. In: 2011 Agile Conference (AGILE), pp. 77–86 (2011)
29. Fox, D., Sillito, J., Maurer, F.: Agile methods and user-centered design: how these two methodologies are being successfully integrated in industry. In: Agile 2008 Conference, pp. 63–72 (2008)
30. Blomkvist, S.: Towards a model for bridging agile development and user-centered-design. In: Seffah, A., Gulliksen, J., Desmarais, M.C. (eds.) Human-Centered Software Engineering — Integrating Usability in the Software Development Lifecycle. Human-Computer Interaction Series, pp. 219–244. Springer, Heidelberg (2006)
31. Chamberlain, S., Sharp, H., Maiden, N.A.M.: Towards a framework for integrating agile development and user-centred design. In: Abrahamsson, P., Marchesi, M., Succi, G. (eds.) XP 2006. LNCS, vol. 4044, pp. 143–153. Springer, Heidelberg (2006)
32. Salah, D., Paige, R.F., Cairns, P.: A systematic literature review for agile development processes and user centred design integration. In: Proceedings of the 18th International Conference on Evaluation and Assessment in Software Engineering, pp. 5:1–5:10. ACM, New York (2014)
33. Teixeira, L., Ferreira, C., Santos, B.S., Saavedra, V.: Web-enabled registry of inherited bleeding disorders in Portugal: conditions and perception of the patients. Haemophilia 18, 56–62 (2012)
34. Teixeira, L., Saavedra, V., Simões, J.P.: Dashboard to support the decision-making within a chronic disease: a framework for automatic generation of alerts and KPIs. In: Magdalena-Benedito, R., Soria-Olivas, E., Martínez, J.G., Gómez-Sanchis, J., Serrano-López, A.J. (eds.) Medical Applications of Intelligent Data Analysis, pp. 160–171. IGI Global, Hershey (2012)
35. Teixeira, L., Saavedra, V., Ferreira, C., Sousa Santos, B.: Improving the management of chronic diseases using web-based technologies: an application in hemophilia care. In: Proceedings of the Conference on IEEE Engineering in Medicine and Biology Society, vol. 106, pp. 2184–2187 (2010)
36. Teixeira, L., Ferreira, C., Santos, B.S., Martins, N.: Modeling a web-based information system for managing clinical information in hemophilia care. In: International Conference of the IEEE Engineering in Medicine and Biology Society, pp. 2610–2613 (2006)
37. Teixeira, L., Ferreira, C., Santos, B.S.: User-centered requirements engineering in health information systems: a study in the hemophilia field. Comput. Methods Programs Biomed. 106, 160–174 (2012)
38. Teixeira, L., Ferreira, C., Santos, B.S.: Using task analysis to improve the requirements elicitation in health information system. In: 29th Annual International Conference of the IEEE Engineering in Medicine and Biology Society, EMBS 2007, pp. 3669–3672 (2007)
39. Teixeira, L., Saavedra, V., Ferreira, C., Simões, J., Sousa Santos, B.: Requirements engineering using mockups and prototyping tools: developing a healthcare web-application. In: Yamamoto, S. (ed.) HCI 2014, Part I. LNCS, vol. 8521, pp. 652–663. Springer, Heidelberg (2014)

Implementation and Evaluation of Interactive Memory-Aid Agent Service for People with Dementia

Seiki Tokunaga[1](✉), Hiroyasu Horiuchi[1], Hiroki Takatsuka[1], Sachio Saiki[1], Shinsuke Matsumoto[2], Masahide Nakamura[1](✉), and Kiyoshi Yasuda[3](✉)

[1] Graduate School of System Informatics, Kobe University, 1-1 Rokkodai, Nada, Kobe, Japan
{tokunaga,horihori,tktk}@ws.cs.kobe-u.ac.jp, sachio@carp.kobe-u.ac.jp, masa-n@cs.kobe-u.ac.jp
[2] Graduate School of Information Science and Technology, Osaka University, 1-5, Yamadaoka, Suita, Osaka 565-0871, Japan
shinsuke@ist.osaka-u.ac.jp
[3] Chiba Rosai Hospital, 2-16 Tatsumidai-higashi, Ichihara, Japan
fwkk5911@mb.infoweb.ne.jp

Abstract. In recent years, a number of reminder systems have been developed to help elderly people with dementia. However, the existing reminder systems lack the sympathetic human-machine interaction.

In this paper, we propose a new reminder service which aims to assist elderly people with dementia using Human Computer Interaction technology. Proposed agent service consists of four components called Care-Module, Virtual Agent user interface (VA), ControllService and Memory Aid Client (MAClient). VA is a promising technology for people with dementia since it can assist a patient based on less-mechanical and (simulated) human-to-human conversation. CareModule is consists of functions that provides the generating the user interface and operation for the VA. The ControllService manages the state of transition and that enables to provide the loosely coupled component among the agent services. Memory-Aid Client (MAClient) visualizes reminder information in a screen, and which provides graphical user interface (e.g., button, list, etc.) to collect responses from a user.

In order to evaluate the feasibility and usability of the proposed agent service, we also conduct the experiment evaluation with actual subjects. Based on the experiment evaluation, we also show the validity of proposed agent service.

1 Introduction

Dementia is a general term to describe a group of symptoms that impairment human memory, communication, and thinking. According to a report in 2015 [6], 46.8 million people are now suffering from dementia in all over the world.

© Springer International Publishing Switzerland 2016
V.G. Duffy (Ed.): DHM 2016, LNCS 9745, pp. 357–368, 2016.
DOI: 10.1007/978-3-319-40247-5_36

Thus, the *home care* for people with dementia becomes more essential, in order to assure the quality of life of the patient. However, sometimes the home care could be a burden to the family or caregivers in a specific context [1].

Moreover, the number of a nursing home is not sufficient for the number of applicants. The labor shortage for the caregivers has occurred based on the social background [9]. Nowadays, some systems have the potential to cover the subset of tasks which caregivers have, in order to complement the lack of human resources [8]. However, to take a proper care of dignity, there are strong needs the Human Computer Interaction (HCI) technology. Because, the mechanical reactions would sometimes impair the dignity of the patient, and decrease the motivation to use the system. If the system could cover the subset of tasks, then the caregivers could focus entirely on making one's own unique contribution.

In this paper, we propose an agent service that provides the voice dialogue and graphical user interface. Our proposed agent service consists of four components called CareModule, Virtual Agent user interface (VA), ControllService and Memory Aid Client(MAClient). VA is a promising technology for people with dementia since it can assist a patient based on less-mechanical and (simulated) human-to-human conversation. CareModule is consists of functions that provides the generating the user interface and operation for the VA. The ControllService provides the loosely coupled component among the agent services. Memory-Aid Client (MAClient) visualizes reminder information in a screen, and provides graphical user interface (e.g., button, list, etc.) to collect responses from a user. VA is a promising technology for people with dementia since it can assist a patient based on less-mechanical and (simulated) human-to-human conversation.

We also implement the agent service based on the proposed architecture. In order to show the validity and feasibility of proposed service, we also conduct the experimental evaluation with actual subjects. The result shows that the both voice dialog with VA and display on the screen (e.g. checklist, images of belongings) are useful for the patients.

2 Preliminary

2.1 Memory Impairment and Memory Aid

The progression of dementia usually begins with mild anterograde amnesia and often involves a variety of behavioral disturbances such as wandering and agitation [2]. People with dementia typically have the following symptoms:

- A decline in memory to an extent that it interferes with everyday activities, or makes an independent living either difficult or impossible.
- A decline in thinking, planning and organizing day-to-day things.
- Initially, preserved awareness of the environment, including orientation in space and time.

To maintain the quality of life of the people with dementia, the care by caregivers or families would become more important. In reality, however, the care is often a burden because of specific features of dementia, including BPSD (behavioral and psychological symptoms of dementia), aggressiveness, wandering, and sleep disturbance [7]. Indeed, it is not easy for general families to always delegate professional caregivers. Hence, there are many cases observed where the families have been *burned out* by the home care.

For this situation, the *assistive technology* is one of the promising solutions, where technologies are introduced to assist the people with dementia and surrounding people.

2.2   Virtual Agent System

The *virtual agent* (VA) is a human-looking animated chatbot program that can communicate with a human user via voice [5]. There are a few studies that adopt the VA for dementia care. Yasuda et al. developed a system where a VA serves as a conversation partner of people with dementia [10].

Our research group has developed a system which exploits a VA as the user interface of the home network system (HNS) [4]. In order to integrate other systems, VA has developed as the Web interface such as say(), smile(), and so on. Hence, the developer could effectively invoke and integrate with other systems. For instance, when some HTTP client invokes http://xxx/agent?say="How are you?", then the VA says "How are you" with text-to-speech technology. Also, VA has the feature of voice recognition to understand what the patients say. Hence, the patient could interact with using voice dialogue. So, we extensively reuse it for the dementia care. The developed VA is internally defined as a finite state machine. The actions include say(), motion(), recognize(), execWebService(). The detailed information can be seen in [4]. VA is a promising technology for people with dementia since it can assist a patient based on less-mechanical and (simulated) human-to-human conversation.

2.3   Goal and Scope of Paper

In this paper, we propose an agent service that provides the voice dialogue and graphical user interface. To achieve the above goal, we try to develop a new agent service that has the potential to provide the heartwarming and intuitive interface. Our proposed agent service consists of four components called Care-Module, Virtual Agent user interface (VA), ControllService and Memory Aid Client(MAClient). VA is a promising technology for people with dementia since it can assist a patient based on less-mechanical and (simulated) human-to-human conversation. CareModule is consists of functions that provides the generating the user interface and operation for the VA. ControllService provides the loosely coupled component among the agent services. Memory-Aid Client (MAClient) visualizes reminder information in a screen, and provides graphical user interface (e.g., button, list, etc.) to collect responses from a user.

We also conduct the experimental evaluation in order to confirm that the people with dementia could interact with proposed agent service.

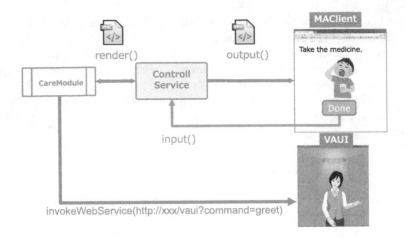

Fig. 1. System overview of agent service

3   Agent Service

3.1   System Architecture

Figure 1 shows the system architecture of agent service. The left of the figure represents CareModule which has the sequence of program execution. In addition to this, CareModule generates HTML data that is rendered on the graphical interface for the patients. We design the CareModule as the tiny program, hence that would apply for the various scenes to care. In order to apply for the various secens to care, we separate CareModule as the tiny program (e.g. greeting cgi, care cgi). The upper center of the Fig. 1 shows the ControllService service which provides the control data transfer between the graphical interface and CareModule. The right of the figure shows the Memory Aid Client (called MAClient) which is the useful interface for the patients. The bottom right of the Fig. 1 represents VA we explained in Sect. 2.2. The MAClient is supposed to be displayed on a touch interface, so that the patient can intuitively interact with the agent service. Moreover, the MAClient can display the images or movies that are quite helpful for the reminder. The MAClient exposes two kinds of API: input() and output(). The input() API displays input GUI components (e.g., list, button, etc.), with which the user can input commands to Agent Service. The output() API displays output GUI components (e.g., text, label, etc.)

The developer could develop the system efficiently because the ControllService provides the independence on each system.

MAClient visualizes reminder information in a screen and provides graphical user interface (e.g., button, list, etc.) to collect responses from a user. The MAClient is supposed to be displayed on a touch interface, so that the patient can intuitively interact with the agent service. Moreover, the MAClient can display the images or movies that are quite helpful for the reminder. When the ControllService. Integrating VA and MAClient, Agent Service provides API that can execute some care using the virtual agent with visualized information. Figure 2 shows the sequence diagram that is the sequence of the agent service. In the following, we show an example of sequence diagram that represents how to remind the patients of taking the medicine with proposed architecture. At first, we have preliminary set the functions to provide the care for the people with dementia. The CareModule invokes the WebAPI which is belongs to the VA. After the invocation of WebAPI, then the VA says the message that "Please take a medicine" (Fig. 3).

Also CareModule generates the HTML to display the button and appropriate message. Then CareModule gives the ControllService service to display the generated HTML. In addition to this, CareModule invokes the render() method to display something. Finally, the MAClient displays the HTML to interact with the patient based on the commands from ControllService.

3.2 Implementation

We implemented the ControllService and agent service as the RESTful Web service. Hence, the developer could develop the software integrated with another web service or system and our proposed service. For example, the ControllService has the above web interface to interact with another system. These WebAPIs enable developers to integrate and manage the UI. Integrating with agent service, the ControllService service could be integrated using render(). The render() methods consumes the HTML format and directly commands to output for the MAClient. The agent service has provided the simple invocation interface such as render() and VA also has each method to behave. We have implemented the proposed service as the following environment.

CareModule Ruby: 2.3.0p0
ControllService Java, Apache Tomcat: 7.0.65, Jersey
VA Java, Apache Tomcat: 7.0.65, Apache Axis2: 1.6.2
MAClient Bootstrap: v3.2.0, jQuery: 2.1.1

4   Evaluation of Agent Service

4.1   Abstract of Evaluation

In this section, we explain the experiment evaluation in order to confirm the system feasibility and usability. We have conducted the experiment at Chiba Rosai Hospital. The goal of the evaluation is to confirm that the patients could interact with the agent service using some interactions (e.g. voice, touch). Especially, we have confirmed the interaction and reactions after the patient used the agent service. Moreover, we show the validity of the possibilities of the adoption of with considering the result of each interface. Seventeen patients participated in the experiment. The age range among the subjects is from forty-six to eighty-four. In the experiment five men were participated and the others were women. And the average score of MMSE [3] among participants is 22.9.

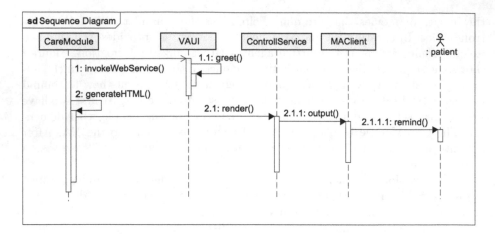

Fig. 2. Sequence diagram of agent service

4.2   Experimental Environment

In the experiment, we have conducted the experiment with five people team. The breakdown of the member is a patient, a caregiver, a recorder, an adjuvant and a system administrator. Figure 4 shows the experimental scene. We deployed the agent service to the Surface Pro 3 which touch panel and a built-in mic. The tablet has connected to the system administrator's device using Wireless LAN. The system administrator controls the agent service and he controls that the operation agent service has started. The subjects interact with agent service in front of the tablet. Among the interaction, the observer conducts the help for the operation and instruction of the subjects. The recorder records the each experimental scene with a video camera.

4.3   Experiment Description

We have explained the feature of agent service, that provides 4 components for the VA and MAClient. Using agent service, we expect the subjects would be feel useful for the people with dementia. However, we have not confirmed that the people with dementia could interact with agent service. In order to validate the evidence, we conduct the experimental evaluation. In the experiment, we focus on the following five points to confirm the feasibility and usability of agent service for patients.

Q1: Can the subjects listen to the speech of what the VA say?
Q1 aims to evaluate that the both voice volume and quality have the feasibility to dialogue for the subjects. In particular, we confirm that the subjects can listen to the speech what the agent says.
Q2: Can the VA system recognize what the subject says? This question aims to validate that the VA system could recognize the speech what the subjects

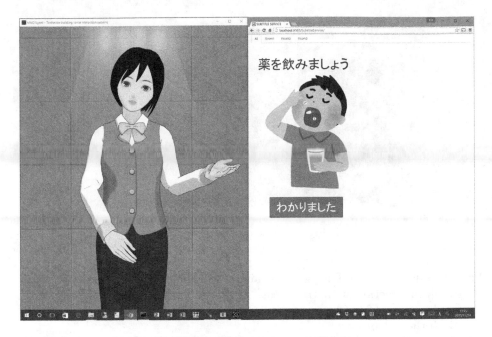

Fig. 3. User interface of agent service

say. We have judged that the voice recognize system have the feasibility for the what the dementia says.

Q3: Does the interface of agent service have an appropriate design?
Q3 aims to judge that the agent service has the appropriate design to display the contents to remind (e.g. display his/her schedules, belongings).

Q4: Can the subjects control the MAClient using touch panel? Q4 aims to confirm that the subjects could control the MAClient using touch screen.

Q5: Does the contents of MAClient have effectiveness for the memory aids?
Q5 aims that verify whether the contents of MAClient helps to understand what the agent says and input assistance. Concretely speaking, the MAClient displays the contents which are expected to remind for the subjects (such as Registration Cards, house key). And we have records that showing above items with image would have effective to understand for the subjects.

4.4 Settings of Experiment

The subjects has conducted the interaction with dementia agent based on the some scenario. In the following, we show the concretely scenario that we have conduced. These scenarios are aimed to verify from the Q1 to Q5.

Preliminary scenario This scenario aims to evaluate Q1 and Q2 through the simple dialogue with agent. We confirm that the subjects could have a voice dialogue with agent after the dialogue.

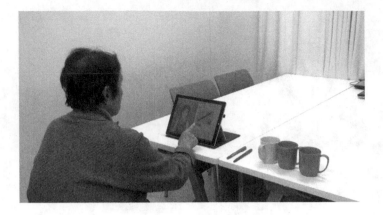

Fig. 4. Scene of experiment

Screen Touch scenario This scenario aims to evaluate that Q3 and Q4 using simple interaction with the agent. After the subjects have dialogue with touch screen of MAClient, we confirm that the subjects could recognize and touch the button.

Check belongings scenario This scenario aims to evaluate the Q5 that has evaluated as the interaction with check list. We suppose this scenario is to confirm the following scene that the subjects go out, then the MAClient displays his/her belongings based on the destination.

(a) represents the checkbox that the user have to have.

Understanding instruction scenario

This scenario aims to evaluate the Q5 that shows the instruction. Specifically, we confirm that whether showing some images on the screen of MAClient was helpful to understand the instruction of what the agent says. In the experiment, we have subjects moves cup or pen with instruction of agent. And then we have compared the case that displays images on the screen or not.

Moreover we have collected the questionnaire from his/her caregiver who has observed the experiment. And we have scored the each evaluation item.

- Q.1 Could the subject recognize the agent? Can he/her talk to the agent?
- Q.2 Could the subject could control the MAClient with a touch screen?
- Q.3 Could the subject understand what the agent says?
- Q.4 Could the subject understand the instruction of agent?
- Q.5 Could the subject offer a response to the instruction of agent?

4.5   Result of Experiment and Discussion

All the subjects[1] have completed the scenario which we have given.

---

[1] We have supported some subjects when they could not recognize the instruction of agent.

Table 1. Result of experiment

No	Sex	Age	MMSE	Q.1	Q.2	Q.3	Q.4	Q.5
1	F	79	20	5	5	5	3	5
2	F	83	16	2	3	3	3	3
3	F	81	25	3	5	5	5	5
4	F	79	16	3	1	2	2	3
5	F	80	25	4	4	5	4	4
6	F	84	27	3	4	4	4	4
7	M	68	29	4	4	5	4	4
8	F	77	26	3	5	5	5	4
9	M	83	26	3	3	3	3	3
10	F	71	24	4	4	5	4	4
11	F	80	15	5	3	5	4	5
12	F	71	24	5	3	5	4	4
13	M	80	16	4	3	4	4	3
14	M	60	25	3	4	5	5	4
15	M	46	27	4	4	5	5	5
16	F	78	29	3	3	3	2	3
17	F	75	19	3	3	3	3	3

Table 1 shows the experiment result. The head of table Q.x corresponds to the above evaluation items. We also figure the coefficient of correlation for the each result of the score. In this experiment, we use Spearman rank correlation because we could not assumption that the result of scores would follow a normal distribution Table 2. * and ** represent the significant level, hence * is the 5 % significant level.

Table 2. Result of experiment: spearman rank correlation matrix

	Age	MMSE	Q.1	Q.2	Q.3	Q.4
MMSE	−0.29					
Q1	−0.32	−0.07				
Q2	−0.22	0.39	0.25			
Q3	−0.42	0.19	0.62**	0.79**		
Q4	−0.43	0.29	0.22	0.66**	0.79**	
Q5	−0.21	0.12	0.56*	0.73**	0.85**	0.60*

Result of Q1: We have some receive the feedback that the speed of speaking is fast. The Table 2 shows that the result of Q.3 is about 4.2 point. We have concluded that the most subjects understand what the agent says. We have thought that this result comes from MAClient performs complementary when the subjects missing what the agent says. The Table 2 shows that correlation of Q.3 and MMSE is 0.19. Next, we have found that there is almost no correlation between understanding of dialogue with Agent and MMSE. This is because the understanding of dialogue relates on the individual body condition, that means some subjects have a weak hearing. Hence, we have to adjust the agent's voice based on the individual body condition.

Result of Q2: All of the subjects could recognize the agent and they could dialogue with agent during the experiment. However, voice recognition system can recognize some subjects speech input voice only. Also, the voice recognize system could not recognize the voice input on the first time. The system could recognize the voice input when the subjects speak twice or more. After the preliminary scenario, subjects alternatively used touch interface as the dialogue interface. Although they speak of the system when the fail of recognition causes no response, they look uneasy. The main reason for the low accuracy of recognition is that a built-in microphone could not pick up the subject's voice. To improve the accuracy of voice recognition, we have to use the directional microphone instead of the built-in microphone.

Result of Q3: All the subjects could recognize the message and button on the screen of agent service. But we gathered feedback from some subjects that they felt the contents on the screen were small. We think that above problems are capable of being coped with resizing the contents on the screen. We also have to adopt the personalized contents size on the screen for the individual. Some subjects could not recognize the button on the screen, and they tend to look for the out of the screen. This is because they are unfamiliar with software button on the screen. Hence, we would like to design the button so as to look like the actual physical button. Moreover, we gathered the comments from a caregiver that if the button has a sound effect, then it would feel better.

Result of Q4: The Table 1, Q2 represents the major of subjects have a lot of trouble to push the button on the screen. Sometimes they push the button too strong, That causes the fail to recognize as the touch event on the device. But most subjects could become familiar with touch sense during the experiment. So they could touch the button on the screen to dialogue with the agent. Table 2 shows that the correlation coefficient between Q.2 and MMSE is 0.39. Above result shows that we could not indicate a significant correlation between them. In addition to this, some subjects who usually use smartphone touched the button on the screen without difficulty. Hence, we have confirmed that whether the subjects could use the contents on the screen strongly depends on that they are familiar with smartphone or tablet.

Result of Q5: We have confirmed that showing the images of objects are effect to the instruction of agent. Concretely speaking, in one case the agent instruct subjects to move the objects with showing the pictures. And another case, the agent instruct subjects to move the objects without showing the pictures. As the result of the experiment, we have confirmed that the almost subjects could move the object accurately. One subject fails to move the object because he becomes distracted by VA. He moves objects without making sure of what it is. In order to prevent the above case, the VA have to behave so as to point to guide the target of the picture on the screen. Moreover, we have confirmed that three subjects look being baffled that the agent only instructs without showing pictures of objects. We also gathered the comments that instruction with the pictures felt easy to understand than without pictures. Based on the results, we have concluded that the instruction with images are useful to understand for the subjects. Next we also have conducted the showing checking list scenario that assumes the subjects go out. In this scenario, the subjects could understand the experiment situation, but they could not touch the checking list. This result comes from two reasons one is the lack of instruction of agent and another reason is unfamiliar with UI for the subjects. The lack of instruction represents that the agent only says "please confirm the belongings", hence, the subjects could not know what to do next. So to cope the above problem, the agent behave to say "please confirm the belongings and also check the buttons". The latter means that the subjects are not familiar with general Web UI checklist. To cope the problem, we have to design the UI so as to understand easily for the subjects.

5 Conclusion

In this paper, we have implemented and evaluated the agent service that provides the heartwarming and careful user interface. We also show the feasibility of the agent service based on the experimental evaluation. Proposed agent service consists of the Virtual agent that provides the rich interface and MAClient provides the flexible interface to display the information to remember. Moreover, we have conducted the evaluation to valid the feasibility of proposed service. The experiment result shows that the VA speaking with voice, touch interaction, and display of captions and images are valid for the people with dementia. Our future work is to improve voice recognition accuracy and to improve the interface based on the questionnaire. Moreover, we have to conduct the long-term evaluation to confirm that the proposed agent service is valid to remind.

Acknowledgements. We are deeply grateful to the subjects and his/her families who participates experiment. We are also deeply grateful to staff of Chiba Rosai Hospital who provides the place of experiment. This research was partially supported by the Japan Ministry of Education, Science, Sports, and Culture [Grant-in-Aid for Scientific Research (B) (No. 26280115, No. 15H02701), Young Scientists (B) (No. 26730155), Challenging Exploratory Research (15K12020)] and Tateishi Science Foundation (C) (No. 2157008).

References

1. Andren, S., Elmstahl, S.: Family caregivers' subjective experiences of satisfaction in dementia care: aspects of burden, subjective health and sense of coherence. Scand. J. Caring Sci. **19**(2), 157–168 (2005)

2. Davis, R.N., Massman, P.J., Doody, R.S.: Cognitive intervention in alzheimer disease: a randomized placebo-controlled study. Alzheimer Dis. Assoc. Disord. **15**(1), 1–9 (2001)
3. Folstein, M.F., Folstein, S.E., McHugh, P.R.: mini-mental state: a practical method for grading the cognitive state of patients for the clinician. J. Psychiatr. Res. **12**(3), 189–198 (1975)
4. Horiuchi, H., Saiki, S., Matsumoto, S., Nakamura, M.: Designing and implementing service framework for virtual agents in home network system. In: 2014 15th IEEE/ACIS International Conference on oftware Engineering, Artificial Intelligence, Networking and Parallel/Distributed Computing. pp. 343–348 (2014)
5. Magalie, O., Pelachaud, C., David, S.: An empathic virtual dialog agent to improve human-machine interaction. In: Proceedings of the 7th International Joint Conference on Autonomous Agents and Multiagent Systems, vol. 1. pp. 89–96. International Foundation for Autonomous Agents and Multiagent Systems (2008)
6. Martin, P., Anders, W., Maelenn, G., Gemma-Claire, A., Yu-Tzu, W., Matthew, P.: World alzheimer report 2015 (2015)
7. Meguro, K., Meguro, M., Tanaka, Y., Akanuma, K., Yamaguchi, K., Itoh, M.: Risperidone is effective for wandering and disturbed sleep/wake patterns in alzheimer disease. J. Geriatr. Psychiatry Neurol. **17**(2), 61–67 (2004)
8. Sakai, Y., Nonaka, Y., Yasuda, K., Nakano, Y.I.: Listener agent for elderly people with dementia. In: Proceedings of the Seventh Annual ACM/IEEE International Conference on Human-Robot Interaction, HRI 2012, NY, USA, pp. 199–200. ACM, New York (2012). http://doi.acm.org/10.1145/2157689.2157754
9. Toda, K.: A background for the labor shortage in care workplace. Kawasaki College Allied Health Prof. **30**, 41–45 (2010)
10. Yasuda, K., Fuketa, M., Aoe, J.: An anime agent system for reminiscence therapy. Gerontechnology **13**(2), 118–119 (2014)

Designing for STEM Faculty: The Use of Personas for Evaluating and Improving Design

Mihaela Vorvoreanu[1(✉)], Krishna Madhavan[2],
Kanrawi Kitkhachonkunlaphat[1], and Liang Zhao[1]

[1] Computer Graphics Technology, Purdue University, West Lafayette, IN, USA
{mihaela, kkitkhac, zhao334}@purdue.edu
[2] School of Engineering Education, Purdue University, West Lafayette, IN, USA
cm@purdue.edu

Abstract. We demonstrate in a case study how we used a qualitative method for user modeling, persona, to evaluate and refine the design of an interactive visual analytics tool. We explain the literature and our methods for building the persona, and its used to (a) evaluate existing design decisions; (b) make new design decisions in order to serve a specific user group, faculty in STEM. We present the results of 24 in-depth, qualitative interviews with STEM faculty. The interviews addressed topics such as daily work, sources of work satisfaction and success, work goals, activities, needs, and difficulties. The results provide an insight into the busy lives of STEM academics and can be useful to other efforts that aim to design for this user group. We discuss how we used these results, presented in the form of a persona, to evaluate existing design decisions and to create new features that would serve this audience.

Keywords: Personas · Scenarios · Use cases · User experience

1 Introduction

User modeling is an important step in user-centered system design. User modeling provides an understanding of users and their behavior patterns that helps design or refine systems and system behavior [14]. Various disciplines of research and practice use different methods for user modeling, but at their core, user models represent synthesized information about user groups. In this paper, we present a case study of modeling users based on qualitative data collected through in-depth interviews. We illustrate the use of this modeling technique known as "persona" [10] with a case study centered around the development of an online interactive platform for knowledge mining and visualization, Deep Insights Anytime, Anywhere (DIA2).

DIA2 is an online platform for mining and visualizing the funding portfolio of the U.S. National Science Foundation (NSF) [22]. NSF is one of the major federal funding agencies in the U.S., with an annual budget of approximately 7 billion USD [27]. The funding rate for the NSF has been about 24 % in the fiscal years 2014 and 2015 [26]. The NSF funds more than 10,000 awards each year [26]. The DIA2 platform was created

© Springer International Publishing Switzerland 2016
V.G. Duffy (Ed.): DHM 2016, LNCS 9745, pp. 369–380, 2016.
DOI: 10.1007/978-3-319-40247-5_37

in response to a competitive call for proposals from an NSF program known at the time as Transforming Undergraduate Education in STEM (TUES) and is funded by the NSF [25]. The TUES program needed a way to understand, visualize and mine their own funding portfolio. Beginning with this need, our interdisciplinary team of researchers and designers created an online platform that would address this problem institution-wide, not only for the TUES program, even though that was our starting point.

DIA2 enables users to interact with data visualizations created from funding data provided by the NSF. In the process of doing so, users can explore, understand, and compare NSF's funding portfolio, as well as identify researchers, NSF programs and program officers by topic, institution, and so on. A detailed description of the system is available in [15]. DIA2 is accessible to the public at www.dia2.org.

DIA2 serves two main user groups: internal NSF staff and external NSF audiences. The first development phase focused on the internal NSF audience. User research and modeling were conducted [34] and an alpha version of the system was developed and evaluated [15, 21, 24]. Once a satisfactory alpha version was launched, the design team proceeded to the second user group, external to the NSF [25]. While there are multiple groups external to the NSF such as journalists, congress and state representatives, etc., we prioritized faculty members who are looking to apply for funding from the NSF. Of these, we focused particularly on STEM faculty, who are the main audience for the TUES program that had funded this project. In this paper, we present our use of the user modeling technique known as persona to understand this user group, and we demonstrate the utility of personas for evaluating existing products and deriving new design requirements.

2   Related Research

2.1   Cooper's Persona: User Research Analysis and Presentation Technique

Personas are an effective technique to understand users that was first introduced in the book The inmates are running the asylum by Alan Cooper [9]. In addition to understanding users, personas are a powerful tool for communication among members of the development team and externally with clients. Cooper developed the persona technique from his experience in the software industry using ethnographic user research to support his goal-directed design methodology [4, 11].

The main idea of persona technique is to conduct in-depth user research to understand users' motivations and behavior patterns, and then create a representation of a composite user to represent the characteristics, goals, and behaviors of real users. Cooper [10] described the construction of persona in seven steps. The first step is to define observable aspects of focus - such as activities, attitudes, and skills. Second, identify the range of each aspect, and where to place each research participant in the range. Third, identify behavior patterns for each cluster of participants. Fourth, perform pattern analysis to reveal characteristics and goals for each cluster. Fifth, refine the analysis to ensure the correctness and the uniqueness of each persona. Sixth, collect more data and create a behavioral narrative for each persona. Seventh, compare and prioritize the personas.

2.2   Arguments for and Against the Utility of Personas

Research on the usage of personas has discussed issues such as personas' accuracy of reflecting user data [8], the engagement of the development team [5, 16], and the appropriate settings for employing personas [32]. While personas are a helpful communication tool, [11, 17, 23], some questions have been raised about the impact of the technique on the end design result [4, 7, 23]. Design practitioners could be mislead and distracted by the abstraction of personas, especially if the personas are not based on in-depth research with users [23]. Blomkvist [4] argued that the persona technique in goal-directed design puts too much effort on the persona creation instead of the real design. Research has found, however, that, when used correctly, personas can be a very effective design tool, but superficial persona approximations that are not grounded in sufficient data merely support communication among designers about the over simplified users without the real consideration of user's personalizing details [23].

2.3   Persona Usage in Industry and Research

A lot of research has supported the idea that personas are an efficient method for developing engagement and enhancing reality when refining techniques. Grudin and Pruitt [16] discussed that personas are a critical method to enhance the efficiency of using scenarios. They pointed out that persona is a medium for communication that helps designers focus on the most crucial aspects throughout the design process. Later research that reflected on the use of personas in the design process also found positive effects on communication and design process [13, 23, 30].

Personas are widely used in various areas of software design such as news website, business interactive services, and educational software [2, 11, 12, 19, 20]. However, in some cases, the modification of the original persona technique is required [1]. Putnam et al. [31] pointed out the use of personas to understand users in different cultural contexts with additional modification of the technique.

Dantin [12] introduced an alternative use of personas as a tool for evaluation. Dantin applied Nielsen's heuristics [28] to the use of persona in order to evaluate the UI of educational applications. Dantin's work indicated the possibility of the use of personas to improve existing design. In this paper, we also demonstrate how personas can be used for evaluating an existing product.

Although personas are commonly used in practice, Idoughi [19] reflected that there are too few implementation guidelines for design practitioners can follow. Previous studies also showed misunderstanding among practitioners about the concept of personas, which rendered the technique ineffective [23]. These conclusions point to the need for elucidating persona building and usage, a need we aim to address with this case study. The remainder of the paper explains the methods we used to collect in-depth qualitative data from a target user group, how we analyzed the data and summarized it into a persona, and how we used the persona to evaluate the existing product version and derive specific design requirements for the subsequent version.

3 Methodology

3.1 Participants

We selected a criterion sample [29] of interview participants who were part of the target audience for NSF, specifically, the TUES program. Therefore, all our participants had to be STEM faculty with an interest in education. We recruited participants at the annual convention of the American Society for Engineering Education, which attracts the particular audience we were targeting. Also, we recruited participants from publicly available lists of researchers who had received awards through the NSF TUES program. We conducted a total of 24 interviews with faculty members. Seven out of 24 participants were females. The participants' age distribution is shown in Fig. 1. Of the participants who revealed highest degree information, 17 had a Ph.D., and one had a Master's degree. Participants held a variety of academic ranks ranging from assistant professor (5), associate (4), full (7) and distinguished (1). Four participants reported holding administrative positions such as dean. Most participants (9) worked in engineering disciplines, followed by Technology (5) and Engineering Education (4).

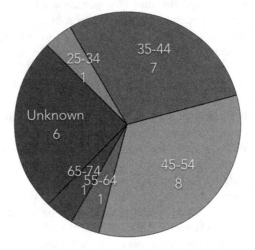

Fig. 1. Interview participants' age distribution

3.2 Procedures

Interviews were conducted with the participants in one of the three ways: in person at the ASEE conference, in person on the researchers' campus, and via Skype. On average, interviews were about 60 min long.

During the interview, the participants were first asked some general questions related to their background, work description, work context, and goals they want to achieve. After finishing gathering general information, the interview started to focus on questions regarding impact and diffusion of educational innovations. The questions were mainly targeted towards understanding their definition of "transformative ideas", how and why they choose certain resources for course preparation, how they stay informed and connected with other professionals, their experience with NSF, and their process of submitting a grant proposal. Afterwards, we described what information DIA2 can provide and asked participants about their attitude towards DIA2. We also asked questions regarding the kind of information they would like to see in DIA2.

3.3   Data Analysis

Affinity diagramming was used to analyze the data. Affinity diagramming is a technique that enables teams to analyze qualitative data together. It requires organizing and grouping ideas and showing common issues and themes in a visual way [3, 18]. The 24 interviews were transcribed into plain text by an external transcription service. The DIA2 UX and development teams read through the transcripts and created work activity notes by recording each single idea on a sticky note. Then, the team members grouped and synthesized ideas into categories. Major findings were discussed and then summarized in the form of a persona. Even though the interview participants' demographics varied, their thinking about issues at hand and their behavior patterns were consistent, which led the team to synthesize data from all 24 interviews into one persona. Had the team noticed remarkably different goals, ways of thinking, and behaviors, we would have had to create more than one persona (Fig. 2).

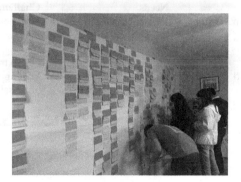

Fig. 2. Affinity diagramming

4   Persona

According to Cooper [10], a persona is a user model derived from motivations and behaviors of real users. The persona encapsulates the synthesized user data into behavior patterns and presents them in the form of a composite character that designers can relate to. Personas support software design by allowing deep comprehension of the users during the design process [20] as well as assisting communications about the design among developers [17]. The persona technique enables designers to empathize with users to a larger extent than nameless, faceless data reports would [10].

In the previous phase of development, the researchers developed personas to represent user groups internal to the NSF [35]. An alpha version of DIA2 had already been launched and tested [15, 21, 24] based on design requirements extracted from the NSF personas. The aim of this phase of research was to further the design of DIA2 to serve the group of STEM academics - a group of target users external to the NSF [25]. The persona revealed specific behavior and motivation patterns of STEM academics, including their goals, needs, and challenges. Then, according to the persona, the researchers developed user scenarios, use cases, and specific design requirements. We present the persona, followed by the design insights derived from this particular persona, in order to illustrate the value of personas in design.

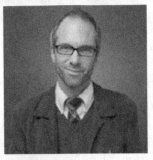

Michael is a 45-year-old associate professor of engineering education at a research university in the Midwest. His focus and heart are in both his teaching and research, but often he must spend much of his typical workday in front of his computer answering emails from colleagues and students. He spends the rest of his busy workday preparing for and teaching courses, working on his research, and in meetings with faculty, research collaborators, and students.

"I want to make a positive impact on my students and others with my research, but busy work days make that difficult."

Goals	Needs	Challenges
• Having an impact on students	• Easy-to-access resources	• Not enough time
• Impacting others with research	• Project collaborators	• Staying up-to-date
• Publishing work and getting grants	• Funding for research	• Finding collaborators that he can trust
• Doing quality work		• Writing a successful grant proposal

Fig. 3. Persona overview

4.1 Persona: Michael Anderson

Figure 3 shows the short version, overview of the persona documentation. A persona report includes a brief overview like the one presented here and an in-depth report. The overview sheet can be easily remembered and even posted in visible locations around the designers' workspace as a continuous reminder of target users and their needs. The persona overview includes a photo, a fictional but realistic full name, and demographics representative of the user group. It also includes a brief description of the persona that focuses on characteristics relevant to the product. A representative quote extracted from the data is also included. This ensures that designers are reminded of the users' voice. The persona overview also includes brief pointers about the most relevant aspects relevant to the design - in this case, goals, needs, and challenges. The persona overview is accompanied by an in-depth report that provides further details about the persona's goals, needs, motivations, behaviors, and challenges. The persona overview serves as a reminder and executive summary of the longer report.

Personas are a product of a design philosophy known as goal-directed design [10]. Goal-directed design is characterized by a focus on helping users achieve broad life and career goals, rather than automating small tasks. This is why the persona must include an understanding of users' goals. In our report, the section on goals was followed by a description of activity and behavior patterns, which lead into a description of the persona's needs and challenges. We present a summary of these insights in the following sections.

Goals.   Two major goals emerged from the interview data: impact and quality work. Michael Anderson's primary goal is to make an impact. He divides this goal into 2 parts: Making an impact on students, and making an impact in his research field. A secondary and related goal for Michael is to produce quality work. Michael assesses the quality of his work by whether it is published and whether it results in research funding.

Activities.   Related to the notion of goals is the issue of what makes Michael feel successful. The top two activities that make him feel successful are research and teaching, followed by meeting and email at the very bottom. However, the activities that take Michael's time are in precisely reverse order, as shown in Fig. 4.

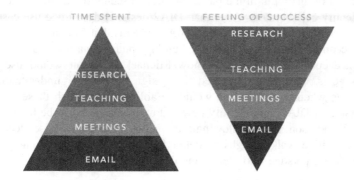

Fig. 4.   Inverse relationship between activities that define success and time spent

Needs and Challenges.   Three main specific needs emerged from the research interviews: finding resources for teaching and research, identifying research collaborators, and securing research funding. For each one of these needs, the persona report includes a description of how Michael Anderson currently goes about accomplishing these tasks, and challenges he encounters while doing so. For example, when identifying research collaborators, Michael's preference is to look within his own network and work with people he knows he can trust. If that is not possible, Michael looks for collaborators at the same institution or in close geographical proximity. He might ask colleagues for referrals or appeal to an administrator, such as a college dean, to help him identify people with the required expertise. Major difficulties emerged when discussing the identification of research collaborators. These were related to the fact that it is difficult to identify collaborators in different academic communities, as these communities tend to be fragmented into specific journals and conferences that Michael might not even know about. This information was very useful to the design team, because it pointed out to the importance of helping Michael reach across academic communities, but also enabling him to be more efficient at doing what he already does - looking for collaborators within his institution.

4.2   Scenarios and Use Cases

Scenarios are a design technique that uses storytelling to envision the use of a future system [6]. In goal-directed design, scenarios describe how the persona would use a future system to accomplish tasks related to their larger goals [10]. The designers use scenarios to understand how users would make use of the product in their natural context and to bridge the research-design gap by beginning to envision specific system features. The common use of the scenario is to guide the design before the creation of a prototype, and an evaluation such as cognitive walkthrough from the user's perspective [23].

The DIA2 design team created user scenarios - stories showing how DIA2 can help Michael Anderson fulfill various tasks. The design team generated two main scenarios. The first scenario was the story of Michael Anderson using DIA2 to help target his funding request to NSF by identifying NSF programs and program officers who have funded research on his topic in the past. The second scenario was his use of DIA2 to help him identify collaborators. After that, DIA2 designer developed use cases, which were detailed step-by-step interactions in DIA2 systems that Michael Anderson might use the to accomplish each scenario. By building both scenarios and use cases, we developed a deeper understanding of how Michael Anderson would use DIA2 to achieve his goals. This process helped the design team better understand the user group, evaluate whether the persona would be able to accomplish these tasks on the existing version of DIA2, and identify new features that needed to be built in order to help Michael Anderson. In the following sections, we describe two user scenarios, use cases, and cognitive walkthroughs in detail for the purpose of presenting how we adapted developed persona into identifying design requirements.

User Scenarios. *Scenario 1: Research funding – identifying NSF programs and program officers.* Michael has an idea for an NSF proposal, but he is not sure what program to submit it to, and what program officer to discuss his idea with. Michael launches DIA2 and begins a topic search in order to identify what NSF programs and officers have supported research on topics similar to his. The topic search helps him to quickly identify relevant program officers, programs, and even other researchers who have been funded in the same area. He is pleased to see that he can read abstracts of funded proposals in his area, but would like to have access to full proposal text, the publications that came out of those awards, and the involved researchers' and program officers' contact information.

Scenario 2: Identifying collaborators. Michael has an idea for an NSF proposal, but needs a collaborator to help him with a specific aspect of the grant – for example, social network analysis. He launches DIA2 and conducts a topic search on social network analysis. The first screen of the resulting search shows the principal investigators

(PIs) and co-PIs who have worked on research related to this topic. He runs the cursor over the dots in the social network visualization to identify some of the names. He then looks at the table on the right-hand side and clicks on several names one by one in order to understand more about the work each person does by reading abstracts of the awards they have received. He would like, however, to see the full award text and resulting publications. He finally identifies a few researchers he would like to contact. He would like to have an easy way to get the people's contact information directly from DIA2.

Use Cases. Based on the scenarios, we created click-by-click stories describing the specific interactions Michael would have with the system in order to accomplish the specified tasks. These detailed descriptions were translated into sketches and wireframes for new system features.

We used the scenarios above for two purposes: to evaluate the current system and understand whether Michael would be able to accomplish the tasks given the current system features; and to derive design requirements for new features we would need to add in order to ensure that DIA2 serves the STEM faculty user group as well as the NSF staff user group. The procedures we used to accomplish these two goals follow the evaluation technique known as cognitive walkthrough, described next.

Cognitive Walkthrough. The cognitive walkthrough is an inspection method for evaluating interfaces [32]. The cognitive walkthrough does not require user input. It is conducted by the design team, who "walks" through the interface as if they were the user attempting to accomplish a specific task. As every step (click), the design team asks a series of questions meant to ensure that the user would know what to do, that there are clear affordances to communicate to the user what to do, and that the user would get some confirmation that they are on the right path to accomplishing the task. The DIA2 team used several of the scenarios developed for Michael Anderson to "walk through" the system. As a result, we learned that the existing features would serve Michael well and help him accomplish the most important tasks. In addition to validating the existing version of the system, the results helped the team identify specific design requirements for features that would improve the system for the STEM faculty user group.

4.3   Design Requirements

We identified six main design requirements for improving DIA2 in order to better serve the STEM researcher user group.

- Improve the social network visualization to make it easier for Michael to understand what it represents and how to use it to identify collaborators.
- Include the ability to contact individuals from DIA2 and send requests for the full text of proposals.
- Speak the user's language (use fewer acronyms and avoid NSF jargon).
- DIA2 should provide recommendations for individuals based on commonalities
  - Commonalities should be transparent (i.e. "X was suggested based on Y")

 – Degrees of connection might be considered as a criterion for recommending individuals, such as:
    People you know or have worked with
    Research you've done or are doing
    What neighborhoods, programs, or communities should (or do) users belong to?
 • Creation of individual profiles that allow customization of research interests so DIA2 can show research news related to those interests
 • Create a marketplace to enable researchers to identify collaborators (i.e. "Looking for collaborators with skills in X, Y, and Z", as well as other postings)

In short, the persona helped the DIA2 team validate the existing design, as Michael Anderson would be able to accomplish the most important tasks on the existing version of the system. At the same time, we used the persona to help generate ideas for new features that would help Michael even more than the existing system version. The team proceeded to prioritize work and resources on the project in order to maximize benefit for both user groups.

5 Conclusion

In this paper, we illustrated the persona method from the field of human-computer interaction for modeling target users using qualitative research. We showed how we created a persona for a specific online tool, DIA2, based on qualitative data collected from 24 in-depth interviews. We presented the persona and explained the parts that went into our persona report, then we explained how the persona was useful to this project for both evaluation and further product refinement. While personas are used often in the field of human-computer interaction, it remains to be seen how the technique can be applied in different design and engineering fields. Future research can explore the use of personas, their advantages and disadvantages in other fields, as well as propose hybrid methods that can combine the depth of qualitative research with the breadth afforded by large amounts of quantitative data.

Acknowledgments.   DIA2 research and design was supported by NSF award 1123108. The authors would like to thank the graduate students who were instrumental in the collection, analysis and reporting of data supporting this paper: Zhihua (Emma) Dong, Kanrawi Kitkhachonkunlaphat, Joshua Sarver, Rachel Whitson, and Liang Zhao.

References

1. Acuña, S.T., Castro, J.W., Juristo, N.: A HCI technique for improving requirements elicitation. Inf. Softw. Technol. **54**(12), 1357–1375 (2012)
2. Adlin, T., Pruitt, J., Goodwin, K., Hynes, C., McGrane, K., Rosenstein, A., Muller, M.J.: Putting personas to work. Paper presented at the CHI 2006 Extended Abstracts on Human Factors in Computing Systems (2006)

3. Beyer, H., Holtzblatt, K.: Contextual Design: Defining Customer-Centered Systems, p. 154. Elsevier, Amsterdam (1997)
4. Blomkvist, S.: The User as a Personality: A Reflection in the Theoretical and Practical Use of Personas in HCI Design (Technical report). Uppsala University, Uppsala (2007)
5. Blomquist, Å., Arvola, M.: Personas in action: ethnography in an interaction design team. In: Proceedings of the Second Nordic Conference on Human-Computer Interaction, pp. 197–200. ACM, October 2002
6. Carroll, J.M.: Making Use: Scenario-Based Design of Human-Computer Interactions. MIT press, Chicago (2000)
7. Chang, Y., Lim, Y., Stolterman, E.: Personas: from theory to practices. In: Proceedings of the 5th Nordic Conference on Human-Computer Interaction Building Bridges - NordiCHI 2008, p. 439 (2008). doi:10.1145/1463160.1463214
8. Chapman, C.N., Milham, R.P.: The personas' new clothes: methodological and practical arguments against a popular method. In: Proceedings of the Human Factors and Ergonomics Society Annual Meeting, vol. 50, no. 5, pp. 634–636. SAGE Publications, October 2006
9. Cooper, A.: The Inmates Are Running the Asylum: [Why High-Tech Products Drive us Crazy and How to Restore the Sanity], vol. 261. Sams, Indianapolis (1999)
10. Cooper, A., Reimann, R., Cronin, D.: About Face: The Essentials of Interaction Design. Wiley Publishing Inc., Indianapolis (2007)
11. Cooper, A.: The Origin of Personas (2008). http://www.cooper.com/journal/2008/05/the_origin_of_personas. Retrieved
12. Dantin, U.: Application of personas in user interface design for educational software. Reproduction **42**, 239–247 (2005). http://dl.acm.org/citation.cfm?id=1082424.1082455
13. Dotan, A., Maiden, N., Lichtner, V., Germanovich, L.: Designing with only four people in mind? – a case study of using personas to redesign a work-integrated learning support system. In: Gross, T., Gulliksen, J., Kotzé, P., Oestreicher, L., Palanque, P., Prates, R.O., Winckler, M. (eds.) INTERACT 2009. LNCS, vol. 5727, pp. 497–509. Springer, Heidelberg (2009)
14. Duffy, V.G.: Handbook of Digital Human Modeling: Research for Applied Ergonomics and Human Factors Engineering. CRC Press, Boca Raton (2008)
15. Elmqvist, N., Vorvoreanu, M., Chen, X., Wong, Y., Xian, H., Dong, Z., Johri, A.: DIA2: Web-based cyberinfrastructure for visual analysis of funding portfolios. IEEE Trans. Visual Comput. Graphics **20**(12), 1823–1832 (2014). doi:10.1109/TVCG.2014.2346747
16. Grudin, J., Pruitt, J.: Personas, participatory design and product development: an infrastructure for engagement. In: PDC, pp. 144–152, January 2002
17. Haikara, J.: Usability in agile software development: extending the interaction design process with personas approach. In: Concas, G., Damiani, E., Scotto, M., Succi, G. (eds.) XP 2007. LNCS, vol. 4536, pp. 153–156. Springer, Heidelberg (2007)
18. Hartson, R., Pyla, P.S.: The UX Book: Process and Guidelines for Ensuring a Quality User Experience, p. 144. Elsevier, Waltham (2012)
19. Idoughi, D., Seffah, A., Kolski, C.: Adding user experience into the interactive service design loop: a persona-based approach. Behav. Inf. Technol. **31**(3), 287–303 (2012). doi:10.1080/0144929X.2011.563799
20. Aquino, Jr., P.T., Filgueiras, L.V.L.: User modeling with personas. Paper presented at the Proceedings of the 2005 Latin American Conference on Human-Computer Interaction (2005)
21. Liu, Q., Vorvoreanu, M., Madhavan, K.P.C., McKenna, A.F.: Designing discovery experience for big data interaction: a case of Web-based knowledge mining and interactive visualization platform. In: Marcus, A. (ed.) DUXU 2013, Part IV. LNCS, vol. 8015, pp. 543–552. Springer, Heidelberg (2013). http://doi.org/10.1007/978-3-642-39253-5_60

22. Madhavan, K., Vorvoreanu, M., Elmqvist, N., Johri, A., Ramakrishnan, N., Wang, G.A., McKenna, A.: Portfolio mining. IEEE Comput. **45**(10), 95 (2012)

23. Matthews, T., Judge, T., Whittaker, S.: How do designers and user experience professionals actually perceive and use personas? Paper presented at the Proceedings of the SIGCHI Conference on Human Factors in Computing Systems (2012)

24. Molnar, A., McKenna, A.F., Liu, Q., Vorvoreanu, M., Madhavan, K.: Using visualization to derive insights from research funding portfolios. IEEE Comput. Graphics Appl. **35**(3), 91–97 (2015). http://doi.org/10.1109/MCG.2015.68

25. McKenna, A., London, J., Johri, A., Vorvoreanu, M., Madhavan, K.: Developing and advancing a cyberinfrastructure to gain insights into research investments: an organizing research framework. In: Proceedings of the 122nd ASEE Annual Conference and Exposition (2015)

26. National Science Foundation, Funding Rate by State and Organization from FY 2014 to 2015 for NSF (2015a). http://dellweb.bfa.nsf.gov/awdfr3/default.asp. Retrieved

27. National Science Foundation, NSF Budget Requests to Congress and Annual Appropriations (2015b). http://www.nsf.gov/about/budget/. Retrieved

28. Nielsen, J.: 10 Usability Heuristics for User Interface Design, 1 January 1995. https://www.nngroup.com/articles/ten-usability-heuristics/. Retrieved

29. Patton, M.Q.: Qualitative Research and Evaluation Methods. Sage, Thousand Oaks (2015)

30. Pruitt, J., Grudin, J.: Personas: practice and theory. In: Proceedings of the 2003 Conference on Designing for User Experiences, pp. 1–15. ACM, June 2003

31. Putnam, C., Kolko, B., Wood, S.: Communicating about users in ICTD: leveraging HCI personas. In: Proceedings of the Fifth International Conference on Information and Communication Technologies and Development, pp. 338–349. ACM, March 2012

32. Rönkkö, K., Hellman, M., Kilander, B., Dittrich, Y.: Personas is not applicable: local remedies interpreted in a wider context. In: Proceedings of the Eighth Conference on Participatory Design: Artful Integration: Interweaving Media, Materials and Practices, vol. 1, pp. 112–120. ACM, July 2004

33. Spencer, R.: The streamlined cognitive walkthrough method, working around social constraints encountered in a software development company. In: Proceedings of the SIGCHI Conference on Human Factors in Computing Systems (CHI 2013), pp. 353–359 (2000). http://doi.org/10.1145/332040.332456

34. Vorvoreanu, M., Dong, Z., McKenna, A., Madhavan, K.: Dealing with data deluge at national funding agencies: an investigation of user needs for understanding and managing research investment. In: Proceedings of CHI 2013 Conference on Human Factors in Computing Systems (2013)

35. Vorvoreanu, M., McKenna, A., Dong, Z., Madhavan, K.: Dealing with data deluge at national funding agencies: an investigation of user needs for understanding and managing research investments. In: Yamamoto, S., Oliveira, N.P. (eds.) HIMI 2015. LNCS, vol. 9173, pp. 140–151. Springer, Heidelberg (2015). doi:10.1007/978-3-319-20618-9_14

Redesign Based on Card Sorting: How Universally Applicable are Card Sort Results?

Jobke Wentzel[1](✉), Nienke Beerlage de Jong[2], and
Thea van der Geest[1]

[1] Department of Media, Communication and Organisation,
University of Twente, Enschede, The Netherlands
{m.j.wentzel,t.m.vandergeest}@utwente.nl
[2] Department of Psychology, Health and Technology, University of Twente,
Drienerlolaan 5, 7522 NB Enschede, The Netherlands
n.beerlage-dejong@utwente.nl

Abstract. Card sort studies can facilitate developers to create an information structure for their website or application. In addition, this human-centered design method provides researchers with insights into the target group's mental models regarding the information domain under study. In this method, participants sort cards, with excerpts of the website's or information source's information on them, into piles or groups. Even though the method lends itself for large numbers of participants, it can be difficult to include sufficient participants in a study to ensure generalizability among large user groups. Especially when the potential user group is heterogeneous, basing the information structure on a limited participant group may not always be valid. In this study, we investigate if card-sort results among one user group (nurses) are comparable to the results of a second (potential) user group (physicians/residents).

The results of a formative card sort study that were used to create an antibiotic information application are compared to the results of a second card sort study. This second study was conducted with the aim of redesigning the nurse-aimed information application to meet the (overlapping) needs of physicians. During the first card sort study, 10 nurses participated. In the second card sort study, 8 residents participated. The same set of 43 cards were used in both setups. These cards contain fragments of antibiotic protocols and reference documents that nurses and physicians use to be informed about the use and administration of antibiotics. The participants sorted the cards in individual sessions, into as many categories as they liked. The sorts of both user groups were analyzed separately. Dendrograms and similarity matrices were generated using the Optimal Sort online program. Based on the matrices, clusters were identified by two independent researchers. On these resulting clusters of cards, overlap scores were calculated (between nurse and resident clusters). Differences are compared.

The results show that overall, residents reached higher agreement than the nurses. Some overlap between categories is observed in both card sort data matrices. Based on the nurses' data, more and more specific clusters were created (which in part were observed in the larger residents' clusters).

Based on our findings we conclude that a redesign may not be necessary. Especially when the target group with the lowest prior knowledge levels of the information domain is included in the card sort study, the results can be

V.G. Duffy (Ed.): DHM 2016, LNCS 9745, pp. 381–388, 2016.
DOI: 10.1007/978-3-319-40247-5_38

translated to other groups as well. However, groups with little knowledge will more likely result in lower agreement in the card sorts. Therefore, a larger sample and/or including participants with low and high knowledge of the information domain is advisable.

Keywords: Card sorting · Re-design · Human-centered design · Information architecture

1   Introduction

Card sorting is a method that is used to establish an information structure for a website or application. In a card sort task, participants sort cards that have excerpts of the information that is to be communicated printed onto them. The resulting sorts (groups of cards) of every participant are compared and analyzed to detect what information topics are related to each other in the eyes of the participants. This method gives insight into the participants' mental models and thus provides a way to create information architectures that meet users' needs [1, 2]. Such an approach may be especially important to take for the development of eHealth applications, which often rely on medical information that is highly expert-driven [3]. Besides patients, health care workers can struggle to process information too. This can be caused by a mismatch between the information and their mental models, causing difficulty in comprehending and applying the information in daily life or clinical practice [4, 5]. Card sorts have been applied with success to create eHealth applications, both for patients and medical professionals [4–6]. In these examples, the human-centered design approach, including card sort studies, enabled a good fit with practice and increased efficiency in information use [7]. One of the possible drawbacks of the card sort approach is that usually a limited number of participants is involved, representing a (often) specific target group. After release, the website or application may prove useful to other user groups as well. This either results in users using an information application that was not designed for them (but possibly works fine), or it forces a re-design. Human-centered design implies certain levels of tailoring of information or features to specific user needs is needed [1]. Following this rationale, developers would need to redesign their application when rolling it out to other groups.

In this paper, we address the question whether a redesign is necessary for different user groups, based on a comparison of card sort results of two user groups. More specifically, we use the case of the information structure of the Antibiotic App, which was driven by a human-centered design approach, including a card sort study among nurses (the main target group) [6]. Physicians and residents (not the app's target group) of the pilot wards who used the app requested to have their own version of the app, quickly after it was introduced onto the wards. To accommodate these new users, a redesign process was started. This process included a second card sort study. In this paper, we describe the analysis of the data of both card sort studies to learn whether card sorting (of identical samples of cards) among different target groups results in substantially different sorts. This study can help researchers and developers decide on who to include in their formative research target groups, and anticipate on the universal applicability of their user-generated information structure.

2 Method

The results of a previous card-sort study with nurses [6] are compared to the results of a later but similar card sort study with a different participant group (medical residents). In the second study, eight residents of the same hospital the nurses in the first study worked at participated. The participants sorted a set of 43 cards with excerpts of medical protocols, reference books, guidelines, and other antibiotic-related information sources printed onto them. In individual settings, every participant created piles or groups of cards that were logical to him/her. The participants were free to create as many groups of cards that they thought was necessary. Prior to participating, participants were instructed about the study's goal and provided their informed consent to participating in the study.

The groups of cards that every participant created were entered in and analyzed with the online Optimal Sort program [8]. In this analysis, a focus was put on the cluster analysis; clusters of cards emerged based on how often two cards were placed together in the same group by the participants. Based on the similarity matrices and dendrograms (tree-like visual representation of clusters, produced by the program), two independent researchers defined the clusters for both participant groups (nurses, residents). The clusters were created by selecting the cards with high similarity (placed together by > 50 % of the participants). Outliers (no participant majority exists for any combination) were placed in the cluster where their similarity scores with the cards are highest. Next, the independent researchers compared the identified clusters to ensure the procedure renders consistent results. The final clusters of both studies (nurses, residents) were analyzed for similarities by calculating an overlap score, based on a similarity calculation applied in card sort analysis; the Jaccard score [9]. In this calculation, the amount of items that occur in both clusters is divided by the total amount of items in both clusters, then multiplied by 100 [9]. An overlap score of 75–100 was considered sufficient to label the two clusters as identical. Scores between 50–75 represent substantial overlap, scores of 25–50 moderate overlap and scores between 0–25 indicate that there is no noticeable overlap. Differences between the clusters are described and interpreted based on the contents of cards that the two participant groups did not agree upon. In the aforementioned analysis, agreement between participants to place two cards in one group was considered, not the similarities between the names participants gave to every pile of cards they created.

3 Results

The similarity matrices and dendrograms of both studies as produced by Optimal Sort can be viewed online via [10, 11].

3.1   Initial Analysis - Dendrograms

Based on the dendrograms, first results indicate that overall, similar groups are created by both participant groups. The dendrograms show that, with a cutoff percentage of 50 %, the nurses' and residents' data both result in 3 overall clusters. Roughly, nurses made a cluster of instructions during/for use (preparation, administration), description or general information, and special cautions or checks. The residents identify similar clusters, but with a separate cluster on dosage instead of cautions or checks, at this very basic agreement level.

3.2   In-depth Analysis – Proximity Matrices

To get more in-depth information on which cards are placed together and thus constitute a cluster, the proximity matrices were analyzed. These analyses resulted in five clusters in the residents' similarity matrix, and seven in the nurses' matrix (see Table 1).

Table 1. Nurses'and residents'cluster overlap scores

Nurse cluster [a] (amount of cards) ↓	Resident clusters [a] (amount of cards) →	Preparation - administration (15)	Particularities in administration (6)	Dose and checks (5)	Particularities – indication (8)	General description (9)
Administration (9)		**50**	7.1	0	0	0
Preparation - dose (11)		**36.8**	13.3	14.3	0	0
Particularities (9)		0	15.4	7.7	6.3	**38.5**
Cautions (6)		0	0	0	**40**	15.4
Type (2)		0	0	0	0	22.2
Side effects (3)		0	0	0	37.5	0
Checks (3)		0	12.5	**33.3**	0	0

[a]Clusters were defined based on similarity matrix scores > 50 %, or highest as possible for outliers.

The researcher provided names for each cluster, based on the cards placed in it. Roughly, the groups of cards that are recognized in both card sort outcomes include a cluster of cards containing information on preparation and administering the medication, cautions, particularities, and general descriptions. The nurses' clusters tend to be more specific (and smaller). Also, the average agreement percentages in the matrices (see outcomes via online display [10, 11]) show that the residents' data results in clearer and stronger clusters. The resident *Preparation and administration* cluster overlaps with the nurses' *Administration* (overlap score 50) and *Preparation- dose* (overlap score 36.8) cluster. However, based on the residents' sorts, dose is associated with some of the checks that need to be done (to adjust proper dosing), and is a separate cluster (*Dose and checks*). The nurse cluster *Particularities* holds information cards that can apply to other categories; the greatest overlap with the residents' clusters is with *General description* (overlap score 38.5), but there is also overlap with *Particularities – indication* (overlap score 6.3), *Dose and checks* (overlap score 7.7), and

Particularities in administration (overlap score 15.4). The nurses' more specific clusters of *Cautions* and *Type* are together with *Particularities* related to the somewhat generic or overarching resident cluster *General description* (overlap scores 15.4, 22.2, and 38.5, respectively).

During the card sort sessions and while analyzing the results it became clear that nurses had a tendency to group cards with information they were unfamiliar with into one group labeled 'for the physician'. The residents did the same with cards that hold information that is (in their eyes) very specific to the nurse tasks.

3.3   Disagreement and Cluster Overlap (Per Participant Group)

Some of the cards showed high disagreement among participants; participants did not agree on which cards the card should be grouped with. To get more insight into this, we checked in the similarity matrices [10, 11] which cards had high (> 50) similarity scores with cards outside their cluster. The residents' data shows that the *Preparation and administration* and *Particularities in administration* clusters (residents) are related, as similarity scores of cards of these two separate clusters range between 12–62 (median 37, mean 37.7). Card 38 (additional checks, belongs to dose and checks cluster) was placed with cards from the *Preparation and administration* cluster often (similarity score median 25, mean 29.1). In addition, card 57 (acute responses, belongs to *Particularities – indication* cluster) is placed with cards from the *Particularities in administration* cluster often (similarity score median 37, mean 33).

The nurses' data shows overall more disagreement; the similarity matrices [10, 11] show that many cards are placed with cards outside their own cluster. In fact, six cards in this matrix were grouped together with every other card by at least one participant. These were the cards 54. Compatibility, 71. Pregnancy, 70. Contra-indications, 73. Interactions, 38. Extra checks, and 39. Blood gas tests. In the residents' data matrix, this (a card being grouped with every other card by at least one participant) did not occur. An overlap between the *Administration* and *Preparation – dose* clusters is observed through the 8 cards of the former category which are placed often (similarity score > 50) with 9 cards of the latter cluster. Many cards of the *Particularities* cluster relate to the cards in *Cautions* (54. Compatibility, 55. Incompatibility, 71. Pregnancy, 68. Kinetic information, 36. Descriptions, 67. Characteristics) or *Type* (68 Kinetic information, 66. CHF advice, 40. Renal insufficiency). The *Checks* cards 38 (Extra checks) and 39 (Blood gas test) are related to the *Caution* cluster. These observations include cards which are placed with another card by at least 50 % of the participants. Smaller overlap (10–50 % agreement) outside the cluster was also observed.

4   Discussion

The results show that overall, similar groups are created by both user groups. However, some subgroups are placed together by nurses but not by residents (e.g., cards on preparation and dose) and vice versa (dose and checks). In addition, the nurse sorts showed less agreement and similarities than the residents' sorts. Regarding the research objective of determining whether re-design is needed, based on card sort results, these data provide useful insights. Especially in medical areas where the target groups have a fairly high level of (formal) training, redesign may not be necessary. Overall, overlap does exist and even when main clusters are not fully equal, subcategories are formed similarly by both groups. If different user groups have mutual understanding and agreement on each other's' (other target groups') tasks and responsibilities, this likely also contributes to universally applicable information structures. A need for redesign may become more urgent when user groups that have less knowledge of the subject wish to start using the application. In other studies, participants who are unfamiliar with the system and its contents created more diverse groups and labels in card sort studies than more knowledgeable and experienced participant groups [12]. Some of the cards were less relevant to the nurses than to the residents (e.g., information on renal insufficiency, kinetic characteristics of the drug), and vice versa (e.g., information on the preparation of an intravenous drug which is done by the nurse). These cards could be seen as a bit 'difficult', as they are not a prominent or relevant part of daily tasks. Interestingly, physicians still grouped all the cards similarly, whereas many difficult or less relevant cards were grouped in very diverse ways by the nurses. An explanation for this could be that residents or physicians are forced to internalize the protocols and reference books to a greater extent than nurses, in order to make save decisions on patient treatment. Nurses, however, mostly perform their regular tasks and only look up the information when something out of the ordinary happens. To accommodate the mental models of the nurses, who, in this case, seem a bit fuzzier than the residents', the information structure should enable cross-referencing to various themes or even include some description of the information structure to facilitate searching.

Possibly, including representatives of the target group with the lowest level of prior knowledge of the information as a participant group in formative card sort studies results in the best chances of universally applicable and comprehensible information structures. However, because participants who have little prior experience with the content need more time and effort to comprehend and process the cards, fewer cards can be used in a study. In addition, it is likely that more participants are needed to be able to identify clusters made by a majority. The reason for this is that there are probably more differences between inexperienced participants' sorts than between the sorts of a sample of participants who are knowledgeable on the subject of the cards that are sorted. In our study, the sorts of both professions were comparable, so designs are based ideally on user studies with both experienced and inexperienced participants. Their precise profession or background may matter less than their experience with the information that is communicated.

In the presentation, we will address the question whether a redesign for different user groups is necessary, based on a comparison of card sort results of our two user groups. Besides the conclusions presented in this paper, we will elaborate in the presentation on the differences between both user groups that we found. In addition, we will discuss how such results have implications for a good comprehension of the tasks to be supported by information applications.

4.1 Limitations

This study suffers from some limitations that need to be taken into account. First, the number of cards used in this study (43) may have been insufficient to enable participants to form various, substantive clusters. In a previous study, samples of 100 cards proved to be about the maximum of cards (if not too much) to sort [12]. Therefore, in this study, fewer cards were used. Likewise, the amount of participants is not high, but not unusual for these types of studies [13]. The ideal amount of cards and participants to include in a study depends on the content (difficulty, variation of cards), and the representativeness of the participant sample. The limited amount of cards allowed us to create the clusters manually (based on the similarity matrices). Bigger samples (of cards and participants) are too complex to analyze manually but they do enable statistical analysis like hierarchical cluster analysis or factor analysis [9].

4.2 Future Work

Possibly, card-sort studies are a low-threshold method to learn whether redesigns are needed. In future studies, the need for additional user studies for a re-design that matches the needs of a new target group can be further investigated. This study shows that in fields with highly protocolled information, inter-professional differences are low. Rather, (job) experience and good understanding of the other target group's tasks and responsibilities might be at play. It is worthwhile to explore to what extent designs can be attuned to information domain novices or experienced users. Our future work will (among other things) further focus on determining the best analytic approach for analyzing card sort data, including in non-web-development settings, as a means of qualitative data structuring [14].

5 Conclusion

Based on our findings, we conclude that card-sorting is a quick method to determine whether a redesign for the information structure is needed for different target groups. However, even when the target groups' tasks differ, results will be more similar with increased participant experience and mutual understanding of the tasks an responsibilities of other user groups. In such cases, redesign is unnecessary. Therefore, if user groups are heterogeneous, and some users may have low levels of information and task experience, it is best to include these users in design studies, regardless of the user target group they represent to ensure the broadest relevance or universal information structure match of the application.

Acknowledgements. We thank the nurses and medical residents of the Medisch Spectrum Twente hospital, in Enschede, the Netherlands, for participating in this study. This study was conducted within the Interreg IVa-funded project EurSafety Heath-net (III-1-02 = 73). This is a Dutch-German cross-border network supported by the European Commission, the Federal States of Nordrhein-Westfalen and Niedersachsen(Germany), and the Dutch provinces of Overijssel, Gelderland, and Limburg. Part of the study was executed within a project (Google Glass For VIPS), funded as a Tech4People 2015 grant by the faculty BMS of the University of Twente.

References

1. Maguire, M.: Methods to support human-centred design. Int. J. Hum Comput Stud. **55**, 587–634 (2001)
2. Morville, P., O'reilly, T.: Information Architecture for the World Wide Web. O'Reilly, Sebastopol (2007)
3. Van Velsen, L., Wentzel, J., Van Gemert-Pijnen, J.E.W.C.: Designing eHealth that matters via a multidisciplinary requirements development approach. JMIR Res. Protoc. **2**(1), e21 (2013)
4. Verhoeven, F., Karreman, J., Bosma. A., Hendrix, H.R.M., van Gemert-Pijnen, L.E.W.C.: Toward improved education of the public about methicillin-resistant Staphylococcus aureus: a mental models approach. Inter. J. Infect. Control **6**(1) (2010)
5. Verhoeven, F., Hendrix, R.M., Daniels-Haardt, I., Friedrich, A.W., Steehouder, M.F., van Gemert-Pijnen, J.E.: The development of a web-based information tool for cross-border prevention and control of Methicillin Resistant Staphylococcus aureus. Inter. J. Infect. Control **4**(1), 11 (2008)
6. Wentzel, J., van Velsen, L., van Limburg, M., de Jong, N., Karreman, J., Hendrix, R., van Gemert, J.E.W.C.: Participatory eHealth development to support nurses in antimicrobial stewardship. BMC Med. Inf. Decis. Making **14**(1), 45 (2014)
7. Wentzel, J., van Drie-Pierik, R., Nijdam, L., Geesing, J., Sanderman, R., van Gemert-Pijnen, J.: Antibiotic information application offers nurses quick support. Am. J. Inf. Control (2016). (in press)
8. Optimal Workshop - Optimal sort. https://www.optimalworkshop.com/
9. Capra, M.G.: Factor analysis of card sort data: an alternative to hierarchical cluster analysis. Proc. Hum. Factors Ergon. Soc. Ann. Meet. **49**(5), 691–695 (2005). SAGE Publications
10. Nurse card sort study results: similarity matrix and dendrogram. https://www.optimalworkshop.com/optimalsort/mrsa-net/68158f/shared-results/ba49d9fe334fe8f3ba780902dc37e6a8
11. Resident card sort study results: similarity matrix and dendrogram. https://www.optimalworkshop.com/optimalsort/mrsa-net/b75e78/shared-results/805474e2179ad3089f370cbb6c73eb58
12. Wentzel, J., Müller, F., Beerlage-de Jong, N., van Gemert-Pijnen, J.: Card sorting to evaluate the robustness of the information architecture of a protocol website. Inter. J. Med. Inf. **86**, 71–81 (2016)
13. Nielsen, J.: Card Sorting: How Many Users to Test (2004). http://www.useit.com/alertbox/20040719html. Accessed 2 March 2015
14. Coxon, A.P.M.: Sorting data: Collection and analysis, vol. 127. Sage Publications, Thousand Oaks (1999)

Work Design and Support

Comparison Knitting Skills Between Experts and Non-experts by Measurement of the Fabric Quality

Kontawat Chottikampon[1]([⊠]), Shunyu Tang[1],
Suchalinee Mathurosemontri[1], Porakoch Sirisuwan[1], Miyako Inoda[1],
Hiroyuki Nishimoto[2], and Hiroyuki Hamada[1]

[1] Kyoto Institute of Technology, Matsugasaki,
Sakyo-ku, Kyoto 606-8585, Japan
ruklongtime@hotmail.com
[2] Osaka Sangyo University, 3-1-1 Nakagaito, Daito, Osaka 574-8530, Japan

Abstract. This research focused on the developing the capacity of knitting skill. The comparison of skill between the experts with non-experts was studied. The movement of arms was measured to investigate the effect of arm movement on quality of knitting fabric. The experiment was carried out with a video camera to record and analyze the differences of the knitting speed and manner in knitting. The quality of the fabric was measured by a loop of fabric to see the consistency of the loop fabric, which is important for beautiful fabrics. The results revealed the procedure used to crochet knitting machines were very different in appearance, knitting and speed. The quality of the fabric was beautiful, similar to the use of the knitting as machine knitting. The main difference between them was only part of the seams.

Keywords: Knitting · Arm movement measurement · Knitting skill · Plain pattern

1 Introduction

The knitting is a process of manufacturing a fabric by inters looping of yarns. Knitting is the second most important method of fabric formation. It can be defined as a needle technique of fabric formation, in which, with the help of knitting needles, loops are formed to make a fabric or garment. Fabric can be formed by hand or machine knitting, but the basic principle remains.

A knitting machine is a device used to create knitted fabrics in a semi or fully automated fashion. There are numerous types of knitting machines, ranging from simple spool or board templates with no moving parts to highly complex mechanisms controlled by electronics. All, however, produce various types of knitted fabrics, usually either flat or tubular, and of varying degrees of complexity. Pattern stitches can be selected by hand manipulation of the needles, or with push-buttons and dials, mechanical punch cards, or electronic pattern reading devices and computers.

© Springer International Publishing Switzerland 2016
V.G. Duffy (Ed.): DHM 2016, LNCS 9745, pp. 391–398, 2016.
DOI: 10.1007/978-3-319-40247-5_39

Manual knitting machines require the knitter to move the specific needles, based on a chart, into pattern position. In this research I study the knitting structure is plain and rib. Plain knit, the basic form of knitting can be produced in flat knit or in tubular (or circular) form. It is also called jersey stitch or balbriggan stitch. A row of latch or beard needles is arranged in a linear position on a needle plate or in a circular position on a cylinder. Rib stitch produces alternate lengthwise rows of plain and purl stitches and as such the face and back of the fabrics are a lookalike. Rib stitch can be produced on a flat rib machine as well as circular rib machine.

2 Experimental

One expert and six non-experts were recorded their movement during knitting process. By all of them used the same material and same pattern in this experiment. Figure 1 shows the knitting process in this study.

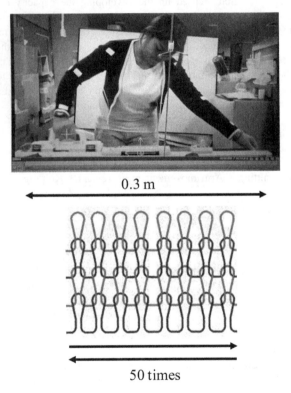

0.3 m

50 times

Fig. 1. Knitting process

3   Results and Discussion

3.1   Knitted Fabrics

Figure 2 shows the final knitting products from the expert and the non-experts. It is difficult to inform which one is poor or good quality by eyes.

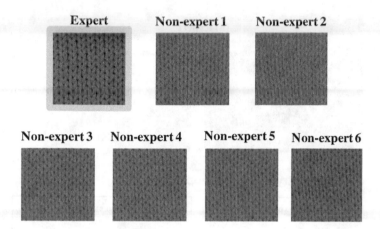

Fig. 2. Photographs of knitting fabrics from the experty and the non-experts

3.2   Quality of Knitted Fabrics

The quality of knitting fabric was observed by the symmetry of knitting loop. The blue line represents the loop of knitting pattern. The length from the center of the curve on the left side to the top curve was measured as well as the right side. In addition, the length from the center of the left curve to right curve was also measured as presented in Fig. 3.

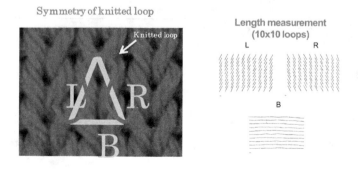

Fig. 3. Observation for the quality of knitted fabrics

3.3   Symmetry of Knitted Loop of the Expert and Non-experts

From Fig. 4(a), it was found that the length of left side and right side of the expert are quite symmetry as show in the length distribution curves. Figures 4(b) to (g) show the result of non-experts. It can be seen that non-expert 2 and 4 showed the symmetry of loop whereas the other revealed the non-symmetry between L side and R side.

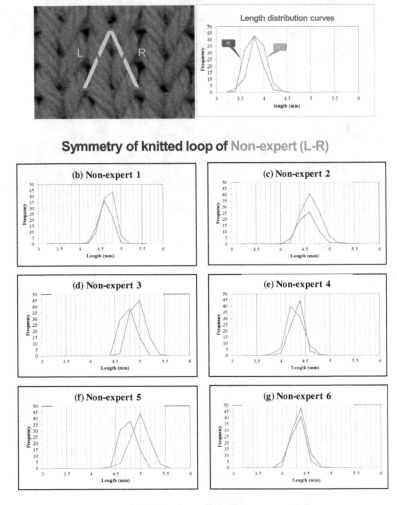

Fig. 4. Symmetry of knitting loop from the expert and the non-experts

3.4 Relative Handle Moving Distance and Times of the Expert and Non-experts

Figure 5 shows the relative handle moving distance and times of expert. The moving distance is in range of −0.3 to 0.3.

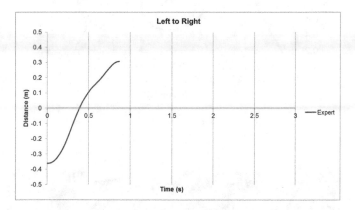

Fig. 5. Relative handle moving distance and times of the expert and non-experts

When compare with non-experts, it was found that the non-experts took longer time for moving the handle from left to right. However, their distances were in the same range as shown in Fig. 6.

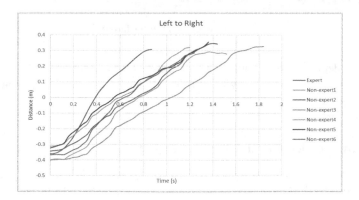

Fig. 6. Movement of the handle from left to right at the knitting of the expert and non-experts

3.5 Relative Velocity and Times of the Expert and Non-experts

Figure 7 presents the relative of velocity and times of the expert. The velocity rapidly increased and droped obviously. The velocity dropped due to the high fiction when handle move pass the fabric as a circle shown in Figs. 7 and 8.

Left to Right expert

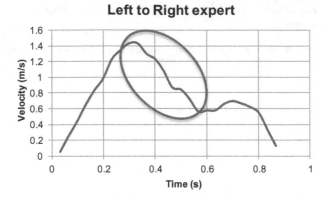

Fig. 7. Relative velocity and times of the expert

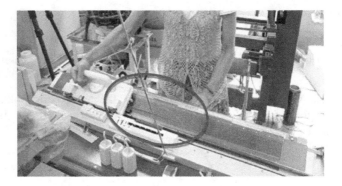

Fig. 8. Position of knitting fabric

Figure 9 depicts the comparison of the velocity between the expert and non-experts. The range of velocity that the handle move pass the fabric of non-expert lower than the expert.

3.6   Relative Acceleration and Times of Expert

For the expert, the acceleration rapidly increased and dropped obviously. Because the high fiction occurred when handle moved pass the fabric, the results of the non-experts are quite different from the expert as presented in Fig. 10. Although, the tendency of them were quite similar, their curves of relationship between time and acceleration did not smooth when compare the expert. When the handle were moved pass the fabric, there is a high variability of acceleration. This may caused the less familiarity of the non-experts. The action of arm movement is also important for forced that propel the handle.

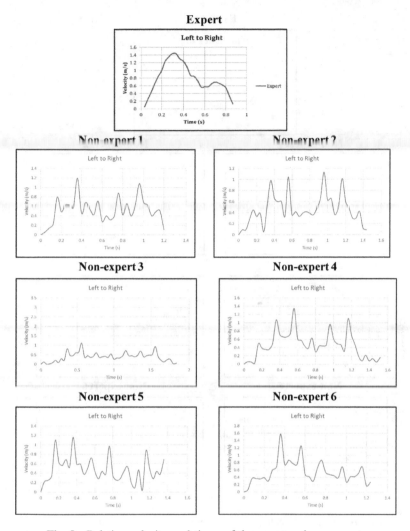

Fig. 9. Relative velocity and times of the expert and non-experts

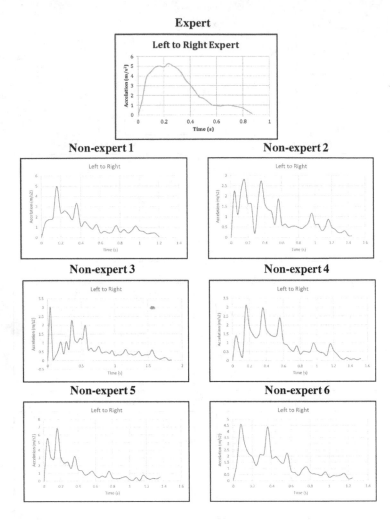

Fig. 10. Relative acceleration and times of the expert and non-experts

4   Conclusion

The comparison of the arm movement analysis between knitting expert and non-experts were reported. The expert showed the highest knitting speed by using the arm moving only. While non-experts used the rotation of body and some non-expert moved their body together with a handle moving to support arm movement because they held a handle incorrectly. That led to the slower knitting speed when compared to the expert. The higher knitting speed affected the bigger area under the knitting loop. For the next experiment, non-experts have to imitate the knitting behavior from the expert especially the arm position and the handle holding position. Then comparing their fabric quality and knitting speed.

Modern Human-Robot Interaction in Smart Services and Value Co-creation

Vincent G. Duffy[✉]

School of Industrial Engineering, Agricultural & Biological Engineering,
Purdue University, Grissom Hall, West Lafayette, IN 47907, USA
duffy@purdue.edu

Abstract. Modern work design must re-examine human-robot interaction and consider ways to effectively utilize emerging industrial capabilities such as collaborative robots and humanoids in the context of usability and our emerging service economy. By incorporating human aspects into technology-based efforts focused on value co-creation, it appears likely that inexpensive collaborative robots and humanoids can serve as integral parts of effective smart service systems designs. Ways to create value through such human-robot interaction are highlighted through recent research. A change in paradigm will need to occur to shift emphasis from 'block the path' to 'design out' when it comes to effective human-robot interaction in the workplace. It is apparent that smart service development will continue through multi-disciplinary initiatives that are human-centered. Usability and other human factors principles will continue to be central to successes. Organizational aspects that recognize fundamental relationships between job satisfaction and service quality can provide a foundation upon which capabilities of humanoids and collaborative robots can be leveraged in modern industrial and smart operations.

Keywords: Value Co-creation · Humanoid · Human-Robot interaction · Smart services · Safety · Operations management · E-Services · Usability · User-centered design · Digital human modeling

1 Introduction

When products are poorly designed, increased business costs include training, user error, poor productivity, reduced sales, increased need for customer support and tarnished corporate image [1, 2]. Capabilities of industrial robots [3] have progressed and show promise beyond traditional assembly and manufacturing, with opportunities for collaboration and education to create value for the service provider and service recipient. Even in most recent books on occupational safety and health [4], the emphasis in regard to industrial robots is on prevention of the interaction between human and robot. A change in paradigm will need to occur to shift emphasis from 'block the path' to 'design out' when it comes to the use of robots in the workplace. System designers will need to consider expected use and design out potential adverse events to avoid potential safety incidents. Modern robots can become an integral part of services provided the human-robot interaction is considered from the usability perspective from the outset.

© Springer International Publishing Switzerland 2016
V.G. Duffy (Ed.): DHM 2016, LNCS 9745, pp. 399–408, 2016.
DOI: 10.1007/978-3-319-40247-5_40

1.1   Value Co-creation

The concept of value co-creation is now widely applied in service systems. Value co-creation can be defined as joint activities of service recipients and service providers to contribute to value that emerges for one or both parties [5]. See Fig. 1. Smart services can be created while turning big data into intelligence following a path that includes identifying useful information and knowledge building.

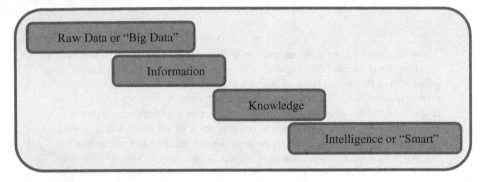

Fig. 1. Human modeling that includes collaborative robots and effective human-robot interaction can provide value for service provider and service recipient by transforming data into intelligence.

1.2   Smart Services

The amount of information available for decision making has grown tremendously in recent years and better knowledge is essential to improved decisions [6]. In fact, one may consider a progression from *raw data* to *information* to *knowledge* and then *intelligence* that has translated to descriptions like "*smart*" in recent systems design initiatives. Industrial managers need research skills. An introduction will be given about Smart Service System Design in Sect. 2 Smart Products and Systems.

1.3   E-Services and Smart Operations

E-Commerce includes business-to-business and business-to-consumer activities for products and services. E-Commerce has grown tremendously in recent years. E-Service is defined as the provision of services over electronic networks such as Internet, without being limited to service organizations and including all enterprises including those that manufacture goods that require development and implementation of sound service practices over electronic networks [7].

In considering smart operations, a brief introduction will be given in the context of smart products. In order to address the use of smart products for services, a range of capabilities of these smart products will be illustrated. As e-services are typically human centered and the smart products exist at the intersection of disciplines, there are opportunities for human factors. Smart operations will be those that can capitalize on such smart products in a systems context.

2 Smart Products and Systems

Information technology is revolutionizing products that were once composed solely of mechanical and electrical parts [8]. In the figure above, intelligence is referred to and gives rise to terms like "smart" to describe capabilities in context of the organizations and how they may benefit. Human factors can contribute as a discipline that considers the interaction between people and the technology. Smart products (see Fig. 2) provide opportunity for more complex systems. Many large complex systems fail to meet stakeholder expectations due to social and organizational complexity of the environment in which the systems are deployed [9]. These will be addressed briefly in the context of human factors fundamentals at the organizational and social level.

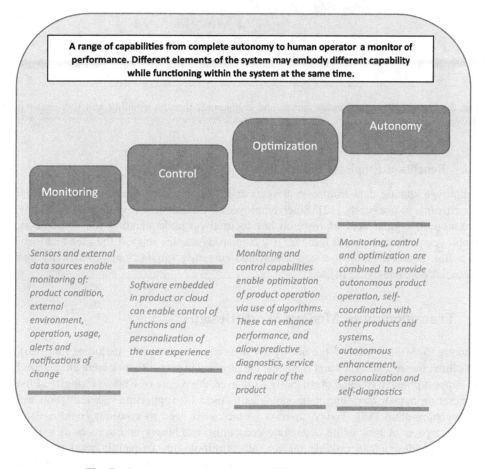

Fig. 2. Smart connected product capabilities (adapted from [8])

2.1   Human Aspects of Smart Service Systems

"Smart devices" exist at the intersection of disciplines. As service systems continue to dominate industrialized economies, it is important to consider these for their potential as service providers. When considering smart things as service providers, a convergence of disciplines is needed [10]. See Fig. 3. Fundamental principles need to be better understood at the intersection of 'sensing and actuating', cognitive, communication and computational fields. Usability is an important aspect of the user experience [11]. It is central to any human-centered devices or systems those devices may be integrated with. The next section will focus briefly on select usability, human error and human factors, including social and organizational aspects.

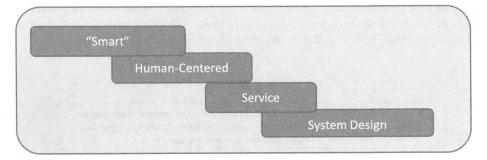

Fig. 3. Opportunities for human factors and ergonomics through usability and user-centered design.

2.2   Benefits of Employee Satisfaction

Employee attitude data from over 8 years and 35 companies were analyzed to draw conclusions in one study [12]. Since employees are ultimately responsible for quality production, a great deal of research has focused on understanding job satisfaction, employee performance and turnover [6]. Numerous studies support the idea that there is a link between employee satisfaction and customer satisfaction, productivity and financial outcomes [13, 14].

3   Transitioning to Modern Work Design

Among 5 Ms considered previously by operations managers, including hu(man), machine, money, materials and methods, the physical aspects of work were emphasized to support productivity and profitability. However, the nature of work is changing. First generation human modeling methodologies focused on supporting risk reduction and injury prevention [15]. Today, there is an increased need to consider cognitive and social aspects of task while leveraging computing machinery and sensors of various types. Job design can provide insight into terminologies frequently used in recent media reports from an organizational perspective such as "big data" and "information engineering". The methods to be presented and their associated principles are presented in support of the development of successful prototypes and applications in the context of these media reports and skills that modern industrial organizations would like new employees to have [16].

Work design previously focused largely at the individual level and overlapped significantly with human factors and ergonomics. Early work by F.W. Taylor, more than 100 years ago now, used motion to film workers to demonstrate how productivity could be improved [6]. It is suggested that large and small businesses can better understand their own internal work environments with modern analytical tools, incorporating the use of computing resources and e-service information available within modern organizations.

Studies have shown the relationships between training and improved performance [17]. Measures such as those outlined in Lee and Duffy [18] can give insight into ways in which to compare before and after training performance in the context of tasks requiring both cognitive and physical aspects of work. *Time Performance Ratio*, *Wrong Answer Rate Ratio*, *Type Rate Ratio* are a few examples [18]. An analysis of other data and information from within or across companies can provide further insight, knowledge and intelligence or "smart" capabilities.

A key objective of this writing is to provide highlight the need for characterizing, analyzing and human modeling for direct application in developing and improving e-services and operations. The service-dominant logic contrasts with traditional goods-dominant logic [19]. The change in paradigm that will need to occur includes a shift in emphasis from 'block the path' to 'design out' strategy in occupational safety-aspects when it comes to the use of robots in the workplace. Human factors and human modeling focusing on user-centered design and usability. Modern human-robot interaction can improve individual and operational outcomes.

4 Modern Industrial Robots and Humanoids in Collaboration

4.1 Changing Paradigm Toward Industrial Collaboration

Boston Dynamics has developed "Petman", an anthropormorphic (human-like) robot designed to test chemical protective clothing [20]. The robot, having some human characteristics will measure if, when and where chemical agents are detected. In this case, chemical sensors are embedded in the "skin" of the robot are intended to identify when chemicals bypass individual protective equipment (clothing). Other chemical-based sensors could be integrated into future robot-human interaction. For instance, wasted food has multi-billion dollar direct economic costs. Sensors that monitor fruit ripeness and meat, fish or poultry freshness in various stages of the supply chain are in development and can contribute toward improved decisions for both retailers and consumers [21].

Until recently, the study of people's relationships and interactions with other (nonhuman) beings has received scant attention from the social sciences [22]. Examples of "Big Dog", a six-legged robot successfully climbing a snow covered hill [23], raise fundamental issues about limits and capabilities for collaboration with robots. Considering these new capabilities recently developed in the robotics community, other potential applications in industrial settings, including collaborative security, are not yet well addressed in service science or occupational safety and health literature.

4.2   Education and Health Services

The "Computers As Social Actors" paradigm was originally presented in human-computer interaction and human-computer studies-related literature [24]. Elements of this framework, applied more recently in education, show feedback from computers and its effect on perceived ability and affect [25]. Researchers in Europe developed a multi-modal tutoring robot. In a recent international workshop, design and implementation principles for human-machine interface are highlighted [26]. In relation to the human modeling community, these researchers highlight real-time capture devices and modeling techniques that are maturing and becoming more accessible to researchers. Al Moubayed and co-authors [27] point out new understandings in human-human conversations.

One major obstacle in the face of exploring the effects of spoken social and affective behavior of artificial embodied entities lies in the multidisciplinary nature of these setups and in the limitations of the different technologies that they involve [27]. As noted by Cassell [28], we, as humans, make complex representational gestures with hands, gaze away and toward one another and use pitch in voice to clarify or emphasize what we are saying. Essentially, there are many non-verbal aspects of our interactions in service and value co-creation that require consideration of potential human-robot interactions that are beyond those previously addressed in the "Computers As Social Actor" paradigm, in order to have effective cooperation and collaboration with these newly available robots.

A recent NSF award for adaptive robotic nursing assistant focuses on support for physical tasks in hospital environments [29]. Oborn and co-authors [30] suggest that the social and technical elements of robots iteratively have and will influence and redefine one another. They highlight the usefulness of a 'service logic' perspective, and that there is a need for increased emphasis on sociological dimensions of using robots, recognizing how social and work relations are reformed during use. Behavior modeling methods and approaches to more natural human-robot interactions, including robot initiating conversation, are highlighted by Masahiro Shiomi and other research colleagues at Advanced Telecommunications Research Institute International in Kyoto, Japan [31]. In one specific application, they used a wheelchair robot they developed in order to support movement of elderly people. They addressed especially 'intention to use' and speaking behavior to convey location related information and speed adjustment based on individual preferences [32].

4.3   "Big Data" and Face Reader in Services

In considering visitor engagement at science centres and museums, Leister and co-authors [33] highlight a four layered assessment framework which emphasizes a

'Scenario layer', a 'Data Collection and Observer layer', an 'Assessment layer' and an 'Assessment Process layer'. Additional insight into best practice in support of interactive technologies in muesums can be found in recent literature by Partarakis, Antona and colleagues at ICS-Forth in Crete [34]. As noted in Leister [33], and in many 'big data' scenarios at this time, most of the data can not be processed automatically and still need human intervention.

An important contribution here [33] is the use of 'face reader' to give objective information that can supplement other modes of information that may be available from the response of the service recipient. Such information could be related to quality of service or satisfaction. Data about emotional response of service providers or service recipients could possibly be retrieved by roaming humanoid service providers that may have direct access to service recipients in collaboration. Variations on Bayesian analyses as outlined in Taylor et al. [35] can be used to advantage in analysis of available data in related applications.

4.4 Eye Tracking Can Assist in Supporting Effective Human-System Interface Design and Human-Robot Interaction

Emotions are an important part of learning and assessment procedures, while measuring emotion is a demanding task [36]. A multi-modal approach can assist in the application of face reader in recognizing response of service recipients. Heat maps showing relative duration of eye fixation and gaze plots showing sequence and locations where participant's gaze lingered, can give insight into user interest under the premise that what people are looking at is related to what they are thinking about [37]. Recent applications in health include prediction of stress recovery in depression cases [38].

Graham and co-authors [39] reviewed literature that considered nutrition label use and utilized eye tracking. Recommendations were made for label enhancement related to nutrition label use. They identified directions for further research and made recommendations in which labels could be modified to improve consumers' ability to use nutrition labels when selecting healthy foods. Eye tracking was also used in combination with word association to assess novel packing solutions in consumer products [40]. Ways to further quantify and model user experience in the context of mobile human-machine interface capitalize on lessons learned in Kansei Engineering and are briefly outlined by Qu and co-authors [41].

5 Conclusions

In summary, the field is wide open. A multi-disciplinary team comprised of individuals contributing from various strategically considered academic specialties can make progress in related research moving beyond traditional human-robot interaction paradigms to support a wide variety of "smart" service related tasks. In this time of greater appreciation for multi-disciplinary research at Federal Agencies and at major Research Universities, you are strongly encouraged to participate.

Acknowledgements. The author wishes to express thanks and appreciation to the following colleagues for participation in related discussions: Mihaela Vorvoreanu, Yuehwern Yih, Barbara Almanza, Jan Schnorr, Rohit Kshirsagar, Debora Steffen, Debra Runshe, Amy Van Epps, Lindsey Payne, Dave Nelson, Chantal Levesque-Bristol, Steve Abel, Shimon Nof, Laura Lynn Henzl, Qing-Xing Qu, Le Zhang, Vivia Wen-Yu Chao, Shefali Rana, Apoorva A. Sulakhe, Nikhil A. Patwardhan and the students of IE556 Job Design in Spring 2016 including Shelley Stites, Kristina Tabar, Kevin Walker, Dina Verdin, William Gerwing, Jeongjoon Boo, Zimeng Liu, Zhanfei Jeffrey Shi, Abigail Tighe and Stephen Murray.

References

1. Dhillon, B.S.: Engineering Usability: Fundamentals, Applications Human Factors and Human Error. American Scientific Publishers Stevenson Ranch, California (2004)
2. Keinonen, T., Mattelmäki, T., Soosalu, M., Säde, S.: Usability Design Methods (1997)
3. Or, C.K.L., Duffy, V.G., Cheung, C.C.: Perception of safe robot idle time in virtual reality and real industrial environments. Int. J. Ind. Ergon. **39**(5), 807–812 (2009)
4. Goetsch, D.L.: Occupational Safety and Health for Technologists, Engineers and Managers, 8th edn. Pearson-Prentice Hall, Upper Saddle River (2015). Computers, Automation & Robots, Chap. 23, pp. 493–496
5. Zhang, L., Tong, H., Demirel, H.O., Duffy, V.G., Yih, Y., Bidassie, B.: A practical model of value co-creation in healthcare service. Procedia Manuf. **3**, 200–207 (2015)
6. Nof, S.Y., Ceroni, J., Jeong, W., Moghaddam, M.: Revolutionizing collaboration through e-Work, e-Business, and e-Service, vol. 2. Springer, Heidelberg (2015)
7. Porter, M.E., Heppelmann, J.E.: How Smart, Connected Products are Transforming Competition. Harvard Bus. Rev. **92**(11), 11–64 (2014)
8. Zewge, A., Dittrich, Y., Bekele, R.: Adapting participatory design to design information system with rural ethiopian community. In: AFRICON 2015, pp. 1–5. IEEE (2015)
9. Medina-Borja, A.: Editorial column—smart things as service providers: a call for convergence of disciplines to build a research agenda for the service systems of the future. Serv. Sci. **7**(1), ii–v (2015)
10. Ardito, C., Buono, P., Caivano, D., Costabile, M.F., Lanzilotti, R., Dittrich, Y.: Human-centered design in industry: lessons from the trenches. Computer **12**, 86–89 (2014)
11. Schneider, B., Hanges, P.J., Smith, D.B., Salvaggio, A.N.: Which comes first: employee attitudes or organizational financial and market performance? J. Appl. Psychol. **88**(5), 836–851 (2003)
12. Hair Jr., J.F., Wolfinbarger, M., Money, A.H., Samouel, P., Page, M.J.: Essentials of Business Research Methods. Routledge, New York (2016)
13. Corporate Leadership Council: Linking Employee Satisfaction with Productivity, Performance and Customer Satisfaction, pp. 1–6 (2003). www.corporateleadershipcouncil. com, http://www.keepem.com/doc_files/clc_articl_on_productivity.pdf. Accessed 1 Oct 2016
14. Parker, D.: Service Operations Management: The Total Experience. Edward Elgar Publishing, Northampton (2012)
15. Duffy, V.G.: Modified virtual build methodology for computer-aided ergonomics and safety. Hum. Factors Ergon. Manuf. Serv. Ind. **17**(5), 413–422 (2007)
16. Demirel, H.O., Duffy, V.G.: Digital human modeling for product lifecycle management. In: Duffy, V.G. (ed.) HCII 2007 and DHM 2007. LNCS, vol. 4561, pp. 372–381. Springer, Heidelberg (2007)

17. Lingard, H.: The effect of first aid training on objective safety behaviour in australian small business construction firms. Constr. Manage. Econ. **19**(6), 611–618 (2001)

18. Lee, B.-C., Duffy, V.G.: The effects of task interruption on human performance: a study of the systematic classification of human behavior and interruption frequency. Hum. Factors Ergon. Manuf. Serv. Ind. **25**(2), 137–152 (2015)

19. Lusch, R., Vargo, S., O'Brien, M.: Competing through service: insights from service-dominant logic. J. Retail. **83**, 5–18 (2006)

20. Nelson, G., Saunders, A., Neville, N., Swilling, B., Bondaryk, J., Billings, D., Lee, C., Playter, R., Raibert, M · PETMAN: A humanoid robot for testing chemical protective clothing. J. Robot. Soc. Jpn. **30**(4), 372–377 (2012). 日本ロボット学会誌

21. C$_2$ Sense (2015). http://www.c2sense.com/. Accessed 10 Oct 2015

22. Serpell, J.A.: Having our dogs and eating them too: why animals are a social issue. J. Soc. Issues **65**(3), 633–644 (2009)

23. Raibert, M.: Dynamic legged robots for rough terrain. In: 2010 10th IEEE-RAS International Conference on Humanoid Robots (Humanoids), p. 1. IEEE (2010)

24. Nass, C., Fogg, B.J., Moon, Y.: Can computers be teammates? Int. J. Hum Comput Stud. **45**(6), 669–678 (1996)

25. Mishra, P.: Affective feedback from computers and its effect on perceived ability and affect: a test of the computers as social actor hypothesis. J. Educ. Multimedia Hypermedia **15**(1), 107–131 (2006)

26. Al Moubayed, S., Beskow, J., Bollepalli, B., Gustafson, J., Hussen-Abdelaziz, A., Johansson, M., Koutsombogera, M., et al.: Human-robot collaborative tutoring using multiparty multimodal spoken dialogue. In: Proceedings of the 2014 ACM/IEEE International Conference on Human-Robot Interaction, pp. 112–113. ACM (2014)

27. Al Moubayed, S., Beskow, J., Beskow, J., Bollepalli, B., Hussen-Abdelaziz, A., Johansson, M., Koutsombogera, M.: Tutoring robots. In: Lopes, J.D., et al. (eds.). IFIP, vol. 425, pp. 80–113. Springer, Heidelberg (2013)

28. Cassell, J.: Embodied Conversational Agents. MIT Press, Cambridge (2009)

29. NSF PFI:BIC Adaptive Robotic Nursing Assistants for Physical Tasks in Hospital Environments, Division of Industrial Innovation & Partnerships, awarded to Popa, D., Wiesman, R., Mor, A., Shin, J., Behan, D. National Science Foundation, Washington, D.C. (2015).   http://www.nsf.gov/awardsearch/showAward?AWD_ID=1534124.   (retrieved 3/15/2016)

30. Oborn, E., Barrett, M., Darzi, A.: Robots and service innovation in health care. J. Health Serv. Res. Policy **16**(1), 46–50 (2011)

31. Shi, C., Shiomi, M., Kanda, T., Ishiguro, H., Hagita, N.: Measuring communication participation to initiate conversation in human-robot interaction. Int. J. Social Robot. **7**(5), 889–910 (2015)

32. Shiomi, M., Iio, T., Kamei, K., Sharma, C., Hagita, N.: Effectiveness of social behaviors for autonomous wheelchair robot to support elderly people in Japan. PLoS ONE **10**(5), e0128031 (2015)

33. Leister, W., Tjøstheim, I., Joryd, G., Schulz, T.: Towards assessing visitor engagement in science centres and museums. In: Proceedings of the PESARO, pp. 21–27 (2015)

34. Partarakis, N., Zidianakis, E., Antona, M., Stephanidis, C.: Art and coffee in the museum. In: Streitz, N., Markopoulos, P. (eds.) DAPI 2015. LNCS, vol. 9189, pp. 370–381. Springer, Heidelberg (2015)

35. Taylor, J.A., Lacovara, A.V., Smith, G.S., Pandian, R., Lehto, M.: Nearmiss narratives from the fire service: a bayesian analysis. Accid. Anal. Prev. **62**, 119–129 (2014)

36. Terzis, V., Moridis, C.N., Economides, A.A.: Measuring instant emotions based on facial expressions during computer-based assessment. Pers. Ubiquit. Comput. **17**(1), 43–52 (2013)

37. Nielsen, J., Pernice, K.: Eyetracking Web Usability, pp. 11–13. Pearson Education & New Riders Press, Berkeley, California (2010)
38. Sanchez, A., Vazquez, C., Marker, C., LeMoult, J., Joormann, J.: Attentional disengagement predicts stress recovery in depression: an eye-tracking study. J. Abnorm. Psychol. **122**(2), 303–313 (2013)
39. Graham, D.J., Orquin, J.L., Visschers, V.H.M.: Eye tracking and nutrition label use: a review of the literature and recommendations for label enhancement. Food Policy **37**(4), 378–382 (2012)
40. Piqueras-Fiszman, B., Velasco, C., Salgado-Montejo, A., Spence, C.: Using combined eye tracking and word association in order to assess novel packaging solutions: a case study involving jam jars. Food Qual. Prefer. **28**(1), 328–338 (2013)
41. Qu, Q.-X., Zhang, L., Chao, W.-Y., Duffy, V.G.: User Experience Design Based on Eye-Tracking Technology: A Case Study on Smart Phone APPs. In: Duffy, V.G. (eds.) Applied Digital Human Modeling and Simulation. Springer (in press, 2016)

Interactive Gestures
for Liver Angiography Operation

Dina A. Elmanakhly[2](✉), Ayman Atia[1], Essam A. Rashed[2],
and Mostafa-Samy M. Mostafa[1]

[1] HCI-LAB, Department of CS, Faculty of Computers and Information,
Helwan University, Helwan, Egypt
[2] Image Science-LAB, Department of Mathematics, Faculty of Science,
Suez Canal University, Ismailia, Egypt
dinaelmanakhly@yahoo.com

Abstract. The main challenge of creating large interactive displays in the operating rooms (ORs) is in the definition of ways that are efficient and easy to learn for the physician. Apart from traditional input methods such as mouse and keyboard, we have developed a multimodal system with two different vision based human-computer interaction (HCI) systems that can simplify the way surgeons interact with the medical images shown on the LCD display. The purpose of this work is to construct a gesture recognition system with a fast, accurate, and easily attainable method. The first system is a laser pointer interaction framework that supports a 2D stroke gesture interface. The recorded laser gestures are recognized using two different algorithms: dynamic time warping (DTW) and one dollar (1$) recognizer. Our experimental results showed that the DTW algorithm performs better with an overall accuracy of 90 %. The second prototype presents an intuitive HCI to manipulate images using freehand gestures. In order to strengthen the gesture recognition process, the system incorporates contextual information to determine the intent of the user of interacting with the large display. Two cameras are used to observe the surgeon's hand movements to continuously determine and monitor what the surgeon intends to perform. Experimental results showed that the system accuracy is 95 % for recognition with the effect of contextual integration.

Keywords: Gesture recognition · Laser pointers · Hand gestures

1 Introduction

Recently, the touchless technique has received considerable attention as one of the promising methods due to its ability to provide a natural interaction between human and computer. Interaction is said to be touchless if there is no contact between the user and any part of the system. For example, the interaction with a Nintendo Wii through its wireless controller is not touchless. Voice based technique, eye gaze, and hand

© Springer International Publishing Switzerland 2016
V.G. Duffy (Ed.): DHM 2016, LNCS 9745, pp. 409–421, 2016.
DOI: 10.1007/978-3-319-40247-5_41

gestures are just a few examples of touchless interactions [1, 2]. There have been several works on touchless interaction that cover different fields, for instance, the medical applications [3].

In the operating room (OR), doctors should minimize the action of touching the surrounding area because of sterilized operation theater. In such situation, the surgeon usually asks another staff member to help him to interact with the display (e.g. zoom in/out images). This way of interaction might lead to some latency and inaccurate decisions between doctor's decisions and actions to be performed by the other member. Thus, several interfaces aiding direct control for the physicians have been developed. Some of these systems depend on voice control devices. However, their use may be associated with obstacles related to misinterpretation of commands, and if there is noise in the room, the error will increase [4]. In other systems, freehand gestures are utilized. The Opect system introduced intangible interface depends on the Kinect device [5]. Although the Opect has a high degree of accuracy, our system is characterized by a low price compared to the Kinect device.

Hepatic angiography is a study of an X-ray of the blood vessels that supply the liver. The procedure uses a thin and flexible catheter that is placed into a blood vessel through a small cut. A trained doctor called an Interventional radiologist usually performs the procedure. In this paper, we present two approaches that will help surgeons in the operating room to interactively control the 3D image on the large screen using pre-set gestures, which can be executed at a distance from the display. One method uses an inexpensive laser pointer with an on/off button and the other one uses freehand gestures.

2   System Overview

The Proposed system aims to help interventional radiologists in the liver angiography operation to control the 3D image (Fig. 1(b)) on the large screen using pre-set gestures (Fig. 1(c)). The system is composed of three cameras and a large screen (Fig. 1(a)). The first method uses one web camera to capture the movement of the laser pointer. The other system uses two web cameras to recognize freehand gestures. The first camera is placed in front of the doctor and the second one is held on a ceiling position.

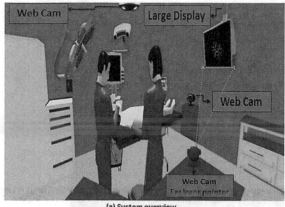

(a) System overview

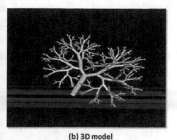

(b) 3D model

	Commands	Gestures	
		Laser pointer	freehand
1	Browse-right Rotate the 3D-modal over Y axis		
2	Browse-left Rotate the 3D-modal over Y axis		
3	Browse-up Rotate the 3D-modal over X axis		
4	Browse-down Rotate the 3D-modal over X axis		
5	Rotate clockwise Zoom-in		-
6	Rotate counterclockwise Zoom-out		-
7	Rotate clockwise increase brightness	-	
8	Rotate counterclockwise Decrease brightness	-	
9	Push forward Zoom-in	-	
10	Pull back Zoom-out	-	

(c) Gestures to browse medical images of the patient

Fig. 1. Proposed system

3 System Details

3.1 Laser Pointer

After the image has been captured by the web camera, it is considered as the input of the laser detection algorithm. Laser spot detection step is performed to identify which one of the detected foregrounds is the actual laser spot. Background subtraction is the most widespread method for detecting the laser spot. In a laser pointer system, most cameras are fixed in their position, thus allowing the use of background subtraction operation to get the foreground object. Frame differencing is the simplest background subtraction technique where a current frame is compared to the previous one in which a significant difference between those frames is identified as the foreground object.

First, the web camera captures the first and the second frames and convert them to grayscale for the process of frame differencing (Fig. 2(b)). Thus, performing frame differencing with the sequential images will output an "intensity image" that needs to be converted into a binary image that provides better information (Fig. 2(c)). However, the thresholded function still needs more enhancement to detect the laser spot. The "Blur" function is performed in order to get rid of the noise and improve the appearance of the laser spot (Fig. 2(d)). Unfortunately, this function will output an intensity image again, so the threshold binary operation is performed for a second time. Fig. 2(e) shows the final threshold image after it's been "blurred".

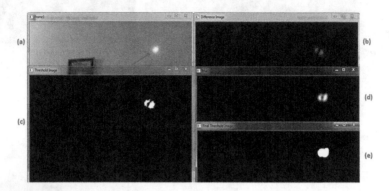

Fig. 2. Background subtraction: (a) Original image, (b) Intensity image, (c) Threshold-binary image, (d) Blur images, and (e) Final thresholded image.

Find contours approach is performed for locating a moving object (i.e. Laser spot). The final threshold binary image is treated as the input image for the tracking process (Fig. 2(e)). First, "findContours" Process is used to find all contours in the binary image where each contour is stored as a point vector (i.e. we search only for the extreme outer contours). Then, we make the assumption that the biggest detected contour is the object we are looking for. The circumscribed rectangle or bounding box has been drawn around the largest contour. Then, the centroid of the rectangle will be the object's final estimated position.

Finally, to recognize the laser gestures, two different algorithms are tested in order to choose the best algorithm for the proposed system. The first algorithm is called dynamic time warping (DTW) algorithm [6]. The second one is called 1$ recognizer algorithm [7].

3.2   FreeHand Gestures

Hand Segmentation. We propose a hand detector that splits into two stages: find the position of the hand only in the first frame, then extract the hue component of the glove color. As, the hue value will be used for further processing.

First, the images are captured with the front camera. The hand region is extracted from the background with the background subtraction method. The hand detection output image is a binary image as the white pixels represent the hand region and the black pixels belong to the background (Fig. 3(a)). Then, "findContours" function is used to find all contours in the binary image. A bounding box has been drawn around the largest contour. Then, the centroid of the rectangle will be the hand's estimated position. However, the subtracted image contains the whole arm region causing a false hand detection as seen in Fig. 3(b).

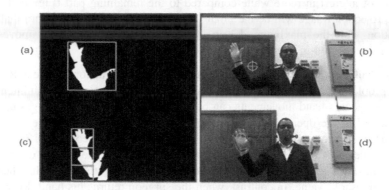

Fig. 3. Hand detection process: (a) and (c) background subtracted images, (b) false detection, (d) true detection.

Therefore, the bounding box width has been reduced to 50 % and the height is divided into three equal parts. The upper part is assumed to be the rectangle that specifies the palm and finger regions (Fig. 3(c)). Then, we calculate again the center of the new rectangle to be the final position of the hand (Fig. 3(d)). Finally, the hue color of the segmented rectangle is calculated in order to be used in the tracking algorithm that depends only on the color that is extracted from the detection stage.

Hand Tracking. The surgeon's right hand is tracked by using a CamShift algorithm [8]. The algorithm works by tracking the hue color value of an object where the color probability distribution for a 2D search window is calculated.

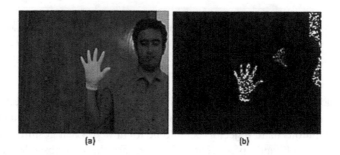

Fig. 4. (a) Test image, (b) Back-projection image

First, we create a hue histogram of an image containing the object of interest (i.e. Surgeon's hand). The hand should fill the image as far as possible for better results. Second, the histogram back-projected image is created. Backprojection image is used to find the object of interest in an image. In other words, it creates an image of the same size as that of our input image (i.e. single channel), as each pixel corresponds to the probability of that pixel belonging to the hand. Therefore, the output image will have our object of interest in more white compared to the remaining part (Fig. 4). Finally, the backprojection image will be the input image to the CamShift algorithm that finds the location with the maximum density. Obviously, when the object moves, the movement is reflected in histogram back-projection image.

Spotting Problem. One of the challenges in gesture interaction in the OR is the spotting problem, the problem of discrimination between intentional and unintentional gestures. Surgeon's hand movements can be divided into two categories: gestures that are performed in the operation mode and the others are performed in the interaction mode. The interaction mode is detected without asking the surgeon to perform a start gesture, we detect it when the surgeon intends to manipulate the images on the large screen by raising his hand up from the patient at a level slightly above the chest that exceeds a threshold value. In contrast, when the surgeon returns his hand down at the patient's level or any level below the level of the chest that means he enters the operation mode and the system is no longer able to recognize any gestures until the surgeon switches to the interaction mode again.

The surgeon's hand movements are divided into periods identical in length, each of them is composed of 20 frames. In practice, we found number of frames = 20 to be adequate. Each period is divided into two segments to merge the second one with the next period in order to make up a gesture. Then, generate a vector representation for this gesture that is classified later through the matching procedure using DTW against a set of templates. The classification results provide information that will enable the system to detect the surgeon's mode. Each two adjunct vectors have a segment length overlap, as shown in Fig. 5.

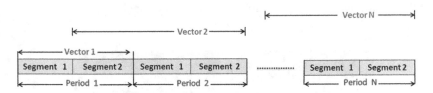

Fig. 5. Illustrations of frame segmentation

In the interaction mode, the surgeon will interact with the system by gesturing in the view of the front camera. However, the start and the end point of the intended hand gesture in a continuous hand trajectory should be identified. Each gesture is recognized by the hand-close and hand-open events that represent the two possible states for the hand. The hand state (open and close) detection is performed by measuring the height of the track window (i.e. the ellipse shape) that is drawn around the user's hand, the size of the track window is updated in each frame (Fig. 6).

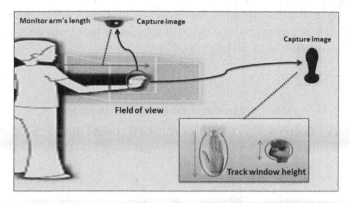

Fig. 6. Image capture with two cameras

Hand Gesture Recognition. In the hand gesture recognition process, a problem of losing information needs to be solved. To overcome this problem, we use two cameras. The trajectory of each gesture is recorded twice, one time from the view of the front web camera and the other time from the view of the ceiling camera in order to make the recognition process easier. The data that is collected from the front camera is used to recognize gestures such as the circle in the two directions and the line with the four directions: up, down, left, and right. The collected data of the ceiling camera recognizes only gestures that are unclear for the front camera (i.e. push-forward and pull-back gestures). It is an important issue to identify when the system starts using the recording data from the ceiling camera. The arm's length is measured in each frame in order to know whether or not the hand is stretched out (Fig. 6). In recognition process, we depend on the 1$ algorithm. This algorithm performs well and achieves good results in differentiating the shape of the gestures (i.e. mouse gestures) at overall accuracy more than 99 % using only a small number of training samples. Take into consideration that we may attempt to increase the number of the command gestures in our system, 1$ classifier is well suited for our situation. In the following section, we conduct a small study to measure the performance of the 1$ algorithm in classifying the shape and the direction of the hand gestures.

4   Primitive Experiment

We have conducted a primitive study for calculating the accuracy of 1$ classifier, we found that the algorithm performs well and achieves good results in differentiating the shape of the gestures, but it also has some limitations. The 1$ can not distinguish gestures whose identities depend on aspect ratios, locations, or specific orientations. This means that separating up-lines from down-lines or left-lines from right-lines is not possible without modifying the conventional algorithm. So, we conducted another study to calculate the accuracy of DTW in recognizing only the directions of the line gestures. We have found that the DTW can achieve 95 % accuracy for the line's direction, Table 1 shows the results for both algorithms. After these two primitive studies, the recognition algorithm in the proposed system depends mainly on two algorithms: the 1\$ for recognizing the shape of the gesture as it gives good results with only a few loaded templates and the DTW to recognize the direction of the line gestures.

Table 1. Detection of the line gesture direction

Gesture	1\$ detection (%)	DTW detection (%)
Left-line	84	100
Right-line	72	88
Up-line	68	92
Down-line	80	100
Push forward	76	96
Pull back	72	92

5   Experiments and Results

5.1   Laser Pointer

The experiment was performed by 15 subjects, there were 5 males and 10 females aged between 19 and 25. The users were asked to stand close to the large display at a distance of 1.5 m (Fig. 7). Each user is asked to use three input ways: the traditional way, i.e. input with a mouse and keyboard, and the laser pointer per each classifier (DTW and 1\$ recognizer) in order to complete tasks as shown in Fig. 8.

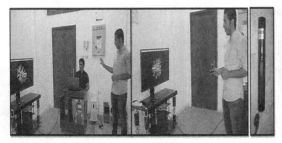
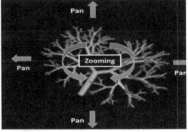
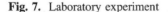

Fig. 7. Laboratory experiment   **Fig. 8.** Laser command mappings

Results and Discussion. Experimental data shows that mouse-based interactions are faster than the laser pointer either with the DTW or the 1\$ (Fig. 9). However, the average time cost to complete the total task with the mouse and the keyboard is just one second faster than that with a laser pointer using the DTW recognizer. Considering that, the latency problem or the slowness of the spot recognition can be solved by using better and faster cameras connections, we are satisfied with the performance of the laser pointer with DTW recognizer relative to the traditional method.

The averaging accuracy of DTW is 89.6 %, it means that the system misinterprets the laser pointer gestures at a rate of 10 %. As shown in Figs. 9 and 10, the laser pointer with the 1$ recognizer including error correction is almost twice as slow as the mouse and the averaging accuracy of 1$ is 75 %. The 1$ can not distinguish up-lines from down-lines and left-lines from right-lines. This explains why the 1$ comes last in the total time results. When the users make mistakes, they need extra time to correct their errors as we give them two trial for error correction.

Figure 11 displays the number of errors for all participants in each session for both algorithms. It is observed that the errors in DTW in session 3 and 4 are much less than those in session 1 and 2 which indicates that a user can be expected to improve in the usage of the laser pointer with the DTW. However, we cannot expect that in the 1$ classifier. There was no discernible difference in user performance between any of the four sessions.

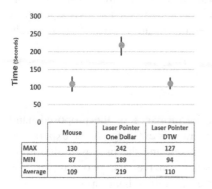

Fig. 9. Time cost in seconds

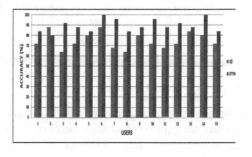

Fig. 10. Accuracy of laser pointer with two algorithms

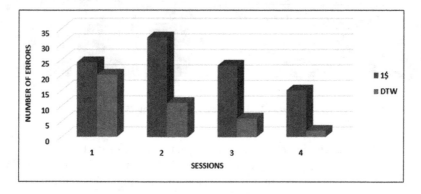

Fig. 11. Number of incorrect gestures recognitions for all participants in each session

The obtained data from participants gestures are then analyzed using an ANOVA test. First, a one-way ANOVA test is performed in regards to the time of the total task for the three input ways. The test indicates that there is a significant difference between the three algorithms ($p<0.05$). However, the ANOVA analysis only indicates that if there is a significant difference between at least one pair of the group means. It does not indicate what the pair or pairs are significantly different. To find which method is of better performance, a Tukey HSD test needs to be performed. A Tukey test is interested in examining mean differences where any two means that are greater than HSD are significantly different. From ANOVA results, the mean values of the three input ways: mouse, 1$, and DTW are M1, M2, and M3, respectively. A post-hoc analysis using a Tukeys HSD test showed that HSD = 13.18, with |M1 - M2| = 109.36, |M2 – M3| = 108.43, and |M3 - M1| = 0.93. Thus, the total time of the 1$ recognizer was significantly larger than those with the other input methods (i.e. no difference was found between the traditional method using the mouse and the laser pointer using DTW recognizer). Second, another one-way ANOVA test is performed in regards to recognition rate (accurracy) of the laser pointer with the two algorithms: DTW and 1$. The test indicates that there is a significant difference between the two algorithms ($p<0.05$). Thus, participants within the DTW method group generated significantly more accurate gestures than the 1$ recognizer.

5.2   Freehand Gestures

Our goal of this experiment was to measure the performance of the proposed hand gesture recognition algorithm, the classification accuracy is evaluated in the experiment using three algorithms: DTW recognizer, 1$ recognizer, and the proposed algorithm. We asked each user to perform a set of movements in the first two minutes (i.e. operation mode). As seen in Fig. 12(a), the user performs hand movements. For example, deals with the patient, talks with a staff member or points to any object. Then for 30 s, the user enters the interaction mode by raising his hand above the chest level next to his/her face (Fig. 12(b) and (c)).

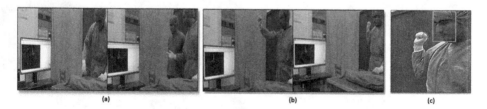

Fig. 12. Laboratory experiment

Results and Discussion. Figure 13 shows the performance of each user in the three algorithms. The averaging accuracy of the proposed algorithm, DTW, and 1$ is 95 %, 84 %, and 80 %, respectively. In the confusion matrix (Fig. 14), the entries of the matrix record the numbers of the gesture predicted as the corresponding gestures.

For example, the numbers in the first row 95 %, 2 %, and 3 % are in the columns corresponding to the gestures circle-clockwise, up-line, and down-line, respectively. It means that the proposed system misinterprets the circle-clockwise gesture at a rate of 5 %. Generally, there are some obvious sources of error in our experiment. For instance, some circle gestures and line gestures are misclassified as down-line, i.e. right-line and left-line. The reason is some users perform lines with a slightly skewness to the down and circles with a very small diameter. So, in these cases the system misunderstands these gestures as down-line. In Push-Forward gesture, the user should perform this gesture with a stretched-out arm, otherwise the system will misunderstand it as a right or left line.

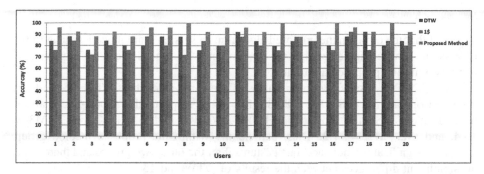

Fig. 13. Accuracy of the three algorithms achieved from the second experiment

	Circle-Clockwise	Circle-Counterclockwise	Left-Line	Right-Line	Up-Line	Down-Line	Push-Forward	Pull-Back	% of the miss
Circle-Clockwise	95%	0%	0%	0%	2%	3%	0%	0%	5%
Circle-Counterclockwise	0%	93%	0%	0%	2%	5%	0%	0%	7%
Left-Line	0%	0%	95%	0%	3%	2%	0%	0%	5%
Right-Line	0%	0%	0%	90%	0%	7%	3%	0%	10%
Up-Line	0%	0%	2%	3%	95%	0%	0%	0%	5%
Down-Line	0%	0%	0%	0%	0%	100%	0%	0%	0%
Push-Forward	0%	0%	2%	5%	0%	0%	93%	0%	7%
Pull-Back	0%	0%	2%	0%	3%	0%	0%	95%	5%
Average Success Rate (True Positive): 94.5%									
Average Misinterpret Rate (False Positive): 5.5%									

Fig. 14. Confusion matrix for the proposed algorithm

Figure 15 displays the number of errors for all participants in each session for each algorithm. In DTW, there is a slight improvement from session 1 to session 3. However, there is no discernible difference in user performance between any of the three 1$ sessions. Furthermore, the number of errors in session 1 and 3 is almost equal. It is

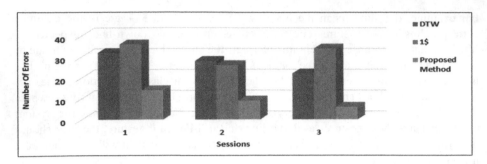

Fig. 15. Number of errors for all participants in each session

observed that the errors in the proposed algorithm in session 3 are much less than those in session 1 which indicates that the performance of the user can be expected to improve with the proposed algorithm.

From ANOVA results, the mean values of the three algorithms DTW, 1$, and the proposed one are M1 = 83, M2 = 80.8, M3 = 94.2, respectively. A post-hoc analysis using a Tukeys HSD test showed that HSD = 3.56, with |M1 − M2| = 2.2, |M2 - M3| = 13.4, and |M3 -M1| = 11.2. Thus, participants within the proposed method group generated significantly more accurate gestures than the other two groups and there were no significant differences between the results of DTW and 1$.

6 Conclusion

A multimodal system with two input modality is introduced in this paper. It provides a good solution to help interventional radiologists in the liver angiography operation to control the 3D image on the large screen using pre-set gestures. Our Future work includes firstly testing the proposed multimodal system in a real-world scenario such as the OR. However, the OR is a very critical place so we need to increase the accuracy of the proposed algorithm. Secondly, extend this work to support multiple users with personalized service.

References

1. Jafari, R., Ziou, D.: Eye-gaze estimation under various head positions and iris states. Expert Syst. Appl. **42**(1), 510–518 (2015)
2. Munteanu, C., Jones, M., Whittaker, S., Oviatt, S., Aylett, M., Penn, G., Brewster, S., Alessandro, N.: Designing speech and language interactions. In: CHI 2014 Extended Abstracts on Human Factors in Computing Systems, Toronto, Canada (2014)
3. Gallo, L., Placitelli, A. P., Ciampi, M.: Controller-free exploration of medical image data: experiencing the kinect. In: Computer-Based Medical Systems (CBMS), Bristol, United Kingdom (2011)

4. Alapetite, A., Andersen, H.B., Hertzum, M.: Acceptance of speech recognition by physicians: a survey of expectations, experiences, and social influence. Inter. J. Hum. Comput. Stud. **67** (1), 36–49 (2009)
5. Yoshimitsu, K., Muragaki, Y., Maruyama, T., Yamato, M., Iseki, H.: Development and initial clinical testing of opect: an innovative device for fully intangible control of the intraoperative image-displaying monitor by the surgeon. Oper. Neurosurg. **10**(1), 46–50 (2014)
6. Myers, C., Rabiner, L.: A level building dynamic time warping algorithm for connected word recognition. IEEE Trans. Acoust. Speech Sig. Proc. **29**(2), 284–297 (1981)
7. Wobbrock, J. O., Wilson, A. D., Li, Y.. Gestures without libraries, toolkits or training: a \$1 recognizer for user interface prototypes. In: Proceedings of the 20th Annual Symposium on User Interface Software and Technology, New York, USA (2007)
8. Bradski, G.R.: Real time face and object tracking as a component of a perceptual user interface. In: Proceedings of IEEE Workshop on Applications of Computer Vision, Princeton, NJ (1998)

Analyzing the Difference Between Floral Materials Water Potential When Cut by Ikebana Experts and Inexperienced Persons

Yuki Ikenobo[1]([✉]), Yuko Hanba[2], Noriaki Kuwahara[3],
and Akihiko Goto[4]

[1] Ikenobo, 248 Donomae-Cho, Nakagyo-ku, Kyoto 604-8134, Japan
hanahana@ikenobo.jp
[2] Centre for Bioresource Field Science, Kyoto Institute of Technology,
Matsugasaki, Sakyo-ku, Kyoto 606-8585, Japan
hanba@kit.ac.jp
[3] Department of Advanced Fibro-Science, Kyoto Institute of Technology,
Matsugasaki, Sakyo-ku, Kyoto 606-8585, Japan
nkuwahar@kit.ac.jp
[4] Department of Information Systems Engineering,
Faculty of Design Technology, Osaka Sangyo University,
3-1-1 Nakakakiuchi, Daito-shi, Osaka 574-8530, Japan
gotoh@ise.osaka-sandai.ac.jp

Abstract. Ikebana is one of the aspects of Japanese traditional culture. Flowers are used for the creation of ikebana, and keeping a completed arrangement in good condition is important. Ikebana arrangements are used for welcoming guests or displayed for a period of several days at exhibitions.

It is thought that floral material cut by an expert lasts longer but this has not been scientifically verified. Therefore this research aims to scientifically calculate and clarify the difference between floral materials cut by ikebana experts and an inexperienced persons, observing the cross section diagram of cut floral materials and their water potential (water retention).

Two kinds of floral material, one generally considered able to absorb water easily and the other generally considered to absorb water with difficulty, were cut by both the ikebana experts and an inexperienced persons, and these materials' cross sections were observed and their water potential (retention) measured.

As a result, material cut by the Ikebana experts showed a tendency for less damage at the cross section and higher water retention than material cut by the inexperienced persons. This was especially pronounced in floral material considered to be difficult in absorbing water. This thus suggested a correlation between the degree of damage seen in cross section and the water potential of floral material.

Keywords: Scissor · Process analysis · Water potential · Cutting speed

© Springer International Publishing Switzerland 2016
V.G. Duffy (Ed.): DHM 2016, LNCS 9745, pp. 422–431, 2016.
DOI: 10.1007/978-3-319-40247-5_42

1   Introduction

Ikebana is one of the aspects of Japanese traditional culture. Flowers are used for the creation of ikebana, and keeping a completed arrangement in good condition is important. Ikebana arrangements are used for welcoming guests or displayed for a period of several days at exhibitions. However, most study of ikebana has been in terms of history or aesthetics and no scientific analysis of movement while arranging or of completed arrangements has been done. Thus it is thought that a scientific approach is needed in order to make clear the whole picture of ikebana.

It is thought that floral material cut by an expert lasts longer but this has not been scientifically verified. Therefore this research aims to scientifically measure and clarify the difference between floral materials cut by ikebana experts and inexperienced persons, observing the cross section of cut floral materials and the water potential (water retention) of cut floral materials.

Two kinds of floral material, one generally considered able to absorb water easily and the other generally considered to absorb water with difficulty, were cut by both ikebana experts and inexperienced persons, and these materials' cross sections were observed and their water potential (retention) measured.

Since cutting floral materials is especially important in ikebana, it is assumed that information about the quantitative evaluation of circumstances of different cutting motions between ikebana experts and inexperienced persons, differences in use of scissors, and how such differences affect cut materials and the condition of materials used in an arrangement will be useful for future teaching methods.

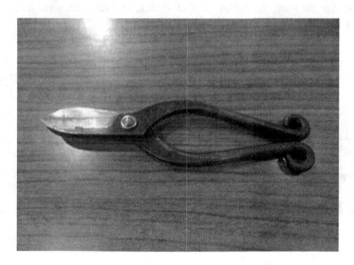

Fig. 1. Scissors "Warabite" (scissor handles in the shape of fern shoots)

2   Outline of Experimental Procedure

2.1   Methods, Conditions, and Floral Material Used

This experiment focused on quantitative evaluation of differences between ikebana experts and inexperienced persons with respect to the motion of cutting floral materials, and quantitative evaluation of the effect on floral materials caused by these differences. Circumstances of cutting motion by ikebana experts and inexperienced persons and cutting speed by ikebana experts and inexperienced persons were measured. Common "warabite" ikebana scissors (with handles in the shape of fern shoots) were used. (Fig. 1) These scissors are different from usual stationary scissors in the absence of a ring or oval-shaped portion for the fingers to pass through. When cutting materials with "warabite" one has to hold the scissors in the hand. To move the upper blade the lower handle is supported and moved by the four fingers other than the thumb; to move the lower blade the upper handle is grasped between the thumb and the palm of the hand.

For measurement of cutting motion and speed, chrysanthemum was used as a softer material, and red budding salix was used as a material harder to cut. Both materials are commonly used for ikebana. On a desk the materials were placed in a frame to prevent change of position during filming, and subjects were asked to cut at the points indicated. The experiment was recorded by high-speed camera (Photoron FASTCAM SA4) at 500 fps. Three points (points 1-3) were marked on the scissors, and two points (points 4 and 5) were marked at both ends of the stick fixed to the material for measuring its rotation. Video of the cutting action was analyzed by TEMA motion analysis software (Photoron), and the speed at each point was measured. A mark was placed at 800 mm from the upper tips of the material in order to assure as much as much as possible the uniform thickness of all stalks, and subjects were instructed to cut at that point (Fig. 2).

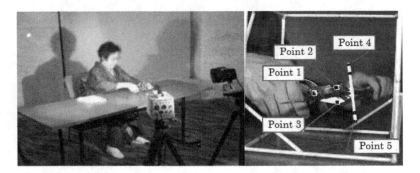

Fig. 2. Conditions for the experiment and the frame used for fixing the cutting position

The general concept of water potential was used for measuring the conditions of a floral material's water absorption. After observation of cut surfaces with the naked eye photographs were taken, and water retention and transpiration amounts were measured. For floral materials, chocolate cosmos and gerbera were used. Generally chocolate cosmos is considered to absorb water with difficulty and gerbera is considered to absorb water more easily. Both materials are regarded as relatively softer materials. Measurements were taken on the 1st, 5th and 9th days after cutting by the subjects.

2.2 Details of the Subjects Participating in the Experiment

Thirty subjects were chosen for the experiment: ten ikebana experts as experienced persons, and twenty undergraduate and graduate students as inexperienced persons. Information on the subjects is as follows:

* Ikebana experts

1. 40 years of experience (69 years old/Female)
2. 33 years of experience (52 years old /Female)
3. 47 years of experience (65 years old /Female)
4. 20 years of experience (37 years old /Female)
5. 40 years of experience (62 years old /Female)
6. 49 years of experience (71 years old /Female)
7. 24 years of experience (44 years old /Female)
8. 40 years of experience (60 years old /Female)
9. 27 years of experience (37 years old /Female)
10. 60 years of experience (84 years old /Female)

* Inexperienced persons

    20 subjects (male and female) with no ikebana arranging experience were chosen, ranging in age from 20 to 49.

3 Results

3.1 Blade Speed When Cutting Flower Materials

Figures 3, 4, 5 and 6 are some instances of blade motion when cutting chrysanthemum and red budding salix by both ikebana experts and inexperienced persons.

Figures 7 and 8 show average blade speed at the moment when stems of chrysanthemum and red budding salix were cut by both ikebana experts and inexperienced persons. Figure 3 indicates that when cutting chrysanthemum the velocity of the blade of experts was faster than that of inexperienced persons. With respect to differences among marked points, blade speed for ikebana experts was faster at point 2 than at point 3, while for inexperienced persons speed was faster at point 3 than at point 2, an opposite result.

Figure 4 shows that the speed of the blade of experts was faster than that of inexperienced persons when cutting red budding salix. Blade speed for cutting red budding salix was faster than for cutting chrysanthemum for both experts and

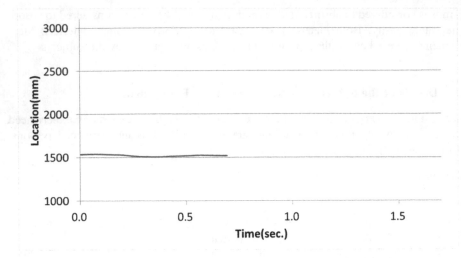

Fig. 3. Blade motion by one of experts (point 1 /chrysanthemum)

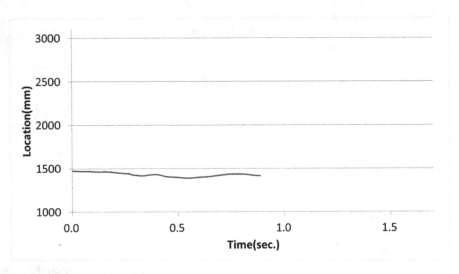

Fig. 4. Blade motion by one of beginners (point 1 /chrysanthemum)

inexperienced persons. However for red budding salix the speed was higher at point 3 than point 2 for both experts and inexperienced persons, a result different from that of chrysanthemum. There was a tendency toward large variation among the blade speeds of the experts.

The results suggest that experts not only cut materials with faster blade speed than inexperienced persons but also that their way of using scissors is different.

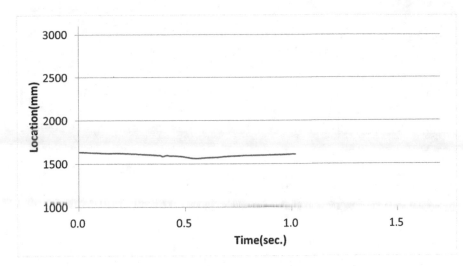

Fig. 5. Blade motion by one of experts (red budding salix) (Color figure online)

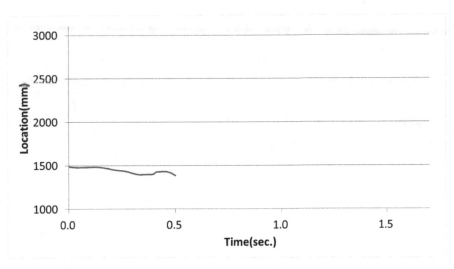

Fig. 6. Blade motion by one of beginner (red budding salix) (Color figure online)

3.2 Condition of the Floral Materials After Cutting

The results of water retention for chocolate cosmos and gerbera are shown in Figs. 9 and 10. Pressure Chamber 600 (PMS Instrument Company) was used for water retention measurement. Water potential is utilized to describe water retention status. Water potential is thermodynamic potential energy, the result of the division of chemical potential by partial molar volume of the water. Water potential, Ψw[Pa] is described in the following equation:

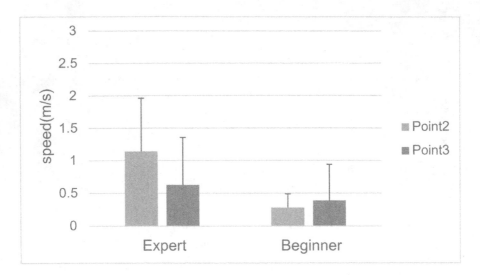

Fig. 7. Blade speed when cutting chrysanthemum

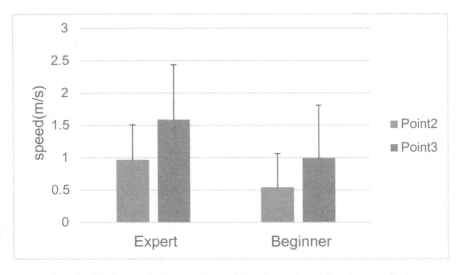

Fig. 8. Blade speed when cutting red budding salix (Color figure online)

$$\Psi_W = \Psi_o + \Psi_m + \Psi_p + \Psi_g$$

Ψo: Osmotic potential
Ψm: Matrix potential
Ψp: Pressure potential
Ψg: Gravitational potential
Water Potential

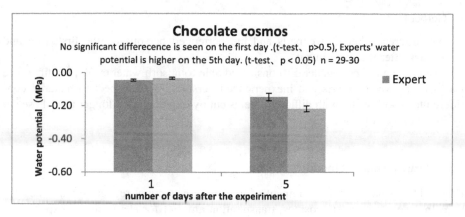

Fig. 9. Water potential of chocolate cosmos

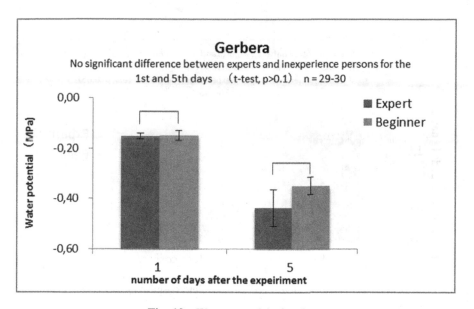

Fig. 10. Water potential of gerbera

- Chocolate cosmos

First day after the experiment: No difference between experts and inexperienced persons

Fifth day after the experiment: Experts' water potential was higher that than of inexperienced persons.

Ninth day after the experiment: No difference between experts and inexperienced persons.

• Gerbera

No difference between experts and inexperienced persons on the first, fifth and ninth days after the experiment.

Concerning material generally considered able to absorb water easily, no difference was seen between experts and inexperienced persons. With respect to material considered to absorb water with difficulty, stems cut by experts lasted longer than those cut by inexperienced persons.

3.3   Transpiration Amount

Figure 11 indicates the measurement of transpiration amount related to water absorption. In case of chocolate cosmos, transpiration amount for stems cut by experts was larger than that of inexperienced persons. With respect to gerbera, no difference was seen.

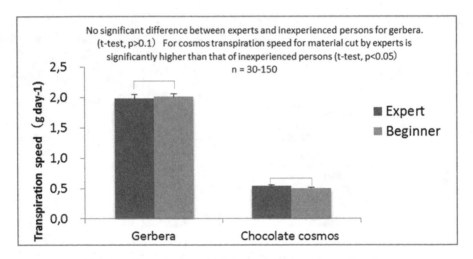

Fig. 11. Transpiration speed for chocolate cosmos and gerbera

3.4   Condition of Floral Materials

In case of chocolate cosmos, material cut by experts was longer lasting. Discoloration and shrinkage of petals were seen in chocolate cosmos cut by experts on the 7th day of measurement. For inexperienced persons the same changes were seen on the 5th day. Also, most of the petals of chocolate cosmos cut by experts had not fallen by the 9th day of the measurement. However for stems cut by inexperienced persons, petals started to fall on the 6th day and petals of many of the sample materials had fallen on the 9th day.

In case of gerbera, no significant change in appearance of the material such as color was observed for materials cut by experts or by inexperienced persons. For gerbera cut by some of the experts stem breakage was noted from the 5th day.

4 Conclusion

Differences in cutting speed and use of scissors were found between experts and inexperienced persons. The cutting speed of experts tends to be faster than that of inexperienced persons. It is possible that when cutting less hard material experts adjust the cutting force with four fingers, while when cutting so-called harder material they use more force applied with the thumb. Therefore this use of two different ways can be considered as a "skill" that experts have. In measurements of water potential, water retention for material cut by experts tends to be longer for chocolate cosmos, a material generally considered to absorb water with difficulty. With respect to gerbera no significant difference was seen between materials cut by experts and inexperienced persons. Internal structure of the materials is not identical; for example, cross section area and configuration or dispersion of vascular tissue are possible factors that might affect water absorption. However, it can be considered that materials considered able to absorb water easily such as gerbera are less likely to be affected by the cutting, while materials considered to absorb water with difficulty such as chocolate cosmos are more likely to be affected.

These results show that by cutting materials quickly in the manner of experts, less damage is done to vascular tissue or other parts of the material, and it can be expected that when a material considered to absorb water with difficulty is placed in water after having been cut quickly, the faster cutting speed will help the material to absorb water more easily and to keep good water retention and good condition of the flower.

From this experiment it was not possible to clarify whether or not differences of cutting speed and use of scissors bring significant difference in water potential. In the case of softer material, however, there seems to be correlation to some extent. I will try to conduct further research with the same materials in the future. The cutting of so-called woody materials (hard materials) will also be a topic for further research. Research will help to clarify the cutting motion and its effects for both experts and inexperienced persons. Based on the results of research, it is expected that an effective way of using scissors will be standardized in teaching manuals, so that beginners can quickly become familiar with use of scissors designed specifically for ikebana and more easily master ikebana skills.

Exploring Risk-Benefit Factors of Electronic Clinical Pathways Regarding Nursing Communication

Tadashi Kanehira[1]([⊠]), Taro Sugihara[1], Muneou Suzuki[2],
Akio Gofuku[1], and Kenji Araki[2]

[1] Okayama University, Okayama, Japan
{pxx24tq8, t-sugihara}@okayama.u-ac.jp
[2] Miyazaki University, Miyazaki, Japan
suzukim@med.miyazaki-u.ac.jp

Abstract. This study explores the influence of electronic clinical pathways (ECPs) on nurses' daily activities, especially nursing communication, in a university hospital. Although an electronic clinical pathway enables medical-treatment processes to be standardized by interacting with different occupations, few studies have been conducted from the managerial perspective. We interviewed a doctor in the Department of Medical Information Systems and eight nurses who make entries and use ECPs. The results of the interview indicated that some nurses learned about the medical processes using electronic clinical pathways. The results also showed that the assessment abilities for patient care could decline, if the nurses failed to incorporate the electronic clinical pathways into their daily routines.

Keywords: Electronic clinical pathways communication standardization risks in nursing practice university hospital risk/benefit factors

1 Introduction

Nurses must work to improve their knowledge and skills to keep up with the rapid advance of medicine. Hospitals, especially university hospitals, now face the difficult situation of understanding the medical-treatment workflow. This can cause a communication problem among the nurses. It is important to manage this problem by efficiently tracking the medical records and providing an atmosphere that encourages communication.

Clinical pathways (CPs) were expected to solve the problem of tracking records. CPs are management plans for medical treatments that display goals for patients, and provide the order and timing of the treatment needed to efficiently achieve these goals [1]. CPs apply the critical-path concept, a project-management scheduling method, to medicine. This approach is intended to improve the quality of the medical-staff activity through processes that delineate standardized medical treatments. CPs were originally conceived to resolve financial issues in hospitals [2]; however, they were gradually adapted to facilitate managerial activities.

© Springer International Publishing Switzerland 2016
V.G. Duffy (Ed.): DHM 2016, LNCS 9745, pp. 432–439, 2016.
DOI: 10.1007/978-3-319-40247-5_43

After they were brought to Japan, CPs were extended past the idea of standardization. If a medical treatment was carried out by various medical staff, standardized processes strengthened the team care by clarifying the respective roles. Risk management was also introduced by standardizing the medical treatments. Medical processes in CPs are fully described when the treatments are conducted. Finally, CPs are used for informed consent by describing the flow for the patient from the beginning to the end [3]. However, studies of the organizational changes that occur after deploying CPs have hardly been conducted.

The purpose of this study is to discuss the influences of electronic clinical pathways (ECPs) on a university hospital. We particularly focused on the issues of nursing communication related to ECPs. We formulated two research questions to clarify the topics covered this study.

RQ1: What kind of benefit/risk factors are shown in the university hospital?
RQ2: How are the factors related to each other?

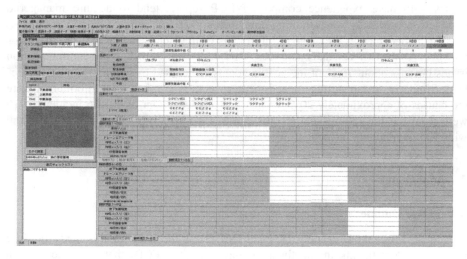

Fig. 1. Electronic clinical pathway interface for medical staff

2   Related Work

2.1   Clinical Pathway Studies

CPs define the optimal sequence and timing of interventions by medical staff, e.g., diagnoses or procedures by doctors or nurses [1]. Conventional studies revealed that CPs have various functions to improve daily activities. A CP improves the delivery of evidence-based care [4, 5, 8], shortens the patient's length of stay [2, 4], reduces the nursing records [5, 8], and improves the patient's education [4]. CPs also facilitate staff-to-staff and staff-to-patient communications [5, 6]. By analyzing the variances in the CPs, nurses learn to differentiate between typical cases and exceptional cases.

CPs have the potential to be both a knowledge-management tool and an education tool for medical staff [7, 9, 16].

2.2 Electronic Clinical Pathway Studies

Paper-based clinical pathways have been integrated into electronic medical records in recent years as ECPs. A few studies on ECP interfaces [10] or implementations [11–13] have been conducted. Balatsoukas and colleagues proposed user-friendly and usable function requirements for ECP implementations [10]. Wakamiya and Yamauchi identified seventeen requirements for ECP implementations based on interviews [11].

ECPs have become useful tools in conveying medical-treatment information to the patient, and sharing patient information in shift reports [14, 15]. However, there are fewer studies about the effects of ECPs and incorporating ECP management into daily activities. Hence, our study group has investigated the effects of ECPs from the standpoint of organizational knowledge management [17]. Sugihara clarified that nurses who have experience composing ECP reports tend to acquire managerial knowledge, especially when training apprentices [17].

This paper enlarges the range of informants from composers to users, and discusses the effects of the ECPs on daily activities. This study focuses on nursing-communication issues because about 70 % of medical incidents are caused by communication failures [18]. Similarly, in Japan, mis-tracked medical records or mis-shared information were the causes of approximately 20 % of medical incidents. Out of 40,156 incidents, 910 were from mis-tracked medical records and 6,508 were from mis-shared information, with 595 overlapping incidents [19].

3 Methods

3.1 Case Outline

We chose Miyazaki University Hospital (MUH) as the field for this study because almost all departments in this hospital have adopted ECPs that combine clinical pathways and electronic medical records; others have merely attempted to use ECPs as prototypes. The input/output devices are stationary computers, personal digital assistants, and smartphones. Nurses usually input vital data, e.g., blood pressure readings, using bedside PDAs, and write long entries, e.g., observation comments, on the computer at the staff station.

MUH is the largest hospital in the Miyazaki prefecture. In a seven-story building with 632 beds, it had 18 departments in 2015. MUH introduced paper-based CPs from 2004 to 2007; they have since converted to ECPs. Almost all of the departments in this hospital employ ECPs.

3.2 Study Design

We employed a case study as an exploratory style. This study consisted of two steps: a semi-structured interview and a modified grounded-theory approach (M-GTA). First, a

30-min semi-structured interview was conducted at MUH; the informants were a doctor and eight nurses. Second, after the interview data was fully transcribed, it was analyzed using the M-GTA. M-GTA, developed in Japan, is an analysis technique for qualitative data [20, 21].

The transcripts were read as many times as possible to identify any commonalities and differences among the data; similar data were classified into the same categories. During this process, when a category was recognized as similar to another one, they were combined into one category. This analysis process was repeated until no new categories could be formed; i.e., until theoretical saturation was reached. The relationship among the categories was depicted by considering the cause-effect characteristics of the comments.

4 Results

4.1 Integrated Categories

Twenty-six concepts were generated by the analysis. These concepts were divided into seven categories.

The first category is reducing the time and effort of keeping medical records. Nurses do not need to rewrite the nursing-care plans for an ECP-adopted patient because the nursing records on the patient's condition already appear in the ECP. Before ECPs were introduced, a nurse had to contact the doctor to find out why a blank record appeared in the medical records.

The second is that the medical process can be learned while composing ECP records. Various medical staff (doctors, nurses, dietitians, etc.) participate in making ECPs. Nurses who make ECPs can learn about the various medical cases through information and knowledge sharing with staff in different roles.

The third is expected spillover effects associated with ECP use. The spillover effect is related to on-the-job training. When a patient begins to receive a medical treatment, senior nurses use ECPs as an orientation tool for apprentices.

The fourth is signs of deterioration caused by ECP use. By reducing the recording time and effort, nurses may lose opportunities to increase their knowledge and skills.

The fifth category is knowledge-acquisition channels for nursing. Nurses acquire knowledge through receiving on-the-job training, reading and writing nursing texts, questioning doctors or senior nurses, and participating in seminars. The process of composing ECP reports provides an opportunity to communicate with doctors and senior nurses.

The sixth involves management policies in the Department of Nursing. The MUH Department of Nursing has introduced various policies to improve the quality of nursing and care; they especially encourage apprentice training. Although these policies have mainly focused on daily nursing activities, some of them have indirectly functioned as practice using the ECPs. For instance, mentoring the apprentices worked as a double-check when inputting ECP records. Moreover, senior nurses were able to convey their knowledge of ECP use, in addition to their nursing methods.

The seventh is an ideal model of the nurse. Some nurses and apprentices have an ideal model of a nurse. The model must possess extensive medical knowledge and skills, be trusted by patients, and be self-disciplined.

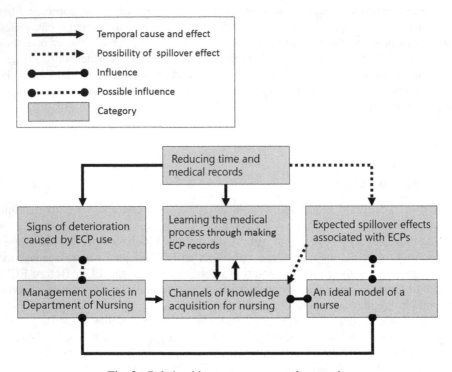

Fig. 2. Relationships among generated categories

4.2   Relationships Among Categories

This section explains the relationships among the categories. Four relationship lines are shown in Fig. 1: (a) a solid arrow, (b) a dotted arrow, (c) a dotted line with round start and end points, and (d) a solid line with round start and end points.

A solid arrow represents temporal cause and effect. For example, since ECPs were first deployed, their role has changed from a cost-cutting tool to a tool for learning the medical workflow, as shown in *Reducing time and medical records* to *Learning the medical process through making ECP records*.

A dotted arrow represents the possibility of spillover effects. For example, nurses suggested that spare time produced by reducing the time for tracking medical records could lead to enriched patient care, as indicated in *Reducing time and medical records* to *Expected spillover effects associated with ECPs*.

A dotted line with round start and end points represents a possible influence of one category on another. ECPs provoked a negative influence when some nurses merely used them to reduce the time for writing medical records. Nurses could lose opportunities to increase their knowledge and skills. MUH has had no incidents, owing to the management of the nursing department; i.e., *Signs of deterioration caused by ECP use* to *Management policies in Department of Nursing* (Fig. 2).

A solid line with round start and end points represents an influence of one category on another. Nurses who have an ideal nurse model want to approach it, so they study hard using the available knowledge-acquisition channels; i.e., *Channels of knowledge acquisition for nursing* to *An ideal model of the nurse.*

5 Discussion

The results of this study indicated that introducing ECPs reduces the time and mitigates the burden of writing medical records. These results are equivalent to conventional studies [18]. Before ECP deployment, it was essential for nurses to contact doctors to know the reason for blank doctor's orders. Basic procedures and medicines are already recorded in the ECPs so the nurses do not need to call the doctor. This effect could signify a reduction in unnecessary communication and fewer overlooked records. One study suggested that the SBAR system (Situation Background Assessment Recommendation) potentially decreases communication failures, which are the leading cause of inadvertent patient harm [19]. From the viewpoint of decreasing unnecessary confirmations, we considered that ECPs are preventing miscommunications.

On the other hand, this benefit has a negative aspect in that nurses lose the opportunities to discuss medical treatments in detail with the doctor. Consequently, the nurses gradually lose opportunities to acquire in-depth knowledge, in terms of assessing a patient's condition through deep communication. This leads to the risk of deterioration for apprentices due to a lack of communication among the staff. Our previous investigation clarified that nurses who made ECP records acquired medical knowledge and learned how to embed ECPs into the workflow by themselves [17]. If an apprentice is faced with a deeply rooted symptom, he/she may overlook the true cause from the outcome on the ECP; an unexpected outcome is difficult to identify in comparison with symptoms of common diseases. Decreasing doctor-nurse communication is equivalent to reducing the opportunities to share knowledge with each other.

However, incidents caused by losing the assessment ability were not observed at the hospital. We consider two probable reasons. The time after deployment is not sufficient to erode the nursing abilities. Another reason is that the chief nurses manage to work around the problem. Therefore, it is essential to conduct a follow-up investigation to uncover the reason.

6 Conclusion

In this paper, we presented a field study from a university hospital, focusing on nursing communication; the subjects make and use ECPs in daily nursing. The results of our study showed that ECPs have both benefit and risk factors. The answers to the research questions are as follows:

RQ1. The benefit factors of ECPs are improved on-the-job training for apprentices, and a mitigated burden of keeping medical records, whereas they risk miscommunications among the medical staff.

RQ2. Ten connections were classified into four major influences; temporal cause and effect, possibility of spillover effects, possibility of influencing each other, and influencing each other. The main results were that a factor related to composing ECP records connects to opportunities for efficiently learning about medical processes. Afterwards, the connections crystallized to channels of knowledge acquisition among the medical staff, especially for the nurses.

Managers and/or engineers in the medical field could consider two possible applications for these results. Medical managers might investigate methods of measuring ECPs' risk factors. Engineers could implement a function to enhance the benefits (e.g., effectively learning the medical processes beyond the boundaries among the medical staff) and reduce the risks (e.g., by promoting communication). However, this study employed interviews to a few nurses and a doctor, as a qualitative approach. We need to follow up with quantitative research, such as questionnaires, to determine the overall trends.

Acknowledgments. Our research was partly supported by the Grant-in-Aid for Scientific Research (21330089, 24330118, 26502008, 15K16168) of the JSPS. We would like to thank the doctor and nurses of Miyazaki University Hospital for their cooperation.

References

1. Every, N.R., Kopecky, S.: Critical pathways: A review. Circulation **101**(4), 461–465 (2000)
2. Zehr, K.J., Dawdon, P.B., Yang, S.C., Heitmiller, R.F.: Standardized clinical care pathways for major thoracic cases reduce hospital costs. Ann. Thorac. Surg. **66**(3), 914–919 (1998)
3. Soejima, H.: Iryō Kiroku Ga Kawaru Ketteiban Kurinikaru Pasu (in Japanese). Tōkyō: Igaku Shoin (2004). Print
4. Renholm, M., Leino-Kilpi, H., Suominen, T.: Critical pathways: A systematic review. J. Nurs. Adm. **32**(4), 196–202 (2002)
5. Campbell, H., Hotchkiss, R., Baradshaw, N., Porteous, M.: Integrated care pathways. BMJ Br. Med. J. **316**(7125), 133 (1998)
6. Vanhaecht, K., Bollmann, M., Bower, K., Gallagher, C., Gardini, A., Guezo, J., Van Zelm, R.: Prevalence and use of clinical pathways in 23 countries—An international survey by the European Pathway Association. J. Integr. Pathways **10**(1), 28–34 (2006)
7. Cabitza, F., Simone, C., Sarini, M.: Knowledge artifacts as bridges between theory and practice: The clinical pathway case. In: Ackerman, M., Dieng-Kuntz, R., Simone, C., Wulf, V. (eds.) Knowledge Management in Action. IFIP, vol. 270, pp. 37–50. Springer, Heidelberg (2008)
8. de Luc, K.: Care pathways: An evaluation of their effectiveness. J. Adv. Nurs. **32**(2), 485–496 (2000)
9. Coffey, R.J., Richards, J.S., Remmert, C.S., LeRoy, S.S., Schoville, R.R., Baldwin, P.J.: An introduction to critical paths. Qual. Manage. Healthc. **14**(1), 46–55 (2005)

10. Balatsoukas, P., Williams, R., Davies, C., Ainsworth, J., Buchan, I.: User interface requirements for web-based integrated care pathways: evidence from the evaluation of an online care pathway investigation tool. J. Med. Syst. **39**(11), 1–15 (2015)
11. Wakamiya, S., Yamauchi, K.: What are the standard functions of electronic clinical pathways? Int. J. Med. Inform. **78**(8), 543–550 (2009)
12. de Luc, K., Todd, J.: E-pathways: Computers and the Patient's Journey Through Care. Radcliffe Publishing, Abingdon (2003)
13. Gooch, P., Roudsari, A.: Computerization of workflows, guidelines, and care pathways: A review of implementation challenges for process-oriented health information systems. J. Am. Med. Inform. Assoc. **18**(6), 738 (2011)
14. Patel, V.L., Kushniruk, A.W., Yang, S., Yale, J.F.: Impact of a computer-based patient record system on data collection, knowledge organization, and reasoning. J. Am. Med. Inform. Assoc. **7**(6), 569–585 (2000)
15. Hyde, E., Murphy, B.: Computerized clinical pathways (care plans). Piloting a strategy to enhance quality patient care. Clin. Nurse Spec. **26**(5), 277–282 (2012)
16. Yang, H., Li, W., Liu, K., Zhang, J.: Knowledge-based clinical pathway for medical quality improvement. Inf. Syst. Front. **14**(1), 105–117 (2012)
17. Sugihara, T., Sakanishi, H., Gofuku, A., Umemoto, K., Suzuki, M., Araki, K.: Potential of electronic clinical pathways as triggers for eliciting implicit knowledge. In: Proceedings of the 41st Annual Conference of the IEEE Industrial Electronics Society (IECON2015), pp. 410–415 (2015)
18. Leonard, M., Graham, S., Bonacum, D.: The human factor: The critical importance of effective teamwork and communication in providing safe care. Qual. Saf. Health Care. **13** (suppl 1), i85–i90 (2004)
19. Japan Council for Quality Health Care.: "iryou ziko joho syu-syu- tou zigyou hiyarihatto 2009–2015", 7 June 2016. http://www.med-safe.jp/mpsearch/SearchReport.action
20. Kinoshita, Y.: Raibu Kōgi M-GTA: Jissenteki Shitsuteki Kenkyūhō: Shūseiban Guraundeddo Seorī Apurōchi No Subete. Tōkyō: Kōbundō (2007). Print
21. Kinoshita, Y.: Guraundeddo Seorī Apurōchi No Jissen: Shitsuteki Kenkyū Eno Sasoi. Tōkyō: Kōbundō (2003). Print

A Study on Development of a Wide Elegant Textile by Using Japanese Traditional Textile Technology of Nishijin-Ori

Masashi Kano[1,2(✉)], Hiro Akaji[1], Akiko Kato[1],
and Noriaki Kuwahara[2]

[1] Kano-ko Co., Ltd., Kyoto, Japan
{masashi,akaji,kato}@kano-ko.com
[2] Kyoto Institute of Technology, Kyoto, Japan
nkuwahar@kit.ac.jp

Abstract. We are trying to express Japanese traditional worldview of Rimpa on our fabric of 150 cm width by using Japanese traditional textile technique of Nishijin-Ori. The dense, exquisite, unique expression of the textile by using shuttle loom will be achieved by using wide rapier loom. Consequently, Nishijin-Ori technique will be the key not only for Kimono, but also for an indoor interior, an interior decoration of a car, and a couture of all over the world, which will rise to great artistic heights.

Keywords: Nishijin-ori · Textile · Fabric · Weaving machine · Design

1 Introduction

As an old establishment among the Nishijin-Ori fabric producers Kano-ko Co., Ltd. has passed traditional skills producing diverse products and elaborate expressions through the 30 cm width fabric used in Obi (Sash for Japanese traditional kimono) down to the current generations. However, as its ability for expression through weaving advanced we faced the limitation due to constrain of 30 cm fabric width. In addition, fabrics with 30 cm width could not be adopted for other products, such as interior decoration or western clothing, which was a problem for its business. Therefore, Kano-ko has been investigating for over several decades the necessity of producing fabric with 100 cm width and above, maximum 150 cm, through its unique weaving technique. But there was hardly any past example of weaving wide fabric using Nishijin technique other than for obi fabric. As knowhow could not be learnt from existing product, engagement with a completely new endeavor was necessary.

Even though we have been weaving 30 cm fabric using shuttle looms for several decades, the fact we never produced wide fabric meant we did not own adequate loom for its production, and it was necessary to start from finding new power loom and weavers. Our first attempt was to modify the loom used in Nishijin to produce neckties. However, in order to weave 150 cm width using the loom with 50 cm by 3 Kama

V.G. Duffy (Ed.): DHM 2016, LNCS 9745, pp. 440–448, 2016.
DOI: 10.1007/978-3-319-40247-5_44

(Kama is the unit used for the pattern contained in the cloth width of patterned fabric) required major modification on the loom such as filling the gaps of fabric between each Kama. The weavers who were using the looms felt it to be an excessive demand. In addition, the aging weavers were extremely reluctant to explore the new challenge in order to produce new type of fabric, leading the project to come to a dead end. For the weavers who have been producing neckties, it was more important to focus on the daily order for neckties, which brings them modest but stable income, than to develop and produce a new innovative fabric.

In order to find a new loom, we expanded our search area to Tango, which is a textile producing town in the northern part of Kyoto. After requesting help from the Tango Textile Industry Association, we discovered a textile production company that possesses looms of every possible width. However, its process and technique was very different from Nishijin style, and its location meant 2 h travel by car between Nishijin and Tango and consequently difficulty in communication, it was not possible in the beginning to prepare environment for starting the production of textile we were searching for.

On the other hand, the demand of market, for instance from apparel makers who use the fabric, began to overtake the preparation of production, and we started to receive requests to use the textile that has not been produced yet because the customer valued the idea. This was the beginning of adoption of our textile to clothes and bags by JUNKO KOSHINO brand run by Ms. Junko Koshino.

In Kyoto, there were many events celebrating 400 years of Rimpa (Rimpa School: one of the major historical schools of Japanese painting) in 2015. Among them was a large event co-sponsored by Kyoto Prefecture and Kyoto City. As a part of large Rimpa exhibition at Kyoto National Museum, a large-scale fashion show produced by Ms. Junko Koshino with invited guests celebrating the 400 years anniversary of Rimpa was being planned. They were looking for fabric to be used for this fashion show. But Ms. Koshino was demanding a fabric that realizes unprecedented bold color and depth. As such textile cannot be found among existing products, they approached the textile business department of Kano-ko.

Therefore, in order to participate in the fashion show of Ms. Junko Koshino, it became necessary to rapidly advance on the production system of wide fabric. Ms. Koshino was wishing for Kanze Water Flow pattern, which is the signature pattern of Rimpa, Rabbit Ear Iris and Thousand Cranes patterns of Ogata Korin and Ivy pattern of Tawaraya Sotatsu.

2 Method

For the realization of these patterns, Kano-ko developed method to produce fabric with 120 cm width. When using rapier loom with 20 cm by 6 Kama, it is not possible to produce expressive fabric that contains our best techniques, we employed shuttle loom with 60 cm by 2 Kama. As it was proven to be possible to realize the effect of blur or shading, which are characteristics of Obi pattern by Kano-ko, environment to start test production was gradually prepared through meetings with weavers, modification and maintenance of looms, revisions of pattern designs (design drawing) which are crucial in Nishijin weaving, and other countless attempts.

The design proposal from the design office required the fabric to express thickness, shading, vivid contrast, crispness, volume and weight, meaning very high standard was demanded on the fabric production. It is common in contemporary Obi production that the parts that are not visible are made cheaply as many expressions has to be included in affordable textile. However, it is absolutely impossible to achieve the innovative fabric with luxurious appearance required by the design office. Therefore, a traditional Nishijin technique called Baikoshi was adopted.

Black lines are base weft threads, red and blue lines are pattern weft threads. Normally, one pattern weft follows one base weft. Here, by weaving in 2 pattern weft threads (they are shown as red and blue in diagram but the same color in reality) after each base weft, it results in more vivid textile (Fig. 1).

Baikoshi is a technique that weaves in 2 (or 3) pattern weft threads after each base weft thread in order to make weave less visible and produce more volume [1]. As it demands considerable amount of work, it is rarely employed today even in Nishijin. But it is also essential for expressing impressive shading, volume and color contrast, it was decided to include Baikoshi technique in the newly developed wide fabric. Through this, black did not appear on surface when weaving blue pattern weft with black warp, showing sharp and vivid blue, resulting in a beautiful fabric as shown in Fig. 2.

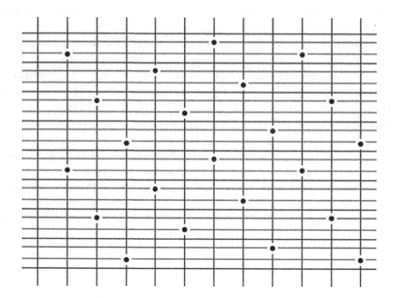

Fig. 1. Weaving structure diagram of Baikoshi technique

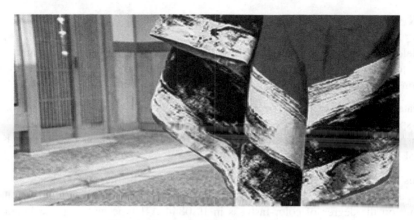

Fig. 2. Example of *Baikoshi* technique

Figure 2 shows an example of design by Junko Koshino woven into a fabric by Kano-ko. Commonly, fabric with pattern that has such subtle blur is produced as print, and even then it is difficult to produce this much sense of depth. In the case of this fabric, blue and silver wefts are woven into black warp. With normal weaving, blue woven with black appears as though the black base color comes through blue, resulting in less sharp blue. The same goes for silver. However, when Baikoshi technique is used, no matter what is the color of warp, base color black appears as black, and any color woven into it will clearly appear as the color of weft without being influenced by the color of warp. This results in superior fabric where the color of weft is vividly expressed. In other words, the color of weft is emphasized by repeating each color twice as in black → sliver → silver → blue → blue.

This is a traditional technique passed on in Nishijin, and not invented by Kano-ko. However, in view of the sever decline in the number of weaver that maintain traditional skill, an attempt to produce fabric that incorporate the top-level techniques of wide twill weave and Baikoshi that are suitable for high-class fabric is extremely rare in the textile industry. For product produced for clothing, it is safe to say this was the first of such production.

Moreover, the wide fabric released this time faithfully reproduced the subtle coloring and atmosphere of original Japanese paintings, which is characteristic of Nishijin-Ori, making it perfect for costume that expressed Rimpa produced to commemorate its 400 years anniversary.

In fact, when seeing the fabric produced by Kano-ko which satisfied the demands other fabric maker could not fulfill, Ms. Koshino said, "I was surprised that they were much closer to my image than I expected", proving that our techniques are surprising even for contemporary apparel makers to whom new things are rarely produced.

3   Result

As yield rate improved by repeating production, we conducted various tests in order to move toward mass production. We used our normally produced Obi fabric as comparison object. Below is the result of this quality inspection.

- Date of Inspection: The 21st of December 2015
- Inspection Subjects: Degree of Color-Fastness/Physical/Performance
- Inspection Institute: General Incorporated Foundation, Kaken Test Center Kyoto Laboratory

Tables 1 and 2 show the result of quality inspection. In the quality inspection test result, among the degree of color-fastness, it either tied to or slightly below the standard number on the degree of color-fastness in JIS0844 A-1 type washing and laundering and the degree of color-fastness to perspiration in JIS0848. Threshold is 2–3, and the gray background cells denote better performance than the comparison object. Table 3 shows the inspection result and differences in relation to the standard number.

However, in case of wool or silk product, it is not considered low-quality if it satisfies 2–3 level. Moreover, the usage of this fabric will be limited to luxury clothing and accessories, meaning heavy-duty factors are not required. It can be concluded that its overall quality perfectly satisfies the standard for usage as textile.

Table 1. Result of quality inspection (Physical)

Fabric	Test Item	Test Method	Length-Wise	Breadth-Wise
Wide	Tear Strength (N)	JIS L 1096 A Method (Cut Strip Method)	1390	2440
	Tear Strength (N)	JIS L 1096 D Method	Above 64.0	Above 64.0

Fabric	Test Item	Test Method	Length-Wise	Breadth-Wise
Obi Fabric	Tear Strength (N)	JIS L 1096 A Method (Cut Strip Method)	470	800
	Tear Strength (N)	JIS L 1096 D Method	60.3	Above 42.9

Table 2. Result of Quality Inspection (Durability / Physical)

		Test Items	Test Method / Fabric No.		Result
Newly Developed Wide Fabric	Degree of Color-Fastness	Light Exposure (Level)	JIS L 0842	Change	Above 4
		Washing (Level)	Color-fastness in JIS0844 A-1 type washing and laundering A-1 Type	Change	5
				Damage	4-5
		Sweat (Level)	Color-fastness to perspiration in JIS0848 (Acid / Alkali)	Change	5·5
				Damage	2·2
		Friction (Level)	JIS L 0849 II Shape	Change	4-5
				Damage	2-3
		Water (Level)	JIS L 0846	Change	5
				Damage	2
		Dry Cleaning (Level)	JIS L 0860 B-2 Method (Petroleum Solvent)	Change	5
				Change	4-5

		Test Items	Test Method / Fabric No.		Result
Common Obi Fabric	Degree of Color-Fastness	Light Exposure (Level)	JIS L 0842	Change	4
		Washing (Level)	Color-fastness in JIS0844 A-1 type washing and laundering A-1 Type	Change	4-5 (4)
				Damage	2
		Sweat (Level)	Color-fastness to perspiration in JIS0848 (Acid / Alkali)	Change	5·5
				Damage	4·2-3
		Friction (Level)	JIS L 0849 II Shape	Change	5
				Damage	4-5
		Water (Level)	JIS L 0846	Change	5
				Damage	3
		Dry Cleaning (Level)	JIS L 0860 B-2 Method (Petroleum Solvent)	Change	5
				Change	5

Table 3. The inspection result and differences in relation to the standard number

Test Item	Standard	Measurement Result	Difference
Washing (Level)	3	2	-1
Sweat (Level)	3	2-3	-1>

4   Future Challenge

The next challenge is to apply Hikibaku technique, which is the ultimate skill in luxury Obi of Nishijin, to complete wide woven fabric using leather. In the limited field of Obi, it is extremely rare to use anything for woven structure itself other than silk, gold or silver thread, or special paper for Hikibaku. However, in the category of decorative products which is the target of wide fabric, leather is a dominant material, leading us not only to explore the combination of fabric and leather, but also to think if we could turn leather into woven fabric, it would become an ideal material. Moreover, by combining this material with gold and silver thread or silk, we hypothesized that it would produce an unprecedented new material.

Hikibaku is a weaving technique that applies Japanese lacquer on Japanese paper made from mulberry tree or oriental paperbush, scatter gold and silver leaves on it, cut it in strips and weave them into a fabric. Our challenge was to weave in leather strips instead of paper strips.

Leather textile that weaves leather strips already exists. However, our challenge is to weave in pattern in this leather textile. This meant instead of printing on leather, pattern is produced through weaving. We know that it is theoretically possible, but it is predicted to be extremely difficult in reality.

If one cuts leather into thin strips and weaves them into fabric, the surface of leather will be hidden by the structure of warp, losing the characteristic texture of leather and will appear as ordinary thread. That does not make an attractive textile. On the other hand, if one uses thick leather strips, it will emphasize the texture of leather but it will also make the weaving pattern rough. Therefore, in order to fully utilize the benefit of leather, the thickness of the strips must be perfectly controlled.

In order to achieve accomplished weaving in leather Hikibaku, we started from weaving Obi fabric with 30 cm width. After long trial, the experienced weaver managed to weave this leather Hikibaku. However, even though Nishijin weaving in unrivaled in its skill for 30 cm width fabric, in order for the fabric to be accepted in the world, it needs at least 1 m width, demanding a totally different approach in everything including threads weavers are not familiar with, new loom, novel weaving structure and Hikibaku technique. For instance, the weaver never makes mistake in the order of Hikibaku strips or its front/back sides when producing 30 cm fabrics. But this occurred when producing 1 m fabrics. Or, each time changing the density of warp and weft, thickness or type of thread, the fabric yield decreased. Solving these problem required time.

Originally, Hikibaku is a technique employed in order to make fabric appear as though gold leaf is applied on its surface, giving it formal character. Its appearance resembled golden folding screen turned into fabric. Golden folding screen is an art form that applies gold leaf on partition wooden boards and painting on them. Formal

Obi using Hikibaku technique is made from weaving thin strips of paper with gold leaf into fabric, then producing pattern by using gold and silver thread for weft, giving it an artwork-like appearance.

Now, among the techniques nurtured in Nishijin, there is a method that gives Hikibaku its optimal appearance. In order to understand this, it is necessary to know the basic structure and texture. That is the difference between plain weave, which is the simplest woven fabric, and twill weave, which is luxurious fabric. Plain weave has the warp : weft ratio of 1:1. If one weaves simply with plain weave, weft obscures the Hikibaku strips and it will not appear on the surface of the fabric. Meanwhile, twill weave has 2:1 ratio of Warp and weft, meaning if one uses Hikibaku technique on it, it has even more warp than plain weave, further sinking Hikibaku into the fabric struc-ture. Therefore, another, about 2/3 thinner, thread aside from warp and weft is woven in us upper layer in order to bind the Hikibaku strips, resulting in vivid appearance of Hikibaku on the surface of fabric. This extra warp is called Betsugarami (Separate entwinement). This means that when using leather instead of normal Japanese paper strips in Hikibaku weaving, it becomes essential to bind the leather Hikibaku with this extra Betsugarami binding warp in order to maximize the material texture of leather. This is a highly specialized process. It is possible only by weavers who mastered Hikibaku technique, and not many textile makers even in Nishijin can produce it.

Fabric using Betsugarami exists for a long time. But as it requires excessive work and cost, and as it is a technique that emphasizes the expression rather than durability of the product that results in delicate textile, it became a declining technique. However, it is an ideal method for weaving depth and limitless expression in fabric with mere 30 cm width. By frequently employing this method, Kano-ko has realized the opulence and beauty radically different from the products of other makers (Fig. 3).

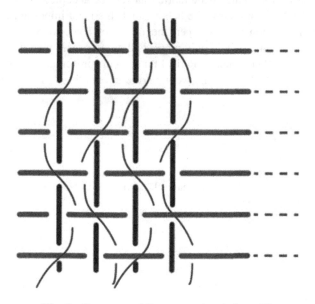

Fig. 3. Structure of Betsugarami technique [2]

Loom that can produce gold brocade fabric for formal Kimono with 1 m width did exist before. But in reality, for producing high-quality fabric, there are only looms for producing 30 cm width fabric, and weavers who possess skill to produce 30 cm width fabric. For instance, loom that weaves low-grade textile has only very short distance between warp beam and cloth fell (suspension), meaning its hold of warp is inadequate and it is more difficult to entwine weft with warp. Furthermore, there are virtually no weavers who weave Hikibaku for wide fabric. Therefore, machine setting for weaving with Hikibaku or knowhow for precise weaving are critically lacking.

Moreover, when weaving Hikibaku into Obi fabric, the movement of loom / weaver is only within 30 cm, but when weaving Hikibaku in wide fabric, it requires 3 times more movement, demanding considerable energy. Even though younger weavers are more fit and have more energy, because they do not have experience in hand-weaving Hikibaku, they make mistakes such as using wrong side of the strip or mixing up thread order. On the other hand, this process requires too much physical burden for older, experienced weavers. Thus, it was extremely difficult to find a weaver who has enough experience but still physically fit. Consequently, it resulted in long-term training of young weavers by experienced weavers, leading to succession of knowhow and future skill transfer.

5 Conclusion

Techniques of Nishjin-Ori were established through refinement after refinement since the 5th century. However, when it is not confined to Obi fabric but fused with a new platform, namely wide fabric, it is self-evident that it will show its strength in usages other than kimono. As the market for kimono, which exists only in Japan, continues to shrink, it is necessary to produce wide fabric that will be accepted in the world in order to pass on the Nishijin techniques. We believe that this is an important mission for us.

During the preparation of this paper, the fabric of Kano-ko was selected for the Maison D'exeption section, which only presents the companies with exceptional skills, of fabric fair Premiere Vision held at Paris, France. This presentation of our fabric drew interests from big fashion brands, and we intend to spread the charm and uniqueness of Nishjin-Ori to the world.

Reference

1. Miyashita, S.: "Manual for Learning Pattern Design Card", Association of Nishijin Pattern Design Card Industry (1995)

The Analysis of Polishing Process of Cold Forging Die in Axial Symmetric Form and Axial Non-symmetric Form

Hidehito Kito[1(✉)], Hiroyuki Nishimoto[1], Akihiko Goto[2], Yuka Takai[2], and Hiroyuki Hamada[1]

[1] Kyoto Institute of Technology, Hashikami-cho. Matsugasaki, Sakyo-ku, Kyoto 606-8585, Japan
h-kito@chukyo-dies.co.jp
[2] Osaka Sangyo University, 3-1-1 Nakagaito, Daito 574-8530, Japan

Abstract. In forging parts production, the die life is important for the production efficiency. If the die is fractured under production accidentally, it may cause a big damage to the productivity. One of die broken mode is a scratch on die surface caused by polishing in order to meet the design. It is for finishing the pre-mature die by polishing. It is required for more skillful craftspeople because the die life depends on damage of scratches. Therefore it is important to succeed their expertise constantly. It takes several years for craftspeople to be the expert on the job training. In this study, in order to accelerate their expertise transferring, we analyzed their expertise in focusing on quality of polishing in a forging part.

Keywords: Skill transfer level · Forging · Die life · Polishing

1 Introduction

Cold forging processing is a method of manufacturing parts that involves inflicting damage on the die used as tool. Therefore, the die life is key to maintaining manufacturing with stability. The mode of damage is of two forms (see Fig. 1). One is breakage in the product's forming area, generally an issue of die construction including press fit rings. The other is frictional wearing of the product's forming area through contact with a processing material, thought to be caused by the surface condition, in other words the way it is polished. Die-making for cold forging is distinguished by hand polishing of the processing part known as product area, which adds greatly to the die life. The polishing work is dependent on a person referred to as "die craftspeople" and though from the past a technical approach has been given trial, the skill has not been fully explicated. This research is aimed at accelerating expertise transfer of expert through analysis of the polishing work.

© Springer International Publishing Switzerland 2016
V.G. Duffy (Ed.): DHM 2016, LNCS 9745, pp. 449–457, 2016.
DOI: 10.1007/978-3-319-40247-5_45

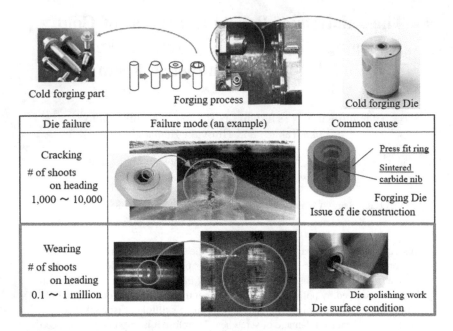

Fig. 1. Die life in a cold forging

2 Polishing Skill of Cold Forging Die

Die manufacturing consists of multiple procedures with machine processing at the core. Generally polishing work is called "finishing process" and comes into play at the end (see Fig. 2). Polishing work has the following two purposes.

- Operation to create a shape that cannot be made by machine processing.
- Operation to draw the surface condition needed for manufacturing of parts.

Even with a polishing process that is treated as a single operation, the craftspeople mentally plans the order for polishing area and the processing method to be used (see Fig. 3). In other words, a single process of polishing work has a procedural design, and the processing method follows the procedural design. Several years is required to learn polishing work. One factor is the ability to work out the procedural design mentioned above. The other requirement is expert operational ability to faithfully implement the procedural design.

In polishing work, some cold forging dies are considered that, even though they are relatively similar in shapes, only specific experts are able polish them. This is thought to be due to the shape and specification of the die, the necessary polishing skill is changed and it demands a new polishing skill that is not an extension of familiar techniques. In this study, we aim to clarify the nature of the new polishing skill demanded in the polishing work of specific dies only the expert can polish by comparing it to the polishing of dies that beginners can also polish [1].

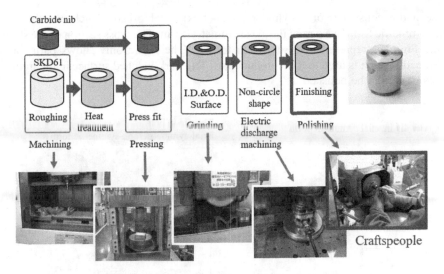

Fig. 2. Cold forging die manufacturing process

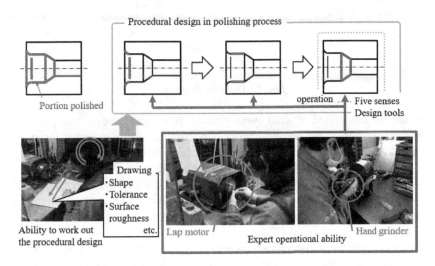

Fig. 3. Ability of craftspeople required to be an expert

3 The Analysis of Polishing Process of Cold Forging Die in Axial Symmetric Form and Axial Non-symmetric Form

3.1 Die Specification

As the die that even a beginner can handle, an axial symmetric shape die consisting of two cylinders in different diameters was chosen. For the die only an expert can polish, in order to make the analysis of the required polishing skill relatively easier, we selected a die that is as close as possible in shape with the die for the beginner. Consequently, we chose a die consisting of a cylinder and a hexagonal prism, which has the axial non-symmetric form in a part of the axis symmetry form. The cross section of die shown in the Fig. 4 is representative subject to testing. The figure only shows parts called carbide nib which is used to form product part. The dark-hatched surface in the figure is the work area to be polished.

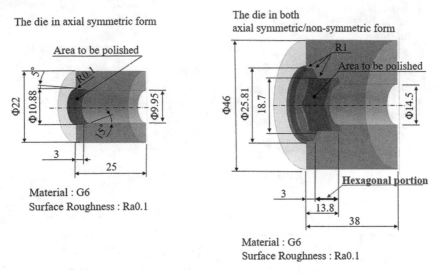

Fig. 4. Die specifications

For the die comprised of axial symmetric form, cutting process was provided by turning machine before the polishing work. On the other hand, the ones comprised of both axial symmetric/non-symmetric form are treated with electric discharge machining. In addition to that, a special-ordered processing jig is used to treat flat surfaces of hexagonal prism for rough-semi finishing. Since cutter marks remain on the cut surface, it needs to be polished at least in the range of 5 μm. Likewise, altered-layers remain on the surface treated with electrical discharge, it also requires removal process with the range of 10 μm.

Commonly, for the polishing of a cold forging die with an axial symmetric shape, the polishing is done after attaching the die to a rotation mechanism called lap motor. For the die chosen for the expert, part of the work cannot be conducted with a lap motor (see Fig. 3).

3.2   Experimental Method

As the purpose of this study is to determine and compare the polishing skill required for the polishing of each die, the focus of the analysis was on the polishing process and the polishing tools used. Moreover, in order to numerically verify the intentions of the workers at each step in the polishing, the dimensional transition of the work area that requires polishing was measured.

The polishing work process and the polishing tools used for analysis should meet the standard. We also selected skilled and experienced workers who are handling test pieces as test subjects. A test subject for the die comprised of axial symmetric form is a skilled male worker with 11 year-experience in polishing work and 6 year-handling-experience of this kind of die. A test subject for the die with both axial symmetric/non-symmetric form is also a skilled male worker with 15 year-experience in polishing work and 10 year-experience in handling this kind of die.

4 Experimental Results

Figure 5 shows the polishing work process of dies in axial symmetric form, the used polishing tools and abrasive grain. Working hours on a representative example are also shown for reference. Work process mainly consists of two parts. One is manual processing around the mouth R0.1 which is not machinery processed. The other is the polishing work on an entire polishing area. In the latter polishing work, the side and the bottom of the cylinder are not separately polished, but polished as continuous plane. The polishing is done after attaching the die to a lap motor.

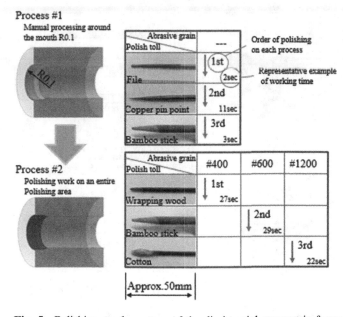

Fig. 5. Polishing work process of the die in axial symmetric form

Figure 7 shows the polishing work done to the die in both axial symmetric/non-symmetric form. Process 1 is the polishing work for the mouth R1 of hexagonal prism for which dimension accuracy should be guaranteed by manual work. Process2 is rough-semi finishing in polishing area excluding the mouth R1 and the side of hexagonal prism. And process3 is final finishing of the entire polishing area. Lap motor was used only in Process 2. Due to its hexagonal shape of the base of the inside, lap motor was used only for polishing of its inscribed circle and manual polishing was applied to the remaining part without rotation. For Process 1 and 3, the work is conducted after gripping the circumference side on the V block. For the polishing work on the V block, the polishing work is conducted with rotating tool attached to the hand grinder. We use copper wire, wrapping wood, bamboo stick and cotton as common polishing tools for both test pieces. Copper wire and wrapping wood are used with the intention of scraping off bumpy surface caused by machine processing. Bamboo and cotton are used as if using its grain as abrading agent to level the surface.

Figures 6 and 8 show distinguishing changes to shape and surface roughness before and after the polishing work in each process. Chamfering process is manually provided in the initial process of Fig. 6. The required surface roughness Ra0.1 is adequately satisfied after the polishing work. Figure 8 shows that R-dimension was maintained according to the required dimension in Process 1. As notable characteristics of work in Process 2, it can be observed that the subject proactively polishes ridgeline in concave shape comprised of hexagonal prism and cylinder. The trace of work can be seen in the vicinity of ridgeline of the inner base. The required surface roughness Ra0.1 is sufficiently met after the work.

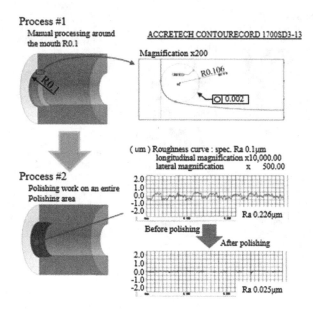

Fig. 6. Shape and surface roughness before and after polishing of the die in axial symmetric form.

It is considered that using rotation is to improve work efficiency in die polishing. It is interesting to note that work-rotating polishing is used together with tool-rotating polishing in the polishing process of the die comprised both axial symmetric/non-symmetric form. It consequently requires many types of polishing tools. Suppose that

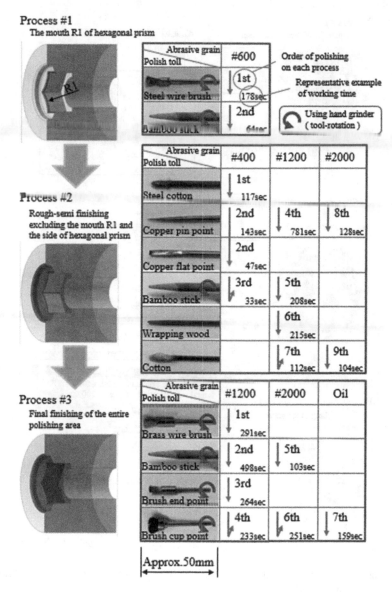

Fig. 7. Polishing work process of the die in both axial symmetric/non-symmetric form

making the work as simplified as possible is a shortcut to acquisition of skills, the number of tools used should be decreased. The reason of using work-rotation simultaneously is thought not to simplify the polishing work but to make it easy to assure quality in terms of roundness and coaxiality. In work-rotation, the subjects should focus on the shape of two-dimensional plane including symmetrical axis. As a result, the work is equally transferred along the direction of circumference. Figure 9 shows differences in movement from subjects' point of view. Looking at work-rotation from

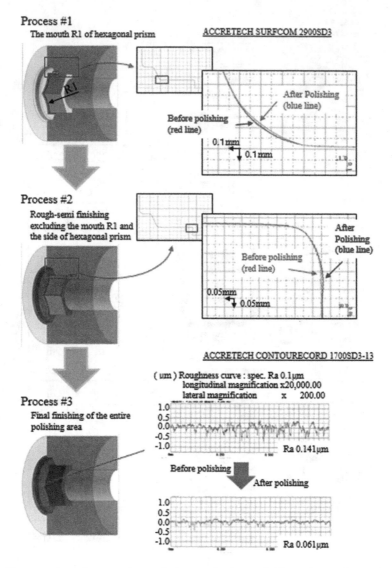

Fig. 8. Shape and surface roughness before and after polishing of the die in both axial symmetric/non-symmetric form.

subjects' point of view, when polishing three-dimensional plane, it can be said that they should focus on only bi-axes with leaving the remaining axis to rotation. It is thought that smaller number of working axis makes it easier to control movement. In other words, it can be thought that the difficulty level increases when handling dies in axial non-symmetric form since it requires tri-axial motion to complete the work. Furthermore, polishing tools used are rotary ones with which a subject needs to be familiar. Craftspeople are required to obtain skills to overcome difficulty in guaranteeing shape accuracy of work range with tri-axial motion.

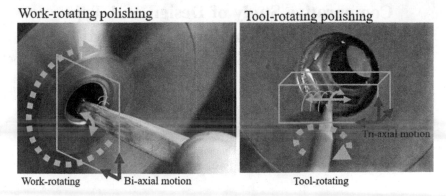

Fig. 9. Differences in polishing motion from subject's point of view

5 Conclusion

The following information was gained by analyzing the polishing of each test piece. For the polishing of the die comprised only of axial symmetric form, even if it is three-dimensional polishing work, the process itself only requires attention on two-dimensional plane because it uses work-rotation. In other words, the work-rotation mechanism along the direction of circumference guarantees the accuracy of the repeated work, and the worker only needs to focus on the movement that follows the contour of two-dimensional plane along the direction of the axis. On the other hand, the polishing work of a die that includes axial non-symmetric form demands the accurate movement in three-dimensional plane. Therefore, it requires a skill that can produce continuously changing shape itself in the three-dimensional space. Moreover, in order to achieve it, it requires the ability to precisely comprehend forms in the three-dimensional space based on the measurement data.

Reference

1. Kito, H., Nishimoto, H., Takai, Y., Goto, A., Hamada, H.: Evaluation approach for measuring the skill transfer level in the forging die polishing. In: Proceedings of the 6th International Conference on Applied Human Factors and Ergonomics AHFE 2015, pp. 5796–5803 (2015)

Comparative Study of Design and Type of Work When Assembling Cardboard Beds for Shelters

Yoshihiro Mizutani[✉], Naoya Yamada, Noriaki Kuwahara,
Kazunari Morimoto, and Hiroyuki Hamada

Kyoto Institute of Technology, Kyoto, Japan
mizutani@jpacks.co.jp

Abstract. When a disaster strikes, it is an international standard to use make shifts beds in shelters but in Japan, refugees are forced to sleep directly on shelters' floor for long periods of time. In recent researches, this type of shelter environment was revealed to lead to different secondary health damages or post-disaster related deaths. However, after the 2011 Great East Japan Earthquake, corrugated cardboard make shift beds began to be used in shelters. Their use can help reduce secondary health damages and improve shelters' environment. From a few hundred to one thousand disaster victims are expected in large scale shelters but corrugated cardboard beds' assembly demand an important work load and it is desirable to install them promptly to prevent evacuees to sleep on the floor as much as possible. It is necessary to plan the optimization of beds' assembly. In precedent cases, beds were installed and assembled with the help of volunteers and there was a tendency for groups to be formed and making assembly a collaborative work. However, the division of labor and cooperative work require time and space and it can be frequently inefficient as the limited manpower, related to the disaster, can be seen as wasted. In this research, we focus on differences in movements for individual work and collaborative work in the process of assembling cardboards beds and use these results to reduce unnecessary movements and to render their assembly and set-up easy and efficient.

Keywords: Temporary bed · Individual work · Collaborative work · Motion analysis · Work efficiency

1 Context and Objectives

Japan is said to be the great country of disaster and since the 2011 Great East Japan Earthquake, various disasters have occurred and when necessary, numerous shelters have been installed. However, it cannot be said that shelters' environment is good for the evacuees as they are forced to sleep directly on shelters' cold floor and living in these conditions for a long period has led to numerous secondary health damages. To improve this situation, cardboard beds for shelters were developed (Fig. 1). This cardboard bed has a simple structure and shape making it easy for anyone to assemble it. Also, they are can be mass produced quickly and at a low price. On the other side,

© Springer International Publishing Switzerland 2016
V.G. Duffy (Ed.): DHM 2016, LNCS 9745, pp. 458–465, 2016.
DOI: 10.1007/978-3-319-40247-5_46

assembling a bed requires quite some time and depending on every person's way of assembly and the use of collaborative work, the time spend assembling the bed could stretch even more. To decrease the burden of the workers, we are aiming to shorten the time necessary by improving the assembly of the cardboard bed and in the first experiment, we have examined efficacy differences between division of work and individual work and in the second experiment, differences between the existing cardboard bed and a newer version with bigger and less parts.

2 Processes in the Standard Assembly of a Cardboard Bed for Shelters

In the first stage, the total of 24 small cardboard boxes are assembled with a diagonal partition of cardboard inserted in each box and then each 4 boxes are inserted in a sleeve. A rectangle is formed by assembling these 3 exterior sleeves for the length and 2 for the width. Two top boards are placed on this rectangle to form the bed. The final product is pictured in Fig. 1.

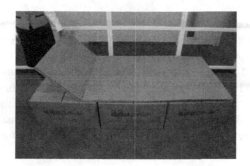

Fig. 1. Cardboard bed for shelters

3 First Experiment

3.1 Content of the Experiment

The experiment was realized indoor with sufficient space. Using unassembled beds, we asked the participants to assembly in order (A) and (B) work type. Work (A) consist in one group of several persons assembling freely the number of beds equal to the number of persons in the group. In Work (B), each person assemble one bed. The work process was recorded on video camera form beginning to end.

This time, we realized this experiment with the following two groups:

- Group 1: 2 participants; in Work (A) 2 persons made 2 beds and in (B) Work, each of the 2 participants made 1 bed each.
- Group 2: 3 participants; in Work (A) 3 persons made 3 beds and in (B) Work, each of the 3 participants made 1 bed each.

3.2   Method of Analysis

To process to the recorded assembly work analysis, we determined the following elements.

The beginning point of the analysis was considered to be "the first time when one touches the cardboard", "the last time one takes their hands of the cardboard" is the final point and one sequence of required time was considered as "entire work time". Situations where "one was waiting without doing nothing" or movements as "holding things and moving" were considered as "wasted time". However, in the case of "one moving and working", it was considered as work time. The time obtained from subtracting "Wasted time" to "entire work time" is considered as "actual work time" and for the work (B), we categorized 12 processes in the method of assembling the cardboard bed (Fig. 5).

3.3   Experiment Results

The results of the analysis of the recorded assembly work are represented in Figs. 6 and 7. Individual work analysis dividing each 12 processes worktime was represented in Table 1.

Furthermore, concerning the Fig. 2, the actual worktime, the wasted time and the entire worktime average are respectively 946.6(s), 230.7(s), 1176.3(s), the deviation is for each 178.8(s), 158.4(s), 22.8(s). For the Fig. 3, the average is respectively 709.8(s), 41.7(s), 751.5(s), and the deviation 50.1(s),15.2(s), 42.6(s). Among the two Work items, we realized the F-test and homoscedastic can't be noticed for the entire worktime only. From this result, we applied Welch test on the entire worktime, for the two other items, we realized the T-test and in every case with $p < 0.05$, statistical difference were observed. Also, in the 12 processes shown on Table 1, "Tidying up" is in itself an unnecessary process.

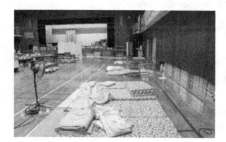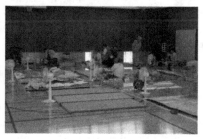

Fig. 2. On On the right, a usual Japanese shelter with bedding directly on the floor or on a thin tatami mat. On the left, a shelter in a Gymnasium where people sleep on the floor

3.4   Discussion

In Fig. 2 as well as Fig. 3, as statistical differences were observed in the entire worktime, the wasted time and the actual worktime, it can be said that the division of

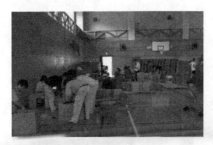
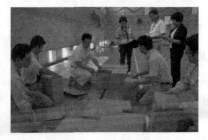

Fig. 3. Volunteers are making beds (collaborative work)

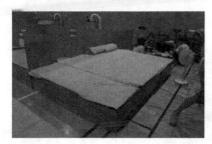
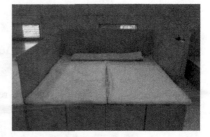

Fig. 4. (a) Completed cardboard bed for a family of 3. (b) Completed bed for two persons.

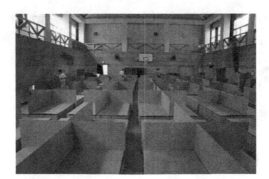

Fig. 5. Beds in a shelter for 100 evacuees

work takes more time to assembly and produces wasted time. If you look closely at each group in Fig. 2, there is a great variation of wasted time between Group 1 and Group 2. In Group 1, the two persons worked resourcefully but on the other side, Group 2 divided complete the work and it can be thought that it is was the source of waiting time. Also, during the individual work phase, 3 of the 5 participants did not use the assembling method thought to be the fastest and had each a different way to

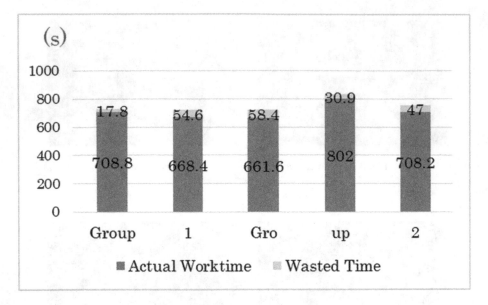

Fig. 6. Analysis results of work (A)

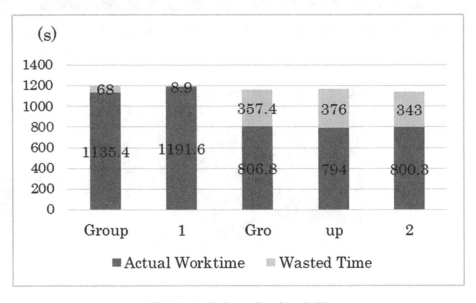

Fig. 7. Analysis results of work (B)

assemble the bed but based on Fig. 3, there is no important variation observable. From this, it appears that during the individual work, the sequence of assembly doesn't not create a great variation in time.

Moreover, observing Table 1, the processes requiring the most time for the individual work are tapping the ends of the box and also inserting the boxes in the exterior sleeves. Also, one of our participants told us the tapping was troublesome which led us to assume that removing the tapping work could lead to decrease substantially worktime.

Table 1. Required time for each process during individual work

Process category	Average of Each Process Time (s)	Deviation	Percentage
Unfolding the cardboard box	63.5	8.0	8.9 %
Closing the bottom lid	49.3	6.0	6.9 %
Taping the bottom lid	143.4	28.0	20.2 %
Turning over the box	37.6	6.7	5.3 %
Inserting the diagonal partition	76.7	11.9	10.8 %
Closing the upper lid	51.8	7.6	7.3 %
Taping the upper lid	126.6	22.0	17.8 %
Putting away the box made	19.4	12.9	2.7 %
Unfolding the exterior sleeve	21.4	4.0	3.0 %
Inserting the boxes in the sleeve	108.2	25.7	15.2 %
Laying over the top boards	8.8	1.7	1.2 %
Tidying up	3.2	6.4	0.5 %
Total	709.8	50.1	

4 Second Experiment

4.1 Experiment Content

The experiment was realized indoor with sufficient space and we used two different types of cardboard beds: the existing type of made with 24 small boxes and a new prototype using 12 larger boxes, half the number of the previous type with one box being the size of 2 small boxes. We asked the participants to make each time of bed alone and we recorded their work from beginning to end. Participants were 5 with four men and one woman and taking into account the effectiveness of the sequence, we separated the participants in two and made them assembly the types of bed in opposite order.

4.2 Method of Analysis

We realized the same analysis as for the first experiment.

Also, we categorized the process of work in 12 processes for every video recordings.

4.3   Experiment Results

The recorded work analysis results are represented in Fig. 8. To show the relation to the time, we choose to represent only results for one person.

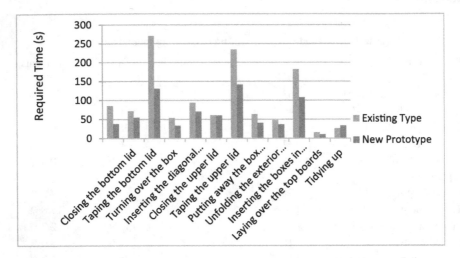

Fig. 8. Comparison of required time for each process by type of cardboard beds

Overall, the new prototype is completed in a shorter required time and in particular processes like tapping both side of the boxes and inserting them in the sleeves dramatically become shorter.

4.4   Discussion

Based on Fig. 4, the new prototype is takes in comparison with the existing type generally less required time, as especially required worktime of tapping or unfolding the boxes is shorter, it can be assumed that with the number of the boxes handled decreasing and the work load also diminished.

On the other side, there are processes showing less improvement such as closing the lid or inserting the diagonal partition, for example, but the new prototype larger boxes are less easy to handle and it can be possible that thicker cardboard used to maintain the bed's strength as the boxes got bigger made assembling the bed harder.

5   Conclusion

For the first experiment, it is usual to think that collaborative work will take a shorter time than individual work but with collaborative work, each process have a different work load and we found that waiting time between processes is more long than with individual work. Rather than the worker trying to work more efficiently, shorten worktime was associated to the reduction of waiting time. Therefore, we found that even with numerous worker, the effective way of shortening worktime was to do all the processes alone.

In the second experiment, we compared work between the existing type and the new prototype of bed using half the number of boxes while being the same bed size. The improved version permitted to cut down by 38 % the worktime. The decreased number of boxes and not their sizes was the reason for this shorten worktime.

In the shelters, there is a great possibility that hundreds of cardboard beds can be installed. As shorter worktime is extraordinary effective, hereafter we want to associate further design and work charge's method improvements with the decrease of worktime in the assembly of the cardboard bed.

The Difference in Micro-deburring Finish Produced by Groove Cutting Method

Mitsunori Mori[1,2(✉)], Tatsuro Nagasuna[1], and Hiroyuki Hamada[2]

[1] Tango-Giken Co., Ltd., Kyoto, Japan
mitsunori-mori@tango-giken.co.jp
[2] Kyoto Institute of Technology, Kyoto, Japan

Abstract. It is ideal to remove micro-bur during the mechanical processing, however, burs in micro level must be removed manually. Moreover, in order to perform an even deburring process, precise angle control of deburring tool and repeatable motion control is necessary, which requires a skilled craftsmanship.

In this report, in order to establish a training method of high-level deburring craftsperson, we will study the difference between skilled and unskilled worker's working process. The research will involve monitoring several workers with different length of experience engaging in the same deburring process of micro-bur, and examine the difference in their working method through eye movement measurement and motion analysis. We will evaluate the data gained from this research and the difference in the time required for the deburring process between the workers of different experience. And with understanding these differences, we will define the process necessary for standardizing the deburring work.

Keywords: Deburring · Eye movement measurement · Motion analysis

1 Introduction

Although there are differences depending on the facility, shape and required precision, the common production process of metal parts involves these 5 steps below.

1. Machine Processing + Deburring
2. Heat Treatment
3. Finishing
4. Surface Treatment
5. Inspection

Among them, #1. is a process that mainly involves cutting and turning, which generate edges and burs that causes functional defects afterwards. It is ideal to remove burs during the machine processing. However, burs in micro level are difficult to remove during the machine processing, meaning it requires manual deburring. Moreover, in order to perform an even deburring, control of deburring tool and repeatable movement are required, which demand advanced craftsmanship.

© Springer International Publishing Switzerland 2016
V.G. Duffy (Ed.): DHM 2016, LNCS 9745, pp. 466–474, 2016.
DOI: 10.1007/978-3-319-40247-5_47

2   Method

2.1   Test Subjects

Test subjects are selected from the workers who have deburring experience. One expert female worker who have worked in the company for 23 years, one non-expert male worker who have worked in the company for 2 years, and one female beginner who even though has worked in the company for 7 years, but has no deburring experience. Table 1 shows each test subject's information.

Table 1. Detailed Information of test subjects

Test Subject	Age	Years of service	Gender	Dominant Hand
Expert	41	23	Female	Right
Non-expert	48	2	Male	Right
Beginner	42	7*	Female	Right

(* An inexperienced person)

2.2   Measuring Condition

Test subjects were instructed to debur a processing object in the same shape. They were given several common deburring tools such as files and grindstones without specifying which tools to use. Table 2 shows the list of deburring tools. The order of work process was not specified as well. Selection of the tools was left to the judgment of individual subject. As shown in the Fig. 1, the part to be deburred is a same-shaped part made of S45C Material. The Measuring location was where the test subjects normally conduct their deburring.

2.3   Measuring Method

Moving images recorded with a video camera was used for work process analysis and movement analysis. Eye movement measurement was conducted with "Mobile Type Eye Mark Recorder EMR-9 (nac Image Technology Inc.)". Figure 2 shows the view during the experiment. Analysis of the test subjects' eye movements/focus points during the deburring was conducted with CCD camera attached to the measurement goggles. The product evaluation after deburring was conducted with a digital microscope VHX-200 (KEYENCE Corporation) for appearance evaluation (in 20 magnification), and "Contour Measuring Instruments SURFCOM 1700DX2 (TOKYO SEIMITSU CO., LTD.) for quality/shape evaluation after deburring. The quality evaluation after deburring was conducted is a separate location that was not disclosed to the test subjects.

Table 2. List of deburring tools.

No	Name	Image
1	Half Round File	
2	Shaping Knife A	
3	Ceramic Grindstone	
4	Shaping Knife B	
5	Shaping File	
6	Flat File (Large)	
7	Ceramic Knife	
8	Flat File(Small)	

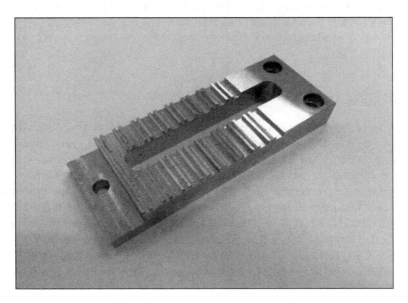

Fig. 1. Object for deburring

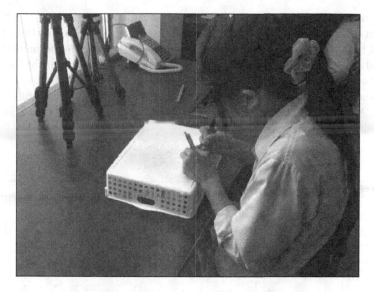

Fig. 2. View from eye movement measurement

3   Result and Examination

3.1   Movement Analysis Result

As shown in Fig. 3, a number was assigned to each section that requires deburring. This numbering was used to analyze the order/tools used for deburring. Figure 4 shows

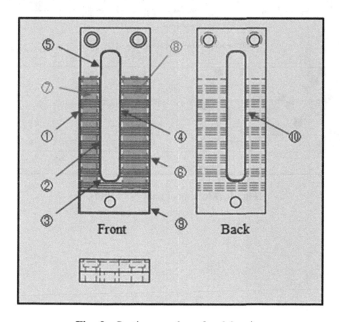

Fig. 3. Section numbers for deburring

the movement analysis of work done by the expert, the non-expert and the beginner. The expert deburred the same section 2.3 times on average, which tends to be lower as compared to the average of the non-expert, which was 4 times. Furthermore, both the expert and non-expert sometime used the same tool that they once finished using, but the average number of times they used the same tool on the same section was 2.1 times for the non-expert as opposed to the 0.5 time of the expert which results in lower tendency. As shown in Fig. 5, the number of palpation done by the expert was 65.3 % less than that of the non-expert.

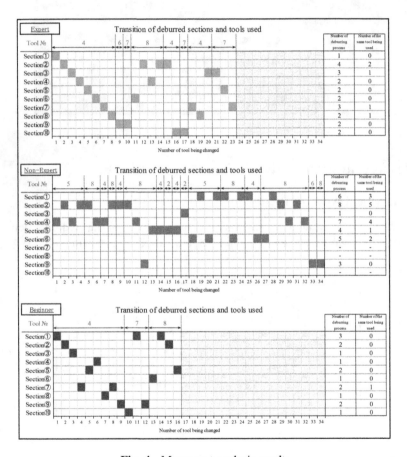

Fig. 4. Movement analysis results

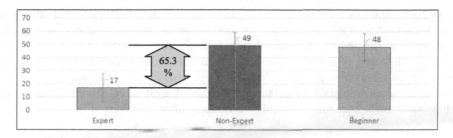

Fig. 5. Number of palpation during deburring process

3.2 Eye Movement Measurement Result

Figure 6 shows the results of eye movement analysis of the expert, the non-expert and the beginner. Even though duration of focus was longest for the expert, she completed the work in more than 45.94 % shorter time as compared to the non/expert and the beginner. Moreover, she had over 10 points less in the result check ratio as compared to the other subjects. Additionally, the expert repeated the 2 steps, namely "checking the shape before deburring" and "focusing on the section to be deburred".

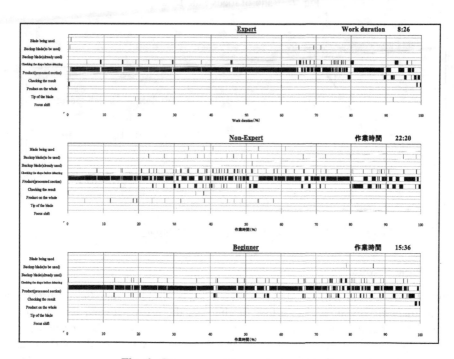

Fig. 6. Eye movement measurement results

In contrast, the non-expert and the beginner showed the tendency to add one more step, namely "checking the result", to these 2 steps. Figure 8 shows this result. The expert conducted the aforementioned 3 steps only after 80 % of the work is completed in 5 out of 6 times. This shows that she emphasizes the certainty of the deburring and evaluates the product quality requirement from the condition of the product at near-completion of deburring, instead of evaluating the effectiveness of deburring through checking the result immediately after deburring (Fig. 7).

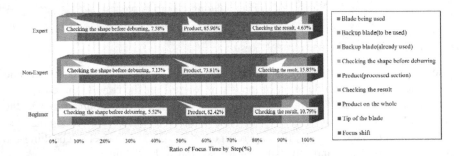

Fig. 7. Ratio of focus time by step

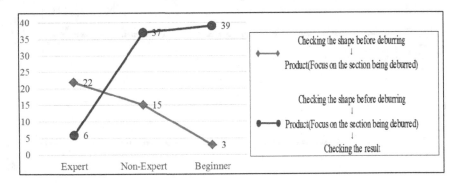

Fig. 8. Numbers of movement repetition according to experience

3.3 Shape Evaluation

Figure 9 shows the results of shape measurement before and after the deburring, as well as magnified pictures. Regarding the burs in the sizes between 0.04–0.06 mm before deburring, the surface after deburring done by the expert and the non-expert were in the state as specified by light chamfering. In contrast, the surface after deburring by the beginner still had burs about 0.04 mm without being removed. On the magnified pictures showing the surface after deburring by the expert and the non-expert display successful deburring. In contrast, the magnified pictures showing the surface after deburring by the beginner show that burs were left partially or continuously.

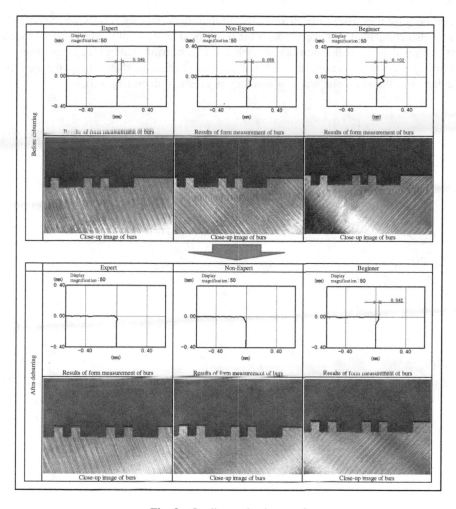

Fig. 9. Quality evaluation result

4 Conclusion

In this research, we conducted the movement analysis, eye movement analysis and quality control during the deburring works done by an expert, a non-expert and a beginner. The result showed that the expert and non-expert have already acquired the ability to produce/assess products that satisfy the required quality standard, despite the differences in their work duration/work process. The expert demonstrated that by acquiring a skill to optimize the deburring process, she could shorten the time spent on "checking the result". Moreover, she is deemed to consider/select the most suitable tools while "checking the shape before deburring" in order to conduct her work with least possible tools and deburring number. In contrast, both the non-expert and the beginner demonstrated that their duration/number of deburring is more than that of expert because they assess the effectiveness of their deburring by "checking the result". It was also concluded that even though the movement analysis of the beginner showed that she displayed smaller number of tools used, deburring number and repetition of deburring the same section, she did not perform deburring that satisfy the quality standard and therefore she was not conduct an effective deburring process.

A Piano Lesson Method Where User Plays the Piano Laying His or Her Hands on the Image of a Model Performer's Hands

Chika Oshima[✉], Kimie Machishima, Katsuki Yamaguchi,
and Koichi Nakayama

Saga University, Saga, Japan
chika-o@ip.is.saga-u.ac.jp

Abstract. We aim that even elderly people with dementia become to live actively with a hobby which provides them a feeling of accomplishment. Playing a keyboard instrument has a high threshold for novice people. Therefore, we proposed a practice method where users can play the piano laying their hands on the image of a model performer's hands. In this paper, we conducted an experiment that ten university students who had no experience or a little experience playing the piano played a musical piece along with the model performance by laying their hands on the CG performer's hands in the mirror. Most students could play the musical piece correctly after playing it only five times. On the other hand, some students hit the wrong keys when the CG model performer hit the key with her mid or ring finger because the model performance was represented like a mirror.

1 Introduction

Most elderly people want to live actively every day even after reaching the mandatory retirement age. Some people enjoy playing golf, fishing, climbing a mountain, playing a musical instrument as a hobby. These hobbies provide the elderly people a feeling of accomplishment. The feeling of accomplishment is effective even for decline of behavioral symptoms of dementia [1,2]. However, some hobbies have a high threshold for novice people.

Although playing a keyboard instrument has a high threshold for novice people, people who practice it hardly is easy to get a feeling of accomplishment. If even people with dementia can try to play the keyboard with a support system/method, they will get a feeling of accomplishment and may live actively every day.

Therefore, we researched what kind of support method enables people with severe dementia to play the piano and get a feeling of accomplishment [3]. We conducted an experiment in which an elderly woman with "higher brain dysfunction" took piano lessons using educational video materials and found that the participant could play the piano as long as she imitated a model performance on

© Springer International Publishing Switzerland 2016
V.G. Duffy (Ed.): DHM 2016, LNCS 9745, pp. 475–483, 2016.
DOI: 10.1007/978-3-319-40247-5_48

a video. We concluded that the participant played the piano with enthusiasm. The number of pitch errors gradually decreased. Moreover, we recognized that she gained a feeling of accomplishment through her utterances and behaviors.

However, the participant complained that it was difficult to find the same key as the key the performer played in the video. Moreover, in one of the lessons, the model performer said the color of the sticker on the key immediately before hitting the key. It was in the same manner as "Lighted Keys [4]" which is a keyboard that lights the key the performer should hit next. In this case, the participant hit most of the keys with her index finger.

Therefore, we present another support method where users can play the piano laying their hands on the image of a model performer's hands. In this paper, we describe this support method and the results of an experiment where ten healthy students tried to play the piano using this method.

2   Reference

There are many systems for healthy people to learn how to play musical instruments. A piano learning support system [5] refers to the key outlined in color and an adequate fingering number that a user should hit in the next timing. "The AR Piano Tutor [6]" also indicates the key that a user should hit in the next timing by a colored rectangle-shaped mark over the real keyboard with the Augmented Reality interface. "Piano Tutor for iPad [7]" and "Piano Marvel [8]" are applications for users who are novice piano learners. These systems show a keyboard on a small picture of a display. These systems have a high-score tracking function. Users can see what key they should hit next on the keyboard and where they made mistakes in their performances. However, it is difficult for elderly novice people to see the small picture on a display and to push the correct key while referring to the fingering numbers. "Family Ensemble [9]" is a piano duo support system that allows parents of novice child to hit keys correctly even with only one finger. Although the system supports only the parent's performance directly, the system was developed on the assumption that the child gets to have the motivation to practice the piano. "The Phantom of the Piano [10]" shows a model performance when a user stops his/her performance.

3   Practice Method of Displaying a Model Performance

3.1   The User's Hands Lay on Hands of the Model Performer

We present a practice method in which a user sets his/her hands on the hands of the model performer. As shown in Fig. 1, a half mirror is placed between an upward-facing 23.8-inch display (EIZO, FORIS FS2434) and an electric keyboard (YAMAHA, NP-30). As shown in Fig. 2, the display represents the model performance made using computer graphics (CG). A user playing the keyboard watches his/her hands laying on hands of the model performer's hands in the mirror. We expected that the user would recognize the key and fingering that he/she should hit simultaneously and successively.

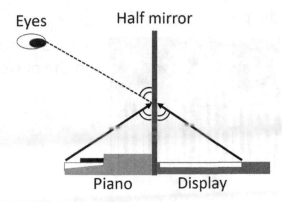

Fig. 1. A half mirror is placed between a display and a keyboard.

3.2 Graphics of Model Performance

The musical piece is a hook-line from "Kawa no Nagare no Yoni (Like a Flowing Stream)," a Hibari Misora song. It is a very famous song in Japan. It consists of eighteen bars.

In our previous research [3], we made a video that a model performer plays a musical piece. If we employ the performer's video to projected in the display, a strain is generated between each key in the video and on the real keyboard.

Therefore, virtual keys and hands of the model performance were made using the computer graphics software, "Blender." Twenty-five frames per one second are generated. The dimension of each key made by Blender is same as the key of the real keyboard that we use in our experiment. The virtual keys and hands were reversed because the video was projected on the display as a mirror image.

Both hands of the model performance were on the keyboard constantly. A contrast between light and shadow on the surface of hands is coordinated according to movement of each finger. This operation allows the user of the system to know which finger will hit a key the next time.

Moreover, the key that the user should be playing displays as red, and the key that the user should play next displays as yellow. The user should release the key when the key returns to white.

The first author made MIDI (Musical Instrumental Digital Interface) data by playing the musical piece with an electronic piano. She played the piece about in one minute. The electronic piano outputs a "Standard MIDI (Musical Instrumental Digital Interface) File (SMF)." The SMF was converted a text file by a software "mft2." In the text file, we can see a hitting time (Note on time) and a releasing time (Note off time). The time when each key or each finger starts to move is assigned by Note on/off time in making each frame of graphics with Blender.

Model performance (CG)

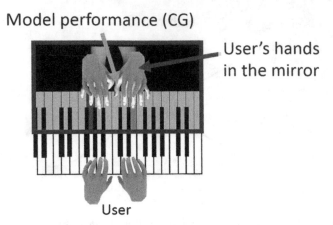

User's hands
in the mirror

User

Fig. 2. The model performance made by computer graphics. (Color figure online)

4 Experiment

4.1 Participants

Ten university students in their early 20 s participated in an experiment. One of them was female. Six participants had no experience playing the piano. Three participants had a littel experience for half a year or one or two years. One participant had taken piano lessons for five years.

4.2 Informed Consent

The participants in this experiment were informed about the intentions of the experiment and the treatment of personal information. Moreover, they were informed that they could withdraw from the experiment at any time and no reward was prepared for them. However, after the experiment, they received one Madeleine. We obtained written consent from them.

4.3 Method

As shown in Fig. 3, the participants ware asked to play a musical piece along with the model performance by laying their hands on the CG performer's hands in the mirror. A headphone output both the sounds of the model performer's and the participants' performances. The participants' performances were recorded by video cameras and a midi editing software (Domino Ver.1.43) to analyze their performance and their mistakes in notes and fingerings. Three participants were asked to set wearable cameras (Pana-sonic HX-A500) on their heads so that we could see what they were watching when they were playing the piano.

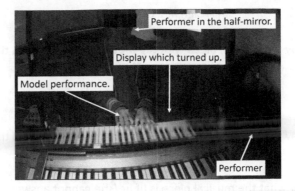

Fig. 3. The participant watches his/her hands laying on hands of the model performer in the mirror.

Figure 4 shows the method of the experiment. Before playing the musical piece, the participants were asked to lay their hands on the hands of the CG's performer. For the model performances, the performer's hands made with CG repeated the hook-line ten times. The first five times, the sounds of their performances and the model performances were not output. The participants may be a little familiar with playing the keyboard because they had been taught playing the keyboard harmonica when they were elementaly school students. We worried that they may try to find each correct key without watching the model performance when they noticed what the musical piece was. For the purpose of the experiment, participants had to depend on the movement of the model performer and the changing colors of the keys to play.

After five times performances, the participants were asked what the piece is. If the participant could not say a correct answer, we asked him/her same question after ten times performances.

The next five times, the sounds of their performances and the model performances were output. After ten performances, the participants played the piece by themselves. It took ten minutes for them to finish playing. We interviewed them regarding what kinds of things confounded them and where they were looking at while playing the musical piece along with the model performance.

4.4   Analysis

We analyzed four of participants' performances; the first, the fifth, and the tenth performances with the model performance, and the last performance without it. We counted correct hitting, extra hitting, and replaying and checked their fingering in each performance.

4.5   Result

Table 1 shows the results of the participants' performances. The number of "wrong" indicates that they played notes that are not in the musical piece

(1) Sign at a consent from

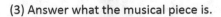

(2) Play the musical piece with the model performance (5 times)
(Sounds are not output.)

(3) Answer what the musical piece is.

(4) Play the musical piece with the model performance (5 times)
(Sounds are output.)

(5) Answer what the musical piece is (if he/she cannot answer it at (3).).

(6) Play the musical piece without the model performance (1 time).
(Sound is output.)

(7)Answer in an interview.

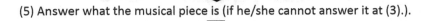

Fig. 4. Method of the experiment.

(extra, replaying). If they could accurately name the title of the musical piece after playing it five times, we marked "5" in the "answer title" and after playing ten times, we marked "10." All of them answered it correctly.

Furthermore, by the mistake of the experimenter, six participants heard a noise when they were playing from the sixth to the tenth time. The noise was other participants' performances collected previously. MIDI data from other participants' performances were input into the keyboard. The "noise" column of concerned participants is indicated by "yes."

Table 1. The results of the participants' performances.

	experience (piano)	answer title	performance 1 (no sound)		performance 5 (no sound)		noise	performance 10 (with sound)		performance 11 (no model)	
			correct	worng	correct	worng		correct	worng	correct	worng
A	no	10	39	23	55	11	no	55	5	–	–
B	no	10	38	8	55	2	yes	55	2	–	–
C	no	10	49	14	55	3	no	47	4	–	–
D	no	10	52	11	56	9	yes	53	7	47	13
E	no	10	53	3	56	0	no	56	0	4	0
F	no	5	55	9	56	1	no	56	1	56	3
G	a half year	5	53	11	55	2	yes	56	1	43	25
H	1 year	10	47	5	55	2	yes	54	1	17^a	25
I	2 years	5	56	1	56	2	yes	51	2	45	15
J	5 years	5	49	18	53	5	yes	56	1	47	3

^{a} means the participant hit some keys with incorrect fingering.

"56" in the column "correct" means that the participants could play all the notes in the musical piece. Participant-I could play all the notes in the first performance in spite of having no prior experience playing the musical instrument. He hit only one extra note. After only five performances, nine participants could play the piece with a few mistakes in pitch and without a mistake in fingering. Moreover, Participant-F could play the piece without the model performance, even though she had no experience playing the piano.

Regarding the fingering, Participant-H mistook six notes when he played the musical piece without the model performance. The others could play with the correct fingerings in all performances.

All participants were told that they were watching the mirror while they played. The images from the wearable cameras showed that the participants had their eyes on the mirror the entire time they played.

Furthermore, four participants reported that they sometimes hit the wrong key when the CG model performer hit a key with his mid finger or ring finger. Figure 5 shows an example of these kinds of mistakes. The upper score shows the model performance. At the last two notes, the performer operated its fingers from the right mid finger (the fingering number is "3") to the left mid finger (the fingering number is "3"). The last note should be the key of A (La) hit with a mid finger. The lower score shows the performances of Participants-D, F, G, and H. They played the key next to A, i.e., G (So) with their ring fingers by mistake.

Model performance

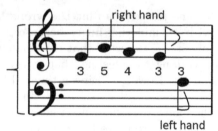

Participant's performance

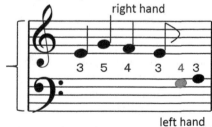

Fig. 5. Confusion of fingering caused by mirror.

5 Discussion

Although the participants had no or little experience playing the piano, almost all of them could hit all the notes of the musical piece correctly after playing it only five times.

We believe there are at least three reasons they were able to play the musical piece easily. First, they only imitated the model performance by laying their hands on the image of a model performer's hands. Second, they were good at hitting keys when the color changed because they were used to playing tapping games. Third, they only needed to focus on one thing, the model performance in the mirror. During the practice stage, a common performer usually needs to see both the keys and a score while he/she is playing. Our system did not give such a burden to the participant.

Participant-I who could play all notes correctly in the first time flattened his fingers and hit the keys. However, in his the ten times performance, form of his hands became round and hit the keys deeply. He got used to keying as well as the hands of the model performance might lead him to the good form of hitting.

Moreover, after playing the piece ten times, Participants-D and F could play the musical piece with the correct fingering without the model performance. The participants practiced the musical piece with the correct fingering because they could see the hands of the model performer. If the keys' color changes are only shown on the display without the hands of the model performer, they could not practice with the correct fingering and some of them might hit all the keys with one finger. We think that the correct fingering encourages a proficiency of playing the piano.

On the other hand, some participants hit the wrong keys when the model performer hit the key with her mid/ring finger because the model performance was represented like a mirror. We expected that the participants gradually come to move their fingers according to a feeling that integrates their fingers into the model performer's fingers. However, being estimated from the participants' mistakes, the participants, first, might catch which finger the model performer hit consciously, e.g. "The model performer used her mid finger to hit the key." Then, they might move their appropriate finger to hit the key. If they practice for long time, they may be used to play the piano with the model performance.

6 Conclusion

In this paper, we presented a practice method in which a user sets his/her hands on the hands of the model performer to play a keyboard with a low threshold. We conducted an experiment where ten healthy students tried to play the piano using this method. They had no or little experience playing the piano. Although the sounds of their performances and the model performances were not output, almost all participants could hit all notes of the musical piece correctly in only five times practice. There are some reasons why users played a musical piece easily. First, they only imitated the model performance by laying their hands on the image of a model performer's hands. Second, they were good at hitting keys when the color changed because they were used to playing tapping games. Third, they only needed to focus on one thing, the model performance in the mirror. On the other hand, the some participants sometimes hit wrong keys when the model performer hit the key with her mid/ring finger.

We aim to develop a practical method that supports elderly people to play a keyboard with a low threshold. The characteristics of elderly people vary. Some have reduced cognitive functioning, a reduction in skilled behavior, some degree of tremor, and/or lose their good eyesight. We will ask for the elderly people to play the keyboard instrument using the practice method in which a user sets his/her hands on the hands of the model performer. Then, we will discuss appropriate supports for them to use the practice method effectively.

Acknowledgment. This work was supported by JSPS KAKENHI Grant Number 15H02883.

References

1. Kolanowski, A., Litaker, M., Buettner, L., Moeller, J., Costa Jr., P.T.: A randomized clinical trial of theory-based activities for the behavioral symptoms of dementia in nursing home residents. J. Am. Geriatr. Soc. **59**(6), 1032–1041 (2011)
2. Machishima, K., Ishii, Y., Oshima, C., Hosoi, N., Nakayama, K.: Personalization techniques of the occupational therapy for people with dementia using daycare, 42th SICE Symposium on Intelligent Systems, F-02 (2015). in Japanese
3. Oshima, C., Machishima, K., Nakayama, K.: Toward a Piano lesson system that gives people with reduced cognitive functioning a sense of accomplishment. In: Antona, M., Stephanidis, C. (eds.) UAHCI 2015. LNCS, vol. 9177, pp. 649–659. Springer, Heidelberg (2015)
4. Casio: Lighted Keys. http://www.casio.com/home
5. Takegawa, Y., Terada, T., Tsukamoto, M.: A piano learning support system considering rhythm. In: Proceedings of International Computer Music Conference, pp. 325–332 (2012)
6. Barakonyi, I., Schmalstieg, D.: Augmented reality agents in the development pipeline of computer entertainment. In: Kishino, F., Kitamura, Y., Kato, H., Nagata, N. (eds.) ICEC 2005. LNCS, vol. 3711, pp. 345–356. Springer, Heidelberg (2005)
7. SmileyApps: Piano Tutor in iPad. http://www.smileyapps.com/
8. PianoMarvel: http://www.pianomarvel.com/
9. Oshima, C., Nishimoto, K., Hagita, N.: A piano duo support system for parents to lead children to practice musical performance. ACM Trans. Multimedia Comput. Commun. Appl. **3**(2), 6 (2007). Article No. 9
10. Oshima, C., Hikawa, N., Nishimoto, K., Inoue, N.: How a piano practice support system should present model performances a pilot study. In: 2006 Proceedings of Information Processing Society of Japan, vol. 72, pp. 71–78 (2006)

The Load Measurement of the Beating Brush in the Second Lining Procedure

Yasuhiro Oka[1(✉)], Yuka Takai[2], Akihiko Goto[2], and Kozo Oka[1]

[1] Kyoto Institute of Technology, Kyoto, Japan
okayas@mac.com, oka@bokkodo.co.jp
[2] Osaka Sangyo University, Osaka, Japan
{takai,gotoh}@ise.osaka-sandai.ac.jp

Abstract. Hanging scroll is a traditional Japanese ornamental art, which includes paintings and calligraphy. Scrolls are unrolled and hung on a wall or in an alcove when displayed and are rolled up and stored in a box. They should hang straight without rippling or warping when unrolled, and be rolled up smoothly and tightly from the bottom when stored. To enable rolling out and hanging scrolls smoothly, the paintings and calligraphy referred to as "main works" are generally backed with traditional Japanese paper and adhered using a paste made from wheat starch. Especially in order to guarantee this flexibility function that enables rolling up smoothly, a type of glue that does not harden after it dries is employed as the adhesive agent for the lining process. But since this glue does not have sufficient adhesive effect, craftsmen employ a traditional technique of pounding the paper with a special "pounding brush" to enhance its adhesive effect. In this study, using pressure measurement films, we considered differences in the techniques of an expert and a non-expert by measuring the pounded area by a brush and the pressure to be applied by pounding with a brush. Through the quantification of the differences of these two subjects, we aim to understand the characteristics of proper pounding technique, to help new craftsmen learn more quickly.

Keywords: Pressure measurement films · Hanging scrolls · Pounding brush

1 Introduction

Hanging scroll is a traditional Japanese ornamental art, which includes paintings and calligraphy. This art works binding method has been playing an important role in decorating the space, with the development of Japanese cultures such as tea ceremony and flower arrangement. Scrolls are unrolled and hung on a wall or in an alcove when displayed as shown in the Fig. 1, and are rolled up and stored in a box as shown in the Fig. 2. Storing the scrolls rolled up protects the artwork inside from exposure to light and air, this method has been recognized as a superior way to preserve paintings and calligraphy from other eras. The preservation method is extremely important for the paintings or calligraphies with high cultural values. In case of repairing the high cultural valued art works bound in scrolls and passed down from ancient or Middle Ages to the present, it usually remove a art work from a scroll and repair the damaged

© Springer International Publishing Switzerland 2016
V.G. Duffy (Ed.): DHM 2016, LNCS 9745, pp. 484–493, 2016.
DOI: 10.1007/978-3-319-40247-5_49

parts and rebind it again. This binding technique is essential method to hand down the precious cultural assets to the next generations. They should hang straight without rippling or warping when unrolled, and be rolled up smoothly and tightly from the bottom when stored. To enable rolling out and rolling up functions smoothly, the paintings and calligraphy referred to as "main works" are generally backed with traditional Japanese paper and adhered using a paste made from wheat starch.

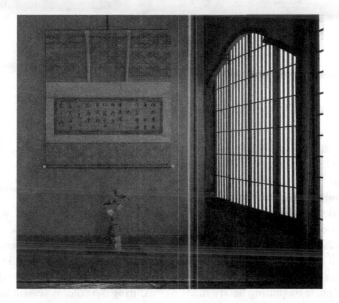

Fig. 1. A Hanging scroll displayed in an alcove with flower arrangement

In order to back-line main works, four layers of paper, called "lining papers," are generally adhered with starch paste. These layers are known as the first, second, third, and final lining papers, in order of proximity to the artwork. *Nakauragami*, or the third lining paper is the name of the layer to be back-lined before adhering the final lining paper, after the work called "*Tsukemawashi*", which applies brocades and silk around the edges of the main work for the purpose of protecting it, as well as for decorations. Depending on quality and size of the base material of the main work, more linings may be applied. In this case, the second and the third lining layers are applied without "*Tsukemawashi*". And the third layer applied in this case is also called "second lining"instead of "third lining". Or sometimes, the final lining paper is applied after "*Tsukemawashi*", without applying the third layer. The Fig. 3 shows the most common type of laminated constitution of binding work, where four layers backing papers were attached to the back side of the main work. Types of Japanese papers and glue, and concentrations of diluted glue used are different for each layer. To enable rolling out and rolling up functions smoothly, it is said that it takes long time to acquire the lining technique.

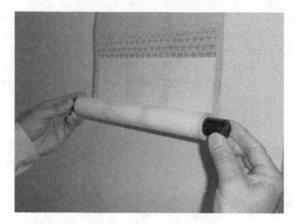

Fig. 2. Rolling up a Hanging scroll

For adhering the first lining layer directly to the back side of the main work, the glue called as "Shin-nori (fresh paste) with strong adhesive properties is used. This glue is made from wheat starch that has been heated and allowed to gelatinize, and then cooled naturally overnight. The purpose of applying the first lining layer is to reinforce the main works from the back side. And in order to prevent ripping and warping, the first lining paper should be adhered firmly with fresh paste. However, since fresh paste has strong adhesive properties, if it is used for the second and later layers, there is a concern that it may spoil the necessary flexibility to be required for a scroll when rolled up and down. Thus, aged paste is used for adhering the second and later layers. The aged paste is made by putting newly made paste during the coldest season in Japan into a pot and sealing it. It is then aged for ten years in a cool, dark place to allow it to ferment. During the fermentation process in the pot, biodegradation advances and the molecular weight of the starch paste decreases, severely weakening its adhesive properties. This weaker aged paste does not stiffen like new paste, even after it has dried. Due to this function, the aged paste is applied for the adhesion of the second and later lining layers, which allows the scrolls to be smoothly rolled up for storage.

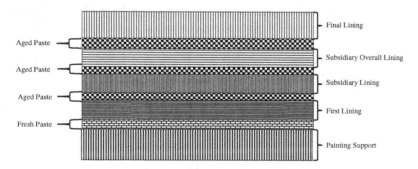

Fig. 3. The Outline of laminated constitution of binding work

For adhering the first lining layer directly to the back side of the main work, the glue called as "Shin-nori (fresh paste) with strong adhesive properties is used. This glue is made from wheat starch that has been heated and allowed to gelatinize, and then cooled naturally overnight. The purpose of applying the first lining layer is to reinforce the main works from the back side. And in order to prevent ripping and warping, the first lining paper should be adhered firmly with fresh paste. However, since fresh paste has strong adhesive properties, if it is used for the second and later layers, there is a concern that it may spoil the necessary flexibility to be required for a scroll when rolled up and down. Thus, aged paste is used for adhering the second and later layers. The aged paste is made by putting newly made paste during the coldest season in Japan into a pot and sealing it. It is then aged for ten years in a cool, dark place to allow it to ferment. During the fermentation process in the pot, biodegradation advances and the molecular weight of the starch paste decreases, severely weakening its adhesive properties. This weaker aged paste does not stiffen like new paste, even after it has dried. Due to this function, the aged paste is applied for the adhesion of the second and later lining layers, which allows the scrolls to be smoothly rolled up for storage.

The aged paste is diluted with water when it is used. Therefore, its adhesive strength is insufficient, and because of that, scroll makers use a traditional technique of pounding the surface of each lining paper with a special "pounding brush," to provide better adhesion. The process of applying glue on the second and later lining papers and pounding on their surface is called "pounding work". When pounding lining papers with a brush, it damages the paper if pounding is too strong, but if it is too weak, it cannot enhance the adhesion property. Moreover, if the entire adhesion surface is not pounded evenly with the consistent strength, it will result in an uneven adhesion state

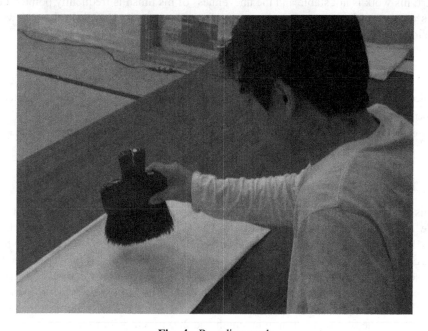

Fig. 4. Pounding work

of the entire surface. And it will eventually cause warping when binding work of a scroll is completed. Same as other traditional techniques, non-experts watch and learn this technique from the movement of experts, so it takes a long time to acquire this pounding technique (Fig. 4).

In this study, using pressure measurement films, we considered differences in the techniques of an expert and a non-expert by measuring the pounded area by a brush and the pressure to be applied by the brush, and the average pressure. The expert and the non-expert were instructed to pound the surface of the pressure measurement films, assuming that the film was a lining paper surface to be adhered. The color of the pressure measurement film changed only on the locations where pressure was applied. From the spots where the color changed, it allowed us to ascertain the differences between the expert and the non-expert, and comparatively analyzed the test results. Through the quantification of the differences of these two subjects, we aim to understand the characteristics of proper pounding technique, to help new craftspeople learn more quickly.

2 Experiment with Pressure Measurement Film

2.1 Subjects

In this study using pressure measurement films, we assigned one expert and one non-expert respectively and instructed them to do the "pounding work". The information of the subjects is stated in the Fig. 1.

The non-expert has been acquiring training of pounding work. But according to the expert, his work is not stable and the unevenness of his finish is frequently pointed out. He is not yet in the stage where he can perform the pounding work in the real work situation (Table 1).

Table 1. Data about the subjects

Subject (age)	Years of Experience	Height (cm)	Weight (kg)	Gender	Dominant Hand
Expert (40)	22	171	72	M	R
Non-expert (27)	6	170	54	M	R

2.2 Pressure Measurement Film

In this study, the pressure measurement film "Prescale" for ultra low pressure LLLW made by Fujifilm Corporation was used. The possible measurement range is from 0.2 MPa to 0.6 MPa. This film consists of two kinds of films, film A and C. Film A, which had a coupler layer, and film C, which had a layer of color developer, were placed together and used for measurement. The mechanism of this film is; when the micro-capsule in the coupler layer is destroyed by pressure, the coupler adheres to the color developer, and then turns to red by chemical reaction (extracted from the instruction manual of "Prescale"). The film was 270 mm in length and 200 mm in width.

2.3 Experiment Method

Both the expert and non-expert were instructed to conduct the "pounding work" on their workbenches in their usual manners. We measured how much pressure was applied by one pounding, and the size of the area of the pounding brush that is used for pounding. In order to obtain the result per each pounding, we asked the subjects to pound the same spot on the workbench repeatedly. During the motion, we inserted a film between the pounding brush and the workbench to take the marks brought by one pounding motion, which was then pulled out after 1 pounding.

Next, the subjects were instructed to pound the entire surface evenly. Based on the standard process of second lining, both subjects started pounding from the right side front, gradually moving the brush in the way shown in the Fig. 5. After the pounded films were scanned and digitalized, they were analyzed by the pressure analysis system FPD-8010 J. The area applied with pressure, pressure load and the average pressure were digitalized according to each pounding. In case the entire surface of a film was pounded, we detected the existence of unevenness visually, and then calculated the pressure load and the average pressure.

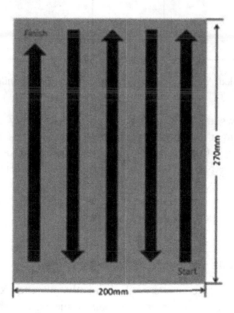

Fig. 5. The outline of motion of brush when pounding entire surface of pressure measurement film.

3   Result and Discussion

3.1   Analysis of One Pounding

The Fig. 6 shows the pressure measurement film pounded by the expert and the Fig. 7 shows that of the non-expert. As shown in these two figures, the expert pounded larger area than the non-expert. Moreover, the area applied with pressure, and pressure load and average pressure obtained by the image analysis are indicated in the Table 2.

Table 2. Comparative analysis between expert and Non-expert about area applied with pressure, pressure load and average pressure by one pounding.

	Pressurized area (mm^2)	Load (N)	Mean pressure (MPa)
Expert	4997	1174	0.23
Non-expert	4101	914	0.22

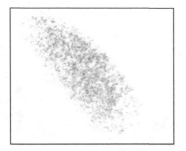   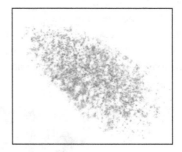

Fig. 6. Trace of Pounded Area by Expert   **Fig. 7.** Trace of pounded area by Non-expert

These results shows that the area the expert could apply the pressure by one pounding for enhancing the adhesive properties is 1.22 times larger than it of the non-expert. Though the difference in the pressures applied by one pounding between the expert and the non-expert is 260 N, no difference in the average pressure between the two subjects was detected. As the result shows, the expert pounded larger area and applied more pressure by one pounding than the non-expert, which enabled him to enhance the adhesive properties efficiently.

3.2   Pounding the Entire Pressure Measurement Film

The Figs. 8 and 9 show the image analysis results for the expert and non-expert respectively. The numbers of poundings of both subjects, and the pressure load and average pressure obtained by the film image analysis are shown in the Table 3.

Although the non-expert showed the higher values in the pressure load and average pressure, the cause of this result was presumed by observing the pounded films shown in the Fig. 8. Generally, the non-expert could not pound evenly; there were some parts where the films remained white, especially in the lower central parts. On the other hand, he pounded the same part repeatedly, which caused that part to turn red. While the image analysis in the Fig. 9 shows that the red spots showing 0.25 N to 0.60 N pressures are distributed evenly in the work done by the expert, the yellow spots showing 0.60 N or more pressures are unevenly distributed in the non-expert's work, especially in the right side of the films as shown in the Fig. 10. And when comparing the number of poundings, while the expert pounded 52 times to complete the pounding on the entire surface, the non-expert needed 88 time to complete his work.

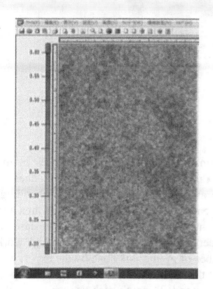
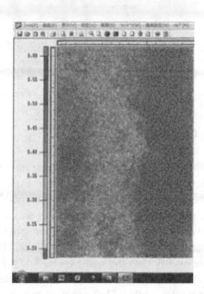

Fig. 8. Analysis after pounded by Expert   **Fig. 9.** Analysis after pounded by Non-expert

3.3   Comparison by the Range Where the Pressure Was Applied

The Fig. 10 shows the pressure distribution chart prepared based on the analysis result.

The differences in the pressures applied on the surfaces of films were observed between the expert and non-expert. While the expert pounded the most of the area with the pressure range from 0.30 MPa to 0.35 Mpa, the non-expert pounded the most of the area with 0.60 MPa or more.

Table 3. Comparison of the number of poundings, pressure load, and average pressure between expert and non-expert.

	Pounding times	Load (N)	Mean of pressure (MPa)
Expert	53	14214	0.40
Non-expert	88	16699	0.47

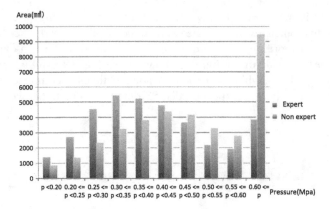

Fig. 10. Pressure distribution chart

4 Conclusion

In this study using pressure measurement films, we verified the differences in the techniques of pounding done by an expert and a non-expert for the purpose of adhesion enhancement, by measuring the pounded area and the pressure applied by pounding. The results showed that the expert was able to enhance the adhesion of larger area and apply more pressure load by one pounding than the non-expert. Thus, in case of enhancing the adhesion in large area, the expert could complete the pounding work more evenly than the non-expert. And the number of poundings done by the expert was less than that of the non-expert. It revealed that the non-expert pounded the same spots repeatedly, while he left some other parts not pounded. Through such unevenness in the adhesion enhancement process, there is a concern that the original function of hanging scrolls which is to hang straight might be impaired.

Also, after pounding works, we interviewed the expert and the non-expert how to grip a pounding brush. While the expert griped the brush with an angle, holding it with upward diagonal angle from fingers to wrist,, the non-expert tended to grip it from side horizontally. Moreover, when asked which part of the bottom of the brush was used, the expert clearly answered that he intentionally used the right side half of the brush when holding it with his right hand. However, the non-expert did not pay attention to which part of the bottom side of the brush he was using during pounding. These differences are presumed to influence the differences in the techniques between the expert and non-expert, so that more discussion is necessary.

The measurement with pressure measurement films is an effective method to evaluate the technique for pounding the adhesion surface evenly. Since this method can visualize the acquired level of technique easily, it is thought to be the effective way to utilize in the instruction manual for new craftspeople in the future.

Acknowledgement. This study received the JSPS Grant-in-Aid of Scientific Research (Kakenhi), #25350327.

References

1. Hayakawa, N., Kigawa, R., Kawanobe, W., Higuchi, H., Oka, Y., Oka, I.: The basic research on the physical property and chemical composition of aged glue. Conserv. Sci. **41**, 15–28 (2002)
2. Hayawaka, N., Kimijima, T., Kyusunoki, K., Oka, Y.: The pounding brush effect on binding work. Focusing Adhes. Property **43**, 9–16 (2004)
3. Nishiura, T.: The adhesive effect enhanced by pounding brush. Sci. Binding Work **30**, 99–107 (1997)
4. Hayakawa, N., Kigawa, R., Nishimoto, T., Sakamoto, K., Fukuda, S., Kimishima, T., Oka, Y., Kawanobe, W.: Characterization of furunori (aged paste) and preparation of a polysaccharide similar to furunori. Stud. Conserv. **52**(3), 221–232 (2007)

A Comparative Study of Instructing Methods Regarding Japanese Bowing

Tomoya Takeda[1]([⊠]), Yuko Kamagahara[2], Xiaodan Lu[1],
Noriyuki Kida[1], Tadayuki Hara[3], and Tomoko Ota[4]

[1] Kyoto Institute of Technology,
Matsugasaki, Sakyo-ku, Kyoto 606-6585, Japan
t.takeda@taste.jp,
luxiaodan0223@gmail.com, kida@kit.ac.jp
[2] Andsmile, 1-1-7 Minamishinmachi Chuo-ku, Osaka 540-0024, Japan
kamagahara0525@gmail.com
[3] University of Central Florida, 4000 Central Florida Blvd. Orlando,
Florida 32816, USA
tadayuki.hara@ucf.edu
[4] Chuo Business Group, 1-6-6 Funakoshi-cho, Chuo-ku, Osaka 540-0036, Japan
tomoko_ota_cbg@yahoo.co.jp

Abstract. We will examine whether a difference emerges between two such teaching methods: a method whereby learners watch a traditional instructional video depicting a situation in which the bowing of an expert is filmed from the side (Group A); versus a method whereby learners watch a video of the movements in the expert's line of sight while bowing (Group B). We could ascertain that the point of vision of the keirei bowing expert was established at approximately three meters in front of her upon the floor, and that she was able to maintain a maximum angle of 30 degrees when bending at her waist. We could discern that the line of sight video had the effect of suppressing $\theta 1$, which had previously been impacted by conformity on the parts of the subjects of Group B to also bend their necks when bending at their waists. Also, we were able to observe several cases in which the angle of test subjects' waists was rectified such as to nearly achieve 30 degrees.

Keywords: Ojigi · Japanese bowing · Japanese hospitality

1 Introduction

The number of foreign visitors to Japan is rapidly increasing. In terms of Japan's tourism resources which pique the interest of people from other countries, there are factors such as its beautiful scenery of nature as an island nation, its rich historical and cultural heritage, and other cultural resources. However, after it was decided that the 2020 Summer Olympics and Paralympics would be held in Tokyo, it seemed to become inevitable that the Japanese way of hospitality– known as "omotenashi"– would also rank as an essential tourism resource. This was especially true because of the attention that would be drawn to lodging facilities like hotels, traditional inns,

© Springer International Publishing Switzerland 2016
V.G. Duffy (Ed.): DHM 2016, LNCS 9745, pp. 494–505, 2016.
DOI: 10.1007/978-3-319-40247-5_50

and bed and breakfasts, as well as dining and drinking establishments from casual eateries to high-end restaurants, and other places visitors are certain to see.

The Japan Tourism Agency is supporting regional pre-emptive initiatives as the "Regional 'omotenashi' Improvement Project Directed at the 2020 Olympics and Paralympics" [1]. Concomitant with this movement, there are also efforts to attract customers by strengthening the spirit of "omotenashi" within the service industry, but in order to do so a proper understanding of "omotenashi" is imperative. The Japan Productivity Center has defined "omotenashi" as "work to provide uncompromisingly heartfelt service while valuing the perspective of customers and/or residents" [2]. "Valuing the perspective of customers and/or residents" can be rephrased as "mutualistic service whereby the provider considers the circumstances of the beneficiary and responds with his or her whole heart," as differentiated from service which is unilateral from the side of the provider only. It can be thought that analogous concepts in other countries such as "hospitality" (the U.S.), 待客之道 (China), and "hospitalité" (France) vary from "omotenashi" on this point of whether the service is or is not mutualistic.

According to research on the degree of cognizance regarding "omotenashi" around the world, at present between 50 % and 80 % of non-Japanese people have heard of the term [2]. However, the increase in foreign visitors to Japan noted previously will bring heightened interest and attention to the Japanese way of customer service. There will presumably be an increase in the number of repeat visitors to Japan moving forward, as well, and as this happens, those visitors' attention will shift in the sense that they will progressively come to think more about how Japanese service differs from the corresponding concepts of hospitality in their own countries. It can be predicted that those foreign tourists will, so to speak, become capable of recognizing the difference in Japanese service.

There has been much debate over the question of what kind of service "omotenashi" entails. But even if we start from the basis of the saying that, "'omotenashi' begins with a greeting and ends with a parting," it seems that we should note the Japanese way of bowing as a first step to studying "omotenashi." The history of bowing being an action of greeting for Japanese people is long, as in the third century Chinese text the Gishi-wajin-den it is recorded that, "When meeting with an important person, Japanese people go to their knees and cast down their heads." Furthermore, the action of casting down one's head, or bowing, has been regarded as showing that one has no enmity toward his or her counterpart, due to the fact that it exposes the back of the head, a point of vulnerability [3].

Bowing is not limited to instances of greeting. It is also performed in various other settings such as to show appreciation or apologize, and is a commonly seen gesture in the course of daily life (Shibata, Takahashi, Gyoba, et al. 2015) [4]. Bowing can be done while standing or while sitting. For both there are multiple classifications according to the angle at which the upper portion of the body is bent. In most settings calling for conventional business etiquette, *eshaku* (15 degrees), *keirei* (30 degrees), and *saikeirei* (45 degrees) are practically being used as the three classifications of bows (Asada 2015) [5]. At the same time, unexpectedly, even Japanese people – who have ample opportunity to learn bowing as a proper manner – are almost exclusively doing so in a self-taught way (Asada, 2015) [5].

As a case study of researching bowing through experimentation, Morishita and Iwashita (1985) [6] reported that as inexperienced persons lowered their heads when bowing there was an intensification in the angle of the curvature of their backs; that in comparison to experienced persons the time of remaining still upon bowing was shorter for inexperienced persons; and that despite their being Japanese, the subjects predominantly bowed in a self-taught manner.

As stated at the outset, there is a movement to attract customers by strengthening the spirit of "omotenashi" within the service industry at this time. It can be thought that the development of an effective method for teaching bowing as a fundamental aspect of "omotenashi" could make a valuable contribution to the advancement of the service industry.

In this paper, we will examine whether a difference emerges between two such teaching methods: a method whereby learners watch a traditional instructional video depicting a situation in which the bowing of an expert is filmed from the side; versus a method whereby learners watch a video of the movements in the expert's line of sight while bowing.

2 Experimentation Method

2.1 Experiment Overview

In order to clarify the difference in terms of impact upon learners' skills levels of the two bowing instruction methods, we divided our subjects – 8 inexperienced persons who had never previously received instruction in the motion of a bow (5 men and 3 women averaging 29.25 years of age, with a standard deviation of 9.69 years) – into two groups of 4 people, "Group A" and "Group B." We set Group A as the group to learn by watching the traditional instructional video depicting the expert bowing from the side, and we set Group B as the group to learn by watching the video showing the movements in the expert's line of sight. We then investigated whether any differences emerged between the levels of mastery achieved by the two groups. With regard to the videos used, these will be discussed in greater detail in Sect. 3, below.

2.2 Measurement Method

As shown in Fig. 1, a marker was affixed at the points of the participants' heads, shoulders, waists, and knees. The motion of each test subject's bow was recorded with a video camera, and the elapsed time as well as the position of the markers was measured.

As the measurement values which were used to gauge the difference in skill between the groups, we adopted the angle from the head to the shoulders to the waist ($\theta1$), and the angle from the shoulders to the waist to the knees ($\theta2$), as calculated based on the measurement data regarding the elapsed time and the positions of the markers.

It has previously been explained that Group A was set as the group to learn by watching the traditional instructional video depicting the expert bowing from the side, and Group B was set as the group to learn by watching the video showing the

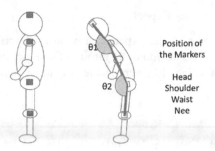

Fig. 1. Position of markers

movements in the expert's line of sight. However, in order to be able to measure any changes in skill level after receiving instruction, prior to viewing their respective videos we recorded each participant from both Group A and Group B performing bows in their own styles.

For the target bow test subjects were to attempt to reproduce, we selected a keirei bow with the lower back bent at a 30 degree angle. Each person performed six bows in total – three bows, punctuated by a break after each repetition, before viewing the assigned video; and three bows, again punctuated by a break after each repetition, after viewing the assigned video.

2.3   Arrangements Concerning Test Subjects

Prior to undertaking the experiment an oral explanation of our purpose and other such information was provided. After acquiring the subjects' consent to participate, we carried out the experiment.

3   Experiment Setup: Creation of the Two Types of Bowing Instructional Videos

In order to compare the effectiveness of the instruction received by Group A and Group B, we prepared two types of instructional videos, one to be utilized by each group. Naturally, we also adopted a keirei bow with the lower back at an angle of 30 degrees for the bows shown in both videos.

For the instructional model who was to act as the expert appearing in the bowing videos, we selected one woman who provides direction on receiving customers professionally. She possesses eight years of experience teaching greeters how to welcome customers at dental clinics and other service-oriented businesses, and we could determine that her level of competency was sufficient for a candidate to serve as the model for these videos.

3.1 Bows Performed by the Expert

The transition of the angles of the expert's previously described bows is depicted graphically below. There is no flexion of θ1 through three trial bows. Also, through the three trial bows θ2 is maintained in a very stable way at an angle of approximately 30 degrees (Fig. 2).

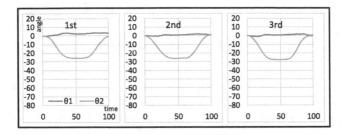

Fig. 2. Transition of angles in bows performed by expert (model from video)

3.2 Instructional Video for Group A

In general, even Japanese people have few opportunities to learn bowing by receiving instruction to improve their technique. More commonly, they would "learn through observing." We therefore created an instructional video for bowing with no verbal explanations, as a reproduction of this context of "learning through observing."

For the instructional video, we recorded a situation in which three keirei style bows were performed, from a lateral point of view (Fig. 3).

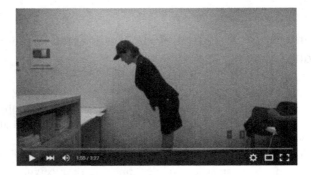

Fig. 3. Image of instructional video for Group A

3.3 Instructional Video for Group B

In order to examine the effectiveness of the instructional method that focused on line of sight for this paper, we employed an "EMR-9 (Eye Mark Recorder-9)" produced by NAC Image Technology, Inc., to measure the movements in the expert's line of sight when bowing. To additionally achieve an instructional video that would enable the expert's point of vision from the side to be understood, we edited in footage to create a two-frame video in which the movements in both frames corresponded with each other. As shown in Fig. 4, below, the sight line positions of the expert's left and right eyes were continuously tracked, and these are indicated in the video by a "+" sign, and a "□" sign, respectively. Also, through confirming by means of the side view video, we were able to verify that an approximately 30 degree angle was accurately being reproduced at the lowest point of the bow, as had been specified in Sect. 2.2.

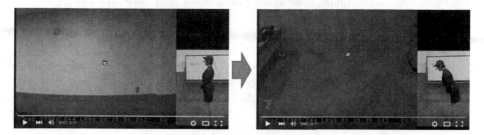

Fig. 4. instructional video for group B (beginning to lowest point of bow)

We ensured a floor surface distance of 300 cm from the expert's feet, when standing, to the surface of the wall opposite her. As a result, we could ascertain that at the lowest point of her keirei style bow, she was looking at a spot approximately 300 cm in front of her in terms of floor surface distance. Various websites report that in general distances such as two meters or three meters should be observed for line of sight focused instruction. Although this kind of guidance is not based on strict definitions of starting points and ending points, and measurement errors can occur depending on whether the subject's eyes are cast down or not, we can say that our results were roughly in agreement. In any case, the expert's point of vision in our finished instructional video for Group B was as shown in the following schematic diagram (Fig. 5).

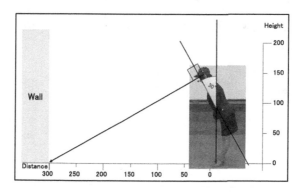

Fig. 5. Schematic diagram

4 Group A Experiment

In this section we will present our measurements regarding the impact that the traditional instructional method whereby learners watched the bowing of an expert as filmed from the side had upon the execution of the bowing sequence by each of the inexperienced participants.

First, the participants performed three bows, with a break after each bow, in a style conceived of by themselves. Then, they viewed the traditional instructional video depicting the expert bowing from the side. Finally, after that they carried out a series of three bows for a second time, once again with a break after each repetition.

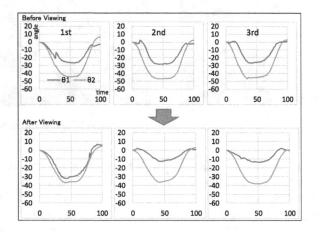

Fig. 6. Test subject A-1: Transition of angles $\theta 1$ and $\theta 2$ in bows before and after viewing video.

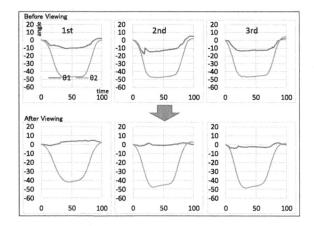

Fig. 7. Test subject A-2: Transition of angles $\theta 1$ and $\theta 2$ in bows before and after viewing video.

4.1   Discussion of Individual Test Subjects

"Test Subject A-1" displayed a tendency of conformity between θ1 and θ2 regardless of whether it was before or after viewing the video. This was manifested through a bending of the neck at the same time bending at the waist occurred. In this regard, as the angle of θ2 became shallow, θ1 did likewise (Figs. 6, 7, 8 and 9).

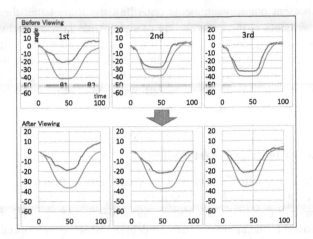

Fig. 8. Test subject A-3: Transition of angles θ1 and θ2 in bows before and after viewing video.

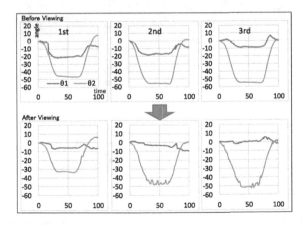

Fig. 9. Test Subject A-4: Transition of angles θ1 and θ2 in bows before and after viewing video.

"Test Subject A-2" showed signs of straightening out θ1 post-viewing, but fundamentally speaking there were no major changes between before and after viewing the video.

"Test Subject A-3" did not demonstrate any pronounced changes between before and after viewing the video.

"Test Subject A-4" showed similarities to Test Subject A-2, in that some indications of straightening out $\theta1$ were discernible post-video, but fundamentally speaking there were no major changes between before and after viewing the video.

5   Group B Experiment

Next, we will present our measurements regarding the impact that the video which showed the movements in the expert's line of sight while bowing had upon the execution of the bowing sequence by each of the inexperienced participants. Again, the participants first performed three bows, with a break after each bow, in a style conceived of by they themselves. Then, they viewed the video depicting the movements in the expert's line of sight. Finally, they carried out a series of three bows for a second time, as before with a break after each one.

5.1   Discussion of Individual Test Subjects

"Test Subject B-1" exhibited a tendency of conformity between $\theta1$ and $\theta2$ before viewing the video, with $\theta2$ reaching a maximum angle of 40 degrees. Post-viewing, the conformity between $\theta1$ and $\theta2$ was reduced. Moreover, in regard to $\theta2$, the maximum angle was improved to the approximately 30 degrees which is appropriate for a *keirei* bow (Figs. 10, 11, 12 and 13).

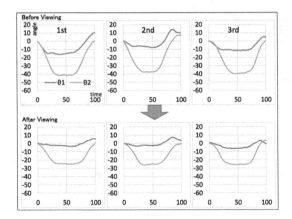

Fig. 10. Test Subject B-1: Transition of angles $\theta1$ and $\theta2$ in bows before and after viewing video.

"Test Subject B-2" did not demonstrate any major changes between before and after viewing the video.

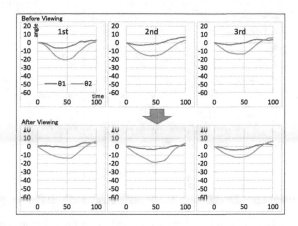

Fig. 11. Test Subject B-2: Transition of angles $\theta 1$ and $\theta 2$ in bows before and after viewing video.

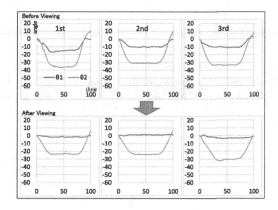

Fig. 12. Test Subject B-3: Transition of angles $\theta 1$ and $\theta 2$ in bows before and after viewing video.

"Test Subject B-3" displayed a tendency of conformity between $\theta 1$ and $\theta 2$ before viewing the video, with $\theta 2$ reaching a maximum angle of 40 degrees. After viewing the video, the conformity between $\theta 1$ and $\theta 2$ was essentially eliminated. Furthermore, with respect to $\theta 2$, the maximum angle was improved to the approximately 30 degrees which is appropriate for a *keirei* bow.

"Test Subject B-4," in spite of demonstrating a tendency of conformity between $\theta 1$ and $\theta 2$ both before and after viewing the video, showed a reduction in the maximum angle of $\theta 1$ post-viewing. Also, the maximum angle of $\theta 2$, which had been from 40 to 45 degrees pre-viewing, was reduced after watching the video and improved to the approximately 30 degrees considered appropriate for a *keirei* bow.

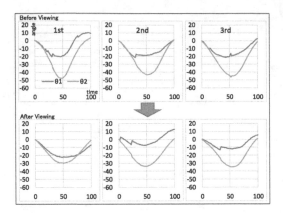

Fig. 13. Test Subject B-4: Transition of angles $\theta 1$ and $\theta 2$ in bows before and after viewing video.

6 General Discussion

6.1 Discussion Regarding $\theta 1$

Figure 14 provide an indication of how $\theta 1$ changed for each test subject after the viewing of his or her video, with Group A set as blue and Group B as red. Also, shown in green is $\theta 1$ of the expert, which is what the transition of the angles should ideally look like. In comparison to Group A, Group B is nearer to that ideal angle.

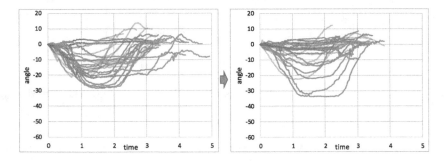

Fig. 14. $\theta 1$ of All test subjects before/after viewing video

6.2 Discussion Regarding $\theta 2$ Before and After Viewing the Video

Figure 15 provide an indication of how $\theta 2$ changed for each test subject after viewing his or her video, with Group A set as blue and Group B as red. Again, shown in green is $\theta 2$ of the expert, which is what the transition of the angles should ideally look like. Both Group A and Group B demonstrated a reduction in terms of maximum angle from pre- to post-viewing. However, we can determine that Group B was the nearer of the two groups to the 30 degree angle considered ideal.

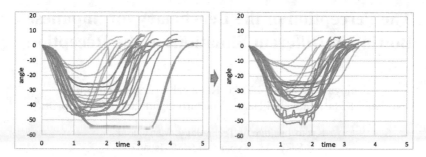

Fig. 15. θ2 of all test subjects before/after viewing video

6.3 Conclusion

During the process of creating the line of sight video, we could ascertain that the point of vision of the keirei bowing expert was established at approximately three meters in front of her upon the floor, and that she was able to maintain a maximum angle of 30 degrees when bending at her waist. Our format verified recent assertions which generally regard two or three meters in front to be an appropriate distance for line of sight focused instruction.

Although the number of test subjects in both groups was relatively small at four people, we could discern that the line of sight video had the effect of suppressing θ1, which had previously been impacted by conformity on the parts of the subjects of Group B to also bend their necks when bending at their waists. Also, we were able to observe several cases in which the angle of test subjects' waists was rectified such as to nearly achieve 30 degrees. By carrying out the present experiment again in the future while further increasing the number of test subjects and further expanding their internationality, the possibility is high that we can establish important findings to rectify the angle more easily than with the existing teaching method of "watch and learn." We intend to pursue this research in much greater depth moving forward.

References

1. According to a presentation by the Japan Tourism Agency on June 17th, 2014
2. Japan Productivity Center. "Investigative Research Project Related to the Promotion of 'The Industrialization of Omotenashi,' Directed at Further Development of the Service Industry" [Bulletin Report]. Japan as an Information and Economy Society – 2011 Infrastructure Development, 8–13 (2012)
3. Japan Manner and Protocol Association. "Lecture Course on Manners that Will Earn Adults Respect (Revised Version)." Japan Manner and Protocol Official Examination Standards Textbook. PHP Research Institute, Inc. 63
4. Gyoba, J., Shibata, H., Takahashi, J., et al.: Subjective impressions of bowing actions and their appropriateness in specific social contexts. Psychol. Res. **85**, 571–578 (2015)
5. Asada, M.: The kind of greetings in communication and bows. J. Wakayama Shin-ai Women's Junior Coll. **55**, 81–84 (2015)
6. Iwashita, N., Morishita, H.: A Consideration of Gesticulation and Posture: Bowing and Greetings. Sci. Phys. Educ. **35**, 823–826 (1985)

The Perception of the Beneficiary for Japanese Bowing in Different Situations at the Reception

Tomoya Takeda[1(✉)], Yuko Kamagahara[2], Xiaodan Lu[1],
Noriyuki Kida[1], Tadayuki Hara[3], Yoichiro Ogura[1], and Tomoko Ota[4]

[1] Kyoto Institute of Technology, Matsugasaki,
Sakyo-ku, Kyoto 606-6585, Japan
t.takeda@taste.jp, luxiaodan0223@gmail.com,
kida@kit.ac.jp
[2] Andsmile, 1-1-7 Minamishinmachi Chuo-ku,
Osaka 540-0024, Japan
kamagahara0525@gmail.com
[3] University of Central Florida,
4000 Central Florida Blvd. Orlando, Florida 32816, USA
tadayuki.hara@ucf.edu
[4] Chuo Business Group, 1-6-6 Funakoshi-cho, Chuo-ku
Osaka 540-0036, Japan
tomoko_ota_cbg@yahoo.co.jp

Abstract. We inspected the effect on the recipient of Japanese bowing (ojigi) in proper keirei style and in one's own style. First, we performed eleven variations of bowing and examined the impression of each bowing. The results were that keirei made the best impression on the recipient. Second, we set up two situations regarding five variations of bowing; absence of any people except the parties (extra 0), and presence of two people (extra 2). Then we examined whether the evaluation for these bowings changed or not depending on the two situations. As for keirei, extra 0 showed a significantly-high score. In "bowing deeply" and "bowing unsteadily," extra 2 showed a significantly-high score. Keirei made the best impression in situations where there were no outside factors. On the other hand, "bowing deeply" could achieve almost the same impression as that of keirei, despite its being in one's own style, in situations such as extra 2.

Keywords: Ojigi · Japanese bowing · Japanese hospitality

1 Introduction

The number of foreign visitors to Japan is rapidly increasing. Since April 2003, when the "Visit Japan Campaign" promotion to attract tourists from abroad was begun by the Ministry of Land, Infrastructure, Transport, and Tourism [1], overseas publicity regarding travel to Japan, domestic infrastructure for the sake of foreign visitors, and other such developments have intensified. Despite the Great East Japan Earthquake in 2011, proliferation of the middle class brought on by a weakened yen and economic growth in various neighboring Asian countries led the number of foreign visitors to

© Springer International Publishing Switzerland 2016
V.G. Duffy (Ed.): DHM 2016, LNCS 9745, pp. 506–517, 2016.
DOI: 10.1007/978-3-319-40247-5_51

jump from a mere 5.24 million in 2004 to 13.41 million in 2014, with forecasts that the number would exceed 19 million in 2015.[1] The government is considering drastically increasing its target of 20 million visitors for the year 2020 to 30 million.[2]

In terms of Japan's tourism resources which pique the interest of people from other countries, there are factors such as its beautiful scenery of nature as an island nation, its rich historical and cultural heritage, and other cultural resources. However, after it was decided that the 2020 Summer Olympics and Paralympics would be held in Tokyo, it seemed to become inevitable that the Japanese way of hospitality– known as "omotenashi"– would also rank as an essential tourism resource. This was especially true because of the attention that would be drawn to lodging facilities like hotels, traditional inns, and bed and breakfasts, as well as dining and drinking establishments from casual eateries to high-end restaurants, and other places visitors are certain to see.

The Japan Tourism Agency is supporting regional pre-emptive initiatives as the "Regional 'Omotenashi' Improvement Project Directed at the 2020 Olympics and Paralympics".[3] Concomitant with this movement, there are also efforts to attract customers by strengthening the spirit of "omotenashi" within the service industry, but in order to do so a proper understanding of "omotenashi" is imperative. The Japan Productivity Center has defined "omotenashi" as "work to provide uncompromisingly heartfelt service while valuing the perspective of customers and/or residents" [2]. "Valuing the perspective of customers and/or residents" can be rephrased as "mutualistic service whereby the provider considers the circumstances of the beneficiary and responds with his or her whole heart," as differentiated from service which is unilateral from the side of the provider only. It can be thought that analogous concepts in other countries such as "hospitality" (the U.S.), 待客之道 (China), and "hospitalité" (France) vary from "omotenashi" on this point of whether the service is or is not mutualistic [2], and we can say that it safely passes as a peculiarly Japanese tourism resource.

There has been much debate over the question of what kind of service "omotenashi" entails. But even if we start from the basis of the saying that, "'Omotenashi' begins with a greeting and ends with a parting," it seems that we should note the Japanese way of bowing (ojigi) as a first step to studying "omotenashi." The history of bowing being an action of greeting for Japanese people is long, as in the third century Chinese text the Gishi-wajin-den it is recorded that, "When meeting with an important person, Japanese people go to their knees and cast down their heads." Furthermore, the action of casting down one's head, or bowing, has been regarded as showing that one has no enmity toward his or her counterpart, due to the fact that it exposes the back of the head, a point of vulnerability [3].

Bowing is not limited to instances of greeting. It is also performed in various other settings such as to show appreciation or apologize, and is a commonly seen gesture in

---

[1] According to Japan Tourism Agency projections and a December 22nd, 2015, news briefing with the Minister of Land, Infrastructure, Transport, and Tourism.

[2] At the first meeting of the "Planning Commission for a Tourist Vision to Support Tomorrow's Japan" (chairperson: Prime Minister Shinzo Abe), which opened on November 9th, 2015, the Government's target of 20 million visitors annually by the year 2020 was raised to in excess of 30 million.

[3] According to a presentation by the Japan Tourism Agency on June 17th, 2014.

the course of daily life [4]. Bowing can be done while standing or while sitting. For both there are multiple classifications according to the angle at which the upper portion of the body is bent. Within standing bows, based on the angle of the bow there are the classifications of eshaku ("greeting bow," 15 degrees), keirei ("respect bow," 30 degrees), saikeirei ("highest respect bow," 45 degrees), and hairei ("worship bow," 90 degrees) [5], or the classifications of eshaku (approximately 15 degrees), keirei (approximately 45 degrees), and saikeirei for the gods and buddhas ("highest respect bow used for the gods and buddhas," approximately 90 degrees) [6, 7], among other ways of classifying. However, in most settings calling for conventional business etiquette, eshaku (15 degrees), keirei (30 degrees), and saikeirei (45 degrees) are practically being used as the three classifications of bows.

At the same time, unexpectedly, even Japanese people – who have ample opportunity to learn bowing as a proper manner – are almost exclusively doing so in a self-taught way [8]. Because of this, bowing without maintaining the correct angle or bowing lightly and repeatedly, et cetera, is often seen. As bows in a self-taught style, the following are commonly observable:

【Tendencies seen in Self-Taught Bowing】

- Errors in execution (too deep/not sustaining proper angle, rushed, not facing directly forward, hands held behind back, premature)
- Excessive movement due to carrying out without adequate preparation (with hesitation, unsteadily, repetitively)
- Repetition in order to correct previous uncompleted attempts
- Errors in knowledge (almost no movement, stiff)

As a case study of researching bowing through experimentation, Morishita and Iwashita (1985) [9] reported that as inexperienced persons lowered their heads when bowing, there was an intensification in the angle of the curvature of their backs; that in comparison to experienced persons the time of remaining still upon bowing was shorter for inexperienced persons; and that despite their being Japanese, the subjects predominantly bowed in a self-taught manner.

In other previous studies, there has also been research from the aspects of what kind of bowing is preferred, and what kind of impression is received. Henmi and Isayama (2010) [10] examined the duration for which pleasure was taken in various types of standing bows, making use of a "standing bow motion stimulus" with the body bent at 45 degrees that was created by three-dimensional computer graphics. Additionally, Shibazaki, Takahashi, Gyoba, et al. (2015) [4] conducted a pair of experiments, one investigating subjective impressions toward the action of bowing, and the other investigating the appropriateness of certain styles in given social contexts.

As stated at the outset, there is a movement to attract customers by strengthening the spirit of "omotenashi" within the service industry at this time. On this point, we have attempted to discover important knowledge as part of "omotenashi" by analyzing the impressions given to other people by bows in one's own style versus proper bows backed by etiquette. In order to verify the impact that the motion of a bow gives to another person in as realistic an environment as possible, while pre-supposing the standing bow of a greeter as seen in the service industry we set not only one-on-one situations in which one individual was bowing and another was being bowed to, but also situations in which other people were present, to measure the impression given according to the skill level of the person bowing. In concrete terms, in Study 1 we had an expert perform eleven varieties of bows ranging from standing bows befitting of a greeter to improper bows in a self-taught style, and evaluated the impressions through responses to a questionnaire. In Study 2, in addition to paring down the eleven types of bows to five, we set two different kinds of environments – one in which other people were present in the place where the action occurred, and one in which they were not – and examined whether the evaluations of the impressions changed.

2 Study 1

2.1 Purpose of Study

The purpose of this study was to investigate the degree to which persons being bowed to had favorable or unfavorable impressions regarding each of various types of bows.

2.2 Method

2.2.1 Creation of the Video Used in the Study

The filming for the video utilized in this study was performed at the entrance of a restaurant which is commonly used for weddings and wedding receptions. For a model to do the bowing in the video, we selected one woman who provides instruction on receiving customers professionally. The model possesses eight years of experience teaching greeters how to welcome customers at dental clinics and other service businesses, and insofar as we could determine that her level of competency was sufficient to serve as the model for the video for this study, we had her perform all of the bows, from what would be conceived of as proper, all the way to those which would be viewed as improper and in a self-taught style. Figure 1 shows the floor layout plan at filming, and an image of the video is shown in Fig. 2.

There were eleven variations of bowing. First, at the entrance of the restaurant, our expert carried out a keirei bow that would be considered suitable for the proper bow of a greeter. Then, we recorded the ten types of bows other than keirei, which are referred to below as "B" through "K," and which would be thought of as unsuitable bows done in a self-taught manner. "B" was a bow with hands behind the back; "C" was a bow while not facing directly forward; "D" was a bow that was too deep; "E" was a bow that was too fast or rushed; "F" was a bow that was stiff; "G" was a bow that was repeated over and over; "H" was a bow with arms swinging; "I" was a bow that was performed unsteadily; "J" was a bow that was almost completely lacking in movement; and "K" was a bow with hesitation.

In choosing bows "B" through "K," selections were made from the categories shown in Table 1, below.

Table 1. Categories concerning selection of bowing variations

Bows regarded as Typical for Students and Young People	
B	Bowing with Hands behind Back
E	Bowing Too Fast
F	Bowing Stiffly
Bows regarded as Typical in Business Settings	
D	Bowing Too Deeply
G	Bowing Repeatedly
J	Bowing with Almost No Movement
Bows considered Impolite regardless of Age and Circumstances	
C	Bowing while Not Facing Directly Forward
H	Bowing with Arms Swinging
I	Bowing Unsteadily
K	Bowing with Hesitation

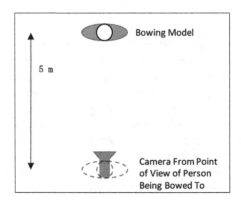

Fig. 1. Image of video used in study 1

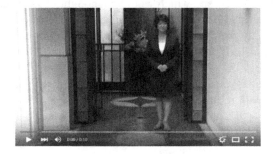

Fig. 2. Image of video used in study 1

2.2.2   Study Procedure

The study was conducted on the web using Google Forms provided by Google Incorporated. Via a survey webform, we evaluated the level of favorability of people's impressions of the bowing they saw after they viewed and listened to the video. For the evaluation method, we used a five point Likert scale, with one representing the worst impression, and five representing the best. We followed a style whereby the eleven types of videos were allocated randomly, and participants were asked to evaluate the videos one by one. As we were adopting an online survey webform that required all questions to be answered, there were no deficiencies in the responses.

2.2.3   Respondents to the Survey

The respondents to our survey were 74 men and women who ranged in age from 20 to 70 years old (mean age: 39.50 years old; standard deviation: 13.59 years). The breakdown of men and women was 46 men to 24 women. Before implementing the survey, we provided an online explanation with respect to the purpose of our study, et cetera, then proceeded after securing consent from individuals willing to participate.

3   Results

Table 2 shows the participants' impressions according to differences in the eleven variations of bowing. From the results of our single-factor variance analysis, with the bowing types set as intrasubject factors, a significant main effect could be detected ($F10,730 = 119.0$, $p < .01$). That is, when using Scheffé's method to perform a multiple comparison test, keirei bowing (4.22 ± 0.86 [mean score $\pm$ standard deviation], as illustrated below) was evaluated the most highly, having a significantly greater value than any other way of bowing. "Bowing stiffly" (3.01 ± 1.00) and "bowing too

Table 2. Evaluations concerning Impressions of Bowing

	$M \pm SD$	n
A Keirei	4.22±0.86	74
B Bowing Stiffly	3.01±1.00	74
C Bowing Too Deeply	3.00±1.11	74
D Bowing with Almost No Movement	2.20±0.91	74
E Bowing Too Fast	2.16±0.99	74
F Bowing Repeatedly	2.04±0.88	74
G Bowing while Not Facing Directly Forward	1.86±0.83	74
H Bowing with Hands behind Back	1.64±0.73	74
I Bowing with Arms Swinging	1.62±0.66	74
J Bowing Unsteadily	1.41±0.60	74
K Bowing with Hesitation	1.08±0.28	74

deeply" (3.00 ± 1.11) were evaluated the next most highly, and they were unified into one subgroup. Another subgroup was formed from the most highly evaluated after that, which were "bowing with almost no movement" (2.20 ± 0.91), "bowing too fast" (2.16 ± 0.99), "bowing repeatedly" (2.04 ± 0.88), and "bowing while not facing directly forward" (1.86 ± 0.83), while another was formed from those that followed, "bowing with hands behind back" (1.64 ± 0.73) and "bowing with arms swinging" (1.62 ± 0.66). The subgroup comprised of "bowing unsteadily" (1.41 ± 0.60) and "bowing with hesitation" (1.08 ± 0.28) was evaluated with the lowest scores Table 2.

4 Discussion

In Study 1, we reproduced keirei bows, which are thought of as proper for professional greeters, and various improper bows of a self-taught style, which in general inexperienced persons are prone to, and upon verifying the impressions to the person receiving the bow, we found that the keirei style generated the most favorable response. The evaluation scores of keirei bows and bows in one's own style had wide disparities; in fact, we found that significant differences were recognizable between keirei and every single type of bow made in a self-taught manner.

One type of mistake which is often made by inexperienced practitioners but which looks correct at first glance is to bow too deeply, so it was of great interest to us that "Bowing stiffly" and "bowing too deeply" obtained the next highest evaluations after keirei. As we have previously noted, due to the fact that bowing is an action which involves the casting down of one's head and therefore leaves the back of the head (a point of vulnerability) exposed, it has been regarded as a way of showing that one has no enmity toward his or her counterpart. Perhaps it is for this reason that the action of lowering the head deeply in and of itself caused the person receiving the bow to harbor a positive impression. Or, since previous research [4] tells us that in a setting where a greeting is made actions that give an impression of elegance are most appropriate, and such factors as the shallowness of the angle or the shortness of the time of remaining still are associated with this impression, it could be that in this case the only difference between keirei and bowing too deeply is corrected simply by making the angle more shallow.

5 Study 2

5.1 Purpose of Study

In Study 2, looking at several types of bows, our objective was to examine how the degree to which the favorable or unfavorable impressions harbored by persons being bowed to would change based on the interposition of other individuals in the place where the bow was performed.

5.2   Method

5.2.1   Creation of the Video Used in the Study

Based off of the results of Study 1, we made a determination to use the five types of bows described below out of the eleven total variations. First, we adopted the bow that was evaluated the most highly (keirei) and the bow that had the lowest evaluation ("bowing with hesitation"). Next, we chose to adopt "bowing too deeply" and "bowing repeatedly," as well as "bowing unsteadily." "Bowing too deeply" was chosen because it is a characteristic tendency to which inexperienced persons are prone, while "bowing repeatedly" was chosen because it is commonly seen in ordinary daily living situations in Japan. Finally, we adopted "bowing unsteadily" because the difference between it and other ways of bowing is very noticeable.

After this, in order to examine changes in the impression held by the recipient of a bow according to the presence of other people where the action takes place, we positioned two individuals as extras presumed to be other customers conversing between the bowing model and the video camera. Then we filmed the situation with the video camera in the same way as carried out in Study 1. In terms of the filming location, we utilized the same restaurant as for Study 1, and we used the video from Study 1 for the case in which there were no extras. We strove to ensure that we could reproduce each of the five types of bows just as they had been performed in Study 1, and we visually confirmed that there were no such differences (Figs. 3 and 4).

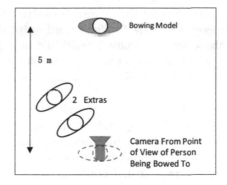

Fig. 3. Study 2 floor layout plan (with extras, from above)

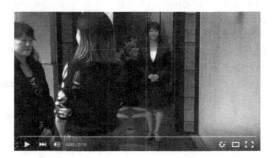

Fig. 4. Image of video used in study 2

5.2.2 Study Procedure

In the same way as with Study 1, we conducted this study on web using Google Forms provided by Google Incorporated. Via a survey webform, we evaluated the level of favorability of people's impressions of the bowing they saw after they viewed the video. For the evaluation method, we used a five point Likert scale, with one representing the worst impression, and five representing the best. That there were five styles of bowing and two cases for each – with the presence of the extras, and without – brought about a sum total of ten types of videos, and the order of presentation for these was random. The format was for the participants to then evaluate the videos one by one. Again, as we were adopting an online survey webform that required all questions to be answered, there were no deficiencies in the responses.

5.2.3 Respondents to the Survey

The respondents to our survey were 60 men and women who ranged in age from 20 to 61 years old (mean age: 38.89 years old; standard deviation: 12.32 years). The breakdown of men and women was 36 men to 24 women. Before implementing the survey, we provided an online explanation with respect to the purpose of our study, et cetera, then proceeded after securing consent from individuals willing to participate.

5.3   Results

First, we examined the reliability of the survey responses through a comparison of the results for Study 2 with those for Study 1. With regard to the disparity between the evaluations concerning the videos for Study 2 which did not feature extras and the mean values for Study 1, we carried out a t-test for two independent between-groups. The results did not show significant differences within any of the five varieties of bowing.

Next, we performed a two-factor variance analysis with both the types of bowing (five levels) and the conditions of having and not having extras (two levels) set as intrasubject factors. We were able to recognize significant mutual interaction through our results ($F4,236 = 9.82$, $p < .01$). From that, we examined a simple main effect. For the videos in which no extras were present, the order from the highest evaluation to the lowest was keirei (4.40 ± 0.89), "bowing deeply" (3.57 ± 0.96), "bowing repeatedly" (2.15 ± 0.80), "bowing unsteadily" (1.37 ± 0.52), and "bowing with hesitation" (1.08 ± 0.42). Between the evaluations of any two styles of bowing, a significant difference could be found. In contrast, while the order of highest to lowest evaluation was the same as it had been for videos which did not include extras, a significant difference was not recognizable between keirei bows and "bowing deeply" in the case of videos which did (keirei [3.97 ± 0.92], "bowing deeply" [3.80 ± 1.01], "bowing repeatedly" [2.23 ± 0.85], "bowing unsteadily" [1.65 ± 0.80], and "bowing with hesitation" [1.23 ± 0.47]).

Finally, we examined the simple main effect for each bowing variation depending on whether there were or were not extras present. Whereas for keirei bowing the results showed a significantly higher value for the video without extras, for "bowing deeply" and "bowing unsteadily," the results showed significantly higher values for the videos with extras. No significant difference based on whether or not there were extras present could be recognized for "bowing repeatedly" and "bowing with hesitation (Tables 3, 4 and Fig. 5)".

Table 3. Questionnaire response results

	Study 1 (n=74)	Study 2 (n=60)
Keirei	4.22±0.86	4.40±0.89
Bowing Too Deeply	3.00±1.11	3.57±0.96
Bowing Repeatedly	2.04±0.88	2.15±0.80
Bowing Unsteadily	1.41±0.60	1.37±0.52
Bowing with Hesitation	1.08±0.28	1.08±0.42

$M \pm SD$

Table 4. Questionnaire response results

	Extras	
	Absent	Present
Keirei	4.40±0.89	3.97±0.92
Bowing Too Deeply	3.57±0.96	3.80±1.01
Bowing Repeatedly	2.15±0.80	2.23±0.85
Bowing Unsteadily	1.37±0.52	1.65±0.80
Bowing with Hesitation	1.08±0.42	1.23±0.47

$M \pm SD$

5.4 Discussion

In Study 2, we verified the impact (or lack thereof) that the presence of other people in a situation in which a bow is offered has upon the impression of the recipient of the bow. Regarding keirei style bowing specifically, when it was performed as a one-on-one exchange from the side bowing to the side being bowed to under the conditions that no one else was between the two parties (extra 0), the recipient evaluated the bow very highly. However, when it was performed under the conditions that two other people were present between the two sides (extra 2), then the bow did not receive as high of marks from the recipient.

On the other hand, there were cases in which extra 2 was actually evaluated more highly than was extra 0 for certain types of the bows considered improper and in one's own style. In this study, "bowing deeply" and "bowing unsteadily" each received significantly higher evaluations under such conditions.

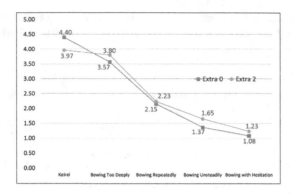

Fig. 5. Evaluation score of each bowing style (simple mean value)

6 General Discussion

Keirei bowing can give the best impression to the recipient in an idealized environment with no outside influences, but we found that in environments in which there are other influences fully conveying the good impression the correct motion gives to the recipient can be difficult. Conversely, we also found that because as stated in the discussion concerning Study 1 even an improper, self-taught styled bow such as "bowing deeply" involves the action of casting down and exposing the back of the head which is a point of vulnerability, and thereby indicates that one has no ill will toward his or her counterpart, under conditions such as those of extra 2 it can acquire approximately the same level of impression as a "correct" bow due to its clearly showing that meaning and intention.

With respect to each of the bows performed in both extra 0 and extra 2 conditions in Study 1 and Study 2, we took great care to ensure the highest possible standard of reproducibility by utilizing an expert, and that reproducibility was used in making strenuous efforts to visually ensure the identicalness of the bows. However, inasmuch as we were dealing with human beings, perfect reproducibility was difficult to achieve. For that reason, we predict that we could complete a more accurate study if moving forward we could carry it out with the heightened reproducibility of extra 0 and extra 2 conditions that would be possible through computer graphics, image compositing, et cetera.

Also, in accord with the promotion of "omotenashi" as part of aiming to make Japan a country which is a travel destination for tourists, the fact that just as "omotenashi" is an idea that is established within Japanese companies, among fellow Japanese people, bowing also is something that is primarily only understood among fellow Japanese people should be kept in mind. As future research, we believe that a study similar to this one which looks at how bowing is being perceived by non-Japanese people is necessary.

References

1. Yoshida, T.: Analysis on the Visitor Arrivals to Japan 2002–2010. Japan Foundation for International Tourism 123–124 (2013 version)
2. Japan Productivity Center. "Investigative Research Project Related to the Promotion of 'The Industrialization of Omotenashi', Directed at Further Development of the Service Industry" [Bulletin Report]. Japan as an Information and Economy Society –: Infrastructure. Development **2012**, 0–13 (2011)
3. Japan Manner and Protocol Association. "Lecture Course on Manners that Will Earn Adults Respect (Revised Version)." Japan Manner and Protocol Official Examination Standards Textbook. PHP Research Institute, Inc. 63
4. Gyoba, J., Shibata, H., Takahashi, J., et al.: Subjective impressions of bowing actions and their appropriateness in specific social contexts. Psychol. Res. **85**, 571–578 (2015)
5. Koga, H.: A Study of Bowing: Four Types of Bow. Kaetsu University Collected Papers, 57–71 (2012)
6. Dictionary of Manners and Social Etiquette. Jiyukokumin-sha Publishing Co., Ltd. 6–7 (2007)
7. Arai, T., Fujita, M., Hara, T., Kuba, K., Yotsui, E.: Analysis of the Relation between the Bow and Customer Satisfaction in Concierge Service (2010)
8. Asada, M.: The kind of greetings in communication and bows. J. Wakayama Shin-ai Women's Junior College, 81–84 (2015)
9. Iwashita, N., Morishita, H.: A Consideration of Gesticulation and Posture: Bowing and Greetings. The Science of Physical Education, 823–826 (1985)
10. Henmi, K., Isayama, H.: Prototype of a System for Adjudicating the Favorability of the Motion of Standing Bows. The Institute of Electronics, Information, and Communication Engineering: Technical Research Bulletin, 47–52 (2010)

Difference of Proficiency in Wooden Tub Manufacturing

Shuhei Yasuda[1(✉)], Keisuke Ono[1], Ryo Takematsu[1],
Mayuko Toyooka[2], Masakazu Aoshima[2], Takeshi Ueshiba[2],
and Hiroyuki Hamada[1]

[1] Department of Advanced Fibro Science,
Kyoto Institute of Technology, Kyoto, Japan
s.yasuda312@gmail.com, ekusiek0223@gmail.com,
takematsu4@gmail.com, hhamada@kit.ac.jp
[2] Fujii Barrel Manufacturing, Sakai, Osaka, Japan
mayufuji7@hotmail.com,
oketarou863@gmail.com, clubman0223@gmail.com

Abstract. Kioke (wooden tub) production, which is a traditional industry, is gathering attention recently because of its great ability for brewing. However, producers of kioke are decreasing year by year, and it may also lead to crisis in oral tradition of production method of kioke resulting from this situation. In this research, the movement of kioke manufacturing was analyzed in order to change the tacit knowledge to explication of knowledge. As a result, there is clearly difference be-tween expert and non-expert, and it could be expressed as values.

Keywords: Wooden tub · Traditional industry · Proficiency · Motion analysis

1 Introduction

Kioke (wooden tub), which is a Japanese traditional product, has started to gather attention again. Kioke is a general term for any cylindrical container made of wood, and it is traditionally indispensable for brewing of sake, soy sauce or miso. In recent years, because of hygienic or cost concerns, it has been supplanted by plastic product. However, because of its many superior properties in production of fermented food, kioke is being reevaluated. The 50 % of the total composition of kioke is formed by fine fibrous cell wall made of cellulose and there are fibrils pores on its woody surface. As these pores become an environment suitable for the existence of microorganism necessary for fermentation, a kioke comes to possess characteristics as fermentation container that cannot be found in other types of containers [1]. Figure 1 shows the structure of a kioke [2]. A kioke has an extremely simple structure consisting of side plates, a base plate and bamboo hoops. The production of a kioke can be roughly divided into the production steps of these 3 parts, and production of each part requires different craftsmanship. However, a large kioke with about the size of 2.3 m diameter and 1.95 m height, which is used for brewing of miso or soy sauce, has a very long life span, 30 to 100 years for miso production and 50 to 150 years for soy sauce production. This makes demand for large kioke unstable. Moreover, plastic products have been

© Springer International Publishing Switzerland 2016
V.G. Duffy (Ed.): DHM 2016, LNCS 9745, pp. 518–525, 2016.
DOI: 10.1007/978-3-319-40247-5_52

supplanting conventional kioke in the recent years, leading to almost total disappearance of kioke producers. Due to this situation, there is a concern among the okeshi, who produces kioke, that the traditional skill may disappear, and it is becoming urgent to conserve the skill and train the next generation of kioke craftsman. Thus, in this research, in order to conserve the skill and pass it on, we will quantify the tacit knowledge involved in kioke production, such as knacks and intuitions, and compared/examined the differences in movement between an expert and a non-expert based on these numbers. In this report, we will present the result in owari (rough splitting) process of cut bamboo, which is an early step in the production of bamboo hoops necessary for holding together a kioke.

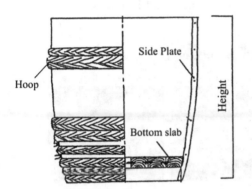
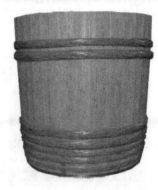

Fig. 1. Structure of kioke.

2 Manufacturing Process

Figure 2 shows manufacturing process of bamboo hoops. The process is roughly classified into 3 works. Those are splitting, plaining and braiding. In splitting process, bamboo is split in suitable width. Splitting process are consists of owari (rough splitting), metori (removing branches) and kowari (fine splitting). After splitting process, a bamboo is plane for the purpose of suitable thickness. The most important thing for making bamboo hoop is stiffness are same in all points in a bamboo. Therefore, workers must adjust for thickness of bamboo with considering about node and other parts. In this process, taper which makes it easier to braid bamboo is also made, and plaining off the corners is conducted. Finally, a bamboo is braided for making hoop. Braiding angle and numbers of bamboo are determined by the size of wooden tub.

Owari (rough splitting) is an initial step in the production of bamboo hoops necessary for holding together a kioke. Figure 3 shows the process of rough splitting. Firstly, make a nick on the edge of a cut bamboo using a hatchet, and tuck an iron stick standing on the ground between this nick. And by pushing this bamboo toward the stick, the bamboo is split in half. The bamboo hoop is produced by splitting the cut bamboo into 6 to 10 pieces after the owari process, go thorough thinning process and then finally woven together. Among these steps, the first owari process particularly demands skill. Normally, there are nodes in a bamboo. Initially, there were branches on nodes. This part of cut bamboo is called metake, is shown in Fig. 4. A metake is harder than other parts, and it becomes an obstacle when weaving a hoop, making its removal necessary. Therefore, at owari process, which is the first step in the production of a hoop, the bamboo has to be cut at right above each metake in order to prepare a homogenous bamboo piece. However, each metake is positioned 180 degree opposite to the one located on the node before, alternating at each node, and moreover they form a spiral throughout a bamboo. This means that when conducting the owari process, the craftsperson has to rotate the bamboo in the direction that he cuts the bamboo against fiber direction between nodes in order to split right above each metake. It is needed to shear the bamboo fiber. Splitting bamboo in perpendicular to direction of fiber is easy, however, it is difficult to shear the fiber and also difficult to tell the method of shear the fiber. Therefore, workers had depended on their knack and intuitions.

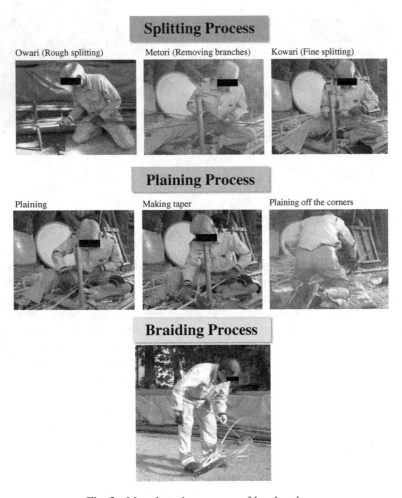

Fig. 2. Manufacturing process of bamboo hoop

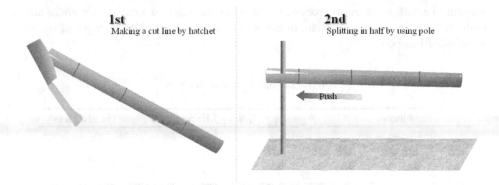

Fig. 3. Process of rough splitting

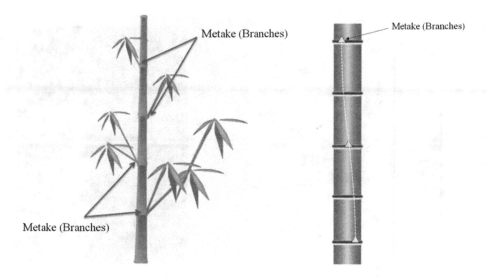

Fig. 4. Structure of bamboo.

3 Experimental Procedure

Table 1 shows the data of the test subjects. The expert is a male with 38 years of kioke production experience, the intermediate is a male with 1 year of experience and non-expert is a male with no experience. Owari process was the object of measuring. Markers were attached to each test subject as sown in Fig. 5, and their movements were recorded using a video camera. Afterward, a moving images analysis software DARTFISH Pro 5.5 (By Dartfish Japan Co., Ltd.) was used to analyze the movement of pushing a cut bamboo toward the iron stick during the owari process. As shown in this Fig. 5, by measuring the d which is the distance from the marker attached to the hands of test subjects and the iron stick, we measured the stroke quantity/pushing speed for each stroke. In addition, quality of owari was evaluated by whether or not a bamboo was cut in a half. After owari process, length of an arc was measured at each nodes and midpoints between nodes. Amount of gap was calculated by divided a length of arc by a radius of bamboo.

Table 1. Biological data of subjects

Subjects	Age	Years of Experience	Handedness
Expert	65	38	Right
Intermidiate	25	1	Left
Non-Expert	28	0	Right

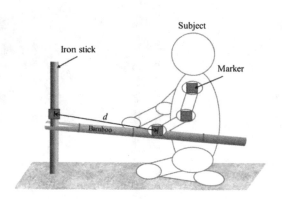 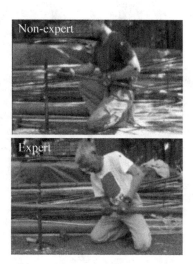

Fig. 5. Attached points of marker

4   Results and Discussion

4.1   Difference in Quality Between the Expert and the Non-Experts

Figure 6 shows amounts of gap of each subject. From the result, expert and Intermediate have slight gaps compared with non-expert. Table 2 shows the average value of gaps of each subject, and the average value of first half and second half are shown respectively. Expert had 2.5 %, intermediate had 2 % and non-expert had 3.9 % gaps as average. Intermediate had the best quality of owari.

There is clearly difference between first half of owari process and second half. In all subjects, amounts of gap in first half is larger than second half. This result means second half of owari process is easier than first half of owari process. A point worthy of special mention is the difference of gaps of first half between experts and a non-expert is larger than second half. It indicates first half of owari process is required for proficient skills.

It is considered that cause of this result is tapered shape of bamboo. In general, diameter of bamboo is gradually decreasing in the direction of the tip. Therefore, around the base of bamboo is harder than around the tip. In the tip of bamboo, the length of arc which is after splitting is not stable because it is easy to change the direction of crack by a little power (Fig. 7).

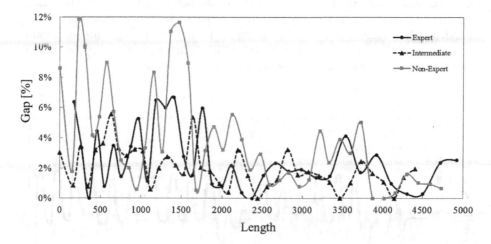

Fig. 6. Relationship between gap and length.

Table 2. Qualty of Owari.

		Expert	Intermidiate	Non-Expert
	First half	3.7	2.7	5.8
Gap, %	Second half	1.5	1.3	2.1
	Average	2.5	2	3.9

4.2 Difference in Movement Between the Expert and the Intermediate

Figure 3 shows the result of strokes measurement, and Table 2 shows the average stroke quantity and average stroke speed of each subject. The vertical axis of Fig. 3 shows the distance from the iron stick to the marker on hand, the horizontal axis shows the time. The amplitude of the line graph represents the stroke quantity, and the gradient represents the pushing speed. Stroke quantity and speed was gained from calculating numbers from the line graph shown in Fig. 5 and averaged. As a result, it was revealed that the stroke quantity of the expert was 0.13 m larger, and his pushing speed was 0.35 m/s faster, than those of the non-expert (Fig. 8).

Moreover, difference in the posture during the owari process was observed between the expert and the non-expert. While the expert was facing the bamboo during owari process, the non-expert turned his body toward the bamboo while working. When the angles made from the bamboo and the front side of the body of each subject were measured, that of the expert was 65°, and that of the non-expert was 27°. This can be inferred that by facing the bamboo, the expert achieved wider movable scope for his shoulders, which made it easier for him to stroke, leading to the larger stroke quantity. However, we believe that there are many other factors influencing the improvement in time and quality of work, needing further study in future (Table 3).

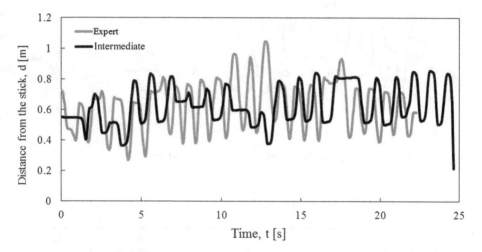

Fig. 7. Relationship between distance from the stick and time

Table 3. Stroke quantity and speed of expert and intermediate

Subjects	Stroke quantity, m	Stroke speed, m/s
Expert	0.37	0.93
Intermediate	0.24	0.58

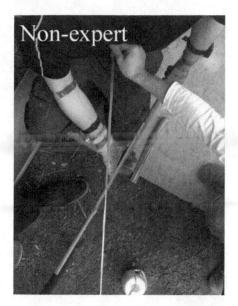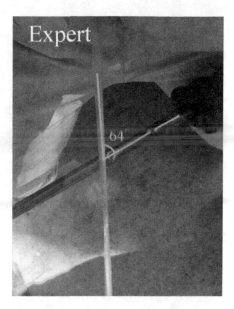

Fig. 8. Difference of positions.

5 Conclusion

In this study, we focused on owari process, which is an initial step in the production of bamboo hoops necessary for holding together a kioke, and examined the difference in movement between the expert and the non-expert. In addition, amount of gap was calculated by divided a length of arc by a radius of bamboo.

As a result, expert had 2.5 %, intermediate had 2 % and non-expert had 3.9 % gaps as average. In all subjects, amounts of gap in first half is larger than second half, and the difference of gaps of first half between experts and a non-expert is larger than second half. It indicates first half of owari process is required for proficient skills.

It was revealed that the expert has larger stroke quantity and faster speed during owari process compared to the non-expert. Moreover, the expert and the non-expert differ in their work posture, and it can be inferred that the expert takes a posture that is easier for him to move his shoulders.

References

1. Ueshiba, T.: The history and development of wooden vat for brewing: wooden vat used in making soy sauce, miso, and rice vinegar. J. Brew. Soc. Jpn. **98**(7), 491–496 (2003)
2. Ishimura, S.: Oke/Taru I. (Foundation) Hosei University Press (1997)

Modelling Human Behaviour and Cognition

A Novel Visualization Environment to Support Modelers in Analyzing Data Generated by Cellular Automata

Philippe J. Giabbanelli[✉], Guru Jagadeesh Babu, and Magda Baniukiewicz

Department of Computer Science, Northern Illinois University, Dekalb, IL, USA
giabba@cs.niu.edu, {z1784615,z1791304}@students.niu.edu

Abstract. In the 'big data' era the attention is often on deriving models from vast amounts of routinely collected data, for example to lear about human behaviors. However, models themselves can produce a large amount of data which has to be analyzed. In this paper, we focus on visually exploring data produced by a type of discrete simulation models known as 'cellular automaton' (CA). In particular, we visualize two-dimensional CA with square cells, which can intuitively be thought of as a grid of colored cells. This type of CA is usually visualized using a slider to display the whole grid at each time of the simulation, but this can make it challenging to see patterns over the whole simulations because of change blindness. Consequently, our new visualization framework uses a temporal clock glyph to show the successive states of each cell on the same display. This approach is illustrated for three classical models using CA: an epidemic (a human health model), sandpiles (a self-organized dynamical system), and fire spread (a geographical model). Several improvements to the framework are discussed, in part based on feedback collected from trained modelers.

1 Introduction

In the 'big data' era, a lot of attention is devoted to processing massive datasets about humans (e.g., Medicare data, hospital discharge data, police calls), by using machine learning or by calibrating and validating digital human models. These models also produce massive datasets to analyze. In particular, they typically produce time series capturing changes from baseline to the end of a hypothetical intervention. While only the last point is seen as the "final result", both modelers and field experts often need to pay close attention to trends in the series. This can inform modelers of potential bugs in the implementation (e.g., identical consecutive pairs may indicate that results are mistakenly registered twice), while informing experts about the human dynamics (e.g., by observing cycles).

Research funded by the Department of Computer Science and the College of Liberal Arts and Sciences at Northern Illinois University.

V.G. Duffy (Ed.): DHM 2016, LNCS 9745, pp. 529–540, 2016.
DOI: 10.1007/978-3-319-40247-5_53

Consequently, many interactive visualizations have been developed for time series generated by simulations (Fig. 1). In this setting, time tends to be either linear (i.e., an ordered collection of time points) or branching (e.g., a simulation splits into 'branches' when there are several possible outcomes or competing hypotheses) [1]. While sliders can straightforwardly navigate through time, they lead to issues such as change blindness (i.e., some differences from one time point to another may be missed). Pixel visualizations [2] or glyphs [3] allow to visualize multiple time series on the same space. Several temporal glyphs have been designed (Fig. 2) and experimentally evaluated for tasks such as detecting peaks of trends [4]. While such innovative visualizations have adopted for simulations in engineering [5] (e.g., automotive, flows), there is a relative paucity of visualization environments for data generated by digital human models.

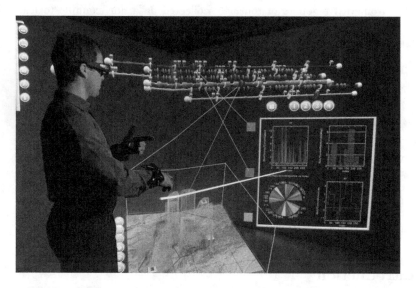

Fig. 1. The EXP V2 environment [6] allows to explore a simulation by hand gestures. *Reproduced with permission from Defense Research and Development Canada, who holds all intellectual rights.*

In this paper, we focus on digital human models implemented as cellular automata (CA). Intuitively, a cellular automaton is a collection of coloured cells on a grid that updates over a period of discrete, fixed time steps based on certain rules defined around neighbouring cells [7]. CA grids and cells can be of different types and shapes. Square and hexagonal cells are most common. CA models are generally one-dimensional (1D), two-dimensional (2D), and three-dimensional (3D), but can have more dimensions as well. There is a vast quantity of research using CA, as it can be applied to study any situation where individual units or cells affect others surrounding them [8]. In this paper, we focus on two-dimensional cellular automata with square cells, while noting that the same

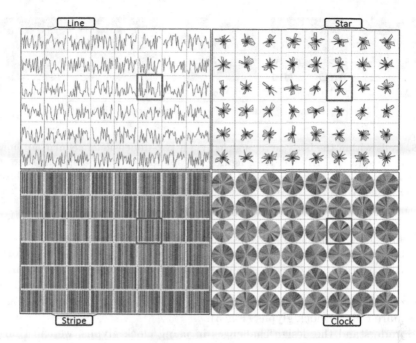

Fig. 2. Fuchs and colleagues compared different temporal glyphs for a dataset with continuous values [4].

principles would apply to other shapes of cells. Such CA are typically visualized by using a slider to move through the grid of states at different time steps (Fig. 3).

Our main contribution is the design and prototype implementation of temporal glyphs for cellular automata. This allows to see multiple time steps rather than going through each one via a slider. Our hypothesis is that this new visualization environment can contribute to providing better analytical capabilities, particularly when designed for the specific needs of modelers.

This paper is organized as follows. In Sect. 2, we introduce our visualization environment and explain how the data is rendered. In Sect. 3, the environment is illustrated for three well-known simulations (i.e., epidemics, sandpile, burning forest). Our hypothesis regarding the usefulness of this framework for modelers is discussed in Sect. 4 based on the feedback obtained from trained modelers. Finally, concluding remarks are provided in Sect. 5 together with a brief overview of future work.

2   Designing the Visualization Environment

Since CA have categorical values, line or star glyphs (Fig. 2; top) are not suitable. Either the stripe or clock glyphs could be used. They encode data values through colours (Fig. 2; bottom), and differ only in their encoding of time as either position (stripe glyph) or angle (clock glyph). Recent experiments found that the

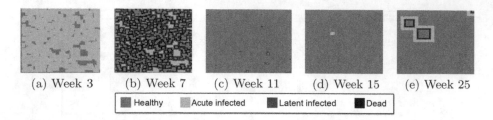

(a) Week 3   (b) Week 7   (c) Week 11   (d) Week 15   (e) Week 25

▓ Healthy   ▒ Acute infected   ■ Latent infected   ■ Dead

Fig. 3. Cells within the body were modeled via a two-dimensional cellular automaton to study the spread of HIV [9]. Each figure corresponds to CA at a specific time step. To visually explore disease progression, the modeler would use a slider and go through the weeks, displaying the CA of each week one after the other.

'clock metaphor' helps with chronological orientation, thus proving better than linear layouts to detect temporal locations, and triangular shapes performed better than rectangular ones to encode colours [4]. This suggests that temporal glyphs with a 'clock' ordering and triangular shapes have potential to support visualizing CA. Since users of CA are particularly familiar with square cells, we used square cells as clock glyphs (Fig. 3).

To understand the design challenges in using clock glyphs, we can think of the well-known pie chart. Having too many slices in a pie chart turns it from a meaningful visualization into an abstract pattern. The number of slices is thus best kept small, for example by collecting small slices within an 'other' category. A clock glyphs with too many data points would thus be like a pie chart with too many categories. This problem is particularly salient in our situation, since each glyph would have to represent the successive states taken by a cell over all time steps of the simulation, and there may be more time steps than could even fit within a circle (i.e., 360 slices). To address this problem, we limited the clock glyph to have either 4, 8 or 16 equal-sized partitions and each partition attempts at displaying the most relevant state within the corresponding segment of the data. This is illustrated in Fig. 4. In Fig. 4(a) we use 8 partitions and there happen to be exactly 8 time steps in the simulation, so each value is mapped to one partition. In Fig. 4(b) there are more values than partitions, so each partition represents the most frequent[1] state among multiple data points. Consequently, the visualization depends on the number of partitions (4, 8, or 16) and on the aggregation method (e.g., most frequent value). Both are set by the user in the current prototype.

Research suggests that "multiple views are particularly helpful in analyzing time-oriented data" [1]. Consequently, another design consideration was to allow working across multiple data representation. Given that the glyphs need a significant amount of space to display each cell, our goal was to have a complementary representation that takes limited space and provides a higher level of

---

[1] If the top frequency is found in multiple states, then ties are solved by picking the first one. For example, if there are 1 'dead', 2 'susceptible', and 2 'infected' then 'susceptible' would be picked.

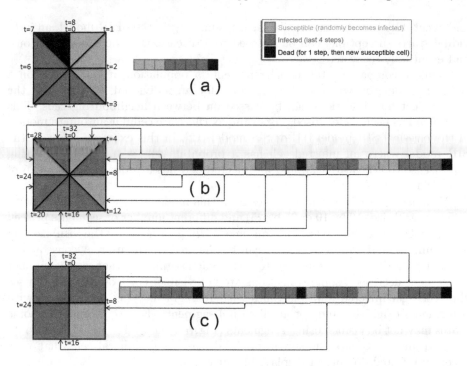

Fig. 4. Data produced by a disease model (top-right: states and transitions) may be entirely visualized if the model is ran for a few time steps (a). As the number of time steps grows, they are aggregated into each of the 8 (b), 4 (c) or 16 possible segments.

abstraction. This was fulfilled by using a flow diagram as secondary view. Flow diagrams are the most common depiction of cellular automata models; that is, a modeler using CA would immediately recognize and know how to interpret a flow diagram. In short, a flow diagram shows each state, and possible transitions between states. Formally, a flow diagram is a directed graph where each state corresponds to a node, and an edge exists from node a to node b if a cell can transition from state a at time t to state b at time $t + 1$. Our prototype automatically generates the flow diagram from the trace file (i.e. dump of simulation data).

3   Application to Classical Cellular Automata Models

3.1   Epidemics

In compartmental modeling, the population is divided into several groups or 'compartments', and then transitions or 'rules' specify the flows. The underlying mathematics are described in details by Hethcote [10]. Compartmental models of epidemics are typically named after the transitions between compartments: for example, in the SIS model an individual starts susceptible, can become infected, and eventually becomes susceptible again; similarly, in the SEIR model, an individual starts susceptible, can be exposed to a disease, then becomes infectious, and eventually recovers.

While a compartmental model represents a population, it can be ran on a cellular automaton where each cell stands for an individual. In this case, the rules reflect how infections can be passed on between neighbouring cells. This approach has been widely used. For example, there are cellular automata models of the classical SIR model [11] or SIS model [12]. In this example, we used the SIR model where an infected cell has a probability $p_i = 0.4$ of transmitting the disease to a healthy cell, and an infected cell has a probability $p_r = 0.5$ of recovering.

Visualizations of simulation traces from this model are shown in Fig. 5, with different grid size (10 by 10 or 25 by 25) and different number of segments per cell (4, 8, or 18). The flow diagram is automatically generated by the visualization environment, and names or colours can be changed by the user. A consequence of displaying the most frequent state within each segment is that, as the number of segment decreases, some transitions are not visible. For example, we can see that cells get infected multiple times with 18 segments (Fig. 5-c), less so with 8 segments (Fig. 5-b), and not at all with 4 segments (Fig. 5-a). Similarly, some states may not be visible: using 4 segments (Fig. 5-d) instead of 8 (Fig. 5-e) would tend to under-estimate the spread of the disease as peripheral cells that were recently infected do not yet display this infection.

3.2   Sandpile

The sandpile model is a vehicle to illustrate the theory of Self-Organized Criticality (SOC), that is, the idea that large interactive systems self-organize into a critical state and that small perturbations in this state trigger chain reactions. Informally, one can build a pile of sand by adding one grain at a time, until reaching a critical point where adding a single more grain causes an avalanche. This model was introduced by Bak and colleagues in 1987 [13]. We implemented the Sandpile model as described by Athanassopoulos and colleagues [14]. There is only one parameter p which applies when two grains are above two empty cells: the configuration either remains as such (with probability p), or both grains fall in the cells below (with probability $1 - p$). In our example, we used $p = 0.5$.

Visualizations of simulation traces from this model are shown in Fig. 6, with different grid size (10 by 10 or 25 by 25) and different number of segments per cell (4, 8, or 18). All visualizations display that grains gradually fall and a stack of filled cell increases from the bottom. This would appear to be too simplified with 4 segments, and perhaps excessively detailed with 18 segments. The visualization with 8 segments could thus offer an interesting trade-off.

3.3   Fire Spread

The mathematical principles of fire spread were summarized by Rothermel in 1972 [15]. Cellular automata have since been abundantly used to model fire

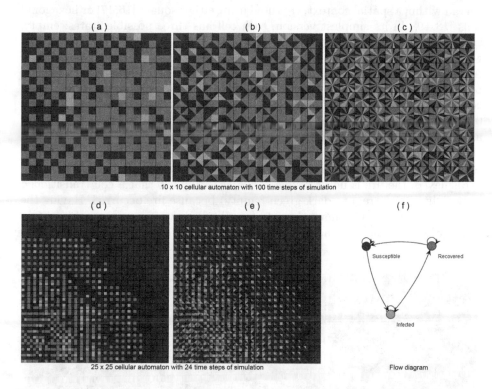

10 x 10 cellular automaton with 100 time steps of simulation

25 x 25 cellular automaton with 24 time steps of simulation   Flow diagram

Fig. 5. Visualization of an epidemic over a 10×10 CA where each cell has 4 segments (a), 8 segments (b) or 18 segments (c). The same model is visualized over a 25×25 CA with 4 (a) or 8 (b) segments. The same flow diagram applies to all simulations and is automatically generated (f).

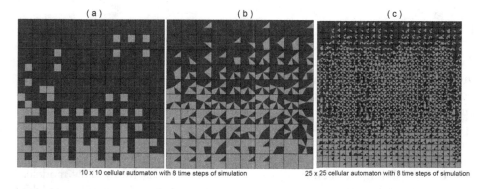

10 x 10 cellular automaton with 8 time steps of simulation   25 x 25 cellular automaton with 8 time steps of simulation

Fig. 6. Visualization of an sandpile over a 10×10 CA where each cell has 4 (a) or 8 (b) segments. The same model is visualized over a 25×25 CA with 8 (c) segments.

spread within a spatial context, captured using either square [16, 17] or hexagonal cells [18, 19]. In its simplest version, each cell has three possible states: empty, tree, or burning. Initially, each cell is empty with probability $p = 0.3$ or a tree with probability $1 - p = 0.7$; the fire is started by picking one cell as burning. At each time step, a tree burns if at least one neighbour is burning, or has a probability 0.001 of spontaneously burning. A burning tree turns into an empty cell after 1 time step, and an empty cell can turn into a tree with probability 0.1. Visualizations of simulation traces from this model are shown in Fig. 7, with a grid of 25 by 25 and different number of segments per cell (4, 8, or 18). In this simulation, no large component formed, thus there were random sporadic and isolated fires. Since the fire lasts only time step and only the most frequent state is displayed, the fire is never visible. Thus, it is implicit that a cell transitioned from light green (tree) to dark green (empty) because fire occurred. Having the most segments (i.e. 18) shows that almost all cells have been occupied by a tree at some point, which is gradually lost as the number of segments decreases.

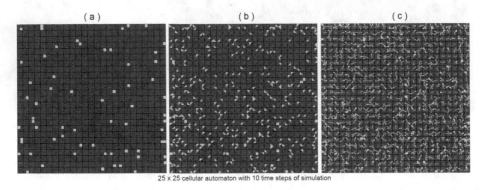

Fig. 7. Visualization of an forest fire over a 25×25 CA where each cell has 4 (a), 8 (b) or 18 (c) segments.

4 Feedback from Modelers

Two trained modelers were contacted to provide feedback on the prototype. On the positive side, the overall idea of avoiding a slider was well-liked. One modeler stated: "I like it a lot because it simplifies visualization of states across timesteps". On the negative side, a modeler reported that it became quite hard to read with a large number of cells or segments per cell. Having 8 segments was considered the most readable version. Several improvements were suggested, falling into three categories. First, even if the motivation for this visualization was to avoid sliding through time, a slider was deemed useful to allow modelers to narrow the range of time steps that are displayed. In other words, modelers agreed that a slider to move through a *single* time step was not as effective as our visualization, but they recommended being able to move through a *range* of time steps. This is in line with the visual information-seeking mantra of starting with an overview, and then having details on demand: narrowing the time range would increase the detail of the cells since their segments would represent a narrower set of values. Using range sliders to narrow the data of interest was also done in the 2-d matrix-based interactive visualization by Song *et al.* [20].

Second, modelers appreciated the flow diagram and offered several way to better link it with the main visualization. For example, hovering over a state or transition in the diagram should highlight all the cells that include that state of transition. Conversely, selecting a cell or group of cells should update the diagram to show only the transitions relevant to the selected cell(s). The idea that selections in one view would affect another view is known as 'brushing', and is essential to work across multiple data representations. Other (interactive) data representations were suggested, such as a stacked bar chart showing the number of cells in each state, which would also update when selecting specific cells.

Finally, the visualization currently displays a summary of the successive values within each cell but leaves it to the user to find relationships between these values. One modeler suggested going further by displaying trends among the values as additional features: "the simulation will generate a temporal data streams (each cell will end up generating a stream of data points), so change analysis (shape, direction and velocity of changes) can be performed to understand how the whole system has impacted the individual cells". Since the colour of the segment already encodes information (i.e. the most frequent state) and all segments must have equal width (as they represent the same amount of time steps), the main possibility to encode additional information is to use the segment's length. This is illustrated in Fig. 8.

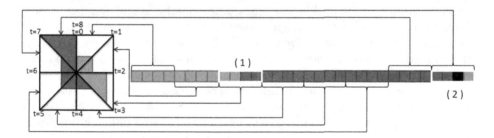

Fig. 8. Segments could have a different length to represent another feature of the data. In this simple example, the length encodes the number of different states present within each segment. All segments are low (since they only have one state) but segments (1) and (2), which encode 2 and 3 states respectively. This encoding helps finding where changes happen in the data.

5   Discussion

There is a growing interest in using visualizations at different stages of the modeling process, ranging from the early conceptual stage [21] to experimentation [6] and the analysis of results. There has been a particular interest for visualizations for cellular automata [22], as it is a widely used modeling approach. In this paper, we focused on the analysis of data generated by a two-dimensional cellular automaton. We presented a visualization in which the successive time steps of the simulation are aggregated and displayed all at once. The resulting visualization allows to see key properties of the models, such as grains of sand falling in a sandpile, or an epidemic spreading. Nonetheless, the visualizations had a number of shortcomings, mostly stemming from the aggregation method and/or the number of segments used within each cell. Two approaches should be explored in future work.

First, we could introduce a customizable weighting, allowing to under- or over-weight certain states for display. For example, consider an epidemic in which individuals start as healthy, get infected, and either recover by being healthy again or die. This scenario has three states (healthy, infected, dead) but they may not be equally important. Indeed, if we are concerned with the spread of the disease, we may want to underweight healthy individuals, give a neutral weight to infected individuals, and over-weight dead individuals. Similarly, in a forest fire, we may be less interested in seeing empty spaces than we are in seeing burning trees. In addition to allowing users to customize the weighting, an interesting research avenue would be to automatically set the weights based on the dynamics of the data. The simplest way would be to perform the equivalent of a histogram normalization, where very frequent states are under-weighted while rare states are over-weighted. However, finding a weighting scheme that best helps modelers understand the dynamics would require performing change analysis on the data as well as structural analysis on the flow diagram.

Second, we could create a large databank of visualizations in which each dataset is visualized using different aggregation methods and number of segments. Then, modelers would assign a score to each visualization based on how informative they find it for a given task. Tasks would be chosen by their relevance to modeling, and by their heterogeneity in terms of the perceptual notions involved. Example of tasks could include identifying cells whose final state is the initial one, localizing a spread, finding clusters of cells in the same state, etc. For example, consider the epidemics described in Sect. 3.1: that same dataset may be rendered with 2 different aggregation methods and 3 different number of segments. For each of the $3 \times 2 = 6$ visualizations, modelers would assign a score from 0 (least useful) to 5 (most useful) expressing the usefulness of the visualization for localizing disease spread. This would generate a relational database consisting of properties of the dataset (e.g. number of states), aggregation method, number of segments, and mean score per specific task. To understand how visualization parameters (i.e. aggregation method and number of segments) affect task performance for a given dataset, we could then mine the relational database by building classifiers [23–25]. We acknowledge that assembling a dataset where modelers judge a large number of visualizations is labour intensive. Nonetheless, having the target audience evaluate the visualizations for a set of task is a routinely performed procedure.

References

1. Aigner, W., Miksch, S., Muller, W., Schumann, H., Tominski, C.: Visualizing time-oriented data - a systematic view. Comput. Graph. **31**, 401–409 (2007)
2. Keim, D.: Designing pixel-oriented visualization techniques: theory and applications. IEEE Trans. Vis. Comput. Graph. **6**(1), 59–78 (2000)
3. Ward, M.: Multivariate data glyphs: principles and practice. In: Handbook of Data Visualization, pp. 179–198 (2008)
4. Fuchs, J., Fischer, F., Mansmann, F., Bertini, E., Isenberg, P.: Evaluation of alternative glyph designs for time series data in a small multiple setting. In: Proceedings of CHI, pp. 3237–3246 (2013)
5. Konyha, Z., Matkovic, K., Hauser, H.: Interactive visual analysis in engineering: a survey. In: Proceedings of the Spring Conference on Computer Graphics, pp. 31–38 (2009)
6. Mokhtari, M., Boivin, E., Laurendeau, D.: Making sense of large datasets in the context of complex situation understanding. In: Shumaker, R. (ed.) VAMR 2013, Part II. LNCS, vol. 8022, pp. 251–260. Springer, Heidelberg (2013)
7. Mago, V.K., Bakker, L., Papageorgiou, E.I., Alimadad, A., Borwein, P., Dabbaghian, V.: Fuzzy cognitive maps and cellular automata: an evolutionary approach for social systems modelling. Appl. Soft Comput. **12**(12), 3771–3784 (2012)
8. Pratt, S., Giabbanelli, P., Jackson, P., Mago, V.: Rebel with many causes: a computational model of insurgency. In: 2012 IEEE International Conference on Intelligence and Security Informatics (ISI), pp. 90–95 (2012)
9. Rana, E., Giabbanelli, P.J., Balabhadrapathruni, N.H., Li, X., Mago, V.K.: Exploring the relationship between adherence to treatment and viral load through a new discrete simulation model of HIV infectivity. In: Proceedings of the 3rd ACM SIGSIM Conference on Principles of Advanced Discrete Simulation, SIGSIM PADS 2015, pp. 145–156. ACM (2015)
10. Hethcote, H.W.: The mathematics of infectious diseases. SIAM Rev. **42**(4), 599–653 (2000)
11. White, S.H., del Rey, A.M., Sanchez, G.R.: Modeling epidemics using cellular automata. Appl. Math. Comput. **186**(1), 193–202 (2007)
12. Fuentes, M., Kuperman, M.: Cellular automata and epidemiological models with spatial dependence. Physica A Stat. Mech. Appl. **267**(3–4), 471–486 (1999)
13. Bak, P., Tang, C., Wiesenfeld, K.: Self-organized criticality: an explanation of 1/f noise. Phys. Rev. Lett. **59**(4), 381–384 (1987)
14. Athanassopoulos, S., Kaklamanis, C., Kalfoutzos, G., Papaioannou, E.: Cellular automata: simulations using matlab. In: Proceedings of the Sixth International Conference on Digital Society (ICDS), pp. 63–68 (2012)
15. Rothermel, R.C.: A mathematical model for predicting fire spread in wildland fuels. In: Research Paper INT-115, U.S. Department of Agriculture, Intermountain Forest and Range Experiment Station (1972)
16. Alexandridis, A., Vakalis, D., Siettos, C., Bafas, G.: A cellular automata model for forest fire spread prediction: the case of the wildfire that swept through spetses island in 1990. Appl. Math. Comput. **204**(1), 191–201 (2008)
17. Karafyllidis, I., Thanailakis, A.: A model for predicting forest fire spreading using cellular automata. Ecol. Model. **99**, 87–97 (1997)
18. Encinas, L.H., White, S.H., del Rey, A.M., Sanchez, G.R.: Modelling forest fire spread using hexagonal cellular automata. Appl. Math. Model. **31**(6), 1213–1227 (2007)

19. Trunfio, G.A.: Predicting wildfire spreading through a hexagonal cellular automata model. In: Sloot, P.M.A., Chopard, B., Hoekstra, A.G. (eds.) ACRI 2004. LNCS, vol. 3305, pp. 385–394. Springer, Heidelberg (2004)
20. Song, H., Lee, B., Kim, B., Seo, J.: Diffmatrix: matrix-based interactive visualization for comparing temporal trends. In: Meyer, M., Weinkauf, T. (eds.) Proceedings of the 2012 Eurographics Conference on Visualization (EuroVis) (2012)
21. Giabbanelli, P.J., Jackson, P.J.: Using visual analytics to support the integration of expert knowledge in the design of medical models and simulations. Procedia Comput. Sci. **51**, 755–764 (2015). Proceedings of the 2015 International Conference on Computational Science (ICCS)
22. Krasnikov, G.Y., Matyushkin, I.V., Korobov, S.V.: Visualization of cellular automata in nanotechnology. Model. Artif. Intell. **3**(3), 98–120 (2014)
23. Crutzen, R., Giabbanelli, P.: Using classifiers to identify binge drinkers based on drinking motives. Subst. Use Misuse **49**(1–2), 110–115 (2014)
24. Crutzen, R., Giabbanelli, P., Jander, A., Mercken, L., de Vries, H.: Identifying binge drinkers based on parenting dimensions and alcohol-specific parenting practices: building classifiers on adolescent-parent paired data. BMC Public Health **15**(1), 1 (2015)
25. Giabbanelli, P., Adams, J.: Identifying small groups of foods that can predict achievement of key dietary recommendations: data mining of the UK national diet and nutrition survey, 2008–2012. Public Health Nutrition (2016)

Changes in Perception of Induced Motion Based on Voluntary Eye Movements in an Attentional Task

Akihisa Hosoya[1(✉)], Hiroto Inoue[1,2], and Nobuji Tetsutani[1]

[1] Tokyo Denki University, Tokyo, Japan
hosoya-tdu@outlook.com, tetsutani@im.dendai.ac.jp
[2] Advanced Institute of Industrial Technology, Tokyo, Japan
inoue-hiroto@aiit.ac.jp

Abstract. Sometimes a static object in video content is perceived to move. This motion illusion has been classified into two types: (1) induced motion and (2) motion capture. The purpose of this paper is to clarify how voluntary eye movements affect perceptions of induced motion and motion capture. By the results of a subjective assessment experiment, it is clarified that induced motion is inhibited by attention in both the horizontal and the vertical directions for reading textual information. It is also clarified that in contrast to induced motion, motion capture is not inhibited by attention. Specifically, motion capture is not inhibited by attention when viewers move their eyes in the same direction as the movement of the background.

Keywords: Motion illusion · Induced motion · Motion capture · Voluntary eye movement · Attention

1 Introduction

Sometimes a static object in video content is perceived to move left when the background moves right, a phenomenon called induced motion. A related type of induced motion, called motion capture [1], occurs when a static object is perceived to move left when the background moves left. Elucidation of these illusions may help lead to elucidation of the visual function. For example, previous research has reported that induced motion is inhibited by attention [2]. Subtitles, annotations, and other textual information in video content will inhibit the perception of induced motion because this textual information captures the viewer's attention.

Japanese text may be written either vertically or horizontally. Vertical writing is a traditional Japanese format and can be seen in samurai drama, anime, manga, and other Japanese content. When attending to or reading vertical Japanese textual information, viewers move their eyes from top to bottom. However, relationships among motion illusions and voluntary eye movements have not been sufficiently studied. The purpose of this paper is to clarify how voluntary eye movements affect perceptions of induced motion and motion capture in an attentional task. We examine the perceptual characteristics of these motion illusions using a subjective assessment experiment.

© Springer International Publishing Switzerland 2016
V.G. Duffy (Ed.): DHM 2016, LNCS 9745, pp. 541–548, 2016.
DOI: 10.1007/978-3-319-40247-5_54

2 Subjective Assessment Experiment

Twenty Japanese individuals aged 19–25 participated in this experiment. The participants watched experimental video content with textual information and features that produce the following two illusions: (1) induced motion and (2) motion capture.

2.1 Experimental Video Content

The experimental video content consisted of a centralized foreground and a dot-patterned background, as shown in Fig. 1. The foreground presented numerical expressions of addition and subtraction equations using single-digit numbers. The size of each character was approximately 0.5°. In the background, the size of each dot was one degree in diameter, and the dot density was 25 percent of the screen size. The background moved UPWARD, DOWNWARD, LEFTWARD, or RIGHTWARD at a velocity of 8°/s, with a frame rate of 60 frames per second. The resolution of the experimental video content, which was presented using a head-mounted display (Sony, HMZ–T3 W), was 1280 × 720 pixels (approximately 45 × 25°), and the foreground was 142 × 142 pixels (approximately 5 × 5°).

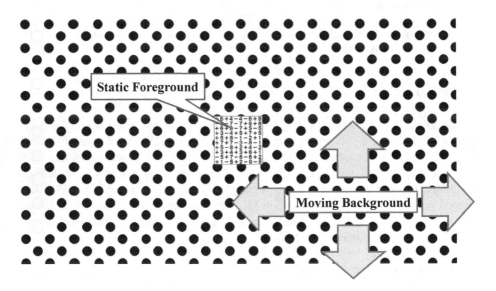

Fig. 1. An example of the experimental video stimuli

2.2 Experimental Methodology

Each time the participants watched the experimental video content, they were instructed to perform one of the following three tasks:

- CALCULATE (Please add and subtract the numbers in the foreground),
- READ (Please read the numbers in the foreground silently), or
- LOOK (Please look at the foreground naturally).

The task of calculating requires attending to the numerical expressions, as opposed to the task of silent reading; by contrast, the task of looking does not require particular attention. In addition, when participants were instructed to CALCULATE or to READ, they did so in one of two directions:

- HORIZONTAL (Please read from upper left to right, as shown in Fig. 2a), or
- VERTICAL (Please read from upper right to bottom as shown in Fig. 2b).

Table 1 shows the combinations of these instructions and the directions of motion of the background. Each participant watched the video content twenty times; the order of the twenty conditions varied for each individual at random.

Figure 3 shows the procedure for this experiment and a typical viewing environment. Participants watched the video content in a seated position on the couch; they then responded to a number of questions related to their impressions of the video content. Figure 4 shows an example of a slide used in the questions. In the example shown, the question relates to perception of the foreground. The experiment was designed so that combinations of responses to the question and the direction of motion of the background would reveal patterns of perception. For example, the perception of induced motion would be identified in participants who responded to choice A in Fig. 4 after having watched video content with a background that moves in the DOWN-WARD direction.

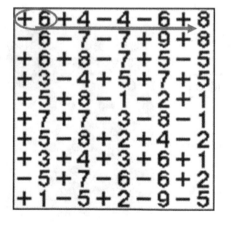

(a) HORIZONTAL

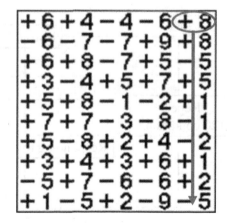

(b) VERTICAL

Fig. 2. Images instructing how to read the numerical expressions in the static foreground

Table 1. Experimental conditions. "Cross direction" indicates the relationship between the direction of motion of the background and the reading direction. For example, the cross direction is SAME when a participant reads in the HORIZONTAL direction and the background moves RIGHTWARD because the instruction of HORIZONTAL means to read in a rightward direction.

No.	Task (Attention)	Reading direction (Voluntary eye movement)	Direction of motion of the background	Cross direction
1	CALCULATE	HORIZONTAL	UPWARD	ORTHOGONAL
2			RIGHTWARD	SAME
3			DOWNWARD	ORTHOGONAL
4			LEFTWARD	OPPOSITE
5		VERTICAL	UPWARD	OPPOSITE
6			RIGHTWARD	ORTHOGONAL
7			DOWNWARD	SAME
8			LEFTWARD	ORTHOGONAL
9	READ	HORIZONTAL	UPWARD	ORTHOGONAL
10			RIGHTWARD	SAME
11			DOWNWARD	ORTHOGONAL
12			LEFTWARD	OPPOSITE
13		VERTICAL	UPWARD	OPPOSITE
14			RIGHTWARD	ORTHOGONAL
15			DOWNWARD	SAME
16			LEFTWARD	ORTHOGONAL
17	LOOK	–	UPWARD	–
18			RIGHTWARD	–
19			DOWNWARD	–
20			LEFTWARD	–

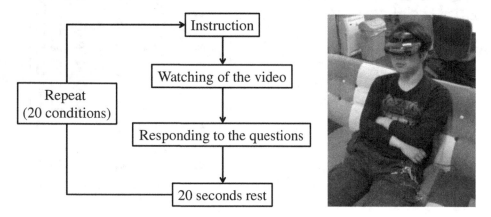

Fig. 3. The procedure for the experiment and a typical viewing environment

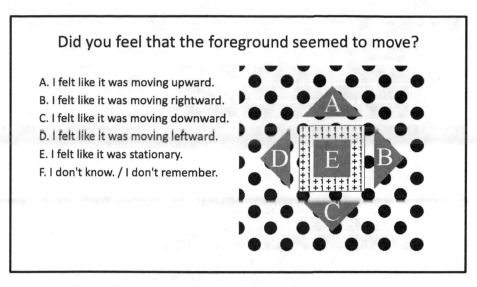

Fig. 4. An example of a slide used in the questions

3   Results and Discussion

Figures 5 and 6 show the proportions of the various responses to indicating the perceived movement of the foreground against the movement of the background. Figure 5 summarizes the responses when the reading direction was HORIZONTAL, and Fig. 6 summarizes the responses when the reading direction was VERTICAL. In these figures, the colors represent the following three categories:

- The black area shows the proportion of responses indicating that induced motion was perceived because the participants responded that the foreground seemed to move in the opposite direction to the movement of the background.
- The three gray areas show the proportion of responses indicating that apparent motion was not perceived.
- The white area shows the proportion of responses indicating that motion capture was perceived because the participants responded that the foreground seemed to move in the same direction as the movement of the background.

Results of Cochran's Q test applied to the relationship between the black areas and the other areas in Figs. 5 and 6 show that perception of induced motion was significantly changed by attentional tasks in all the combinations of conditions ($p < 0.05$). We can therefore conclude that induced motion is inhibited by attention. This result is similar to that found in previous research [2]. In addition, it was revealed that this phenomenon occurs in both the horizontal and the vertical directions for reading textual information.

In contrast, the results of Cochran's Q test applied to the relationship between the

546   A. Hosoya et al.

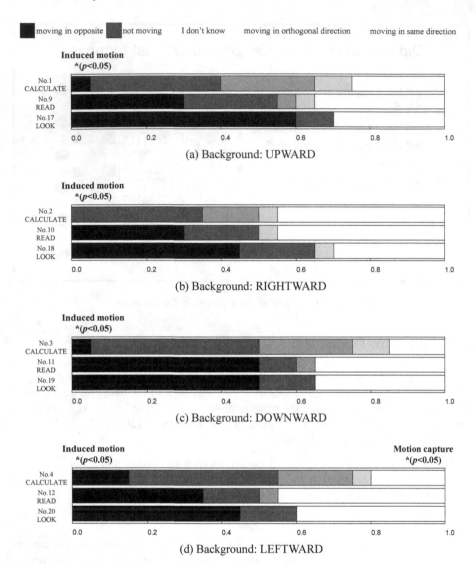

Fig. 5. Proportions of responses indicating perceived foreground movement against the movement of the background when reading direction was HORIZONTAL. The condition numbers refer to the descriptions given in Table 1.

white areas and the other areas in Figs. 5 and 6 show that perception of motion capture was significantly changed by attentional tasks in only two conditions, as shown in Figs. 5d and 6b ($p < 0.05$). Therefore, it was revealed that motion capture is not always inhibited by attention and that voluntary eye movements do affect the perception of motion capture. Specifically, in this experiment, motion capture was not inhibited by

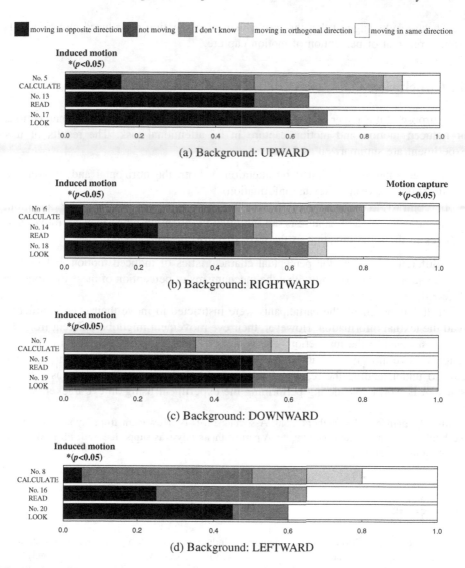

■ moving in opposite direction   ■ not moving   ■ I don't know   □ moving in orthogonal direction   □ moving in same direction

Fig. 6. Proportions of responses indicating perceived foreground movement against the movement of the background when reading direction was VERTICAL. The condition numbers refer to the descriptions given in Table 1. The proportions of responses for LOOK (Nos. 17, 18, 19, and 20) are used in both Figs. 5 and 6 because a reading direction for LOOK was not specified.

attention when the participants moved their eyes in the same direction as the movement of the background. This result contrasts with that for induced motion: during calculating, no participants perceived induced motion when the direction of reading and of movement of the background were the same, as is shown in Figs. 5b and 6c (conditions No. 2 and No. 7).

These results suggest that the mechanism of perception of induced motion is different from that of perception of motion capture.

4 Conclusion

The purpose of this paper is to clarify how voluntary eye movements affect perceptions of induced motion and motion capture in an attentional task. The results of this experiment are summarized as follows:

- Induced motion is inhibited by attention in both the horizontal and the vertical directions for reading textual information.
- In contrast to induced motion, motion capture is not inhibited by attention. Specifically, motion capture is not inhibited by attention when viewers move their eyes in the same direction as the movement of the background.

The difference between the perceptual characteristics of induced motion and motion capture suggests the possibility that the mechanisms of perception of these illusions are different.

In this experiment, the participants were instructed to move their eyes in order to read the textual information. However, their eye movement might be different from the direction given in the instruction. The authors of this paper did not measure the participants' eye movements with an eye tracker. Eye tracking data may be an important clue to understanding the results of this experiment in detail. Therefore, as a future study, it is worth considering performing the experiment using an eye tracker.

Acknowledgement. The authors thank Associate Prof. N. Kuwahara from Kyoto Institute of Technology for his valuable comments. A part of this study was supported by JSPS KAKENHI Grant Number 15K12130.

References

1. Murakami, Ikuya: Motion capture changes to induced motion at higher luminance contrasts, smaller eccentricities, and larger inducer sizes. Vision. Res. **33**(15), 2091–2107 (1993)
2. Sashino, K., Inoue, H., Tetsutani, N.: Inhibition of illusory motion based on attentional task. In: Proceedings of the International Workshop on Advanced Image Technology, Os, vol. 32, p. 87 (2015)

A Comparison of Processing Time and Strike Position Between Experts and Non-experts of Sheet-Metal Repair

Shigeru Ikemoto[1], Hiroyuki Hamada[1], and Yuka Takai[2(✉)]

[1] Kyoto Institute of Technology, Kyoto, Japan
ikeikel489@gmail.com, hhamada@kit.ac.jp
[2] Osaka Sangyo University, Osaka, Japan
takai@ise.osaka-sandai.ac.jp

Abstract. Repairing a car is a constantly evolving process. Such a task is individualized and is performed using hand. Analyzing the processing behavior of car repair experts can play an important role in improving the training procedure for craftspeople in this field. The goal of this study is to develop a learning system for car mechanics by examining the techniques used by craftspeople. In this study, the striking motion of an expert's hammer during the sheet-metal molding process in an automobile repairing process was analyzed and compared with those of non-experts. As the first step, the study attempted to examine the characteristic motions of experts performing such a task. Using a three-dimensional digital motion analysis equipment, we measured the movement of skilled and unskilled individuals while repairing cars by using the sheet metal molding process. The results showed that the total time spent for 'hammering,' 'others,' and 'total work time' by the experts was significantly shorter compared to the time spent by non-experts. Furthermore, experts were able to complete the task with one hammer. Additionally, experts used a lower number of strikes compared to non-experts as the hammering time increased.

Keywords: Sheet metal repair · Motion capture · Processing time

1 Introduction

Sheet metal molding is a technique whereby a human or machine introduces a metal mould into a thin metal sheet in order to transform the metal into the desired shape. In the context of automobile repair, this technique is utilized to return the automobile body back to its original shape. Each repair always bears some differences and may not be optimal. Therefore, a flexible approach should be taken to optimize the procedure under various circumstances. Furthermore, a significant amount of time is required to acquire an expert level of skill. Sheet metal molding for automotive repair is not sufficiently covered in vocational colleges and similar institutions. Therefore, non-experts must acquire skills through companies or union training, and textbooks outlining the process. As a result, each trainee develops their own and unique understanding of the process. In the context of declining birth rate, aging population, diminishing number of engineers, and retirement of many highly skilled individuals,

© Springer International Publishing Switzerland 2016
V.G. Duffy (Ed.): DHM 2016, LNCS 9745, pp. 549–558, 2016.
DOI: 10.1007/978-3-319-40247-5_55

it is feared that the current method of skill acquisition will be threatened by the shortage of experts in the near future. One way to address this issue is to utilize a motion analysis technique using a three-dimensional motion capture system. Motion analysis is already utilized in many forms of skill acquisition [1–8] and is regarded as an effective way of acquiring skills. Suzuki and Furuta clarified moving forms in hand sewing known as *Unshin*, a Japanese cultural skill, using a motion analysis computer system [1]. Murata and Iwase described the characteristics of baseball pitches from skilled pitchers by using a three-dimensional cinematographic analysis [2]. Hayashi and Yanagisawa showed skilled techniques for cutting cucumbers and carrots by using a video motion analysis system [3]. Digitization and characteristic evaluation of an expert's motion were also performed using a three-dimensional motion measurement system for the following activities: a nail strike [4], burner's work in glass processing [5], chest compression movement in lifesaving first aid [6], jump phase in a downhill race [7], and transfer care in elderly nursing [8] etc.

In this context, the objective of this study is to develop a sheet metalwork learning system for non-experts. In particular, the study focuses on clarifying the motion characteristics of experts when performing such a task. Experts and non-experts were filmed performing such a task and the differences in the process behavior and hammer striking position were examined.

2   Methodology

2.1   Outline of the Experiment

The fender of an automobile was repaired by workers by using a sheet metal working technique. The work was recorded using a video camera and a three dimensional motion measurement system. Then, the results were analyzed.

2.2   Experimental Facility

The experiment was carried out in March, 2015 at the Nara Auto Body Repair Association Training Facility. At the training facility, there was a booth with an automobile servicing lift. All measurements were carried out in this booth.

2.3   Participants

Participants were ten craftspeople involved in automobile repair in the Kinki Region. Those with ten or more years of experience were classified as experts and those with less than three years of experience were classified as non-experts. There were five expert participants and five non-expert participants. Table 1 presents the relevant details of the participants. Participants were informed that their work would be recorded and that the results of the analysis would immediately be made available to the public. Non-expert 5 had no work experience but did possess relevant background knowledge, working on a daily basis in the field of automotive paint repair.

2.4   Materials and Tools

Tools used in the experiment included a wooden hammer (hammer A, 213.3 g), three metal hammers (hammer B, C, D, weighing 433.4 g, 296.5 g, and 240.7 g, respectively), and three forming dollies (dolly A, B, C). Figure 1 displays these tools. The object of metalwork was the right front fender of a Corolla Fielder (Toyota Motor Corporation), shown in Fig. 2. The fender press line was dented with a heavy object (indicated by the red circle in Fig. 2), and the dent was defined as the object of repair.

Table 1. Participant information.

Participants	Career (years)	Height (cm)	Weight (kg)	Dominant hand
Expert 1	23.0	178	78.0	Right
Expert 2	19.0	170	60.0	Right
Expert 3	16.0	177	65.0	Right
Expert 4	15.0	164	84.0	Right
Expert 5	10.9	172	82.0	Right
Non-expert 1	2.5	181	80.0	Right
Non-expert 2	2.1	171	68.0	Right
Non-expert 3	1.9	175	60.0	Right
Non-expert 4	0.8	179	70.0	Left
Non-expert 5	0.0	184	64.0	Right

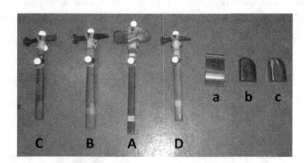

Fig. 1. Hammers and dollies

2.5   Experimental Process

The participants were directed to repair the fender, which had been fixed to a real car, using the tools that we had prepared for them in advance. Participants were asked to repair the fender to a state that was ready for the next processing (puttying), and the decision on when this level had been reached were left up to them. However, it should be noted that a time limitation was imposed to finish the task such that the participants had to abandon the process if the task exceeded 30 min.

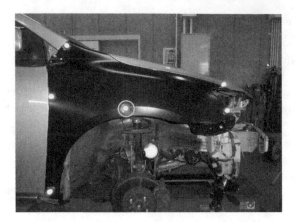

Fig. 2. Fender panel (Color figure online)

2.6   Recording Procedure

Infrared responsive markers were placed on 20 locations on each participant's body, five of them on each hammer, and the other five on the fender, and then set as targets. A coordinate collection was performed with a MAC 3D System (Motion Analysis Corporation) equipped with an optical, three-dimension, and automated analysis device. The sampling frequency was set at 120 Hz. Figure 3 illustrates the recording setup. The frame of reference was set to the left-right movement of the participant on the x-axis, forward-backward movement on the y-axis, and up-down movement on the z-axis. Three video cameras were used to record the movement of the participant, concurrently.

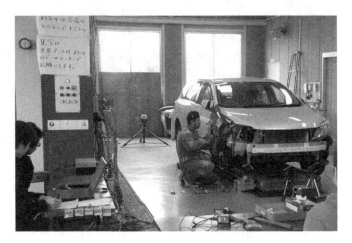

Fig. 3. Recording setup

2.7 Analysis

An analysis of the task was performed using the recorded video. In addition, the use of the hammer was also investigated. The position of the blow to the fender when using the hammer was measured through the three-dimensional motion analysis. The test was performed to investigate the differences between experts and non-experts. The level of significance was set at 5 %.

3 Results

3.1 Work Time

The task was divided into four processes: (1) Hammering using tools, (2) judging by hand, (3) judging by eyes, and (4) Others. Table 2 presents the work times for each process. The experts spent a significantly less amount of time compared to non-experts on hammering, others, and total work time, non-experts 2 and 3 were not able to complete the task during the allotted 30-min period. In contrast, experts 4 and 5 were able to complete the task within 5 min. The 'others' aspect of non-expert work time was long, and an examination of the details reveals that non-experts spent a significant amount of time on placing the dolly before hammering.

Figure 4 shows the distribution of work processes for hammering, judging by hand, judging by eye, and others, totaling one hundred percent. Experts, as compared to non-experts, spent a smaller proportion of their time hammering and a greater proportion of their time checking their work by hand.

3.2 Hammering Time

Figure 5 shows the hammering time for hammers A through D. All experts used just one hammer to carry out the task. On the contrary, non-experts used two or three types of hammers. No experts chose to use the wooden hammer A.

3.3 Strike Position

Figure 6 show the strike positions for expert 4 (the expert with the shortest hammering time), expert 1 (the expert with the longest hammering time), non-expert 1 (the non-expert with the shortest hammering time), and non-expert 2 (the non-expert with the longest hammering time), respectively. The black dots represent where the fender was struck, and the grey dots show the placement of the infrared markers. Compared to the strike positions of experts 1 and 4, the strike positions of non-experts 1 and 2 are broader in range. The same trend was observed for the other participants. The majority of strikes made by expert 4 were not on the press line where the dent was placed, showing that the repair work was performed by striking around the dented area.

The hammer strike count is presented in Table 3. Expert 4, who had the shortest hammering time, also recorded the least number of strikes. Experts recorded a significantly lesser number of strikes compared to non-experts.

Table 2. Work time results

Participant	Hamme-ring (s)	Judge by hand (s)	Judge by eyes (s)	Others (s)	Total work time (s)
Expert 1	408.5	77.1	0.0	111.0	596.6
Expert 2	322.7	430.2	23.4	233.9	1010.2
Expert 3	192.5	33.5	0.0	83.7	309.6
Expert 4	90.0	34.1	2.9	89.4	216.5
Expert 5	120.6	23.5	0.0	128.6	272.8
Non-expert 1	348.9	69.2	18.3	229.6	666.0
Non-expert 2	1149.8	114.6	4.6	607.0	1876.1
Non-expert 3	796.7	142.7	34.9	879.3	1853.5
Non-expert 4	364.5	184.7	0.0	201.2	750.4
Non-expert 5	742.8	366.2	2.3	407.9	1519.3
Expert Avg.	226.9	119.7	5.3	129.3	481.1
Non-expert Avg.	680.5	175.5	12.0	465.0	1333.1

(*:p<.05)

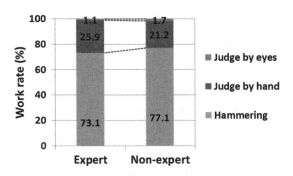

Fig. 4. Work rate (Color figure online)

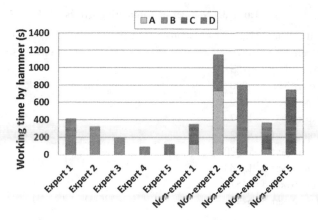

Fig. 5. Working time by hammer (Color figure online)

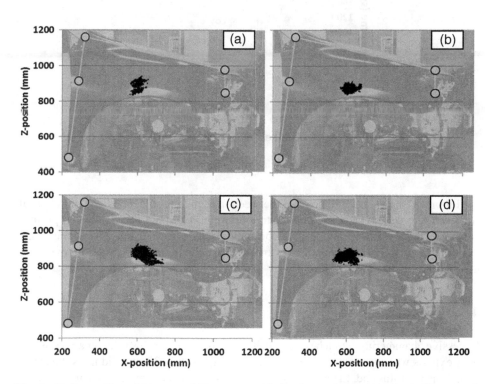

Fig. 6. Strike position of (a) expert 4 (the expert with the shortest hammering time), (b) expert 1 (the expert with the longest hammering time), (c) non-expert 1 (the non-expert with the shortest hammering time), and (d) non-expert 2 (the non-expert with the longest hammering time)

Table 3. Number of hammering strikes

Participants	Number of hammering strikes (times)	Avg.	S.D.
Expert 1	4271	3340	1534
Expert 2	5125		
Expert 3	3800		
Expert 4	1509		
Expert 5	1997		
Non-expert 1	8092	9224	4312
Non-expert 2	11920		
Non-expert 3	15183		
Non-expert 4	4451		
Non-expert 5	6477		

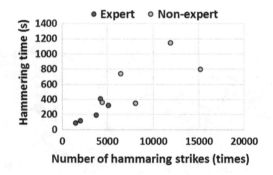

Fig. 7. Relationship between hammering time and strike count (Color figure online)

Figure 7 shows the relationship between hammering time and the number of strikes. There was no significant correlation between the expert and non-expert groups. However, there was a strong positive correlation for the participants as a whole group ($r = 833$, $p = .00278$) showing a clear trend where the number of strikes increased as the hammering time increased.

4 Discussion

Excessive hammering stretches the metal, causing it to lose its characteristics. Non-experts who were not able to complete the task within 30 min did not suffer from time constraint. Instead, the dents that they created while attempting to repair the target dent also needed to be repaired. As a result, the number of areas to be repaired became too high and recovery was impossible. Although non-expert 1, who had the shortest hammering time among non-experts, had a hammering time of approximately 60 s, which is less than the time spent by expert 1 (the expert with the longest hammering time) the strike count of non-expert 1 was almost twice that of expert 1. Further, as shown in Fig. 7, there was a trend toward an increase in the number of strikes as hammering time increased. This observation indicates that spending more time on the task does not result in completion of repairing. The short repairing time taken by experts is because of their ability to concentrate one every blow of the hammer.

Figure 4 also shows that experts spent the majority of their time on validating their work, implying that they place great importance on this part. Differences in movement during the validation phase were apparent between experts and non-experts. Experts attempted to check the change of the fender in its entirety by standing up and changing their positioning. In contrast, non-experts focused only on the changes in front of them, the use of their hands was limited, and their field of vision did not extend to the whole fender.

5 Conclusions

With the objective of investigating the characteristics of how experts perform metal-work during an automotive repairing process, the work of experts and non-experts was analyzed. The results of the experiment indicate the following points:

1. The hammering time, others, and total work time of experts was significantly shorter than that of non-experts.
2. Experts completed the task by using only one hammer.
3. Experts used a significantly less number of strikes than non-experts, with the number of strikes increasing as the hammering time increased.

Acknowledgments. This work was supported by Kinki Aria Auto Body Repair Association, Nara Prefecture Auto Body Repair Association, Osaka Prefecture Auto Body Repair Association, Protorios Inc. and JSPS Kakenhi Grant Number 26882052.

References

1. Suzuki, A., Furuta, S.: A study of motion analysis of hand-sewing with a computer system - a comparison in the motion of Unshin between skillful and unskillful subjects. Jpn. J. Ergon. **30**(5), 323–329 (1994)
2. Murata, A., Iwase, H.: On skillful pitch of baseball pitchers - comparison of pitching motion between skilled and nonskilled pitchers. Jpn. J. Ergon. **36**(6), 299–309 (2000)
3. Hayashi, T., Yanagisawa, Y.: Comparison of the movement of knives cutting food between experts and non-experts by motion analysis techniques. J. Cooking Sci. Jpn. **37**(3), 299–305 (2004)
4. Sano, S., Ueda, T., Terada, T., Izumi, Y., Nishijima, S.: Fundamental study of evaluation method of nailing by the 3D motion analysis for improving the skill. J. Life Support Eng. **20**(1), 3–8 (2008)
5. Umemura, H., Ishikawa, J., Endo, H., Abe, K., Matsuda, J.: Analysis of expert skills on burner works in glass processing. Jpn. J. Ergon. **47**(4), 139–148 (2011)
6. Okada, M., Kayashima, S.: Motion instruction of first aid chest compressions using pseudo-reference and its evaluation, Trans. Jpn. Soc. Mech. Eng. Ser. C **79**(800), 1090–1101 (2013)

7. Mazzola, M., Aceti, A., Gibertini, G., Andreoni, G.: Aerody-namics and biomechanical optimization of the jump phase in skiing, through a simulation-based predictive model. In: Proceedings of the 5th International Conference on Applied Human Factors and Ergonomics AHFE 2014, pp. 7245–7254 (2014)
8. Liao, M., Yoshikawa, T., Goto, A., Ota, T., Hamada, H.: Effect of care gesture on transfer care behavior in elderly nursing home in Japan, digital human modeling. Appl. Health Saf. Ergon. Risk Manag.: Ergon. Health **9185**, 174–183 (2015)

Analysis of the Thought Process for Choosing a Suitable Kimono for a Customer by an Expert

Kumiko Komizo[1]([⊠]), Noriaki Kuwahara[1], Kazunari Morimoto[1], and Takashi Furukawa[2]

[1] Kyoto Institute of Technology, Kyoto, Japan
kkumikok@gmail.com
[2] Hishiken Co. Ltd., Kyoto, Japan

Abstract. Currently in Japan the opportunities for wearing a kimono have decreased, e.g., for graduation, weddings and other special days.. One of the major causes for this is that there are strict kimono rules. Among the established rules for a kimono we need, first of all, to choose one that is appropriate for the occasion.. Additionally, such things as the "season," "texture of the material" and "color" must also be considered. Still further, it is necessary to pair a kimono with a suitable *obi* (sash). At present, when kimonos are no longer worn on a daily basis, it is difficult to determine what constitutes a "suitable kimono." Together with complex rules, it is difficult to choose a kimono and *obi*. In this research, we first surveyed the thinking of consumers about kimonos in order to clarify why they no longer wear kimonos. A further objective was to have experts in "kimono wearing" clarify their thought process when selecting a suitable kimono.

Keywords: Kimono · *Obi* · Protocol analysis · Algorithm

1 Introduction

When statistics relating to the kimono are seen, it can be said that the kimono industry is in a state of steady decline,. For example, 1975 is called the golden age of the kimono industry. Designating the amount of Japanese style clothing sold throughout the country in that year as 100, in 2011 the total of income derived from, kimono and *obi* sales had fallen to 20. Further, when looking at the frequency with which kimonos and *obi were purchased*, in 1975, we find that a new kimono was purchased 1 every 5 years and an obi, 1 every 3 years. However, in 2011 this had declined to the purchase of a new kimono only once every 49 years and an *obi* once every 56 years. [1]. This alienation from kimonos is not only a problem for those involved in the kimono industry but it is also a serious problem for the continuation of Japanese traditional culture.. Among the reasons for this are the difficulty of putting on a kimono, its functionality, cost, and social acceptance.. However, these are not the only problems, it must not be forgotten that kimonos have very strict rules. A kimono and *obi* have "established norms", to which we have to add the need to match them to the season and

© Springer International Publishing Switzerland 2016
V.G. Duffy (Ed.): DHM 2016, LNCS 9745, pp. 559–567, 2016.
DOI: 10.1007/978-3-319-40247-5_56

situation. In general it can be said there are four types of kimono, those for formal wear, semiformal wear, streetwear and everyday use. For example, when attending a wedding party as a guest, we have to wear a semi-formal kimono, such as a Houmongi or Iro-Tomesode. The type would also change depending on whether one was single or married, as well as the status of the wedding location. There is also a rule regarding the "pattern" incorporated into a kimono. For example a morning glory pattern can only be used in summer, and not in other seasons. Still further, the color of the kimono and the *obi* is also important in kimono selection. There is the joy of making people feel cool simply by observing someone who is wearing a cool-appearing kimono. Should you make a mistake in this regard you will be considered unrefined. The "material" and "feel" of a kimono and an *obi* are also important. For example, strict rules dictate that kimonos of "Ro" are for midsummer, and in May, one must wear "Hitoe." While following these rules, we have to choose a kimono and an *obi* which "look good on the person." This is called the "selection" of a kimono. Furthermore, in a situation like the present when many people no longer wear kimonos, people don't know whom to consult about kimonos and selecting one which looks good. In light of this situation, we established a hypothesis that this is the cause of becoming alienated from kimonos. Therefore, as indicated in Fig. 1, we are considering the development of an automated system for matching a kimono with an *obi*. First of all, we input such things as the season of the year and the place that a consumer wears a kimono together with his or her preference for a kimono and an *obi*. We further input the consumer's facial picture.. Based on this data, and in accordance with the consumer's taste and rules for matching a kimono with an *obi,* it is possible to recommend a kimono and an *obi* that looks good on the consumer. The first thing we did with our present research is to determine the attitudes of contemporary persons toward Japanese dress. Based on this attitudinal research we clarified the reasons for their alienation from kimonos. Next, in order to clarify the developmental elements necessary to automate the selection of a kimono with an appropriate *obi,* we analyzed the thinking and protocols of kimono professionals regarding the consumer's selection of a kimono. As a result we have been able to clarify the thinking process of kimono professionals as they select "suitable kimonos." (Table 1)

Table 1. The major types of kimono and *obi*

	Kimono types	Obi Types
Formal	Uchikake, Kurotomesode	Maru-obi
Semi-formal	Irotomessode, Houmong, Iromuji, Furisode	Fukuro-obi
Street costume	Komon,Tukesage	Nagoya-obi
Everyday clothing	Wool, Light cotton	Nagoya-obi, Hanhaba-obi

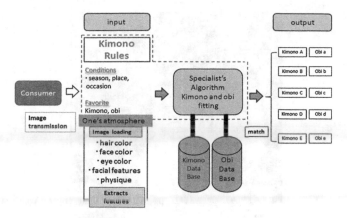

Fig. 1. Summary of a system for selecting a kimono and *obi*

2   Experimental Methods and Conditions

2.1   Attitude Survey

We performed a survey of attitudes toward kimonos through the use of a questionnaire. A total of 52 Japanese women (average age 41.2 years old (SD: 19.8)) cooperated with our research, including students and housewives. We further divided this number into two groups, comparing one group with the other. The first group of 20 young people was composed of those in their teens and 20's whose average age was 22.0 years old (SD: 2.9) The second group of 32 middle-aged and elderly was composed of those in their 30's up through their 80's whose average age was 53.2 years old (SD: 15.6). The questionnaire was divided into five levels of evaluation and asked such questions as: (1) Do you like kimonos? (2) Do you want to wear kimonos more? (3) How many kimonos and *yukata* (summer kimonos) do you have? (4) How often do you wear kimonos in a year? (5) Can you put on a kimono by yourself? (6) What are the reasons why you don't want to wear a kimono? These first few questions were centered on Japanese dress. Next, in order to inquire about the subject's knowledge of kimonos we asked: (7) Do you have confidence in matching a kimono with an *obi*? (8) Who advises you regarding matching a kimono with an *obi*? (9) Can you understand the various "kinds" of kimonos as well as the "rules" for wearing them? (10) Do you understand the appropriate kimono "patterns" to match the season? (11) Do you understand the appropriate kimono "material" to match the season? (12) Do you know the color that best suits you?

2.2   Protocol Analysis

The subject was a man at Kyo Yuzen Company who selects kimonos for consumers on a daily basis. He chose a "suitable" kimono for a female model. To learn more about the content of his thought process we had him complete a questionnaire about his selection methodology. The assumption was that the kimono would be worn for "a meal with one's boss." The location was the exhibition room of Kyo Yuzen Sales Company in Kyoto (Fig. 2).

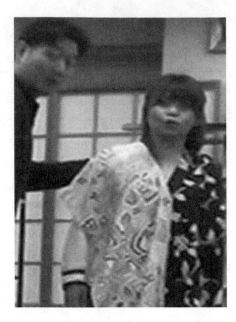

Fig. 2. Choice of a kimono by an expert

2.3   Data Collection and Analysis Method

At that time, the protocol analysis was conducted by asking the model to dictate the things that they see and hear, which influence them to choose a particular kimono. Based on the data, we analyzed the specialist's train of thought and behavior, and revealed the thought process of a specialist when "choosing" a kimono.

3   Results

3.1   Attitude Survey

(1) "Do you like kimono?" 90 % of young people and 94 % of middle-aged and elderly answered "Yes". (2) "Do you want to wear kimono more? 75 % of both young people and middle-aged and elderly both answered "Yes". (3) "How many kimono and *obi* do you have? Young people averaged 1.6 each, and middle-aged and elderly people averaged 25.3 each but became 11.0 each after excluding those who wear kimono as part of their occupation. The number of *obi* owned by young people was 1.7 each, and 43.9 each for middle-aged and elderly people. After excluding those who wear *obi* as part of their occupation, the number became 7.8 each. (4) "How often do you wear kimono in a year?" Young people answered 2.2 times, and the middle-aged and the elderly answered 23.0 times. Those who wore a kimono as part of their occupation were included, and the figure became 6.1 times after they were removed. (5) "Can you wear kimono by yourself?" 10 % of young people and 53 % of middle-aged and the elderly answered that they could. (6) As for reasons why they don't want to wear a kimono, from both

young people and the middle-aged and elderly many answered "I don't know how to dress myself" and "there are no places to which I can wear it" (Fig. 3). (7) "Do you have confidence about arranging the kimono and obi?" Less than 10 % of young people and the middle-aged and elderly answered "Yes" (Fig. 4). (8) "Who advises you on the arrangement of the kimono and *obi*?" Popular answers were "my mother" for young people, and 'the kimono shop attendant' for the middle-aged and elderly (Fig. 5). (9) "Can you differentiate the type and rank of a kimono?" 85 % of young people answered "No" (Fig. 6). (10) "Do you understand the design of a kimono, and what seasons are acceptable to wear them?" 70 % of young people answered that they didn't know (Fig. 7). (11) 85 % of young people also answered that they didn't know what the material used to make a kimono is (Fig. 8). (12) "Do you know which colors suit you?" 45 % of young people answered that they didn't know (Fig. 9),

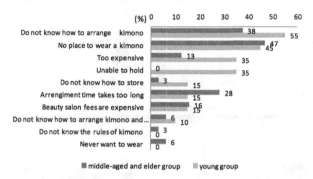

Fig. 3. Reasons why you don't want to wear a kimono?

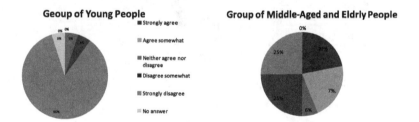

Fig. 4. Do you have confidence about arrangement with kimono and obi?

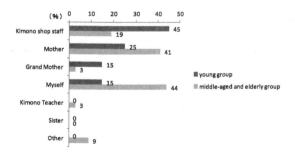

Fig. 5. Do you have confidence about arrangement with kimono and obi?

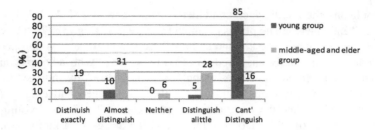

Fig. 6: Can you differentiate the "type" and "rank" of a kimono?

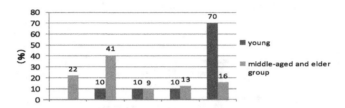

Fig. 7. Do you understand the design of a kimono, and what seasons are acceptable to wear them?

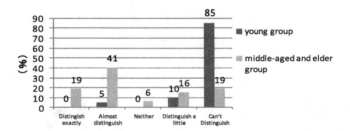

Fig. 8. Do you understand the design of a kimono, and what seasons are acceptable to wear them?

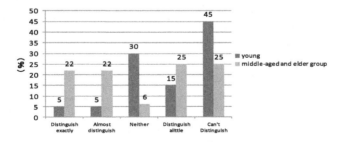

Fig. 9. Do you know which "colors" suit you?

3.2 Protocol Analysis

We performed a questionnaire to an expert about their methods of choosing kimono. When asked "What do you look at in a model (customer) when arranging a kimono?", the expert answered "body type", "height", "hair color" and "facial impression". As for the color of the model's hair, the expert answered that the "the length of the hair", "straightness", and "waviness" are used as a reference. The expert said that the "face color" and "eye color" are also looked at. For the model's facial impression, facial

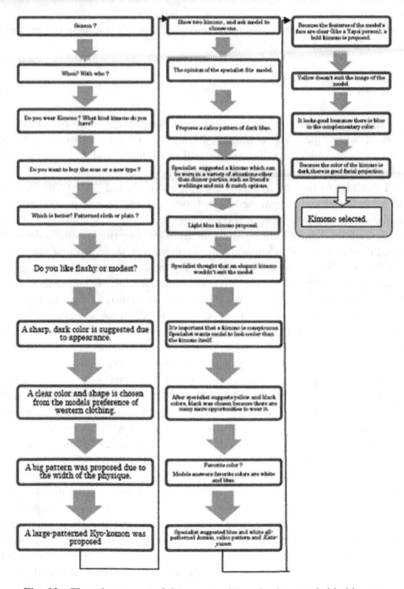

Fig. 10. Thought process of the expert when selecting a suitable kimono.

features like whether they have a dark or pale facial complexion are used as a reference. When asked "what kind of kimono do think would look good on this model as a first impression?", the expert answered that based on his impression from the model's "facial projection", that a navy blue or charcoal gray color would be suitable When asked "will the kimono be more suitable for the model in a pale or dark color?", the expert answered that after considering the model's "chubby face" and "facial projection", that a dark color would be more suitable. When asked "Would you recommend either an expensive or inexpensive kimono to the model?", the expert answered that since the model had "knowledge about kimono", he would recommend an expensive one. Also, when the expert chooses a kimono, what he values the most is that "the person who wears the kimono is the main actor, and my job is to help the person wear the kimono with confidence" (Fig. 10).

4 Discussion

It is clear that the separation from kimono is becoming severe, even by looking at the number of times people wear a kimono throughout the year. However, from this experiment we were able to see that people still like kimono and want to wear it more often. The reasons for which we thought this separation from kimono was occurring, such as "I don't know how to arrange a kimono and *obi*", and "I don't understand the rules of kimono" were only mentioned a few times. This can be interpreted that most do not rise above the consciousness of a consumer, by leaving *obi* adjustment up to the kimono dressing teacher or kimono store. In addition, as many youths answered that they do not have confidence in kimono and *obi* alignment, there is a fear that they may choose a kimono that does not follow the Japanese garment rules and go to an unsuitable place wearing it. If there is an algorithm for the *obi* alignment, then one could choose a kimono and *obi* by themselves, so automation is very important. This time we revealed a specialist's thinking process to see how a specialist chooses a "suitable kimono". Since there were many answers for a counselor for kimono and *obi* selection as the 'kimono store attendant', we used our kimono selection expert as a 'kimono store attendant' for the protocol analysis in this study. First with the expert, we inquired about the "season" to wear a kimono, and situations such as "with who" and "where". After that, we asked "What kinds of kimono do you have?". We expect this was asked because unlike a western-style dress, a kimono must be coordinated with an *obi*.. Furthermore, the expert was asked whether a kimono with "extensive patterns" or "plain" was better, and his "likes' such as a "flashy" or "modest" kimono. For the first time, the expert proposed a kimono of "dark color" and "sharp color" based on the appearance of the model. This is because the expert "was able to understand the customer's preferences from the western clothing the model was wearing". Next, as the model's "physique is transversely large", the expert proposed "big patterns" charcoal-gray color and a *Kyo-komon* of a large lotus pattern. The expert then proposed a yellowish-green kimono covered extensively in patterns, and allowed the model to choose from a selection of two. Furthermore, he suggested a dark blue kimono completely covered with a calico pattern. After thinking of "different uses and mixing & matching opportunities' other than dinner parties, the expert proposed a light blue kimono. The model did not understand the reason, but was told an elegant kimono would not be suitable. A kimono in which "the model shined" more was important, and the expert wouldn't propose anything unsuitable because he wanted someone to look "cool" in a kimono. He then suggested a light yellow and black cloth with patterns, but recommended the black kimono with many opportunities to be worn. Next, the expert asked a model for her favorite color, and the model answered white and blue. The expert finally suggested a blue and white all-patterned *komon*, calico pattern and *Kata-yuzen*. Afterwards, he added that the reason he chose this kimono was that the model had clear "facial features", and due to the dark color of the kimono, her facial projection would be great. Based on this, experts will be able to determine by means of a simulation the "rules" for wearing a kimono based on such things as the season and the situation. Next, they will be able to determine the proper kimono patterns based on the model's physical features. Further they will be able to determine the kimono's "color," "flashiness" and "brilliance" based on the model's looks. It also suggests the selection of a kimono that harmonizes well with the model's face. Along the way it suggests thought given to the selection of a kimono based on such things as the model's likes, easy coordination with items already in her possession, and non-selection of things that are similar to items she already has.

As a result of the above, there is a possibility of constructing a system, using this algorithm, that incorporates the rules for Japanese dress, the consumer's tastes, along with the selection of a kimono "suitable for that person". Further, in the future it will be possible to employ this system to select an algorithm for *obi* selection. We expect this to assist the automation of matching a suitable kimono with an *obi* for the consumer.

Reference

1. Yokoyama, T.: The demand for japanese clothing and management of obi weaving in the nishijin production area. J. Jpn Soc. Silk Sci. Technol. **21**, 23–29 (2003)

A Fundamental Study on Differences in Heart Rates During Creative Work and Non-creative Work

Tatsuo Nakagawa[1,2(✉)], Hiroto Inoue[2,3], and Shigeomi Koshimizu[2]

[1] Technicol Inc., Tokyo, Japan
t.nakagawa@technicol.co.jp
[2] Advanced Institute of Industrial Technology, Tokyo, Japan
{inoue-hiroto,koshimizu}@aiit.ac.jp
[3] Tokyo Denki University, Tokyo, Japan

Abstract. We sought to clarify how creative and non-creative work influence R-R intervals. Clearly different patterns of R-R intervals were found between creative and non-creative work, with heart rate quickening during creative work and recovering during subsequent rest periods. The differences between median R-R intervals during creative work were significantly and positively related to feelings of stress, with most coefficients of greater than 0.7 (reaching as high as 0.840; $P < 0.001$). In contrast, the differences between R-R intervals during non-creative work were not significantly correlated with feelings of stress, and the maximum coefficient did not exceed 0.3. Therefore, it appears that variability of median R-R intervals can be used to effectively predict feelings of stress when people engage in creative work but not when they engage in non-creative work.

Keywords: Heart rate variability · Wearable sensing · Stress response

1 Introduction

In Japan, the mental health of the general population is receiving increasing attention. A more pertinent statistic here would be to cite statistics regarding mental stress in Japan, such as the prevalence of high stress among workers. Indeed, in December 2015, Japanese companies with more than 50 employees were required by law to test the mental stress levels of employees [1]. Mental stress is typically subjectively screened for using questionnaires. More recently, research has indicated that heart rate variability (i.e., intervals between R waves, or R-R interval, which relates to activation of the autonomic nervous system), salivary amylase, and various other biological data can serve as accurate indicators of mental stress, which has led to the development of methods of testing stress based on these data [2–4].

Mental stress may decrease when workers actively engage with their work. For example, workers who find it difficult to engage in menial work may experience less mental stress when engaging in creative work. Therefore, we consider that metal stress may be related with work type. However, the relationship between work type and biological indicators has not been studied sufficiently—it is not clear how these data

© Springer International Publishing Switzerland 2016
V.G. Duffy (Ed.): DHM 2016, LNCS 9745, pp. 568–575, 2016.
DOI: 10.1007/978-3-319-40247-5_57

differ between work types, such as creative and non-creative work. In this paper, we define the meaning of creative work that persons have to consider method and solution for task by him/herself. Also, we define non-creative work that person does not have to consider method and solution for task by him/herself and is required to perform just according to some rules. Thus, the purpose of this paper was to clarify how creative and non-creative work influence R-R intervals.

2 Experimental Methods

Eighteen individuals aged 21–24 participated in this experiment. Participants were explained ethical guideline and agreed with the contents. Written informed consents were obtained from all participants. Participants were asked to try four tasks (A–D), as shown in Fig. 1. Task A was termed the "marshmallow challenge" [5], and involved having participants build the tallest structure they could using uncooked dried spaghetti noodles; an entire marshmallow had to be held at the top of the structure. Task B was called "binding", and required participants to assemble triangles by binding dried noodles with kite strings together as much as possible in the time allotted. Task C was "calculating", wherein participants added together 3-digit numbers, and Task D was "spot the difference", wherein participants had to identify an anomalous character out of a hundred identical characters. Both tasks had to be performed as much as possible in the time allotted. Task A was considered to require the most creativity out of the four tasks because participants who perform Task A to be required to consider the method and solution by him/herself. Also, Tasks A and B were craftworks requiring manual dexterity, while Tasks C and D were simple, repetitive tasks that did not require creativity.

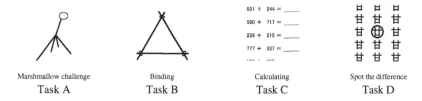

| Marshmallow challenge | Binding | Calculating | Spot the difference |
| Task A | Task B | Task C | Task D |

Fig. 1. Task contents

The participants attempted each task three times per day, as shown in Fig. 2. The time allotted for each task was 30 min in total. First, participants were instructed on how to perform one of the four tasks. Then, the participants took a rest, wherein they sat with both eyes closed for 3 min. After this, the participants performed the task for 6 min as the first attempt. Each attempt comprised two periods of 3 min (former and latter); when the latter period began, a timekeeper began a countdown in 1-min intervals (e.g., "last 3 min", "last 2 min", and "last 1 min"). After the 6-min attempt, participants again took a rest with both eyes closed in a sitting position. The participants repeated this procedure for two more attempts. During all task attempts and rests, participants' R-R intervals were recorded with a wearable heart rate meter (Uniontool, WHS-1).

Upon completing all attempts of the day, the participants responded to a self-assessment questionnaire with the following format:

- Did you experience a feeling of "stress" during the 1st/2nd/3rd attempt?

Eleven different words appeared within the quotation marks (e.g., "stress", "fatigue", "tension"). The ordering of the quoted words changed each day at random. The participants selected one of five responses to the questions, as follows.

| | 0 min. | 3 min. | 6 min. | 9 min. | 12 min. | 15 min. | 18 min. | 21 min. | 24 min. | 27 min. | 30 min. |

Day 1 Task A

Period 1	Period 2	Period 3	Period 4	Period 5	Period 6	Period 7	Period 8	Period 9	Period 10
Rest	The 1st attempt		Rest	The 2nd attempt		Rest	The 3rd attempt		Rest
With closed eyes		With countdown	With closed eyes		With countdown	With closed eyes		With countdown	With closed eyes

Day 2 Task D

Period 1	Period 2	Period 3	Period 4	Period 5	Period 6	Period 7	Period 8	Period 9	Period 10
Rest	The 1st attempt		Rest	The 2nd attempt		Rest	The 3rd attempt		Rest
With closed eyes		With countdown	With closed eyes		With countdown	With closed eyes		With countdown	With closed eyes

Day 3 Task B

Period 1	Period 2	Period 3	Period 4	Period 5	Period 6	Period 7	Period 8	Period 9	Period 10
Rest	The 1st attempt		Rest	The 2nd attempt		Rest	The 3rd attempt		Rest
With closed eyes		With countdown	With closed eyes		With countdown	With closed eyes		With countdown	With closed eyes

Day 4 Task C

Period 1	Period 2	Period 3	Period 4	Period 5	Period 6	Period 7	Period 8	Period 9	Period 10
Rest	The 1st attempt		Rest	The 2nd attempt		Rest	The 3rd attempt		Rest
With closed eyes		With countdown	With closed eyes		With countdown	With closed eyes		With countdown	With closed eyes

Fig. 2. Example of a timetable. The task order was randomly determined for each individual. The columns depict Periods 1–10 (repeated rests and attempts)

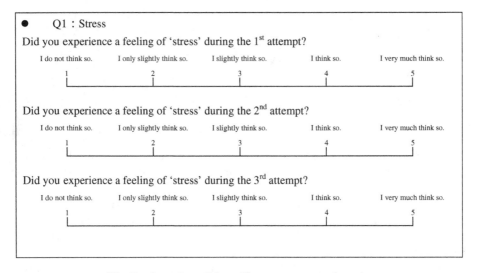

- Q1 : Stress

Did you experience a feeling of 'stress' during the 1st attempt?

I do not think so.	I only slightly think so.	I slightly think so.	I think so.	I very much think so.
1	2	3	4	5

Did you experience a feeling of 'stress' during the 2nd attempt?

I do not think so.	I only slightly think so.	I slightly think so.	I think so.	I very much think so.
1	2	3	4	5

Did you experience a feeling of 'stress' during the 3rd attempt?

I do not think so.	I only slightly think so.	I slightly think so.	I think so.	I very much think so.
1	2	3	4	5

Fig. 3. A portion of the self-assessment questionnaire

5. I very much think so.
4. I think so.
3. I slightly think so.
2. I only slightly think so.
1. I do not think so.

These choices have an ordinal relationship. Figure 3 shows the response format of the five choices.

3 Results and Discussion

3.1 Differences in R-R Intervals Between Resting and Work

Figure 4 shows examples of time-series datasets of R-R intervals. The stepped lines in the figure show the median R-R intervals in each period. Figure 5 shows box plots of the medians of all participants; the horizontal axis shows each period.

Figure 4a shows one participant's time series of R-R intervals in Task A. For example, the median R-R interval in Period 1, wherein the participant took his/her first rest, was 724 ms. Then, the median R-R intervals in Periods 2 and 3, wherein the participant made the first attempt to complete Task A, were 643 and 616 ms, respectively. As can be seen, they were lower than the median R-R interval in Period 1, with differences of 81.0 and 108 ms, respectively. The median R-R interval in Period 4, wherein the participant took his/her second rest, increased to 686 ms. As shown in Fig. 4a, this pattern was observed for the subsequent periods. In contrast, there were no clear differences in R-R intervals between rests and attempts in Task D, as shown in Fig. 4b. The difference in medians between Periods 1 and 2 for Task D was only 8.50 ms, even though the results in Fig. 4a and b are derived from the same participant. We noted these same two patterns depicted in Fig. 4 in some of the participants. The results of Task B were similar to those of Task A, while the results of Task C were similar to those of Task D.

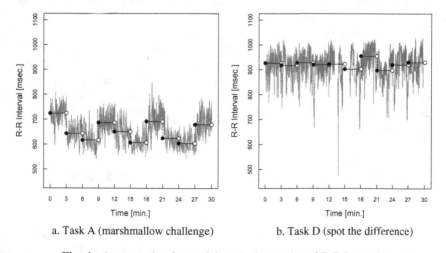

a. Task A (marshmallow challenge)   b. Task D (spot the difference)

Fig. 4. An example of a participant's time series of R-R intervals

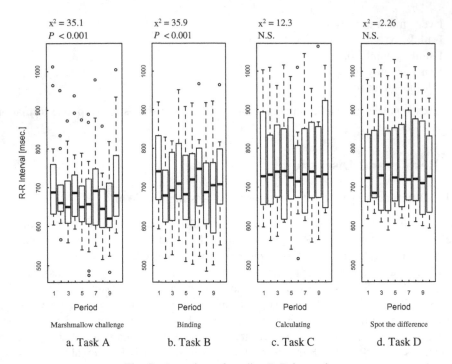

Fig. 5. Box plots of median R-R intervals

Figure 5a shows distributions of medians in each period across all participants, and is in line with the abovementioned patterns. Figure 5a shows that the median R-R intervals during attempts at Task A tended to be lower than were those during the rests. The Friedman test indicated that the medians significantly differed among the periods in Fig. 5a ($P < 0.001$). We also noted significant differences in Fig. 5b ($P < 0.001$). Specifically, participants' R-R intervals were quicker during their attempts at the craftworks (e.g., Tasks A and B) compared with resting. In contrast, the medians did not significantly differ among the periods in Tasks C and D, as shown in Fig. 5c and d.

Notably, the median R-R intervals in Fig. 5a were lower than were those in Fig. 5c and d, even during the rest (i.e., Period 1) before the first attempt at Task A. For example, the median R-R intervals in the first rest in Fig. 4a and b were 724 and 927 ms, respectively, with a difference between them of 203 ms. Overall, our results indicated that participants' heart rates did not quicken when attempting simple work such as Tasks C and D.

3.2   Correlation Between Variability of R-R Intervals and a Feeling of Stress

Figures 6 and 7 show the scatterplots of the correlations (Spearman's rank correlation ρ) between variability in R-R intervals and a reported feeling of stress. In these figures, the horizontal axes show differences in median R-R intervals between Period 1 and the periods when participants attempted the tasks, while the vertical axes showed the strength of the feeling of stress based on questionnaire responses.

According to Spearman's rank correlation analysis, the variability in median R-R intervals in Task A had strong positive correlations with feelings of stress; all of these correlation coefficients were greater than 0.7, with the highest coefficient being 0.840 ($P < 0.001$), as shown in Fig. 6. The means ($\pm$ SD) of the differences in Fig. 6a and b were -58.1 ($\pm$ 86.8) and -58.6 ($\pm$ 87.8) ms, respectively. More specifically, participants did not appear to report a feeling of stress when their R-R intervals quickened by approximately 150 ms; this rate is the means minus SD. In this way, we can predict the strength of the feeling of stress according to heart rate variability when individuals engage in relatively creative tasks such as the "marshmallow challenge".

In contrast, we observed no significant correlations between variability in median R-R intervals in Task D and feeling of stress; indeed, the highest correlation coefficient was no more than 0.3. The mean differences in Fig. 7a and b were approximately zero: -1.50 ($\pm$ 48.0) and -0.595 ($\pm$ 46.3) ms. It must be noted that, as shown in Fig. 8, the strength of the feeling of stress during attempts at Task D was comparable with that during attempts at Task A. However, the heart rate variability in the simple tasks did not significantly correlate with a feeling of stress; thus, it is difficult to estimate feelings of stress based on heart rate variability when the individuals are attempting simple tasks.

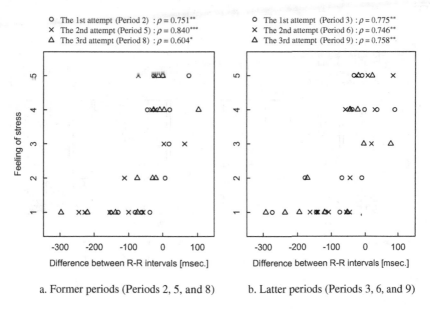

a. Former periods (Periods 2, 5, and 8)   b. Latter periods (Periods 3, 6, and 9)

Fig. 6. Correlations between variability in R-R intervals and feelings of stress in Task A (marshmallow challenge).

Overall, feelings of stress are not likely to be predicted by median R-R intervals for Tasks C and D. However, it is possible that the conditions of the initial rests influenced the R-R intervals during each attempt, and therefore would influence the above-mentioned correlation analysis results.

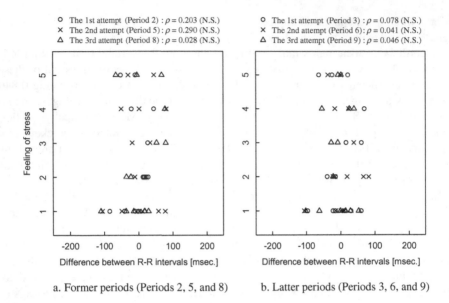

a. Former periods (Periods 2, 5, and 8)   b. Latter periods (Periods 3, 6, and 9)

Fig. 7. Correlations between variability in R-R intervals and feeling of stress in Task D (spot the difference).

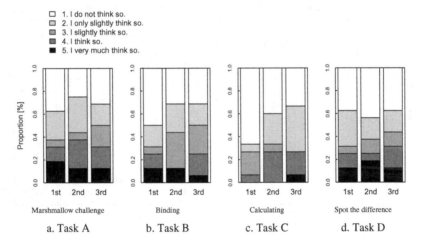

Fig. 8. Strength of feeling stress in each Task (spot the difference).

4   Conclusion

The purpose of this study is to clarify how creative and non-creative work influences heart rate variability. We found that patterns of R-R intervals differed noticeably between creative and non-creative work, with the heart rate quickening during creative work and recovering during the subsequent rest. Additionally, the variability in median R-R intervals in creative work was strongly and positively related to feelings of stress (with most correlations being > 0.7 and the highest being 0.840; $P < 0.001$). These results suggest that it is possible to predict feelings of stress according to heart rate variability when people are engaged in creative work. In contrast, variability in median R-R intervals in non-creative work was not significantly correlated with feelings of stress (with the highest coefficient being no more than 0.3).

Acknowledgement. We thank Associate Prof. N. Kuwahara from Kyoto Institute of Technology and Prof. N. Tetsutani and Mr. S. Ohhara from the Tokyo Denki University for their valuable comments. A part of this study was supported by JSPS KAKENHI Grant Number 15K12130.

References

1. Ministry of Health, Labour and Welfare, Japan, Outline of the Act for Partial Revision of the Industrial Safety and Health Act. http://www.mhlw.go.jp/english/policy/employ-labour/labour-standards/dl/140711-01.pdf
2. Izawa, S., et al.: The application of saliva to an assessment of stress: Procedures for collection and analyzing saliva and characteristics of salivary substances. Jpn. J. Complement. Altern. Med. 4(3), 91–101 (2007)
3. Takatsu, H., et al.: An evaluation of the quantitative relationship between the subjective stress value and heart rate variability. IEEJ Trans. Electron. Inf. Syst. 120-C, 104–110 (2000)
4. Ohsuga, M., et al.: Quantitative evaluation of stress responses. Jpn. J. Ergon. 29(6), 353–356 (1993)
5. Wujec, T.: The marshmallow challenge. http://marshmallowchallenge.com/TED_Talk_files/TED2010_Tom_Wujec_Marshmallow_Challenge_Web_Version.pdf

A Study of Eye Movement Analysis
for Investigating Learning Efficiency
by Using a Highlighter Pen

Hiroki Nishimura[(⊠)], Kazumasa Shibata, Yuki Inazuka,
and Noriaki Kuwahara

Kyoto Institute of Technology, Kyoto, Japan
arc-nnlervmenve@arc-edu.com,
shibataka3hiro160moon@gmail.com,
y.inazuka0124@gmail.com, nkuwahar@kit.ac.jp

Abstract. For learners including elementary, junior high school and high school students, acquiring an ability to solve various types of questions in every subject is one of the most important learning objectives.

This study verified the effects of a highlighter on the process of information processing in solving questions. Marking with a highlighter pen, as a means of organizing information, can have effects on the improvement of academic performance by the visual effects as well as through marking works.

Therefore, changes in the number of eye movements as well as visual fixation duration of learners were measured to verify the visual effects of marking with a highlighter pen.

Keywords: Highlighter pen · Memory · Attentional capacity · Academic performance

1 Introduction

In recent years, there has been increasing attention to cognitive and learning sciences that study learning process and problem-solving process of various learning students including elementary, junior high school and high school students.

Cognitive science in learning is a study that aims to scientifically understand deep learning and the process of information processing to promote effective and efficient learning for learners. Thus, a concrete method needs to be developed to help learners recognize necessary information for problem-solving in learning.

Currently, various types of tests including entrance and regular examinations are conducted to measure academic performance of learners. However, it is critical for learners to acquire, understand and recognize necessary information correctly from given questions in any form of examinations.

Daniel Kahneman argues that humans possess two different systems of thinking for decision-making. 1)

The first system is called Fast (System 1), thinking driven by intuitive and emotional value evaluation. The second system is known as Slow (System 2), thinking

© Springer International Publishing Switzerland 2016
V.G. Duffy (Ed.): DHM 2016, LNCS 9745, pp. 576–585, 2016.
DOI: 10.1007/978-3-319-40247-5_58

based on logical and rational value evaluation. The complementary interaction between these two different value evaluations enables humans to recognize and process various information and to make decisions. In intuitive decision-making by Fast (System 1), humans match new information with existing learning experience, retrieve a range of associated information and make decisions unconsciously and automatically based on associated information. Sophisticated Fast (System 1) combines accurate information instantaneously and builds a new information network for problem-solving. However, wrong and little input or non-existing input in past experience can easily result in simplistic thinking, which creates biases and errors. In contrast, thoughtful decision-making by Slow (System 2) can be seen as a statistical thinking that makes rational decisions by consciously recognizing implications of information.

In other words, despite having the two different systems of thinking for information processing and decision making, humans tend to rely on intuition of Fast (System 1) for value evaluation, automatic and unconscious thinking, rather than Slow (System 2) that generates excessive stress in the process of information processing. This tendency has been one of causes for errors.

For this reason, information analysis and decision making skill are also required to solve questions in various daily examinations for learners including elementary, junior high school and high school students.

Thus, attention has been given to general highlighter pens used by learners in order to help learners organize information accurately and make right decisions by enhancing problem-solving skill. Highlighter pens are used to highlight important points and to draw attention with vivid and bright colors so as to improve learning efficiency.

To examine the effect of marking with a highlighter pen, there have been studies dealing with visually favorable fluorescent colors, its impacts on memory2), as well as how proper marking in sentences influence key word searching. 3)

However, it has been unknown how marking with a highlighter pen for different purposes would influence attentional capacity, cognitive capacity and memory ability and what changes marking would bring to the process of information processing and eye movements of humans.

Card advocates Model Human Processor, a simplified and approximated model of the process of information processing of humans, consisting of perceptual, cognitive and motor processors. 4) When learners process information (and solve problems), information is input through sensory organs including eyes and ears and stored in the visual image store. Learners repeat the process of matching input information with long-term memory and answering selected responses to solve various problems. When problems are recognized visually, marking with a highlighter pen can limit the amount of visual information input and ease cognitive load.

Therefore, with the focus on perceptual system in Model Human Processor, this study verified the effects of marking with a highlighter pen on eye movement patterns by measuring changes in the number of eye movements and visual fixation frame rate.

2 Experimental

2.1 Test Subjects

The test subjects were 2nd and 3rd grade junior high school students who study at a cram school. Table 1 shows data of the test subjects. All test subjects have normal eyesight with naked eyes. Students with glasses are not included in the test subjects so as not to interfere the measurement of eye movements.

Table 1. Grade, number of tests subjects, ratio of male and female students

Grade	Male students	Female students	Number
2nd grade junior high school students	1	2	3
3rd grade junior high school students	10	7	17
Total	11	9	20

2.2 Experimental Details

Questions on third person singular present S and tense (present, past and future tense) of English were prepared with and without marking respectively.

First, 10 questions on third person singular present S and tense (Both without marking) were presented in turns to the test subjects. Then, 5 questions on third person singular present S (with marking) were given, followed by 5 questions on tense (with marking). At the end, 10 questions on third person singular present S and tense (both without marking) were presented in turns to the test subjects. The purpose of this experiment was to verify how marking with a highlighter pen would influence eye movements. It can be expected that there would be changes in answer time and the number of eye movements to key points and clues of questions if marking is related to problem-solving. Thus, the number of eye movements and fixation duration on each item were measured when the test subjects answered each question.

2.3 Experimental Conditions

Each question was projected one by one on white board (140 cm W x 80 cm H), using a projector. Once the test subjects answered a question, next question was projected on the white board. The tests subjects sit at a distance of 130 cm from the white board. A chin rest was also used to fix the head of the test subjects to minimize influences on the eye movement measurement by preventing inadvertent movements of the upper body and neck. Figure 1 shows the picture of the chin rest.

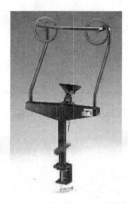

Fig. 1. Chin rest, interacoustics

Mobile Eye Mark Recorder EMR-9, eye-tracking analysis system made by NAC image technology, was used for the measurement. Figure 2 shows the picture of the device.

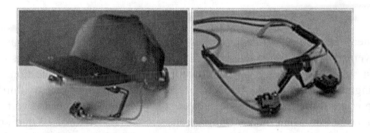

Fig. 2. Eye tracking analysis system: product name Mobile Eye Mark Recorder EMR-9

2.4 Experimental Questions

Figure 3 shows the question on third person singular present S without marking while Fig. 4 presents the one with marking. The question on tense without marking is shown in Fig. 5, and the one with marking is provided in Fig. 6.

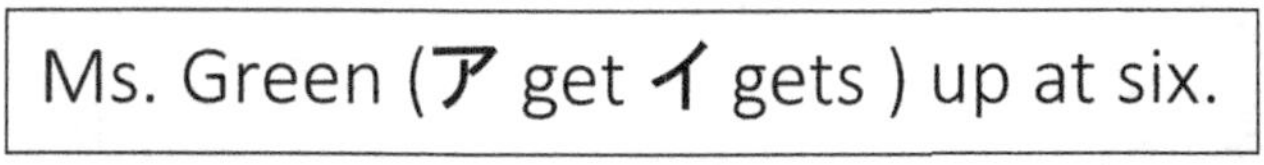

Ms. Green (ア get イ gets) up at six.

Fig. 3. Third person singular present S: example without marking

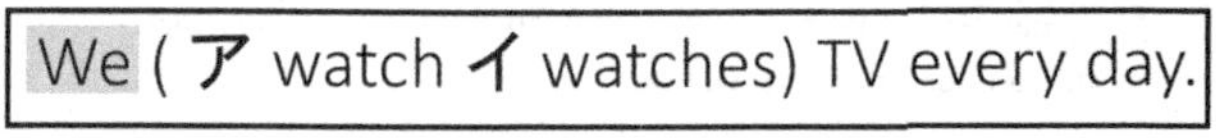

We (ア watch イ watches) TV every day.

Fig. 4. Third person singular present S: example with marking

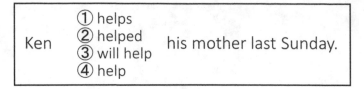

Fig. 5. Tense: example without marking

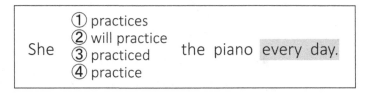

Fig. 6. Tense: example with marking

3   Results

3.1   Visual Fixation Frame Rate on Each Item

Fixation items in each question were categorized into subject, verb, times and others, and the average fixation frame rate on each item (60 frames per second) was measured for all test subjects. Figures 7 and 8 show the frame rate result of questions on third person singular present S and tense respectively. In the questions of third person singular present S, the frame rates on subject, a key item to answer, and verb, choices of answer, were low when the test subjects answered C (2ⁿᵈ half of 10 questions) that was presented after A (1ˢᵗ half of 10 questions) and B (10 questions with marking).

The questions of tense showed the similar result of low frame rate on times, a key item to answer and verb, choices of answers.

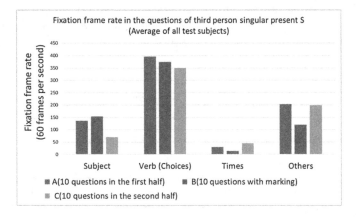

Fig. 7. Fixation frame rate (Third person singular present S) (Color figure online)

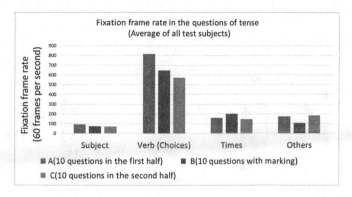

Fig. 8. Fixation frame rate (Tense) (Color figure online)

3.2 The Ratio of Fixation Frame Rate on Key Item

In the questions of third person singular present S, the ratio of frame rate on subject, a key item to answer, to the total frame rate was confirmed to further investigate fixation duration on each item. Figure 9 shows its result. The value of C (10 questions in the 2nd half) that was given to the subjects after B (10 questions with marking) was lower than that of A (10 questions in the 1st half).

Figure 10 shows the result for the tense questions. As is the case with third person singular present S, C (10 questions in 2nd half) presented the lower value. Meanwhile, B (10 questions with marking) showed the highest value in the questions of both third person singular present S and tense.

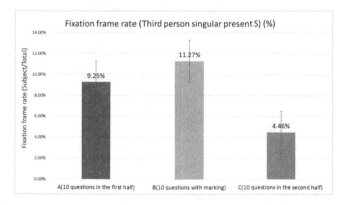

Fig. 9. Fixation frame rate on key item (Third person singular present S) (Color figure online)

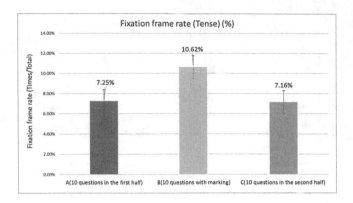

Fig. 10. Fixation frame rate on key item (Tense) (Color figure online)

3.3 Comparison of High and Low Academic Achieving Students(the Number of Eye Movements)

Figures 11 and 12 show the number of eye movements of the top two and bottom two students in the test result for third person singular present S and tense respectively. In the number of eye movements in the question of third person singular present S, the top two test subjects made the fewer eye movements than the bottom two in all sections, A (10 questions in the 1st half), B (10 questions with marking) and C (10 questions in the 2nd half).

Likewise, in the questions of tense, the top two showed the fewer eye movements than the bottom two.

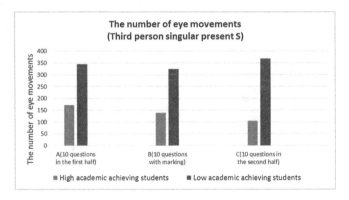

Fig. 11. The number of eye movements in high and low academic achieving students (Third person singular present S). (Color figure online)

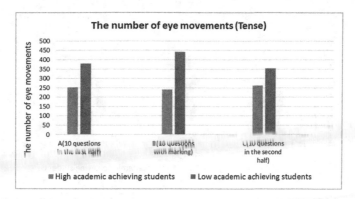

Fig. 12. The number of eye movements in high and low academic achieving students (Tense) (Color figure online)

3.4 Comparison of High and Low Academic Achieving Students (Fixation Frame Rate)

Fixation frame rate on each item in question sentences (subject, verb, times, others and unrelated objects) was verified for the top two and bottom two test subjects. The results for third person singular present S and tense are provided in Figs. 13 and 14 respectively. In the question of third person singular present S, the ratio of frame rate on subject, a key item to question, to the total frame rate was verified. In the questions of tense, the ratio of the frame rate on times to the total frame rate was examined.

In the questions of third person singular present S, the top two test subjects recorded lower frame rate than the bottom two in A (10 questions in the 1st half). However, the top two showed a tendency of higher frame rate than the bottom two in B (10 questions with marking) and C (10 questions in the 2nd half).

In the questions of tense, the top two test subjects recorded higher frame rate than the bottom two in A (10 questions in the 1st half), B (10 questions with marking) and C (10 questions in the 2nd half).

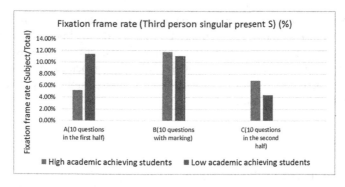

Fig. 13. Fixation frame rate of high and low academic achieving students (Third person singular present S). (Color figure online)

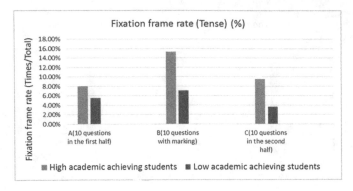

Fig. 14. Fixation frame rate of high and low academic achieving students (Tense) (Color figure online)

4 Discussion and Conclusion

In this study, effects given to eye movements in processing information (and solving problems) by marking with a highlighter pen were verified by experiments using questions of third person singular present S and tense.

The result of fixation frame rate for all test subjects showed that frame rate on a key item and choices of answer was low when the test subjects answered C (10 questions in the 2nd half) that was given after B (10 questions with marking). For this reason, it can be assumed that marking with a highlighter pen has potential to shorten time to reach an answer.

The comparison of high and low academic achieving students showed the fewer eye movements and high fixation frame rate on key word item among the top students. This suggests that the top students have a tendency of processing information fast to recognize key word and reaching an answer after double-checking. In contrast, the bottom students presented more eye movements and the lower fixation frame rate on key word item. It can be assumed that key word searching led to more eye movements and lower fixation frame rate, which resulted in the fewer number of correct answers among low academic achieving students.

This experiment was conducted in an environment where unrelated items projected on the screen were also in the view of the tests subjects. By the improving experimental environment and increasing the number of test subjects, further analysis will be performed to verify the effects of marking with a highlighter pen in the future. Furthermore, effects of marking on information searching will be examined by analyzing brain activities including cerebral blood flow.

References

1. Kahneman, D.: Thinking Fast and Slow
2. Suzuki, K., Ohuchi, H.: The effect of marking by the fluorescent color. Proc. Conf. Japan Ergon. Soc. **38**, 500–501 (2002)

3. Kuwahara, N.: A Study on Learning Effects of Marking with Highlighter Pen: Japan Ergonomics Society
4. Card, S.K., Moran, T.P., Newell, A.: The Psychology of Human-Computer Interaction, pp. 24–90. Taylor & Francis, London (1983)

The Research of Airport Operational Risk Alerting Model

Mei Rong, Min Luo$^{(\boxtimes)}$, and Yanqiu Chen

China Academy of Civil Aviation Science and Technology, Beijing, China
{Rongmei, luomin, Chenyq}@mail.castc.org.cn

Abstract. This research determines ten key modules affecting the airport operational safety, including vehicles and aircraft scratching, runway incursion, the runway unseaworthiness and so on. Then, we design 165 airport operational risk monitoring indicators using the system and job analysis method, fault tree analysis method, expert brainstorming etc. These indicators can be divided into three levels including incidents level, the other occurrences level and process monitoring level.

Based on risk management theory, safety performance management theory, the Heinrich's Law and the 2011-2014 years' data of a certain airport group, we set the weight of each level indicator and the severity value of each indicator, and establish the operational risk warning model. This model is verified to be applicable through three months data collection, calculation and risk warning of two airports.

Keywords: Operational risk alert model · Risk monitoring indicator · Safety performance management · Heinrich's law

1 Introduction

Modern safety management theory emphasizes the safety management should focus on active management rather than passive management. At present, the safety level of airport in China is always evaluated through high consequences indicators like incident rate. This "ex-post" evaluation method makes the regulator and airport focus on the occurrence of incidents rather than the risk management capability and prevention capacity. For the airport, no accident does not mean the risk level is low. Therefore, in addition to the accidents or incidents, the airport also should pay close attention to the state of the operational process. If we can take the active management, monitor the safety risk factors or the state of operational state and alert staff to take measures before accidents or incidents, airport operational safety can be promoted. This is the highest goal pursued by airport safety management work.

This research designs airport operational safety risk monitoring indicators based on the risk management theory and safety performance management theory. And then builds the operational risk warning model. This model can monitor the airport safety risk and help the airport detect the abnormal events or unacceptable risk early, take appropriate risk management measures promptly, in order to avoid the occurrence of accidents or incidents.

© Springer International Publishing Switzerland 2016
V.G. Duffy (Ed.): DHM 2016, LNCS 9745, pp. 586–595, 2016.
DOI: 10.1007/978-3-319-40247-5_59

2 The Establishment of Airport Operational Safety Risk Monitoring Indicators

The airport operational safety risk monitoring indicators are not limited to high consequence (safety results) indicators; also include low consequence (operational process) indicators to reflect the operation state and safety management indicators. Therefore, the indicators can systematically and scientifically evaluate the safety state of an organization, and the results can reflect the safety results while expose the problems in the process of operation and management.

2.1 The Method of Designing Safety Risk Monitoring Indicator

(1) The method of designing low consequence (operational process) indicators

The method of designing low consequence (operational process) indicators includes the following two categories.

• Forward analysis method

The first step of forward analysis method is to decompose and analysis system and processes, then identify the hazards may lead to the unusual process, further deduce unusual activities or status, until the final consequences of danger (As Fig. 1.). Then the abnormal activity or status can be designed as low consequence indicators. The analysis methods from the hazards to the dangerous consequences include the event tree analysis (ETA), hazard and operability analysis (HAZOP), What-if analysis, etc.

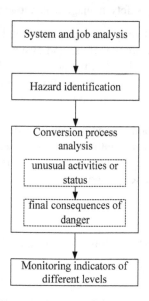

Fig. 1. Forward analysis method

- Reverse analysis method

Inverse analysis method is defined from the dangerous consequences (such as runway incursion etc.) to the beginning state. To analysis the unsafe activities or status, and the direct and indirect causes. Then the abnormal activity or status can be designed as low consequence indicators (As Fig. 2.). The analysis methods from the dangerous consequences to the hazards include the fault tree analysis (FTA), Reason model, SHELL model, etc.

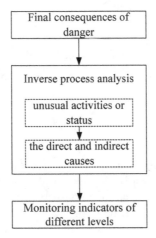

Fig. 2. Reverse analysis method

(2) The method of designing safety management indicators

Design of safety management indicators can be carried out in accordance with the safety management system elements method and system elements method.

Safety management system elements method means that we can design indicators to measure the implementation and construction of the SMS's 12 elements. For example, in view of management commitment, we can design the indicator "safety committee attendance rate".

The system elements method means that we can design indicators to elements of system including responsibility, authority, procedures, tools/method, personnel, implementation, control and effect. For example, in view of implementation of the safety inspection work, we can design the indicator "safety inspection work completion rate".

2.2   The Design of Airport Operational Safety Risk Monitoring Indicators

This research first identifies ten key modules that can influence airport operation risk, including the runway unseaworthiness, navigation facilities failure, obstacle clearance excessive, runway incursion, flight area perimeter intrusion, vehicles and aircraft scratching, FOD, bird strike, hidden load and hazards of non-stop flight construction.

Then, we analyze the possible hazards of the ten key modules, establish the low consequences indicators through the forward analysis method and the safety management indicators based on the system elements method. We also design the high consequence indicators through analyzing China civil aviation incidents standard terms associated with the ten key modules. Specific process is as follows:

(1) The design of the low consequences indicators and the safety management indicators

• Initial design

We design the low consequences indicators and the safety management indicators based on the ten key modules firstly.

• Airport survey

We go to an airport, organize the relevant experts to analyze the applicability of indicators. Then, we revise the risk monitoring indicators.

We develop the ten key modules risk monitoring indicators questionnaire after the initial risk monitoring indicators are formed, and collect 12 airports questionnaires.

• Revise and improve the indicators

The returned questionnaires are analyzed. We analyze the airports disagreement based on the principle of majority and the final low consequences indicators and safety management indicators are formed.

Take the vehicle and aircraft scratching module for example, part of the low consequences indicators and safety management indicators final formed are as shown in Table 1.

Table 1. Part of the vehicles and aircraft scratching module's low consequences indicators and safety management indicators.

Type	No	Safety Risk monitoring indicators
	1	The incidence of the infield vehicle driver speeding driving
	2	The incidence of the staff failing arrived at the designated location
	3	The incidence of the infield vehicle violations through the "stop" sign
	4	The incidence of passenger bridges operators' illegal operations
	5	The failure rate of passenger bridges
	6	The major change rate of key personnel
	7	The completion rate of safety training program
	8	The qualified rate of safety training

(2) The design of the high consequences indicators

The standard terms of incidents and occurrences associated with the ten key modules are identified based on the China "Civil aircraft incidents standard" and "Civil aviation occurrences sample". These incidents and occurrences identified formed the ten key modules related high consequence indicators.

Take the vehicle and aircraft scratching module for example, the high consequence indicators associated with this module include: The incidence of aircraft and aircraft, vehicles, equipment and facilities scratching that damage the aircraft; the incidence of aircraft and aircraft, vehicles, equipment and facilities scratching.

(3) Integrating various types of safety risk monitoring indicators

We integrated all the indicators to form the various types' indicators including high consequences indicators, low consequences indicators and safety management indicators associated with the ten key modules. Through the survey of the two airports, the safety risk monitoring indicators are analyzed, screened and improved; finally 165 airport operational risk monitoring indicators are established.

3 The Establishment of Airport Operational Risk Alerting Model

3.1 Principle

(1) Risk assessment principle

Safety risk is the combination of possibility and severity of the consequence or outcome from an existing hazard or situation.

On the basis of hazard identification and analysis, risk assessment evaluates the possibility of risk and the harm degree. Comparing with the safety standards, it can measure the risk level, and help us to determine whether to need to take corresponding measures. According to this principle, the key step of risk assessment is the comprehensive assessment of the likelihood and the severity of risk events, and then it needs to establish an acceptable level of safety standards.

The principle of risk assessment can provide theoretical foundation and concrete ideas for the airport operational risk alerting model.

(2) Heinrich's Law

Heinrich's Law was provided by Herbert William Heinrich in 1931. It became known as that in a workplace, for every accident that causes a major injury, there are 29 accidents that cause minor injuries and 300 accidents that cause no injuries. Because many accidents share common root causes, addressing more commonplace accidents that cause no injuries can prevent accidents that cause injuries.

Although this analysis will vary by the improvement of aircrafts' reliability and the management ability, it still illustrates the inevitable link between accidents and safety. Heinrich's Law is a warning for us. It shows that any accident has a reason and previous signs. On the other side, it tells us safety can be controlled, and the disaster can be avoided, It also gives us a method of safety management, which is finding and controlling the symptoms before bad consequences.

The Heinrich's Law can be used to prove the importance of lower-consequence indicators, and to establish the index of various indicators' severity.

(3) Safety performance management

The basic principle and methods of safety performance management is elaborated more in "safety management manual (ICAO's Doc9859), it propose the indicators for monitoring and evaluation organization safety status should include not only high consequence indicators, but also include low consequence indicators, and it gives the setting methods of safety performance indicators' target and alert level.

We use one incident rate per million flights at the airport as an example.

(1) Alert level setting

The alert level for a new monitoring period (current year) is based on the preceding period's performance (preceding year), namely its data points average and standard deviation. The three alert lines are average + 1 SD, average + ? SD and average + 3 SD.

(2) Alert level trigger

An alert (abnormal/unacceptable trend) is indicated if any of the conditions below are met for the current monitoring period (current year):

− Any single point is above the 3 SD line;
− 2 consecutive points are above the 2 SD line;
− 3 consecutive points are above the 1 SD line.

When an alert is triggered (potential high risk or out-of-control situation), appropriate follow-up action is expected, such as further analysis to determine the source and root cause of the abnormal incident rate and any necessary action to address the unacceptable trend.

3.2 The Airport Operational Risk Alerting Model

According to the above principle and the characteristics of the airport operation, the research needs these six steps to set up integrated Airport Operational Risk Alerting Model.

(1) Establish the layer of risk alerting model

The risk alerting model has three layers at least in our research as Fig. 3. The bottom layer calculate the different modules' risk that needs to use the indicator including high consequence indicators and low consequence indicators, the middle layer synthesize all modules' risk as one index for single airport, and finally, the upper layer synthesize all airport' risk as one index for an airport group.

(2) Assignment the severity weight of different indicators' corresponding event

Based on the principle of risk evaluation, safety risk is the combination of possibility and severity of the hazard. In our research, the possibility is the frequency of the happening, but the severity of the event needs to be standard uniformed and quantified.

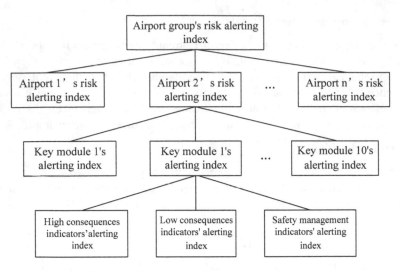

Fig. 3. Airport group risk alerting index model

Based on the China "Civil aircraft incidents standard" and "Civil aviation occurrences sample", the experts give different score according to the influence degree of the possible consequences. The score range is showed in Table 2.

Table 2. The severity weight range of various indicators

Risk Indicators rank	Severe flight incidents	General flight incidents and ground incidents	Occurrence/safety management corresponding event	Low consequence corresponding event
severity weight	[3,4)	[2,3)	[0.5,2)	[0.1,0.5)

(3) Define the severity coefficient of indictors

According to Heinrich's Law, the frequency of the events is 1:1/29:1/300:1/1000, we define the reciprocal of the frequency as severity coefficient, which means the severity coefficient of severe flight incidents, General flight incidents and ground incidents, Occurrence/safety management corresponding event and Low consequence corresponding event is 1000,35,3and1respectively. Use this method, we collect and analyze one airport group data from 2011-2014 to adjust the coefficient suitable for the real operation. Finally, we get the coefficient of severity is 4600:460:10:1

(4) Calculate monthly different modules' risk score

The modules' risk score is the sum of the indictors' corresponding events risk score.

(5) Calculate monthly risk index of single airport I

I = the sum of different modules' risk score/air traffic movements.

(6) Calculate monthly risk index for airport group Is

I_s is the average of all members of airport group risk index.

3.3   Example

The research picks two airport data for analysis, the actual operation data are collected from Aug to Oct, 2015. After calculating, the research gets the result as Table 3 shown.

Table 3. Monthly risk index of single airport

Month	Airport	Severity	Air traffic movements (thousand)	Risk
Aug.	A	222.2	8.773	25.33
	B	117.8	17	6.93
Sep.	A	150.2	6.385	23.52
	B	134.6	11.3	11.91
Oct.	A	155.4	6.378	24.37
	B	118.2	11.5	10.28

If we want to set the alert line or section, we need the data before the Aug. Thus, we give the virtual severity and risk index of airport A from Jan to Jul as Table 4 shown.

Table 4. Virtual Severity and Risk Index of airport A from Jan. to Jul

Month	Severity	Risk
Jan.	135.8	20.33
Feb.	192.0	24.52
Mar.	114.7	17.56
Apr.	188.0	28.96
May.	129.4	20.36
Jun.	170.2	26.78
Jul.	155.9	19.65

According the setting methods of safety performance indicators' target and alert level:

The average of airport A is 23.08, and the SD is 4.38, and

Average + 1 SD = 27.46;

Average + 2 SD = 31.84;

Average + 3 SD = 36.21.

The research assumes that the risk below 27(including 27) for green zone, 27-32 for yellow zone, 32-37 for orange zone, and above 37(including 37) for red zone. Based on the different zone, the research draw the Aug., Sep. and Oct.'s risk index as Fig. 4 shown.

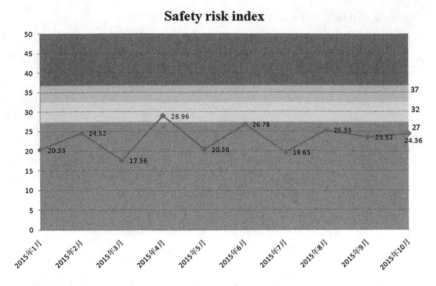

Fig. 4. Airport A's safety risk index

Use the same method, the research can draw the Aug., Sep. and Oct.'s severity as Fig. 5 shown.

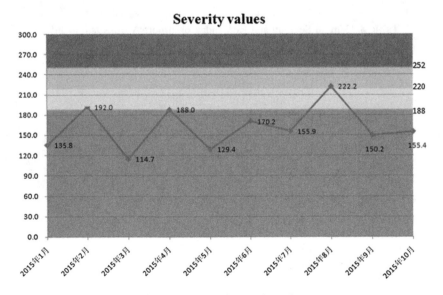

Fig. 5. Airport A's severity values

4 Conclusion and Recommendations

In summary, this research establishes the airport operational safety risk indicators based on the safety risk management theory and safety performance management theory. The airport operational risk alerting model is also established based on the Heinrich's Law, risk assessment principles and historical data of an airport group. This model is verified to be applicable through three months data collection, calculation and risk warning of two airports.

On the one hand, this research can be used of the more comprehensive scientific assessment of airport operational risk and warning to find the abnormal events or unacceptable risk to take preventive measures timely. On the other hand, it can also help to improve airport information reporting standards, in order to obtain more comprehensive operational process data.

References

1. ICAO. ICAO Doc9859 《Safety Management Manual》 Appendix 6 to Chapter 5 (2013)
2. Safety Management System and Safety Culture Working Group. Guidance on Hazard Identification. ECAST (2012)
3. Mei, R., Yanqiu, C., Yuan, Z.: The theory and method of safety performance management. Aviat. Saf. 17(1), 266–285 (2014)
4. Gang, L.: The study on airport safety risk identification and alerting. Doctoral thesis of Nanjing University of Aeronautics and Astronautics (2008)
5. Ruigang, Z.: The study of aviation risk assessment. Master thesis of Southwest Jiaotong University (2001)

Eye Movement Analysis for Expert and Non-expert in Japanese Traditional Culture of Tea Ceremony - From the View Point of Japanese Hospitality, "Omotenashi"

Tomoya Takeda[1], Yuki Miyamoto[2], Xiaodan Lu[1], Kayo Okuhira[2],
Noriyuki Kida[1], and Tomoko Ota[2(✉)]

[1] Kyoto Institute of Technology, Matsugasaki,
Sakyo-ku, Kyoto 606-6585, Japan
T.takeda@taste.jp
[2] Chuo Business Group, 1-6-6 Funakoshi-cho,
Chuo-ku, Osaka 540-0036, Japan
Promot1@gold.ocn.ne.jp

Abstract. The Japanese traditional culture of tea ceremony is sometime employed as a way to learn the spirit of "Omotenashi" that is a particularly Japanese form of hospitality. Because when conducting a tea ceremony, care and concern toward the attendants (the guests) are considered to be important. In tea ceremony, there are many states of mind that is important when receiving the guests at the ceremony, such as "Seven Rules of Rikyu", "Harmony, Respect, Quietness and Simplicity" or "Treasure Every Meeting, For It will Never Recur". Especially, attitudes that "the host must prepare thoroughly for the guests, stage a pleasant experience" and "the guest enjoys the preparation of the host" are important. In "Omotenashi", the side providing the service and the side receiving the service are equal, and the guest and the host (the one who invites guest) are also equal in tea ceremony. In our research, we study the lines of sight of the their guest to tea ceremonies and analyze the difference between experts and non-experts in order to learn the spirit of "Omotenashi" from tea ceremony. In this report, we focused on the eye movement of the guest. As the experiment method, we attached an eye movement measurement device to each guest (the side receiving the hospitality), and measured from the moment of tea preparation to just before the moment the guests drank their tea.

Keywords: The way of tea · Omotenashi · Eye movement · Expert · Non-expert

1 Introduction

Tea ceremony, which is considered to be the representative of Japanese traditional culture, is used as one of methods to learn the spirit of "Omotenashi" that is a particularly Japanese form of hospitality. That is because when conducting a tea ceremony, care and sympathy shown toward one's guest is considered to be the most

© Springer International Publishing Switzerland 2016
V.G. Duffy (Ed.): DHM 2016, LNCS 9745, pp. 596–603, 2016.
DOI: 10.1007/978-3-319-40247-5_60

important. In tea ceremony, there are attitudes, such as "Treasure Every Meeting, For It will Never Recur" that are crucial when hosting guests.

Especially, attitudes that "the host must prepare thoroughly for the guests, stage a pleasant experience" and "the guests enjoy the preparation of the host" are important. In "Omotenashi", the side that is providing the service and the side that is receiving the service are equal, and the guest and the host (the one who invites guest) are also equal in tea ceremony.

Moreover, there are many types of utensils (tea things) that are used for tea ceremony. Many of them are specific to tea ceremony, and the ways they are used are also unique.

Originally, tea ceremony (Sado) was called "Chato" or "Cha no Yu". The name "Sado" was adopted in early Edo period, and it is used until today. The ultimate aim of tea ceremony is the sense of harmony between the host and the guest. Therefore, elements such as tea things, chiefly among them the tea bowl, or hanging scroll with Zen wisdom hang in the alcove of tea room are more than just individual artworks. Rather, they are parts that constitute the whole, and the passing time of tea ceremony itself is regarded as a total work of art. The traditional Japanese act of boiling water, prepare tea and serve it, and the style and art based on this act, is considered to be a particularly Japanese "Omotenashi". In tea ceremony, the host that is holding the ceremony invites guests after careful preparation, and the guests are expected to understand the intention of the host, behave appropriately to the situation and show gratitude. In other words, they create pleasant space by the host and the guests becoming one. This "reciprocity of the host and the guests" is also called "unity of the hosts and the guests".

In our series of research, we study the lines of sight of the guests invited to tea ceremonies and those of their hosts and analyze the difference between experts and non-experts in order to learn the spirit of "Omotenashi" from tea ceremony. In this report, we focused on the eye movement of guests. In this report, we focused on the lines of sight of the guests in order to measure the difference between expert and non-expert when they are on the side that is receiving "Omotenashi", i.e. the side of the guests. As the experiment method, we attached an eye movement measurement device to each guest, and measured from the moment of tea preparation to just before the moment the guests drank their tea.

The reason why we focused on the eye movement is because the line of sight is considered to be more important than action in people. As acknowledged in proverb "The eyes are as eloquent as the mouth", eye movement is said to makes various impressions on others as one of non-verbal communication. In tea ceremony, the guests and the host are always in equal position, and on the whole, ceremony is conducted in silence. Therefore, line of sight is considered to be established as one of non-verbal communication. By analyzing these lines of sight, we will be able to understand the difference in Omotenashi of an expert and a non-expert, and we will be able to enjoy Omotenashi, based on the spirit of tea that aims to "Treasure Every Meeting, For It will Never Recur".

2 Research

2.1 Purpose

Research the eye movements of the expert and the non-expert who are acting as guests in a tea ceremony, and clarify their difference.

2.2 Method

2.2.1 Production of video footage to be analyzed.

The expert who is in the video is a male expert who is an instructor of tea ceremony. The other participant in the video is a beginner in tea ceremony. The expert participant in the video has 30 years experience in instruction of tea ceremony. He was evaluated as to have sufficient skill to be the expert participant in this video. Figure 2 shows the layout during the filming. A still image from the video is shown in Fig. 3.

The procedure for the research is Furo Usucha Tatemae (Furo Usucha Technique of tea preparation) from Ura Senke, which is the leading school of Japanese tea ceremony. It starts from picking up a tea ladle, taking tea from tea caddy and putting tea in tea bowl, and ends at making tea with tea whisk and serving it to the guest. (Table 1).

Table 1. Procedure of Preparing Tea in Furo Usucha Technique (Excerpt)

Content of Action	
1	Action of picking up a tea ladle with right hand.
2	Action of picking up a tea caddy with left hand, opening its lid with right hand while holding the tea ladle in the same hand, and putting the lid in front of right knee.
3	Action of changing the way one holds the tea ladle, scooping tea from the tea caddy and putting it in a tea bowl.
4	Action of closing the tea caddy and putting back the tea caddy and the tea ladle in their original position.
5	Action of scooping hot water from a teakettle with a dipper, pouring the right amount of hot water into the tea bowl, pouring back surplus hot water into the teakettle and gently place back the dipper on the teakettle (Kiribisyaku)
6	Action of picking up the tea bowl, preparing tea with a tea whisk and putting the whisk back to the original position.
7	Action of turning the tea bowl so that the correct side is facing the guest, and placing it with right hand to Joza (fixed position).
8	Action of receiving the greeting from the guest.

Based on the procedure shown in Table 1, it was classified into 6 steps in order to analyze eye movement analysis. 1 is the act of taking hot water from a teakettle. 2 is the act of pouring hot water into a tea bowl. 3 is the act of making tea with a tea whisk. 4 is the act of holding a tea bowl. 5 is the act of the guest holding the tea bowl. And 6 is the act of the guest drinking tea. (Table 2). This procedure was conducted by both the expert and the non-expert. When the host part was performed by the expert, the non-expert performed the part of guest and her eye movement was analyzed. In turn, when the host

Table 2. Process in Eve Movement Analysis

	Content of Action
1	Action of taking hot water from teakettle.
2	Action of pouring hot water into a tea bowl.
3	Action of making tea with a tea whisk.
4	Action of holding a tea bowl.
5	Action of the guest holding the tea bowl.
6	Action of the guest drinking tea.

Table 3. Classification of focal points of the guest part

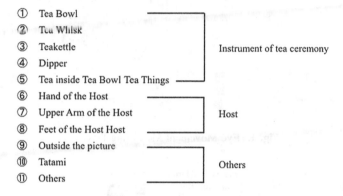

① Tea Bowl

② Tea Whisk

③ Teakettle ————————— Instrument of tea ceremony

④ Dipper

⑤ Tea inside Tea Bowl Tea Things ———

⑥ Hand of the Host

⑦ Upper Arm of the Host   Host

⑧ Feet of the Host Host

⑨ Outside the picture

⑩ Tatami   Others

⑪ Others

part was performed by the non-expert, the expert performed the part of guest and his eye movement was analyzed. Furthermore, area classification was conducted in order to identify the focal points of the eyes for the study of the eye movement, as shown in Table 3 (Figs. 1 and 4).

2.2.2   Research Procedure

Both the expert and the non-expert performed the role of the guest for 6 times and each time the eye movement of the guest part was measured. The eye movements of the test subjects were recorded on the video filmed by the eye movement measuring device. This video was played frame by frame, and the focal point of the guest in each frame was studied. (Table 3) After this focal point study was conducted from the beginning to the end of the video, a focal points graph data where the horizontal axis is time and the vertical axis is focal point were produced. With these graphs, the difference in the eye movements between the expert playing guest and the non-expert playing guest was researched.

2.3   Result

Table 4 is the eye movement of the expert playing the guest part. The expert did not only focus on the preparation of tea, i.e. the phenomenon in front of him, but also paid

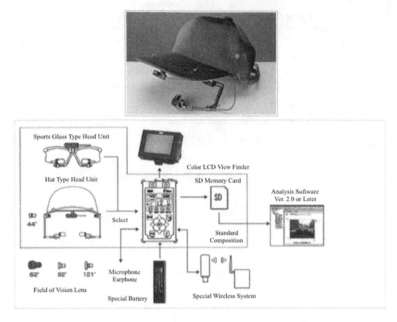

Fig. 1. Eye Movement Measuring Device

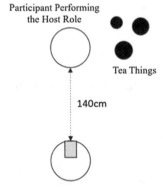

Fig. 2. Positions During the Research

attention to the tea things. In tea ceremony, the selection of the things is an important component of "Omotenashi". Therefore, it can be said that the expert feels the whole room in total as the space, and its atmosphere, while receiving hospitality, and he became one with the person preparing tea.

Table 5 is the eye movement of the non-expert playing the guest part. The non-expert focused only on the moving parts of the person preparing tea. This can be considered that she was merely following the gestures and hands movement of the person preparing tea.

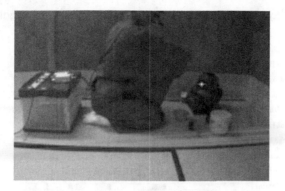

Fig. 3. Still from Study Video of Expert (1)

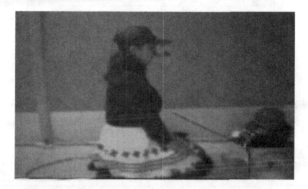

Fig. 4. Still from Study Video of Non-expert (2)

Next, we will discuss the step (1) and (2) as the comparison of each step. One of the etiquettes of tea ceremony is called "Sekiiri". In this, the convention is for the guest to look at and appreciate the decoration in alcove or the tea things in front of him/her. The lines of sight of the expert show that he was following this etiquette and paid attention to the teakettle or the tea things around the kettle. On the other hand, the focal point of the non-expert was recorded to be on the tatami floor at first. This suggests that she was more concerned about the rule that "One should not step on the edge of tatami" than the etiquette. The reason why you cannot step on the edge of tatami is that because the edge is considered to be the "face" of tatami in Japan. Each sheet of tatami has a pattern with vertical stripes called "Tatamime". Each of this Tatamime is about 1.5 cm, and in tea ceremony, the position of tea things is determined in relation to this Tatamime. Moreover, some tatamis have the family crest of the host on its edge. Therefore, as the crest represents the house of the host, stepping on it is considered to severely disrespect the ancestors of the host.

Following will discuss the step (3) and (4). In these steps, the expert elegantly observed the flow of procedures, and at the same time paid attention to the tea things being used. However, the non-expert paid attention to each procedure for too long, and it appears that she was trying to learn the correct movement, in other words the efficient and beautiful movement of the hands of the host.

Table 4. Eye Movement Data When the Expert Was Performing the Guest

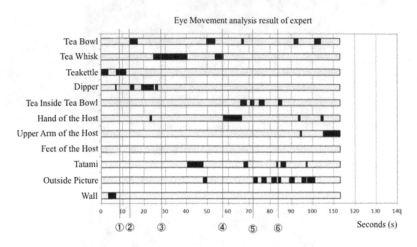

Table 5. Eye Movement Data When the Non-Expert Was Performing the Guest

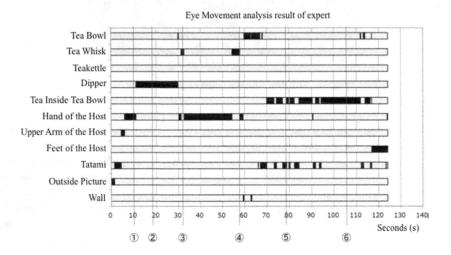

Lastly, steps (5) and (6) will be discussed. Before drinking the tea offered by the host, the expert naturally focused in order of, on inside the tea bowl (tea) → tatami → tea bowl → hand, for two rounds. The non-expert also naturally focused in order of, on inside the tea bowl (tea) → tatami → inside tea bowl (tea) → hand, and repeated it. Both the time it took in mixing tea with tea whisk and the time it took to pass on the prepared tea inside the tea bowl over tatami were longer then expert.

3   Discussion

When the expert was performing the role of guest, he focused not only on the movement of the host, but also on the tea things such as teakettle or tea whisk. The non-expert however focused only on the movement of the host. This led us to conclude that for the expert, tea things would also be important factors in enjoying a tea ceremony. On the other hand, the non-expert appeared to enjoy only the movement of the host. As the result of this research, the important element in enjoying a tea ceremony for the expert is not to focus only on the movement of the host, but also to appreciate the tea things, tea bowl or tea-set being used in the ceremony.

In tea ceremony, one can enjoy all the "five senses", namely sight, hearing, smell, touch and taste, in a tranquil space.

Utensils, hanging scroll or the tea things please the "sight", the sound of cracking charcoal, tea whisk cleansing or whisking tea please the "hearing", the smell of incense, charcoal and tea please the "smell", the surface of the tea bowl pleases the "touch", and the tea and sweets please the "taste".

In Japanese "Omotenashi", one can receive deeper hospitality by the guest and the host being in the equal position and sharing knowledge and education.

In future, we will research "Omotenashi" in tea ceremony, which is Japanese traditional culture, even deeper by measuring the lines of sight on the side of the host.

References

1. Tanko Text New Edition Temae-Hen 5, Tankosya, pp. 34–35 (1986)
2. Isao, K.: Japanese Omotenashi seen from tea ceremony, Shinkumi, pp. 20–22 (2015)
3. Masako, S., Mayumi, T.: Creation by both the host and the guest, Japanese Omotenashi seen from tea ceremony, Jinzai Kyoiku. Pract. J. Hum. Resor. Dev., pp. 52–55 (2014)
4. Masako, S.: Discussion on the inter-relationship between host and guest in tea ceremony (1), Hospitality. Jpn. Hospitality Manage. J., pp. 127–132 (2003)
5. Masako, S.: Discussion on the inter-relationship between host and guest in tea ceremony (2), Hospitality. Jpn. Hospitality Manage. J., pp. 141–148 (2004)

Automatic Imagery Data Analysis for Diagnosing Human Factors in the Outage of a Nuclear Plant

Pingbo Tang[1(✉)], Cheng Zhang[1], Alper Yilmaz[2], Nancy Cooke[3],
Ronald Laurids Boring[4], Allan Chasey[1], Timothy Vaughn[5],
Samuel Jones[5], Ashish Gupta[2], and Verica Buchanan[3]

[1] Del E. Webb School of Construction, Arizona State University,
Tempe, AZ, USA
{tangpingbo, czhan139, achasey}@asu.edu
[2] Department of Civil, Environment and Geodetic Engineering,
The Ohio State University, Columbus, OH, USA
{yilmaz.15, gupta.637}@osu.edu
[3] Human Systems Engineering Program, Arizona State University,
Mesa, AZ, USA
{Nancy.Cooke, ncooke, Verica.Buchanan, vbuchana}@asu.edu
[4] Idaho National Laboratory, Idaho Falls, ID, USA
ronald.boring@inl.gov
[5] Palo Verde Nuclear Generating Station, Tonopah, AZ, USA
{Timothy.Vaughn, Samuel.Jones}@aps.com

Abstract. Nuclear power plant (NPP) outages involve maintenance and repair activities of a large number of workers in limited workspaces, while having tight schedules and zero-tolerance for accidents. During an outage, thousands of workers will be working around the NPP. Extremely high outage costs and expensive delays in maintenance projects (around $1.5 million per day) require tight outage schedules (typically 20 days). In such packed workspaces, real-time human behavior monitoring is critical for ensuring safe collaboration among workers, minimal wastes of time and resources due to the lack of situational awareness, and timely project control. Current methods for detailed human behavior monitoring on construction sites rely on manual imagery data collection and analysis, which is tedious and error-prone. This paper presents a framework of automatic imagery data analysis that enables real-time detection and diagnosis of anomalous human behaviors during outages, through the integration of 4D construction simulation and object tracking algorithms.

Keywords: Human factors · Computer vision · Construction automation · Project control · Nuclear plant

1 Introduction

Nuclear power plant (NPP) outages involve maintenance and repair activities of a large number of workers in limited workspaces, while having tight schedules and zero-tolerance for accidents [1]. During a typical outage, more than 2,000 workers will

© Springer International Publishing Switzerland 2016
V.G. Duffy (Ed.): DHM 2016, LNCS 9745, pp. 604–615, 2016.
DOI: 10.1007/978-3-319-40247-5_61

be working around the NPP [2]. Expensive delays in maintenance projects (around \$1.5 million per day ode delay) require tight outage schedules (∼20 days) [3]. Any accidents or incidents can cause risks in collaborative field operations and unwanted wastes and delays.

Human factors play critical roles in busy workspaces that have high safety and productivity requirements. Improper design of site layouts and workspaces can force the workers to waste time on acquiring materials and tools for completing their work [1, 4]. Improper arrangements of workplaces can cause awkward positions of human bodies that reduce the productivity and increase the risks of occupational diseases [5, 6]. In addition, cluttered site conditions and occlusions can influence the capabilities of workers in recognizing potential risks on job sites [7–9]. When workers work simultaneously across multiple areas of a job site, their activities can rely on each other, or compete for limited workspaces and resources. Human errors, such as miscommunications between workers in crowded job sites, can cause unnecessary waiting of workers for collaboration activities or resources, or unexpected sharing of spaces and resources that reduces the productivity of scheduled tasks [10]. Comprehending and diagnosing human factors issues in outage processes and workspaces is thus important for proactive control of outage operations through real-time adjustment of resource allocations, and for improving the design of outage workspaces and processes as long-term solutions.

Existing methods and technologies used for outage control and human-factor analysis could hardly achieve real-time monitoring and analysis of outage processes. Such methodological limitations impede engineers from understanding certain details about how human factors contribute to the inefficiencies, accidents, and incidents observed during outages. In current practice, an Outage Control Center (OCC) has human individuals who observe multiple places across an outage jobsite and who exchange data and information with multiple groups of outage participants for coordination purposes [1]. Manual field data collection and analysis, including video data collection and interpretation, highly rely on the experiences, intuition, and cognitive capabilities of human individuals to achieve reliable and timely outage process monitoring and control. For busy and crowded jobsites of outages, a manual approach could hardly guarantee zero-errors and observation of all critical spatiotemporal details that are relevant to waste of time and resources, as well as risks that involve correlated operations at multiple locations.

This research proposes an automated multi-sensor-based outage control framework that enables effective detection and diagnosis of human behaviors that cause inefficiencies and risks in outage processes. In this framework, detection algorithms automatically detect objects that include workers, building elements, equipment, materials, equipment, and building structures from image sequences collected in the fields of views of cameras. Object tracking algorithms then monitor motion and changes of the detected objects for deriving construction progress and spatiotemporal relationships between workers, objects, and construction activities. A spatiotemporal comparison algorithm then automatically compares the as-designed construction progress and expected spatiotemporal relationships among workers, objects, and activities against the object recognition and tracking results for identifying discrepancies and dangerous spatiotemporal relationships that can cause accidents. Finally, human behavior modeling methods and anomaly detection algorithms will collectively diagnose human behaviors (e.g., very long waiting, frequent travels without much progresses, activities out of the order as specified in the schedules) that cause a majority of risks of delays and accidents. The authors expect that this integrated outage control framework will not only improve the safety, productivity, and quality of current outage project, but also provide sufficient data for future outages to reduce excessively long planning stage of an outage project.

2 Background Research and Literature Review

Figure 1 shows an overview of the envisioned outage control process that integrates advanced technologies in order to enable proactive control of an outage composed of large number of rapidly executed processes interwoven in both spatial and temporal domains. The overall process has three stages: (1) the inspection stage "discovers" parts of the nuclear plant that need maintenance before and during the outage, and generates a to-do list; (2) in the following scheduling stage, the to-do list generated by the inspection stage triggers the development of an outage project schedule (before the outage) and the update of that schedule (during the outage); (3) the execution stage will carry out the scheduled maintenance activities, under continuous monitoring and adjustment of engineers for ensuring the productivity and safety of the outage processes. This overall process is a loop of "outage control" during the outage, because information and data gathered from the field will guide outage participants to adjust their activities and resource allocation for minimizing the risks of delays and accidents/incidents, while maximizing the productivity.

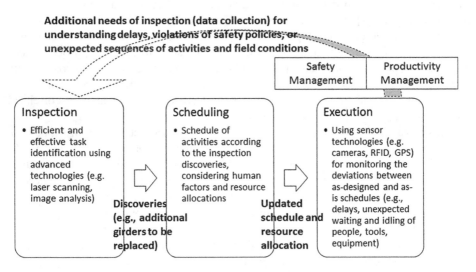

Fig. 1. Overview of the loops of outage control and technologies potentially useful

Within this loop of outage control, human factors issues play critical roles. As shown in Fig. 2, three major elements interact with each other and form various human-related problems in outage control. Quality of communication and collaboration between outage participants determines the performance of teamwork in terms of the timeliness, comprehensiveness, and responsiveness to changes in schedule, field conditions, and availability of resources. Communication protocol designs and team organizations involve considerations about human behaviors related to expressing their needs, perceiving messages from others, and psychological mechanisms related to collaboration behaviors within and between groups of outage participants. Interactions between project engineers and coordinators with field tasks generated based on maintenance needs are critical for improving the schedule updating process according to the field needs. Cognitive capability and behaviors of field engineers, coordinators, and people in the OCC determine the timeliness and effectiveness of schedule updates. On the other hand, various outage participants interact with the workspaces of tasks within outage processes while completing these tasks. The cognitive and physical conditions of human individuals can vary in different environments, because different environments pose different physical and environmental stresses to human individuals.

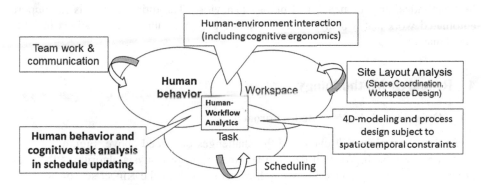

Fig. 2. Overview of human-related factors in nuclear plant outage control

Previous studies in the domains of civil and construction engineering, computer vision, cognitive science, and geospatial analysis have demonstrated the potential for automating the monitoring of human behaviors within engineering workflows, though serious barriers still exist. Computer vision algorithms can extract features from videos in order to detect and track objects across multiple videos taken at different locations [11]. However, when the number of objects increases, the computational complexity and reliability of tracking objects having interwoven trajectories become unacceptable [12]. Some civil engineering applications share the same needs and job site environments as nuclear plants, and computer vision technologies tested in civil engineering applications have the potential to support NPP operation and maintenance activities. For example, construction engineering researchers have examined automatic spatial data collection techniques, such as 3D laser scanning, for automated workspace modeling and management [13, 14]. The authors believe those methods can also assist in the management of NPPs. To date, such civil engineering studies have mostly focused on deriving spatial information for progress monitoring and quality control [13, 14]. Limited studies were devoted to comprehending how behaviors of workers produce bottlenecks and risks in construction workflows in packed workspaces, such as the ones in outage control.

3 Scientific Objectives

The scientific objectives of the presented study include: (1) Establish real-time object/human tracking and spatiotemporal analysis methods for automatically comparing the productivity and expected arrangements of field activities against as-planned schedules and field operation rules related to safety and productivity; (2) Establish human factors modeling methods for automatically detecting anomalous human behaviors that cause risks and inefficiencies in the field, such as unexpected trajectories of workers that cause inefficient collaborations between the OCC, satellite outage centers, NPP workers, and maintenance service providers. The authors expect that addressing these scientific objectives will assist automated and proactive outage control based on more timely and detailed spatiotemporal information from the field related to field activities, environments, and human behaviors. The ultimate goal is to support automated work status analysis and automatic pending support notifications in NPP maintenance.

4 Research Methodology

4.1 Overview of the Proposed Approach

The proposed project will overcome the challenges described above. Figure 3 shows the overall approach. We will develop automatic image analysis algorithms that can process 3D imageries collected by depth cameras, such as the Kinect sensor, to track 3D motions of human and equipment in packed workspaces, as well as process 2D imageries collected by electro-optical cameras to track the changes across large and open job sites. Image analysis algorithms would enable reliable workflow surveillance, as well as detailed analysis of interactions among outage participants. The outputs of the imagery analysis algorithms will represent the real-time status of various elements (human, objects, and spatiotemporal relationship among them) within outage workflows. Comparing real-time status against the as-planned status of workflow will reveal inefficiencies and risks. Such a comparison has two aspects:

1. "Workflow Performance Analysis" focuses on assessing the productivity of various activities and spatiotemporal relationships among these activities. Anomaly in certain activities can cause delays which may propagate into stoppages in workflows. Comparing the real-time schedule against the as-planned schedule can help decision makers to update the schedule and avoid waste. In some cases, decision makers also have safety concerns related to improper spatiotemporal relationships between activities (lifting using a crane would prohibit having a human below the crane).

2. "Human Performance Analysis" focuses on assessing the trajectories of people and interactions among them. Unexpected long interactions and trajectories can cause inefficiencies. Improper design and arrangement of equipment and workspaces can also cause inefficiencies and risks related to human factors. Thus, an awareness of anomalies related to human factors will guide decision makers in improving the design of the OCC.

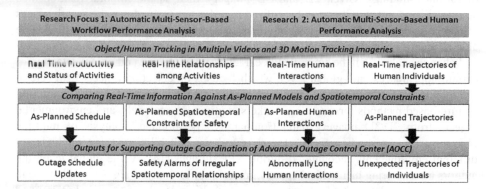

Fig. 3. Overview of the automatic imagery analysis framework for NPP outage control

4.2   Real-Time Object/Human Tracking and Spatiotemporal Analysis

This part of the computational framework involves the following elements: (1) Real-time and robust algorithms that reliably track human, equipment and environmental objects across multiple videos and monitor their changes (e.g., motions, addition, and removal); (2) Real-time assessment of the progress and productivity of individual activities, based on object/human tracking results. The approach is to match both the features of human/objects/activities (colors, shapes), and their spatiotemporal relationships, with contextual human/objects/activities (objects or human individuals having similar spatiotemporal contexts) in order to identify corresponding human/objects in multiple imageries. The purpose is to reduce the search space of corresponding human individuals or objects in multiple imageries, while improving the reliability of human/object tracking. The paragraphs below describe these methods in detail.

Tracking location changes, additions, and removal of human or objects relevant to maintenance activities is important for understanding the progress of the work. For example, movements of construction equipment and tools indicate active workspaces and additions or removals of building components indicate the progress of installations. Frequent motions of people in certain areas indicate how active workspaces are in terms of human activities. The challenge here is how to ensure the comprehensiveness, robustness, and computational efficiency of human/object tracking in cluttered environments while determining changes of objects. A typical NPP outage site could have numerous moving people and objects within cluttered environments. Tracking large numbers of people or objects while considering occlusions and clutters in busy workspaces could be unreliable and thus require large amounts of computing time and memory with the use of conventional object tracking methods [6]. When multiple objects in the workspaces have similar appearances (e.g., similar machines, similar ductworks, etc.), reliable object tracking becomes even more difficult.

In this research, we use depth cameras, such as Kinect sensors, for capturing 3D objects and their motion in smaller spaces (e.g., imaging range < 10 m), and using high-resolution cameras for tracking objects in large and open spaces, such as on roofs of turbine buildings. Given 2D and 3D imagery data, spatiotemporal relationships among objects and activities will be utilized in order to narrow down the search spaces of object tracking, and to correct ambiguities caused by similar objects; we will then be able to identify added and removed objects. Specifically, two levels of object tracking and change analysis will be employed: local level, which focuses on object detection of certain appearances, and global level, which focuses on detecting objects with certain spatiotemporal relationships to contextual objects. At the local level, we are examining feature-based methods for detecting workers, equipment, materials, and environmental objects from 2D/3D imagery data. Comparative performance analysis of multiple object tracking methods are expected to reveal the suitability of these methods for different environments encountered during NPP outages [14]. At the global level, the authors are exploring hierarchical spatiotemporal pattern analysis algorithms that group spatiotemporal relationships among objects at multiple levels of details (LODs), and match spatiotemporal relationships at multiple LODs to constrain the object tracking algorithms for reducing the search space. Figure 4 shows spatial relationships matched across multiple imagery data sets in order to identify corresponding lines extracted from different images.

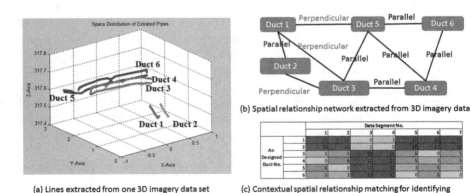

(a) Lines extracted from one 3D imagery data set

(b) Spatial relationship network extracted from 3D imagery data

(c) Contextual spatial relationship matching for identifying lines having similar spatial contexts as corresponding ducts in other 3D imagery data sets

Fig. 4. Matching spatial relationships between objects for associating lines from different imagery data sets when dislocations, additions, and removals of ducts occur.

4.3   Automatic Workflow and Human Performance Diagnosis Through Comparing Field Observations and as-Planned Activities

This part of the computational framework involves the following elements: (1) Algorithms that automatically compare the observed maintenance activities and their spatiotemporal contexts against the expected ones for revealing anomalous activities that indicate inefficiencies and risks in outage processes; (2) Algorithms that automatically compare the observed human behaviors against the expected ones for identifying anomalous interactions between human individuals and environmental conditions that indicate how human performance influences the productivity and safety of an outage. Outputs of these algorithms collectively provide observations that assist the OCC in detecting and addressing possibly improper team arrangements and behaviors, as well as observations that assist safety engineers in detecting unsafe human motions and time-wasting human activities, such as abnormally long conversations between human individuals in areas where progress lags behind, or unexpected trajectories of workers that are long and not following the safe and productive paths as expected by the OCC.

Given the human/object tracking results, the algorithm can then assess the status of individual activities. The objective is to associate object tracking and change detection results with specific activities in the outage schedule, and then determine the "resource consumption status" (number of workers and equipment used) of those activities and real-time progress. Specifically, to assess the status of an activity (e.g., lifting a girder to the roof), the authors acquired the location, needed resources, and expected progress information of the assessed activity from the as-planned schedules. Detailed motions of construction activities in a 4D (3D geometrics plus time dimension) simulation environment further reveal how spatiotemporal arrangements of maintenance activities within outage workspaces influence the productivity and safety of field operations. Figure 5 shows a conceptual 4D simulation: two jobsites working in parallel are sharing one safety inspector and one material/tool storage place; the time needed for a cycle of checking out materials/tools, safety checking, working, and checking out materials/tools again can fluctuate as uncertainties exist in human behaviors, field conditions, and availability of the safety inspector and storage place shared by two job sites.

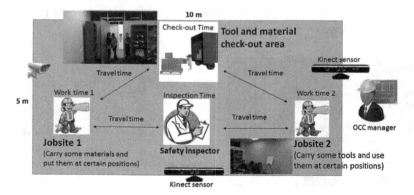

Fig. 5. A 4D simulation example: one safety inspector shared by two job sites

A 4D simulation will generate random numbers about the amounts of time needed for each step in those cyclic processes using the average and variance information of productivity based on historical productivity data, and execute workflows with steps that have uncertain durations for predicting the most likely productivity of the whole process. Simulation models can help engineers predict the "as-planned" waiting time of workers for the safety inspector and the material/tool storage area, considering uncertainties in the durations of traveling and working.

Assuming that the real-time schedule would have similar activities and relationships among them as the as-planned schedule, the authors are examining an algorithm that compares the location information of activities in the as-planned schedule against the object tracking results from imaging sensors (depth cameras and CCD cameras) that are pointing to those locations in the field. Specifically, the algorithm will match the detected objects, including workers, equipment, building elements, and materials, against the resource information in the as-planned schedule. Such matching between imagery data and as-planned schedules associates objects in the as-planned schedule with objects detected in imagery data. Given such data-schedule associations, the authors are testing an algorithm that automatically uses the "addition" events of building elements for progress monitoring (e.g., counting the number of elements installed against the as-planned progress), and then use the activity durations derived from imagery data to calculate the productivity.

In order to achieve real-time 2D/3D imagery data analysis for detecting anomalous interactions between people and anomalous trajectories, the authors are using object-tracking algorithms in recognizing roles of people on outage job sites, and analyzing motions of these people that indicate interactions between them. Specifically, this research focuses on lifting operations around turbine buildings and cooling towers. The authors are designing a field experiment that has crane operators, helpers, NPP safety personnel, and field supervisors wear different vests and hard hats to indicate their roles, and uses the spatial contexts of people and communication frequencies between certain people for checking the tracking results. Figure 6 shows a test case of tracking multiple people and inferring their social relationships based on the time periods shared by them in a scene observed by a camera. The research team is using this tested algorithm for recognizing roles of outage participants and individuals who have close collaboration relationships with each other in outage processes. Such information can help the OCC diagnose how interactions among people influence the productivity of outage.

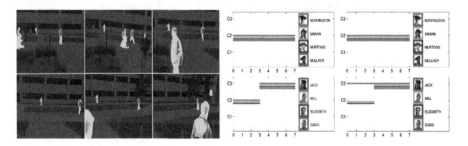

Fig. 6. Tracking multiple people in an outdoor scene (left); inferred relationships (right)

Given the tracked motions and gestures of people, the authors will be applying a pattern classification approach that uses example images having behaviors labeled (e.g., talking, nodding) for "training" the classifier. The trained classifier will then take new images for automatically classifying motions and gestures as various interactions. Comparing the frequency, time and durations of those interactions against the baseline model will reveal anomalous interactions.

Another part of the studied computational framework is to analyze the trajectories of individuals in identifying unexpected motions. The motion tracking results capture the motions of workers staying at a place to complete a task, and the trajectories and velocities of movements of workers across workspaces. The authors plan to compare the trajectories' information (paths, speeds, frequencies of travels) against the expected trajectories based on the literature review and interviews. Anomalous motions will involve trajectories significantly different from expected trajectories, unexpectedly frequent travels, and movements having speeds significantly slower or faster than as-planned speeds. This information will assist human factors scientists in under-standing how the arrangement of working environments influences worker efficiency and safety. In addition, the human motions and posture analysis information from the OCC will also assist human factors engineers to design better control centers that improve the efficiency and effectiveness of OCC personnel (e.g., better table size, computer and control panel design for improved human performance).

The last part of the computational framework will be conducting spatiotemporal relationship analysis among multiple activities and objects in order to assess improper spatiotemporal arrangements that could lead to incidents or accidents. Currently, this part of research is in the planning stage, the authors plan to transfer the object tracking and change detection results into simulation models of job sites. The real-time pro-ductivity information derived by human/object tracking algorithms would be the input for updating the as-planned schedule into the real-time schedule. The movements of equipment, workers, and other objects would produce a safety simulation model for predicting likely clashes between objects, and alert us risky relationships (e.g., crane above a human). Safety manuals of outage list all types of improper spatial arrange-ments in the field as "risky relationships".

5   Results of Experimental Design and Workflow Simulation

The authors have designed an indoor experiment to test the proposed computational framework described above for automatically identifying inefficiencies in field work-flows and anomalous human behaviors. Figure 5 shows the layout of the room for testing the human/object tracking and imagery analysis algorithms. This figure also shows the locations of two Kinect sensors and one camera for observing the scene. Figure 7 shows the simulation model designed by us for serving as the as-designed process. The representation of this simulation model follows the specification defined in [15]. A comparison of the automatic imagery data analysis results and the simulation results will validate the technical feasibility of the proposed computational framework.

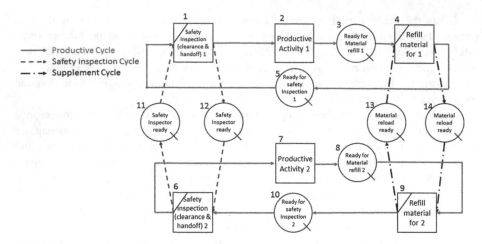

Fig. 7. Process simulation model for testing the proposed computational framework

6 Conclusion

This paper presents a computational framework that enables automatic imagery data analysis for diagnosing human factors in the outage of a nuclear plant. The literature review and preliminary studies conducted by the authors revealed the technical feasibility and potential of this computational framework. Future studies will be carrying out the experiments and field data collection during real outages for improving and validating this computational framework.

Acknowledgement. This material is based upon work supported by the U.S. Department of Energy (DOE), Nuclear Engineering University Program (NEUP) under Award No. DE-NE0008403. DOE's support is acknowledged. Any opinions and findings presented are those of authors and do not necessarily reflect the views of DOE.

References

1. St. Germain, S.W., Farris, R.K., Whaley, A.M., Medema, H.D., Gertman, D.I.: Guidelines for Implementation of an Advanced Outage Control Center to Improve Outage Coordination, Problem Resolution, and Outage Risk Management. Idaho National Laboratory, Idaho Falls (2014)
2. Wilson, C.: when the outage workers come to town - nuclear energy institute. In: News Arch. Nucl. Energy Inst. (2014). http://www.nei.org/News-Media/News/News-Archives/When-the-Outage-Workers-Come-to-Town. Accessed 25 Feb. 2016
3. Roadtechs: Nuclear outage list. In: Interact. Site Travel. Contract. (2016). https://www.roadtechs.com/nukeout.htm. Accessed 26 Feb. 2016

4. Wang, C., Zhang, J., Yu, H., Dai, S.: Marine nuclear power plant human error analysis and protective measures. In: Long, S., Dhillon, B.S. (eds.) Proceedings of the 14th International Conference on Man-Machine-Environment System Engineering. LNEE, vol. 318, pp. 33–42. Springer, Heidelberg (2010). http://link.springer.com/chapter/10.1007/978-3-662-44067-4_4

5. Ray, S.J., Teizer, J.: Real-time construction worker posture analysis for ergonomics training. doi:10.1016/j.aei.2012.02.011

6. Seo, J., Han, S., Lee, S., Kim, H.: Computer vision techniques for construction safety and health monitoring. Adv. Eng. Inform. 29, 239–251 (2015). doi:10.1016/j.aei.2015.02.001

7. Carbonari, A., Giretti, A., Naticchia, B.: A proactive system for real-time safety management in construction sites. Autom. Constr. (2011)

8. Mitropoulos, P., Memarian, B.: Team Processes and Safety of Workers: Cognitive, Affective, and Behavioral Processes of Construction Crews (2012)

9. Mitropoulos, P., Namboodiri, M.: New method for measuring the safety risk of construction activities: task demand assessment. J. Constr. Eng. Manag. 137, 30–38 (2011). doi:10.1061/(ASCE)CO.1943-7862.0000246

10. Boring, R.L., Griffith, C.D., Joe, J.C.: The Measure of human error: direct and indirect performance shaping factors. In: 2007 IEEE 8th Hum. Factors Power Plants HPRCT 13th Annual Meeting, pp. 170–176. IEEE (2007)

11. Berclaz, J., Fleuret, F., Turetken, E., Fua, P.: Multiple object tracking using K-Shortest paths optimization. IEEE Trans. Pattern Anal. Mach. Intell. 33, 1806–1819 (2011). doi:10.1109/TPAMI.2011.21

12. Teizer, J., Vela, P.A.: Personnel tracking on construction sites using video cameras. Adv. Eng. Inform. 23, 452–462 (2009). doi:10.1016/j.aei.2009.06.011

13. Turkan, Y., Asce, M., Bosché, F., Haas, C.T., Haas, R.: Toward Automated Earned Value Tracking Using 3D Imaging Tools, vol. 139, pp. 423–433 (2013). doi:10.1061/(ASCE)CO.1943-7862.0000629

14. Yang, J., Arif, O., Vela, P.A., Teizer, J., Shi, Z.: Tracking multiple workers on construction sites using video cameras. Adv. Eng. Informatics. 24, 428–434 (2010). doi:10.1016/j.aei.2010.06.008

15. Martinez, J.C., Ioannou, P.G.: General-purpose systems for effective construction simulation. J. Constr. Eng. Manage. 125(4), 265–276 (1999). http://doi.org/10.1061/(ASCE)0733-9364(1999)125:4(265)

Constructing a Decision-Support System for Safe Ship-Navigation Using a Bayesian Network

Ruolan Zhang[(⊠)] and Masao Furusho

Graduate School of Maritime Sciences, Kobe University, 5-1-1 Fukae-Minami,
Higashinada, Kobe 6580022, Japan
156w204w@stu.kobe-u.ac.jp,
furusho@maritime.kobe-u.ac.jp

Abstract. In a complicated sea environment, a ship needs experienced sea-farers to steer it safely. Advancements in technology have not fundamentally reduced the number of accidents at sea. In deep-seated research and analysis of accident causes, human factors will always have an obvious or potential impact. Maritime transport is an arduous industry. Workers' willingness to engage in seafaring occupations is gradually decreasing. This is an irreversible trend. The seafarer shortage and the seriousness of the safety situation are seemingly irreconcilable. To address this situation, the automation of ship equipment and intelligent decision-making must be accelerated. Autonomous decision-making is a basic step toward intelligent or unmanned navigation. The purpose of this paper is to construct a human-in-the-loop decision-support system for safe ship navigation, to minimize the impact of human factors, to reduce the accidents that occur because of poor human decision-making, and to ensure the ship will navigate safely at sea. This presupposes that a reliable decision-support system can be constructed. It requires relatively accurate predictions, based on past experience and objective accident-probability statistics. A Bayesian network can be used for risk and accident predictions. Therefore, the principles of a Bayesian network can be used for collision avoidance, and also for decisions on other sea conditions during a voyage. This paper discusses the prospects of an intelligent decision-support system to ensure reliable navigation safety, using a decision-support systematic approach, with a Bayesian network.

Keywords: Decision support system · Navigation · Bayesian network · Decision-making · Human factors · Ship safety

1 Introduction

In recent years, great oceanic powers have proposed future maritime strategy objectives. The next generation of intelligent maritime transports has already triggered a new upsurge in research. For example, Japan has proposed an E-navigation strategy. Hasegawa et al. [1] have specifically described intelligent ship-navigation systems for the future. Europe has unmanned ship research organizations based on smart networks, e.g., the European-Union-funded Maritime Unmanned Navigation through Intelligence

V.G. Duffy (Ed.): DHM 2016, LNCS 9745, pp. 616–628, 2016.
DOI: 10.1007/978-3-319-40247-5_62

in Networks (MUNIN) project. Rødseth and Burmeister [2] discuss some of the key challenges for unmanned ships in existing navigational-aid conditions. Intelligent ship designs have been envisioned by large companies, e.g., autonomous navigation research from Rolls-Royce PLC in the merchant ship field.

Objectively speaking, in the ancient merchant-shipping industry, the speed of automation research and development, even the unmanned process of maritime transportation systems (MTS), is very slow, compared with Google and other Internet and automotive companies. However, considering the risk of maritime transport and the monotony of the crew's work, intellectualization and automation should have greater development prospects in the MTS field. A research approach that draws on road transportation systems is necessary, especially in maritime transport safety and other important areas.

Trucco [3] used a Bayesian belief network—a specific extended application—for marine-traffic risk assessment. In his discussion, Trucco integrated human and organizational factors, using a Bayesian network to support hazard identification and assessment. This model had good risk-assessment support for a human involved in the situation, but it did not integrate a decision support system. When a ship encounters a dangerous situation, this model cannot play the role of decision support. This study intends to further use the Bayesian network approach to construct decision-support systems for handling complicated hazards in a sea environment.

In other areas, e.g., medical care quality, Ltifi [4] used Dynamic Decision Support Systems in the healthcare domain (MDDSS). Ltifi used the Knowledge Discovery from Databases (KDD) process technique in Dynamic Bayesian Networks (DBN), and proved that it can be used in a complex system when the situations are dubious and/or the raw data are complex structures. Lepreux [5] described a methodological process for the design and evaluation of a Human-Machine interactive system in an industrial railway context. In the maritime transportation field, Abu-Tair [6] presented a practical solution for obstacle (e.g., target ship) detection and collision avoidance, mainly for Unmanned Surface Vehicles (USVs). Perera [7] used a fuzzy-logic-based parallel decision-making (PDM) module and a Bayesian-network-based module to present a collision-avoidance system (CAS) at sea. It could handle multiple parallel collision-avoidance decisions, regarding several target-ship collisions. The decisions are executed as continuous handling actions to avoid complex collision situations at sea.

Seafarers at sea have their own unique traditions. To develop the features of this work, the same content was repeated extensively, which has been proved to be an appropriate and simple approach to automation. However, the complete ship navigation operation must have sufficient experience to deal with unexpected accidents or emergency situations. Before an accident, the officer of the watch (OOW) must have the ability to cut off the line caused by the accident. Therefore, based on experience and collected data, using Bayesian methods to make predictions, we can construct a decision-support system to help the OOW judge the danger and make decisions, before the accident, to achieve the safe navigation of the ship.

2   Reliable Decision Support System

Since "Preventing Collisions at Sea" was added to the International Maritime Organization (IMO) regulations, the proportion of accidents caused by human factors has increased year by year. For many accidents, an in-depth analysis has always found a human-factor impact. When conducting a comprehensive assessment on the safe navigation of a ship, Furusho [8] summarized four factors of safe ship navigation, according to the MTS characteristics: Man, machines, media, and management. Human factors are an important part of ship safety. The authors of this article also pointed out in a previous paper [9] that when constructing the basis for next-generation ship-navigation safety, a human (OOW) should be at the core position and at the top decision-making layer in collision avoidance. Therefore, when constructing a reliable decision-support system, the presupposition is to achieve autonomous ship-collision avoidance with automatic navigation.

2.1   Decision Pyramid

Safe ship navigation requires an operating system composed of two departments: the bridge and the engine room. (This is also called a conventional or traditional operating system). This operating system needs an automatic identification system (AIS), electronic chart display and information system (ECDIS), global positioning system (GPS), and a series of sensors to receive the navigation-environment information, estimate and operate the ship according to the OOW's experience and skills, and avoid collisions or other difficulties. According to the previous discussion, it is necessary to design a next-generation reliable and compatible artificial-intelligence decision-making pyramid system. Figure 1 shows the Bayesian methods of artificial intelligence decision-support systems, which comprise the decision-making pyramid: OOW, Bayesian network method (BN Process), Operating System, Physical Environment, and Navigation Environments.

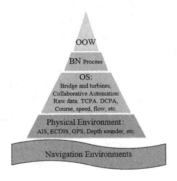

Fig. 1. Decision pyramid for safe navigation

2.2 Safe Ship Navigation Process

For safe ship navigation using the decision-making process of the pyramid, the structure needs all aspects of technology research support, e.g., sensors collecting the ship's environmental information, turbine reliability, ship maneuverability, steering stability, training of the Bayesian network nodes and structures, etc.

The physical environment of the ship includes the ship's structure, anti-shear properties, stability, pressure stability, balance stability, etc. Another part is the performance of various sensors, including the AIS, ECDIS, GPS, depth sounder, etc. The navigation environment information is received by sensors; environment information can include the performance data of the ship itself, sea-state information, and the target-ship information. The specific classifications are shown in Table 1.

Table 1. Navigation environment information

Own ship	Service life of the navigational equipment, error range; Service life of the navigational sensors, error range; Steerage performance (rudder effectiveness), stability, damage stability, etc.; Course, speed, draft, ballast situation, nature of cargo; Etc.
Environment	Position of the shore, reefs, offshore platforms; visibility; Flow, direction of flow, flow rate; wind, wind direction, wind speed; temperature, etc.; Etc.
Target ships	Ship name, call sign, maritime mobile service identity (MMSI), IMO code, kind of ship, length, width, etc.; Latitude, longitude, heading, range itineraries, speed, etc.; Ship status, draft, destination, estimated time of arrival (ETA), etc.; Etc.

Navigation-related data can be automatically calculated by the operating system, according to the relevant IMO navigation regulations. For security, the information can be submitted to the operating system to select the steering operation. Guo et al. [10] compared the cerebellar model arithmetic computer (CMAC) neural network, the fuzzified CMAC, the bang-bang CMAC, and several of the more common methods of ship steering. The proposed multiple-fuzzy CMAC (MFCMAC) algorithm adopts the advantages of each mode and yields better control performance than each algorithm by itself. Under difficult circumstances, if the normal collision-avoidance operation cannot be completed, the navigation environment is extreme, or there is no trained data support, a Bayesian network (BN) can help avoid the collision based on the collected information of the past. When the available data do not allow the Bayesian network to make a complete decision, or past data on encountering the current situation is too sparse, the decision cannot be made. The OOW must complete the operation before the hazard occurs. Many complex situations are encountered at sea. The main objective of this paper is focused on how to make a collision-avoidance decision when one's own ship and the target ship constitute the hazard-encounter situation.

With the data and structure trained by the BN, the system will support more conditions for automatic hazard prediction and decision-making. Finally, approaching the top of the decision pyramid, there will be less need for human participation in the decision-making. In the end, the human (OOW) could be replaced, and the necessary decision support and ship manipulation could be done remotely. This is an inevitable trend for the automated safe navigation of ships and autonomous decision-making processes.

3 Using Bayesian Networks to Support Decision-Making

On February 7, 2006, the Japanese body of maritime safety submitted a document to the Maritime Safety Committee of the International Maritime Organization (IMO) [11]. This document (MSC/81/18-1) presented how to use Bayesian network modeling in a formal safety assessment. The Bayesian network uses the past data as well as human factors. (The human (OOW) involved in the ship handling will generate a new data node, which will directly influence the exactness of the system prediction.) A Bayesian prediction, using a method that combines the objective and subjective information, can handle abnormal situations, recognize unknown conditions, or reasonably predict an unexpected emergency situation, by monitoring and then supporting the appropriate decision.

3.1 Definition of a Bayesian Network

A Bayesian network is a mathematical graphical prediction model based on probabilistic reasoning (a type of statistical model) that represents a set of random variables and their conditional dependencies via a directed acyclic graph (DAG). The Bayesian network provides statistical predictions, not only with reference to the objective data, but also to subjective information. At present, the Bayesian network does not have a universally accepted definition. In 2001, "Jensen" stated that a network with conditional independence and d-separation that satisfies the following four conditions is called a Bayesian network:

  I. There is a set of variables $V=\{Xi\}$, i=1,2,...,n, that correspond to nodes; between the nodes is a set of directed edges E;
 II. Each variable takes a finite number of discrete values;
III. Using the nodes and the variables corresponding to the directed edges between the nodes, construct a directed acyclic graph $G = (V, E)$;
IV. Each stage of Xi and its parent node set $\prod_i$, corresponds to a conditional probability distribution table $p(x_i|\pi_i, G)$, and satisfies $p(x_1,x_2,...,x_n) = \prod_{i=1}^{n} p(x_i|\pi_i, G)$.

3.2 Bayesian Probability and Prediction

Good predictions can help decision makers make reliable decisions. A Bayesian probability is derived from Bayesian statistics. If a hazard occurs, depending on the extent the OOW is trusted (this is usually a subjective probability), the OOW (or system), based on prior knowledge and existing observational data (trained data), uses probabilistic methods to predict the risk and make decisions. Note $D = \{x1 = x1,$ $X2 = x2,..., Xn = xn\}$ of the observed sample, in which X is an event variable, and x is the variable state or variable weights. Parameter θ is the prior probability of the occurrence of event X $[\theta = P(x \mid \xi)]$ and $P(\theta \mid \xi)$ is a probability function, in which ξ is the prior experience of the OOW.

The Bayesian probability can be stated as follows: Given a prior probability $\theta = P$ $(x \mid \xi)$ and an observed sample D, seeking an operation step of $n + 1$ times, the probability of occurrence of event $Xn + 1$ is $P(Xn + 1 = xn + 1 \mid D, \xi)$. According to the stated Collision Regulations of the International Convention and the Predetermined Decision-Making System Ship Collision-Avoidance model, Bayesian methods can be used to construct a basic prediction sample; the process is shown in Fig. 2.

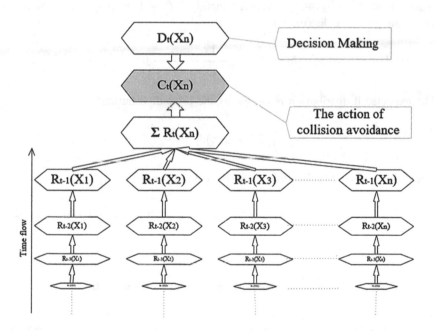

Fig. 2. Part of a sample flowchart for collision avoidance

Here, $R_t(X_n)$ represents the probability of collision risk encountered in ship navigation, and corresponds to $P(\theta \mid D, \xi)$; $R_{t-1}(X_n)$ represents the prior probability of $R_t(X_n)$, and corresponds to $p(\theta \mid \xi)$. According to the Bayesian formula, the posterior probability of formula $p(\theta \mid D, \xi)$ can be calculated by a prior probability $p(\theta \mid \xi)$:

$$P(\theta \mid D, \xi) = \frac{P(\theta \mid \xi)P(D \mid \theta, \xi)}{P(D \mid \xi)} = \frac{P(\theta \mid \xi)P(D \mid \theta, \xi)}{\int P(\theta \mid \xi)P(D \mid \theta, \xi)d\theta}.$$

In the prior probability ($\theta \mid \xi$), a known sample D is conditionally independent of each event X. According to the ship sailing conditions and conforming to the international regulations for preventing collisions, the operation of variable X is only considered as a binary distribution. p ($\theta \mid$ D, ξ) = $\theta^h (1 - \theta)^t$, in which h is the number of occurrences of the event in a sample D, and h + t = n.

Hypothesis. If a prior probability satisfies a β distribution, according to the distribution of the conjugate-distribution principle, the posterior probability is also a β distribution.

$$P(\theta \mid \xi) = \beta(\theta \mid r_h, r_t) = \frac{\Gamma(r)}{\Gamma(r_h)\Gamma(r_t)} \theta^{r_h - 1}(1 - \theta)^{r_t - 1},$$

where $r_h > 0$, $r_t > 0$ is a β-distribution parameter, and prior experience is determined by nature itself. $R = r_h + r_t$. Gamma Function Γ (x + 1) = $x\Gamma$ (x), Γ (1) = 1.
   Then, the posterior distribution

$$p(\theta \mid D, \xi) = \beta(\theta \mid r_h + h, r_t + t) = \frac{\Gamma(r + n)}{\Gamma(r_h + h, r_t + t)} \theta^{r_h + h - 1}(1 - \theta)^{r_t + t - 1}.$$

The expected β distribution is known by the prior distribution:

$$\int \theta \beta(\theta \mid r_h, r_t)d\theta = \frac{r_h}{r}$$

Then, the predicted probability of the Bayesian formula:

$$P(X_{n+1} = x_{n+1} \mid D, \xi) = \int \theta P(\theta \mid D, \xi)d\theta = \int \theta \beta(\theta \mid r_h + h, r_t + t)d\theta = \frac{r_h + h}{r + n}.$$

3.3   Case Study: Decision Analysis Before a Cargo Ship Collision

In specific cases, a particular feature is the key to causing an accident. This section selects a representative collision case study. According to the relevant experience of the OOW and fully estimating the sea conditions at the time, we use the previous discussion of Bayesian methods to help the OOW make navigation decisions before the collision.

This accident occurred 930 km off the east coast of Kinkazan Island, Ishinomaki City, Miyagiken. The source of this accident is the Japan Transport Safety Board [12]. Ship A—cargo ship NIKKEI TIGER—and ship B—fishing ship Hori Sakae Maru—collided, caused a serious accident leading to 13 people missing from the fishing ship. Figure 3 shows the three-minute relative position before the two ships collided, and a schematic diagram of their relative course. (Appendix A shows the two ships' navigation tracks before and after the collision.) The OOW of ship A lacked navigation experience and was not familiar with the international navigation regulations. In the process of collision avoidance, as ship B's green light (starboard lights) became visible, he incorrectly steered to port (left); then, he sharpened the angle of his turn (by $10°$, twice). This is the direct reason for the collision.

Hypothesis: The probability that the OOW saw the green light is $P_{(G)}$. Upon seeing a green light, the ship should maintain its speed and course. The probability of keeping watch is $P_{(K|G)}$ and the probability of a safe pass is $P_{(S|K,G)}$. The probability of a turn to port is $P_{(T|G)}$ and the probability of a collision is $P_{(C|K,T,G)}$. The specific structure is shown in Fig. 4. According to the hypothesis and using the Bayesian prediction method, the following conditional probability table can be obtained. $K = 0$ indicates that the OOW of ship A saw the green light and did not keep watch. $T = 0$ indicates that he saw the green light and did not turn to port. $P_{(C=0)} = 0.9$ indicates a "strong" likelihood of a ship collision; $P_{(C=0)} = 0.1$ indicates a "weak" likelihood of a ship collision.

3.4   Application of a BN to a Human-in-the-Loop Decision-Support System

Academic research applying Bayesian methods to practical applications is extensive; e.g., macro-economic trends, financial risk management, intelligent user interfaces, information filtering, automatic vehicle navigation, medical care, economic prediction, speech-recognition text classification, etc. Depending on the different areas, there are different interpretations of the Bayesian network; e.g., Bayesian belief networks and dynamic Bayesian networks.

The core idea is to use the prior distribution and add sample information to infer the posterior distribution. The prior portion may be according to long-term experience in

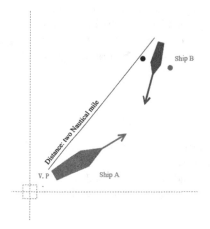

Fig. 3. Relative positions before collision

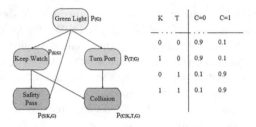

K	T	C=0	C=1
0	0	0.9	0.1
1	0	0.9	0.1
0	1	0.1	0.9
1	1	0.1	0.9

Fig. 4. Examples of BN probability

terms of human activity. It also can be judged by the decision-makers' past common sense. It can also be applied to the OOW. Because of the experience, knowledge structure, individual differences in quality, and other reasons, the OOW would construct his own judgments and predictions in a certain kind of situation. A general prediction will always contain uncertain elements, as in the definition of information theory. In this paper, entropy is borrowed to describe the uncertainty prediction factors. This study uses Bayesian methods and Bayesian networks to construct an autonomous human-in-the-loop decision-support system. Prediction and assessment may encounter various problems when the ship sails, including human involvement in ship manipulation, the conditional probability of the OOW making decisions, etc.

4   Constructing the Decision-Support System

The Bayesian network is the core of the decision-support system for the ship's safety navigation. Therefore, constructing a reasonable and reliable Bayesian network is the most significant work of this article. It can be approached from the definition of Bayesian networks. A Bayesian network consists of two parts: the structure (directed acyclic graph) and the parameters (conditional probability distribution table). To establish a Bayesian network model, first, the model must be given an index to predict, and collected examples of the corresponding data. Then, a predictive model is built based on the index and example data. The predictive model can be used to predict the new situation.

4.1   Index System for Risk Prediction

According to the actual ship-navigation conditions, the risk index is divided into four levels: decision-making risk D [t], the factor index, the direction index, and the basic event index. The first three indexes are defined as random discrete variables; the last stage can be discrete or continuous. The specific classifications are presented in Table 2.

Table 2. Decision-making risk index

First level	Second level	Third level	Fourth level
	Human Factors $(H_1[t])$	Operational errors $(H_{11}[t])$	Professional skill level $(H_{111}[t])$
			Attainment $(H_{112}[t])$
			Work attitude $(H_{113}[t])$
			Character flaw $(H_{114}[t])$
			Hobby, alcoholism, etc. $(H_{115}[t])$
		Illegal operations $(H_{12}[t])$	Lazy $(H_{121}[t])$
			Habitation $(H_{122}[t])$
			Job competition $(H_{123}[t])$
			Money trading $(H_{124}[t])$
		Personnel relations $(H_{13}[t])$	Concept difference $(H_{131}[t])$
		Working pressure $(H_{14}[t])$	Commercial requirements $(H_{141}[t])$
	Process Factors $(P_2[t])$	Process defects $(P_{21}[t])$	Dereliction of duty $(P_{211}[t])$
			Supervisor absences $(P_{212}[t])$
		Poor supervision $(P_{22}[t])$	Negligence $(P_{221}[t])$
			Lack of staff $(P_{222}[t])$
	Systemic Factors $(S_3[t])$	System completeness $(S_{31}[t])$	Operation is not continuous $(S_{311}[t])$
			Abnormal module $(S_{312}[t])$
		System security $(S_{32}[t])$	Abnormal backup system $(S_{321}[t])$
			Data transmission error $(S_{322}[t])$
		System interruption $(S_{33}[t])$	Signal interruption $(S_{331}[t])$
			Part out of control $(S_{332}[t])$
			Sensor loss $(S_{333}[t])$
			Section break $(S_{334}[t])$
			Physical damage $(S_{335}[t])$
		System failure $(S_{34}[t])$	Completely lost $(S_{341}[t])$
	Outside Factors $(O_4[t])$	Ship $(O_{41}[t])$	Hull damage $(O_{411}[t])$
			Fire $(O_{412}[t])$
		Sea environment $(O_{42}[t])$	Aground $(O_{421}[t])$
			Rough waves $(O_{422}[t])$
			Off course $(O_{423}[t])$
			Tornado $(O_{423}[t])$
		Target ship $(O_{43}[t])$	Miscommunication $(O_{431}[t])$
			Error message received $(O_{432}[t])$

(Continued)

Table 2. (*Continued*)

First level	Second level	Third level	Fourth level
			Error avoidance action ($O_{433}[t]$)
			Urgent situation ($O_{434}[t]$)
			Collision risk ($O_{435}[t]$)
		Terrorist attack ($O_{44}[t]$)	Life threatened ($O_{441}[t]$)

4.2 Process of Training the Structure and Parameters

Constructing a Bayesian network consists of two parts: (1) Defining the variables; (2) training the structure and parameters. Generally, these two tasks are executed sequentially; then, during construction, the following two aspects must be compromised.

On the one hand, to achieve sufficient accuracy, a sufficiently large and rich Bayesian network model must be constructed; on the other hand, the maintenance costs and the complexity of the probabilistic reasoning should be considered. For a complex model structure, the complexity of the probabilistic reasoning is also higher, which often affects the efficiency of the Bayesian network. In fact, the establishment of a Bayesian network often involves running the two processes iteratively, with repeated interaction.

The first main task is under the guidance of domain experts: Selecting the appropriate variables for the research questions field. In some cases, it also requires a certain strategy: Selecting an important factor from the variable provided by the expert. The second task is to construct the key node of the Bayesian network. The main objective is to build a directed acyclic graph and provide the distribution parameters for each node, where each node corresponds to a conditional probability-distribution table (CPT). Under normal circumstances, there are two different ways to construct a Bayesian network:

1. The completed study. In this approach, the structure and parameters of the Bayesian network are subjectively defined by people. Experts in the field determine the Bayesian network variables, the structure, and specify the distribution parameters. This Bayesian network is constructed entirely under the guidance of experts. Due to the limitations of the experts' knowledge, the data from the constructed Bayesian network may greatly deviate from what occurs in practice.
2. Partial learning. In this approach, the node variables of the Bayesian network are subjectively defined by people. The Bayesian network structure and parameters are learned through extensive training with the data. This is a completely data-driven approach, with strong adaptability. The evolution of artificial intelligence, data mining, and machine learning makes this approach possible. Learning the structure and parameters of a Bayesian network from the data, is a direction for future research.

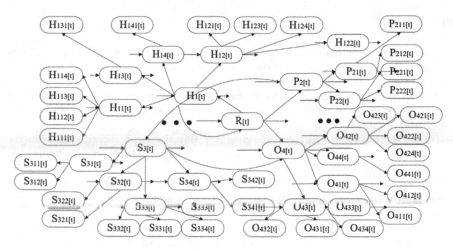

Fig. 5. Vertical view of the Bayesian network model for risk prediction

4.3 Construction of the Bayesian Network Prediction

Figure 5 shows the Bayesian network prediction model for decision support used for safe ship navigation, according to the characteristics of decision-making and risk assessment. The index system is optimized, with participation and abundance from expert knowledge.

5 Conclusion

Bayesian networks can fully utilize the dependency information between variables to make predictions. The purpose of this paper was to draw experience from Bayesian networks successfully applied in other science fields, and utilize them to do risk prediction of ship navigation, and build a navigation decision-support system. This paper, with the OOW at the center and the top layer of decision-making, elaborated on the advantage of Bayesian methods to quantify in terms of human factors, the importance of added experience and past relevant knowledge to the prior information. We constructed a decision-support pyramid system based on Bayesian network prediction, to enhance the safe navigation of ships at sea.

The core of the decision-making pyramid system was a Bayesian network process. Bayesian networks are constituted by the defined variables and the training composition of the structure parameters. From Bayes' theorem, this paper discussed in detail a variety of situations that could be encountered in ship navigation. To define these nodes for different risk conditions, a directed acyclic graph is given for each parameter position based on a Bayesian network for each stage of the corresponding conditional probability-distribution table. Finally, we displayed the fundamental vertical view of the Bayesian network model for risk prediction.

References

1. Hasegawa, K., Shigemori, Y., Ichiyama, Y.: Feasibility study on intelligent marine traffic system. In: Fifth IFAC Conference on Manoeuvring and Control of Marine Craft (MCMC 2000), pp. 327–332 (2000)
2. Rødseth, Ø.J., Burmeister, H.C.: Developments toward the unmanned ship. In: Proceedings of the International Symposium on Integrated Ship's Information Systems–ISIS, vol. 201, pp. 30–31 (2012)
3. Trucco, P., Cagno, E., Ruggeri, F., et al.: A Bayesian belief network modelling of organizational factors in risk analysis: a case study in maritime transportation. Reliab. Eng. Syst. Saf. **93**(6), 845–856 (2008)
4. Ltifi, H., Trabelsi, G., Ayed, M.B., et al.: Dynamic decision support system based on Bayesian networks application to fight against the nosocomial infections. arXiv preprint (2012). arXiv:1211.2126
5. Lepreux, S., Abed, M., Kolski, C.: A human-centred methodology applied to decision support system design and evaluation in a railway network context. Cogn. Technol. Work **5**(4), 248–271 (2003)
6. Abu-Tair, M., Naeem, W.: A decision support framework for collision avoidance of unmanned maritime vehicles. In: Li, K., Li, S., Li, D., Niu, Q. (eds.) ICSEE 2012. CCIS, vol. 355, pp. 549–557. Springer, Heidelberg (2013)
7. Perera, L.P., Carvalho, J.P., Soares, C.G.: Intelligent ocean navigation and fuzzy-Bayesian decision/action formulation. IEEE J. Oceanic Eng. **37**(2), 204–219 (2012)
8. Kum, S., Fuchi, M., Furusho, M.: Analysing of maritime accidents by approaching method for minimizing human error. In: Proceedings of IAMU AGA-7, Globalization and MET, Part 2, pp. 392–409 (2006)
9. Ruolan, Z., Masao, F., Xinjia, G.: A predetermination decision-making system for Auto-mated ship navigation and collision avoidance. In: Asia Navigation Conference, pp. 387–393 (2015)
10. Guo, C., Ye, Z., Sun, Z., et al.: A hybrid fuzzy cerebellar model articulation controller based autonomous controller. Comput. Electr. Eng. **28**(1), 1–16 (2002)
11. Maritime Safety Committee: Consideration on utilization of Bayesian network at step 3 of FSA. 81st Session (2006)
12. Japan Transport Safety Board. http://www.mlit.go.jp/jtsb/ship/rep-acci/2014/MA2014-6-5_2012tk0037.pdf

Author Index

Printed in the United States
By Bookmasters